Maternal/Newborn
Plans of Care
Guidelines for
Planning and
Documenting Client Care

Maternal/Newborn Plans of Care Guidelines for Planning and Documenting Client Care
Second Edition

Marilynn E. Doenges, MA, RN, CS
Clinical Specialist Psychiatric/Mental Health Nursing
Author/Private Practice
Instructor, Beth-El College of Nursing
Colorado Springs, Colorado

Mary Frances Moorhouse, RN, CCP, CCRN, CRRN
Author/Consultant, TNT-RN Enterprises
Colorado Springs, Colorado

 F. A. DAVIS COMPANY · Philadelphia

F. A. Davis Company
1915 Arch Street
Philadelphia, PA 19103

Printed in the United States of America

Last digit indicates print number: 10   9   8   7   6   5   4   3

Publisher, Nursing: Robert G. Martone
Nursing Acquisitions Editor: Joanne DaCunha
Production Editor: Marianne Fithian
Cover Design: Steven R. Morrone

As new scientific information becomes available through basic and clinical research, recommended treatments and drug therapies undergo changes. The authors and publisher have done everything possible to make this book accurate, up to date, and in accord with accepted standards at the time of publication. The authors, editors, and publisher are not responsible for errors or omissions or for consequences from application of the book, and make no warranty, expressed or implied, in regard to the contents of the book. Any practice described in this book should be applied by the reader in accordance with professional standards of care used in regard to the unique circumstances that may apply in each situation. The reader is advised always to check product information (package inserts) for changes and new information regarding dose and contraindications before administering any drug. Caution is especially urged when using new or infrequently ordered drugs.

Library of Congress Cataloging-in-Publication Data

Doenges, Marilynn E., 1922–
    Maternal/newborn plans of care : guidelines for planning and documenting client care / Marilynn
E. Doenges, Mary Frances Moorhouse. —2nd ed.
        p.   cm.
    Rev. ed. of: Maternal/newborn care plans. c1988.
    Includes bibliographical references and index.
    ISBN 0-8036-2668-1 (alk. paper)
    1. Maternity nursing.   2. Pediatric nursing.   3. Perinatology   4. Nursing care plans.
I. Moorhouse, Mary Frances, 1947–   . II. Doenges, Marilynn E., 1922–   Maternal/newborn
care plans. III. Title.
    [DNLM: 1. Maternal-Child Nursing.   2. Infant, Newborn, Diseases--nursing.   3. Patient Care
Planning.   WY 157.3 D651m 1994]
RG951.D64   1994
610.73'678—dc20
DNLM/DLC   94-6574
for Library of Congress   CIP

This book is dedicated:

To our husbands, Dean Doenges and Jan Moorhouse who are still supporting and cheering us on.

To our children Nancy (Jim) Daigle, David (Monita), Jim, Barbara (Bob Lanza), and John (Holly Sponaugle) Doenges; and Paul and Jason (Ellaina) Moorhouse,
and grandchildren, Jennifer and Jonathan Daigle, Matthew and Tyler Doenges, Nicole and Kelsey Doenges; and Alexa Moorhouse, who provided us with first hand knowledge about this subject.

To our mothers and fathers who encouraged us to dream.

To the FAD family for their support and friendship and for making us a part of the family, our great appreciation.

Special thanks to our editor, Robert Martone; production director, Herb Powell; and the rest of the Production Department who survived our changes; and to Ruth deGeorge who relayed messages so well.

Thanks also to the staff of the Memorial Hospital Library, who so promptly provided us with articles we requested.

and

Finally this book is dedicated to the student and practitioner who daily face the challenge of caring for the maternity client, her newborn and family in a rapidly changing healthcare environment.

CONSULTANTS FOR SECOND EDITION

Janet R. Kenty, MSN, RN
Visiting Lecturer
University of Massachusetts-Dartmouth
Dartmouth, Massachusetts

Carolyn Dagrosa, PhD, RN
Nurse Research
Department of Research and Development
Women and Infants Hospital
Providence, Rhode Island

Belinda Strickland, RN, MSN
Instructor, Maternal/Newborn
Beth-El College of Nursing
Colorado Springs, Colorado

Joan E. Bierchen, RN, EdD
Chair, Library Committee
St. Petersburg Junior College
St. Petersburg, Florida

Fran Martin, RN, PhD
Assistant Professor
Maternal-Child Nursing
University of Southern Mississippi
School of Nursing
Hattiesburg, Mississippi

Ginna Wall, MN, RN
Clinical Faculty
University of Washington Medical Center
Seattle, Washington

Sarah E. Whitaker, MSN, RNC
Instructor
University of Texas
College of Nursing and Allied Health
El Paso, Texas

CONTRIBUTORS FOR FIRST EDITION

Mary Barabe, RNC
Women's Health Care Nurse Practitioner
Penrose Community Hospital Birth Center
Colorado Springs Medical Center
Colorado Springs, Colorado

Susan Bennett, RN, ACCE
Nursing Director, Prematurity Prevention Program
Memorial Hospital
Colorado Springs, Colorado

Martha Reid Brown, RNC, BS
Neonatal Staff Instructor
Women & Infants Hospital of Rhode Island
Providence, Rhode Island

Sandra Conant, MS, RN
Parent/Child Clinical Specialist
Boston University School of Nursing
Boston, Massachusetts

Susan Craw, RN
Staff Nurse
Women's Center
Humana Hospital-Mountain View
Thornton, Colorado

Dorothy Crowder, RN, MS, CCE
Associate Professor, Maternal-Child Nursing
Virginia Commonwealth University
Medical College of Virginia School of Nursing
Richmond, Virginia

Carol A. Dabek, MS, RN
Staff Instructor, Nursing Education
Women & Infants Hospital of Rhode Island
Providence, Rhode Island

Carolyn Dagrosa, RN, PhD
Nurse Researcher
Department of Research and Development
Women & Infants Hospital of Rhode Island
Providence, Rhode Island

Marilynn E. Doenges, MA, RN, CS
Clinical Specialist Psychiatric/Mental Health Nursing
Author/Private Practice
Instructor, Beth-El College of Nursing
Colorado Springs, Colorado

Julie Christina Fortier, RN, BSN, MS, PhD
University of Maryland
School of Nursing
Baltimore, Maryland

M. Lynne Francis, MS, RN
Director of Nursing Education
Women & Infants Hospital of Rhode Island
Providence, Rhode Island

Wendy D. Gerhardt, BSN, RN, MS
Certified Nurse Mid-Wife Program
University of Minnesota
Minneapolis, Minnesota

Carolyn Cooper Hames, MN, RN
Assistant Professor
Coordinator, Parent-Child Health Nursing
Department of Nursing
University of Rhode Island
Kingston, Rhode Island

Linda Harrison, RN
Labor/Delivery Nurse
Memorial Hospital
Colorado Springs, Colorado

Janet R. Kenty, RN, MSN
Visiting Instructor
University of Massachusetts - Dartmouth
Dartmouth, MA

Patricia C. Kiniry, MS, RN
Formerly, Assistant Professor
University of Rhode Island
Kingston, Rhode Island

Rebecca Lassan, RN, PhD
Associate Professor
Rhode Island College
Providence, Rhode Island

Patricia McGaffigan, RN, MS
Instructor
School of Nursing
Boston University
Boston Massachusetts

Gwendolyn Edmonds McGaugh, RN, BSN, OBNP
Staff Nurse, Women's Clinic
Oklahoma Teaching Hospital
Oklahoma City, Oklahoma

Susan Rush Michael, MS, RN
Assistant Professor
University of Nevada, Las Vegas
Las Vegas, Nevada

Mary Frances Moorhouse, RN, CCP, CCRN, CRRN
Author/Consultant, TNT-RN Enterprises
Colorado Springs, Colorado

Rebecca F. Murray, RN
NICU Nurse (Retired, MOT)
Colorado Springs, Colorado

Cindy G. Plant, RNC
Nursery Clinical Educator
Memorial Hospital
Colorado Springs, Colorado

Alice Salter, RN, MS
Assistant Professor
School of Nursing
Salem State College
Salem, Massachusetts

Rachael F. Schiffman, MS, RN
Assistant Professor
Rhode Island College
Providence, Rhode Island

Judy Setchell, RNC, BS
Nursing Manager, OB/GYN Services
Lovelace Medical Center
Albuquerque, New Mexico

Andrea Laura Tatkon-Coker, RN, MSN
Consultant
Cedar Springs, Iowa

CONSULTANTS FOR FIRST EDITION

JoAnne Broadus, RN, MSN
Assistant Professor
College of Nursing
University of South Alabama
Mobile, Alabama

Patricia Contrisciani, RN, EdD
Professor of Nursing
Delaware County Community College
Media, Pennsylvania

Andrea Hollingsworth, RN, BSN, MSN
University of Pennsylvania
School of Nursing
Philadelphia, Pennsylvania

Marcia London, RN, MSN, NNP
Associate Professor
Beth-El College of Nursing
Colorado Springs, Colorado

Rebecca F. Murray, RN
NICU Nurse (Retired, MOT)
Colorado Springs, Colorado

Emma Nemivant, RN, MEd, MSN
Assistant Professor
College of Nursing
University of Illinois
Chicago, Illinois

Sally B. Olds, RN, MS
Associate Professor
Beth-El College of Nursing
Colorado Springs, Colorado

Celeste R. Phillips, RN, EdD
Director of Professional Relations
Borning Corporation
Spokane, Washington

KEY TO ESSENTIAL TERMINOLOGY

CLIENT ASSESSMENT DATA BASE

Provides an overview of the more commonly occurring etiology and coexisting factors associated with a specific maternal/newborn diagnosis as well as the signs/symptoms and corresponding diagnostic findings.

NURSING PRIORITIES

Establishes a general ranking of needs/concerns on which the Nursing Diagnoses are ordered in constructing the plan of care. This ranking would be altered according to the individual client situation.

DISCHARGE GOALS

Identifies generalized statements that could be developed into short-term and intermediate goals to be achieved by the client before being "discharged" from nursing care. They may also provide guidance for creating long-term goals for the client to work on after discharge.

NURSING DIAGNOSES

The general problem/concern (Diagnosis) is stated without the distinct cause and signs/symptoms, which would be added to create a diagnostic statement when specific client information is available. For example, when a client displays increased tension, apprehension, quivering voice, and focus on self, the nursing diagnosis of Anxiety could be stated: Anxiety, severe, related to threat to self-concept as evidenced by statements of increased tension, apprehension; observations of quivering voice, and feelings of inadequacy.

In addition, diagnoses identified within these guides for planning care as actual or high risk can be changed or deleted and new diagnoses added, depending entirely on the specific patient information.

MAY BE RELATED TO/POSSIBLY EVIDENCED BY

These lists provide the usual/common reasons (etiology) why a particular problem may occur with probable signs/symptoms, which would be used to create the "related to" and "evidenced by" portions of the *client diagnostic statement* when the client situation is known.

When a high-risk (formerly "potential") diagnosis has been identified, signs/symptoms have not yet developed and therefore are not included in the nursing diagnosis statement. However, interventions are provided to prevent progression to an *actual* problem.

DESIRED OUTCOMES/EVALUATION CRITERIA—CLIENT WILL

These give direction to client care as they identify what the client or nurse hopes to achieve. They are stated in general terms to permit the practitioner to modify/individualize them by adding time lines and individual client criteria so they become "measurable." For example, "Client will appear relaxed and able to discuss feelings within 24 hours."

ACTIONS/INTERVENTIONS

Activities are divided into independent and collaborative and are ranked in this book from most to least common. When creating the individual plan of care, interventions would normally be ranked to reflect the client's specific needs/situation. In addition, the division of independent/collaborative is arbitrary and is actually dependent of the individual nurse's capabilities and hospital/community standards.

RATIONALE

Although not commonly appearing in client plans of care, rationale has been included here to provide a pathophysiologic basis to assist the nurse in deciding about the relevance of a specific intervention for an individual client situation.

CONTENTS

INTRODUCTION

One of the most significant achievements in the healthcare field during the past 20 years has been the emergence of the nurse as an active coordinator and initiator of client care. Although the transition from helpmate to healthcare professional has been painfully slow and is not yet complete, the importance of the nurse within the system can no longer be denied or ignored. Today, the nurse designs nursing care interventions that move the whole client toward a positive outcome and optimal health.

The current state of the theory of *nursing process, diagnosis,* and *intervention* has been brought to the clinical setting to be implemented by the nurse. This book gives definition and direction to the development and use of individualized nursing care for women during the childbearing years, and their families. Therefore, this book is not an end in itself, but a beginning for the future growth and development of the profession.

Professional care standards, along with physicians and clients, will continue to increase expectations for nurses' performance as each day brings advances in the struggle to understand the mysteries of normal body function and human response to actual and potential health problems. With this increased knowledge comes greater responsibility for the nurse. To meet these challenges competently, the nurse must have up-to-date physical assessment skills and a working knowledge of pathophysiologic concepts concerning the common changes occurring during pregnancy and birth and the conditions or diseases that may have an impact on the outcome. This book is a tool, a means of attaining that competency.

In the past, plans of care were viewed principally as learning tools for students and seemed to have little relevance after graduation. However, the need for a written format to communicate and document individualized client care has been recognized in all care settings. In addition, governmental regulations and third-party payor requirements have created the need to validate the appropriateness of the care provided, as well as the need to justify staffing patterns and monetary charges for client care. Thus, although the student's "case studies" were too cumbersome to be practical in the clinical setting, the client plan of care meets the above identified needs. The practicing nurse, as well as the nursing student, will welcome this text as a ready reference in clinical practice.

The primary focus of this book is on wellness, with inclusion of common health problems that impact on the maternity client and her newborn as well as plans of care identifying general considerations for the high-risk maternity client who presents with less common health problems. This book is designed for use in the maternal/newborn setting, serving as a guide for nurses who plan and promote healthcare for the maternity client and her family. The plans are organized by stages of pregnancy and address specific conditions and diseases in each stage for easy reference. *Rationales* (which not only state why an intervention is important, but also provide related pathophysiologic information, when applicable) enhance the reader's understanding of the intervention. This information also serves as a catalyst for thought in planning and evaluating the care being rendered.

Chapter 1 examines current issues and trends and their implications for the nurse caring for the couple in the childbearing and early newborn phases. Trends in healthcare such as cost containment, shortened hospital stays, home care, and increased use of alternative birth centers are examined in light of possible effects on the delivery of maternity care. An overview of cultural, community, sociologic, and ethical concepts impacting on the maternity nurse in a variety of healthcare settings is included. The importance of the nurse's role in cooperation and coordination with other healthcare professionals is integrated throughout the plans of care.

Chapter 2 reviews the historical use of the nursing process in formulating plans of care and discusses the nurse's role in the delivery of that care. Nursing diagnosis is discussed to assist the nurse in understanding its role in the nursing process.

In Chapter 3, a nursing-based assessment tool is provided to aid the nurse in identifying nursing diagnoses. A sample client situation with individual data base and corresponding plan of care are included to demonstrate how to adapt the nursing process theory to practice. Finally, evaluation and documentation are addressed to complete the nursing process cycle.

Chapters 4 through 6 provide plans of care that include information from multiple disciplines to assist the nurse in providing holistic care for the client or couple during the prenatal, intrapartal, and postpartal phases within the community or acute care setting. Chapter 7 addresses the care of the newborn. Assessment guides incorporating the pertinent and customary questions to be asked of the client are included for each phase. Each plan includes a client assessment data base (presented in a nursing format) and associated diagnostic studies. After the data base is collected, nursing priorities are sifted from the information to help focus and structure the care provided. *Discharge goals* are listed to identify which general goals should be accomplished in situations in which care is expected to be terminated and not simply to progress to another stage. The nursing diagnoses contain "related to" and "evidenced by" statements that provide an explanation of client problems or needs. Desired *client outcomes* are stated in behavioral terms that can be measured to evaluate the client's progress and the effectiveness of care provided. The interventions are designed to promote problem resolution.

A decision-making model is used to organize and prioritize nursing interventions based on the nurse acting independently or collaboratively within the health team. No attempt is made to indicate whether independent or collaborative actions come first, because this must be dictated by the individual situation. Inclusion of rationales for the nursing actions will assist the nurse in deciding whether the interventions are appropriate for an individual client. A bibliography follows the text to allow for further reference and research as desired.

This book is designed to be a ready reference for the practicing nurse as well as a catalyst for thought in planning and evaluating care. Students will find the plans of care helpful as they learn and develop skills in applying the nursing process using nursing diagnoses in the maternal/newborn setting.

As a final note, this book is not intended to be a procedures manual, and efforts have been made to avoid detailed descriptions of techniques or protocols that might be viewed as individual or regional in nature. Instead the reader is referred to an actual procedures manual or a book covering standards of care if detailed direction for these concerns is desired.

CHAPTER 1

TRENDS AND ISSUES IN MATERNAL/NEWBORN CARE

In considering trends and current issues in maternal/newborn nursing care, one must look to the overall trends and restructuring within the healthcare industry. The impetus to restructure healthcare is due in part to the rapidly rising cost of healthcare delivery, the increasing numbers of uninsured or underinsured consumers, the need for allocation of resources, and liability concerns. Additionally, increased technologic advances, the needs of special populations, greater consumer participation in decision making, expanded roles for the healthcare professional, managed care, and ethical issues will also affect the way in which obstetrical care will be provided in the future. Nurses must become aware of these influences and be actively involved in formulating policies and standards of care so that care continues to be provided at a high level of quality.

The Changing Healthcare Environment

HEALTHCARE COSTS

Healthcare expenditures continue to rise. The National Leadership Coalition for Health Care Reform figures estimate that healthcare in the United States was a $756 billion industry in 1991, and, if not controlled, could reach $1.2 to $1.3 trillion by 1995. At this rate, without change, the cost of healthcare would reach between $2.1 and $2.7 trillion by the year 2000. Public Law No. 98-21 changed the method of payment for federally subsidized healthcare for inpatient services from a cost-based retrospective payment system to a prospective payment system based on 467 diagnoses or diagnostically related groups (DRGs). Most states are considering options to similarly curb Medicaid reimbursement. All types of nongovernment payors of healthcare are pursuing various methods of cost containment, including managed care and special incentives for the consumer and/or provider. The majority of plans include precertification, early discharge, outpatient care, and some home care. Cost containment programs are having a significant impact on obstetrical care. Private insurers often mandate discharge within 24 hours of routine vaginal delivery or 72 hours for uncomplicated cesarean birth.

ALLOCATION OF RESOURCES

Data are still being gathered regarding what impact the DRG prospective payment system is having on hospital costs for high-risk mothers and infants. Although some states have modified payment structures for high-risk services in certain perinatal centers, not under the reimbursement system, a national restructuring may be necessary for equitable treatment. "Rationing" of healthcare dollars or allocation of resources may mandate the limitation of services and therapy modalities provided to preterm infants based on predetermined guidelines such as gestational age and/or birth weight, and so forth. Studies now in progress by the division of Maternal and Child Health of the U.S. Department of Health and Human Services may provide the data for such a restructuring to ensure that perinatal programs caring for the high-risk client are not unduly compromised. In 1991, the American Nurses Association, with the support of other nursing organizations, presented an *Agenda for Health Care Reform,* in which they propose "delivering primary healthcare in community-based settings," "consumer responsibility for personal health, self-care, and informed decision making," and "utilization of the most cost-effective providers to include certified nurse midwives and nurse practitioners," among other proposals. This agenda affects how care would be delivered to all clients, and most certainly to maternal/newborn clients.

UNDERSERVED/UNINSURED

The current healthcare delivery system has resulted in large populations of underserved and uninsured individuals. Some of these persons are uninsured by choice, such as young adults who may choose to budget their healthcare dollars elsewhere, believing that at this stage of their lives they will not need healthcare services. Others are not offered healthcare insurance by their employers or cannot afford the cost of monthly premiums. Even those with insurance may find their policy does not provide maternity benefits. Lack of preventive and primary care for infants and women of childbearing age has contributed to a lack of decline in fetal mortality rates and to the increased cost of care for infants with special needs. Preconception counseling as well as prenatal and perinatal care for all women is necessary to effect change in these areas. Nurses can play a primary role in providing leadership, client education, counseling, and screening.

LIABILITY CONCERNS

The increasing frequency of litigation has had an impact on the way in which maternity care is practiced. Heightened concern for fetal safety during the labor process has increased the use of invasive fetal monitoring, diagnostic testing, and even cesarean birth. These practices may create a conflict between cost-conscious third-party payors and the client's desire for a "natural" birthing experience. Although the need for services and providers has increased, the crisis in liability insurance has caused a decline in the availability of general practitioners and specialists, who are choosing to discontinue obstetrical services because of the high cost and difficulties of carrying liability insurance. The demand for healthcare providers in obstetrics *will* continue in the future. Where practice acts permit, certified nurse midwives (CNMs) can fill a vital role in providing the professional comprehensive care that mothers and infants deserve in a rapidly changing healthcare environment. In addition, plans to restructure healthcare are also recommending tort reform. Currently, some providers require clients to agree to mediation in the event of an untoward outcome. This may control insurance costs, and these savings can then be passed on to the consumer.

ADVANCES IN TECHNOLOGY

Complex technologic advances and scientific discoveries have altered the scope of maternity care. For instance, genetic research and engineering have expanded the scope of prenatal testing to include an ever-increasing number of diagnoses and interventions. Management of infertility problems now includes in vitro fertilization and surrogate parenting. New pharmaceuticals have frequently been successful in controlling premature labor. Clients with high-risk pregnancies can often be monitored at home, rather than in the hospital, using sophisticated communication systems linked to central computers or laboratories in large medical centers. Some women with long-standing severe health problems are successfully conceiving and delivering viable infants. Advances in ultrasonography have enabled surgeons to operate on the developing fetus for select problems. Increasingly sophisticated methods for assessing fetoplacental well-being are available to detect problems during a high-risk pregnancy. Neonatal intensive care units are equipped and staffed to provide life support to premature infants who previously would never have survived. With these advances come additional concerns, ethical dilemmas, and higher costs.

SPECIAL POPULATIONS

The trend of immigrants to locate in specific urban areas and their desire to retain ethnic and cultural identity has created large numbers of clients and families with diverse backgrounds and needs. Problems related to healthcare in these populations include language barriers, lack of knowledge or understanding, and unique health beliefs or practices that influence behaviors adopted during the prenatal, intrapartal, and postpartal periods. In addition, there has been an increase in health-related problems, particularly with foreign populations, owing to lack of immunizations, exposure to communicable diseases, poor health and hygiene habits, the carrier status of diseases, and variations in immune systems. Nurses need to enhance their cultural awareness and to be adaptable, creative, and knowledgeable in dealing with the needs of these clients, their family members, and communities as a whole.

Increasingly, women are electing to postpone childbearing until completion of certain educational, personal, or professional goals, thereby entering childbearing as "elderly" primigravidas, who may have some increased risk for complications during the prenatal, intrapartal, and postpartal periods. For these women, who thus far have been able to control events in their lives, a crying baby, breastfeeding problems, and infant care tasks can be overwhelming. Unfortunately, these clients may not be recipients of agency referral or support services that are afforded to many other high-risk groups. With proposed shorter hospital stays, such clients may have a difficult time adapting to new mothering roles. However, these women may have increased problem-solving skills related to their work and life experience that can help them to adjust to this new situation. The nurse may be instrumental in helping these clients cope positively, by creating and/or implementing a comprehensive plan of care to include home visits and/or timely telephone calls. In addition, the nurse may be involved in establishing or teaching community-based parenting/postpartal classes to meet the needs of the family.

Not only are nurses caring for older maternity clients in greater numbers, but they also continue to care for large numbers of adolescents. Adolescent pregnancy, with its identifiable physical and emotional risks, affects approximately 1 million teenagers, their families, and significant others. In creating and implementing a plan of care for the adolescent, the nurse must recognize that this client's developmental needs may interfere with her cooperation, necessitating alternative approaches toward the goal of optimal maternal and fetal well-being. Whether the adolescent chooses to terminate the pregnancy, or carry the pregnancy to term and either keep the infant or relinquish the baby for adoption, an educational program must include information about family planning methods, sexually transmitted diseases, and infant care/parenting, as applicable.

The incidence of sexually transmitted diseases (STDs) tends to remain high, particularly among adolescents, age 15 to 19 years. Researchers report that the high rate of STDs is related to a lack of treatment, drug use, multiple sex partners, and unsafe sex practices. Such infections may have a negative impact on the outcome of a pregnancy and/or future childbearing capabilities. The incidence of chlamydia and gonorrhea infections remains high, yet cases of syphilis and HIV/AIDS are reaching epidemic proportions and, therefore, creating much concern among healthcare workers as well as the population in general. A new technique for locating the AIDS virus in the blood may help doctors predict if a baby born to an HIV-infected mother will eventually develop the disease. Ongoing research may lead to the establishment of new vaccines to protect the fetus from such threats as herpes, cytomegalovirus (CMV), and AIDS.

Current mortality trends indicate that HIV/AIDS is now one of the five leading causes of death in women of reproductive age. Because women infected with HIV are the major source of infection for infants, these trends in AIDS mortality in women forecast the impact of AIDS mortality in children as well. Such statistics have tremendous economic implications for the healthcare delivery system in terms of meeting the physical and emotional needs of affected mothers, infants, and families. Primary prevention through health education programs aimed at the primary and secondary school level may be the most effective means to reduce the impact of this health problem.

These same approaches are being used to deal with the problem of substance abuse, which continues to have a significant effect on the prenatal well-being of the mother and her offspring. Cigarette smoking, alcohol and prescription/street drug use have far-reaching short- and long-term effects. The National Institute on Drug Abuse estimates that 15% of American women between the ages 15 and 44 years (or 8 million women) are currently substance abusers, and this number is increasing. The National Association for Perinatal Addiction Research and Education predicts that as many as 375,000 infants may be affected each year by their mother's drug abuse during pregnancy. Cocaine use and abuse, particularly among women between the ages of 15 and 25 years has increased dramatically in recent years, and it has had a significant impact on women during the childbearing years, increasing perinatal morbidity and mortality. Researchers are now beginning to examine both short- and long-term effects of maternal cocaine use on the pediatric population and the impact that such effects will have on the education system.

It is imperative that the healthcare system develop methodologies that will facilitate identification of substance abuse in the prenatal client and to establish protocols for primary, secondary, and tertiary treatment. Use of the media to educate the public about the dangers of substance use, particularly during pregnancy, is critically important. Prenatal programs must focus on educating the at-risk client about the dangers of substance abuse during pregnancy and must establish therapeutic networks between identified abusers and prenatal healthcare providers. Social policy must address who should pay for the healthcare and education required by the substance-abusing mother and her infant.

CONSUMER PARTICIPATION

The self-care focus of the 1960s and 1970s is being sustained by the push to contain healthcare costs. This approach requires the client to be assertive, to seek necessary information to make informed decisions, and even to assume some primary care functions, including monitoring physiologic status and the performance of diagnostic tests. This may be in direct conflict with the individual client's cultural/religious beliefs, expectations, and practices. It is the responsibility of the nurse to be attuned to the client's needs in general and to recognize and incorporate these specific issues into the plan of care as appropriate.

As consumers become increasingly sophisticated in their approach to maternity care, they have some expectations for specific labor, delivery, and postpartal experiences, such as a family-centered approach to childbirth and reduced medical interventions. Such sophistication, together with strong economic incentives to provide lower-cost alternatives to hospital care, has promoted the rapid development of alternative birth centers (ABCs) throughout the country. Such centers allow women with low-risk, uncomplicated pregnancies to give birth in a home-like setting. The need to rely on complex technology to monitor the progress of labor and fetal well-being is not in harmony with this environment. The nurse working in an ABC must philosophically accept the mission, goals, and objectives of the center and possess a broad base of clinical experience in prenatal care as well as labor and delivery. Preparing the family for discharge from the birth center within 12 hours after delivery also requires the nurse to demonstrate comprehensive skills in needs assessment and health education for the postpartal family. An integral component of such a program involves home follow-up assessments of both mother and infant at specific intervals during the early postpartal period. A plan of care provides documentation to facilitate the transition from the birth center to the home or community setting.

Similarly, mothers seeking obstetrical care within the acute hospital setting are increasingly experiencing a shorter stay of less than 2 days (more often 12 to 24 hours) after delivery. The nurse must be prepared to provide a thorough needs assessment and to create a comprehensive plan fostering self-care. Follow-up home care, parenting and infant care classes, and health promotion programs are anticipated components of the nurse's role in providing support to the client and her family after discharge. This role may involve spending some time with the client in an inpatient setting as well as in the client's home or in a community setting. Regardless of the setting, many new mothers experience some degree of anxiety and ambivalence in the first few days at home alone. These women can benefit from additional teaching and assistance provided by a qualified nurse provider.

EXPANDING ROLES FOR THE HEALTHCARE PROFESSIONAL

In an effort to contain costs and avoid duplication of services, hospitals are regionalizing obstetrical/perinatal units and defining the responsibilities of each agency based on its categorization as a Level I, II, or III/IV (primary, secondary, or tertiary) facility. Such regionalization may force separation of families when a high-risk situation requires the hospitalization of the prenatal client and/or the birth of a preterm infant. Such a crisis presents unique challenges to the nurse, who may function as an information link between the larger medical center and the absent family.

The complexity of new technology and of new approaches to obstetrical care has placed enormous demands on the nurse providing care. Nurses are actively involved not only in the technologic aspects of care, but also in the educational process of the client and family members. The rapidly changing knowledge base requires constant updating of information. Continuing education through formal classwork, workshops, seminars, and professional reading is essential. Improved clinical practice skills for the advanced care of mothers and infants, particularly those in a high-risk category, must be ongoing. Nurses will be the link between the client/family and the physician.

A trend that causes concern is the public's increasing reliance on house or lay midwives. This is due in part to the consumer's desire for providers who will respond to requests for a more personal, neutral, and nonintervening approach. By virtue of their educational background, scope of practice, standards of care, and access to resources (such as medical consultation), CNMs are better qualified to provide individualized, safe client care than lay midwives. However, without the support of physicians, legislators, and third-party payors, the acceptance of CNMs will be delayed, limiting the client's options and forcing clients to continue to choose between licensed physicians and lay midwives.

MORAL/ETHICAL CONCERNS

Advances in technology have created many moral and ethical dilemmas for the obstetrical nurse. Many more infants with extremely low birth weights are now surviving, raising issues of quality of life versus sanctity of life for the offspring and parents. Long-term effects of prematurity can lead to severe lifelong physical and mental disabilities. The physical, emotional, and financial burdens on the family can result in increased family discord, divorce, and child abuse, as well as physical and psychologic illnesses.

Unhealthy family interactions leading to physical/emotional abuse are not restricted to families with premature infants. Official U.S. government statistics indicate that 1 in 10 women are abused by the man with whom she lives. Often, abusive episodes increase or occur for the first time during pregnancy, particularly if the male member of the couple has an immature personality and weak ego identity. The nurse can play a major role in assessing the adequacy of available support systems and identifying and intervening with families in crisis.

The expanding field of genetics, which comprises research, screening, engineering, and counseling, raises many moral, legal, and ethical concerns for the individual and society. Society may mandate genetic screening prior to marriage, as has been done in some foreign countries. Serum/amniotic fluid analysis or chorionic villi sampling for the detection of specific genetic or congenital disorders may be voluntary, or it could become state or federally mandated as phenylketonuria (PKU) screening is at present. Nurses in expanded roles are becoming increasingly involved in genetic counseling and education and are dealing with more sophisticated consumers, who are aware of the effects of teratogens and hereditary disorders. Unresolved issues regarding the rights of the fetus, in vitro fertilization, surrogate parenting, and abortion persist.

Additionally, women of childbearing age now have increased options related to family planning with Food and Drug Administration (FDA) approval of the simple, effective implant contraceptive, levonorgestrel (Norplant), which effectively prevents pregnancy for up to 5 years. In addition, results of animal laboratory studies at the National Institutes of Health report success with the development of a long-acting contraceptive vaccine for women that was developed using genetic engineering. Such a vaccine would prevent fertilization of eggs by sperm rather than interfere with the development of a fetus after conception. The issues of women's reproductive rights related to abortion will continue to create intense conflict. In Europe, women have access to RU486, an oral drug that safely accomplishes a first-trimester abortion without need for surgical intervention. As yet, this controversial drug has not received FDA approval. Access to legal abortion has been shown to reduce maternal and infant mortality in that it reduces unwanted and high-risk pregnancies, especially among low-income women and adolescents.

Of equal or even greater concern is an alarming trend for physicians to refuse to administer care to individuals who have communicable diseases, particularly those who are HIV-positive. Nurses are also increasingly concerned about the need to protect themselves from possible contamination from certain communicable diseases. Diseases such as herpes, AIDS, hepatitis B, and syphilis are all potentially transmitted via blood products and body fluids. However, the use of universal precautions can provide adequate safeguards when appropriately implemented. The nurse also has a role in educating the client, family members, peers, and the community about modes of transmission in order to correct misconceptions and reduce inappropriate fears.

It is essential for healthcare providers to have objective support through peer support groups or counselors to help in dealing with these issues and potential conflicts. In many cases, the answers are not clear-cut, but discussion provides an opportunity to share feelings and approaches in coping with such dilemmas.

Summary

Nurses electing to care for the maternity client and her family face many exciting challenges created by increased technologic advances, expanded nursing roles and responsibilities, and increased consumer participation in decisions having an impact on the family. The professional nurse takes individual responsibility for ensuring that his or her clinical skills and theoretical framework keep pace with these changes, to meet the needs of individuals, families, and society as a whole.

CHAPTER 2

NURSING PROCESS: PLANNING CARE WITH NURSING DIAGNOSES

There is a growing awareness that nursing care is a key factor in client survival, and in the maintenance, rehabilitative, and preventive aspects of healthcare. Publication of the American Nurses Association (ANA) Social Policy Statement (1980), which defines nursing as the diagnosis and treatment of human responses to actual and potential health problems, in combination with the ANA Standards of Clinical Nursing Practice (1991), has provided impetus and support for the use of nursing diagnosis in the practice setting. The prospective payment plans, movement from acute care (hospital) to community settings, alternative birth centers, home health services, the development of specialty standards of care, and other changes in the healthcare system have given rise to the need for a common framework of communication and documentation. Such a framework assures continuity of care for the client who moves from one area of the healthcare system to another. Evaluation and documentation of care are important parts of this process.

Nurses have visionary ideas for delivery of quality care to all clients. Often, turning those ideas into action seems an exercise in futility, as what appears easy in theory becomes difficult in practice. Because of hectic schedules, many nurses believe that time spent writing plans of care is time taken away from client care. In reality, the delivery of quality care involves planning and coordination. We believe that as the nurse works with nursing diagnosis and learns the etiology and defining characteristics of clients' conditions, outcomes become apparent and interventions for attaining these outcomes become clear. Plans of care, properly written and used, provide tools for evaluation of client care, guidelines for documentation, and direction for continuity of care among nurses and other healthcare professionals.

Nursing Process

The term *nursing process* was introduced in the 1950s, but it has taken many years to develop national acceptance of the process as the framework for nursing care. The concept is adapted from the scientific approach to problem solving and requires the skills of (1) assessment, including focus assessments (systematic collection of data relating to clients and their problems), (2) problem identification (analysis and interpretation of data), (3) planning (choice of solutions, prioritizing, and goal setting), (4) implementation (putting the plan into action), and (5) evaluation (assessing the effectiveness of the plan, and changing the plan as indicated by current needs). Although nurses use these terms separately, they are actually interrelated and form a continuous circle of thought and action, providing an efficient method of organizing thought processes for clinical decision making. Nursing process is now included in the conceptual framework of most nursing curricula and is accepted in the legal definition of nursing in most nurse-practice acts.

To use this process, the nurse must demonstrate fundamental abilities of knowledge, intelligence, and creativity, as well as expertise in interpersonal and technical skills. The following are some *critical assumptions* for the nurse to consider in the decision-making process:

- The client is a human being with worth and dignity.
- There are basic human needs that must be met. When they are not met, problems arise requiring interventions by another person until the individual can resume self-responsibility.
- The client has a right to quality health and nursing care delivered with concern, compassion, and competence and focusing on wellness, prevention, and restoration.
- The therapeutic nurse-client relationship is a critical element in this process.

Nursing Diagnosis

Nurses have struggled for years to define nursing by identifying its parameters, with the goal of clarifying the professional status of nurses. To this end, nurses have been meeting and conducting research to develop nursing diagnoses. The North American Nursing Diagnosis Association (NANDA) has accepted the following working definition:

"Nursing diagnosis is a clinical judgment about individual, family, or community responses to actual and potential health problems/life processes. Nursing diagnoses provide the basis for selection of nursing interventions to achieve outcomes for which the nurse is accountable."

Nursing diagnosis provides a framework for using the nursing process. Although nursing diagnosis is only one component of nursing practice, it provides a common language for identifying client problems, nursing interventions, and evaluation tools. This common language is important for several reasons. It promotes communication between nurses, shifts, units, and alternative care settings. It provides a base for clinicians, educators, and researchers to document, validate, and/or alter the nursing process. As nurses begin to use nursing diagnoses on a daily basis, they become more familiar with the value of the diagnoses in the communication process.

Nursing diagnosis, as the crux of the nursing plan of care, focuses attention on certain areas and is the prime determinant of the style of nursing care to be delivered. Nursing actions have often been based on such variables as signs and symptoms, test results, and medical diagnosis. Nursing diagnosis is a uniform way of identifying, focusing on, and dealing with specific client problems and responses. The affective tone of the nursing diagnosis can shape expectations of the client's response and influence the nurse's behavior toward the client. For instance, if the nurse sees the client as noncompliant, the nurse's attitudes and behavior may reflect anger and mistrust, and judgmental decisions may be made that do not accurately treat the client's problem. However, accurate diagnosis of a client's problem (e.g., Altered Compliance related to medication side effects) can become a standard for nursing practice, understood by all who are using the plan of care, and thus can lead to improved delivery of care.

The nursing diagnosis is as precise as the data will allow because it is supported by the immediate data collected. It communicates the client's present situation and reflects changes as they occur. It is necessary to seek, incorporate, and synthesize all the relevant data and make the diagnosis statement meaningful to provide direction for nursing care. The nurse needs to be aware of biases that may interfere with reaching an accurate diagnosis. Keeping an open mind to numerous possibilities and not becoming preoccupied with a single symptom or thought facilitates this process. For example, when identifying a cue of restlessness in a client, the nurse may infer that the client is anxious. The nurse may believe that the restlessness is only psychologically based, overlooking the possibility that it is a physiologic response.

Planning Care

Medicine and nursing, as well as other health disciplines, are interrelated and therefore have implications for one another. This interrelationship should allow the exchange of data, the sharing of ideas and thoughts, and the development of plans of care that include all data pertinent to the individual client and/or family.

The plan of care contains not only the actions initiated by medical orders, but also the written coordination of care given by all related healthcare disciplines. The nurse becomes the person responsible for coordinating these different activities into a functional plan, which is necessary to provide holistic care for the client. Independent nursing actions are an integral part of this process. Collaborative actions are based on the medical regimen as well as on suggestions or orders from other disciplines involved with the care of the client. In this book, collaborative actions in conjunction with other disciplines are identified to assist the nurse in choosing appropriate interventions for the individual client and setting. The educational background and expertise of the nurse, the standing protocols, and the area of practice (rural or urban, acute care or community care settings) can influence whether an individual intervention is actually an independent nursing function or requires collaboration.

The written plan of care communicates the past and present health status and needs of the client to all members of the healthcare team. It identifies problems solved and those yet to be solved, approaches that have been successful, and patterns of client responses. The plan of care documents client care in areas of liability, accountability, and quality improvement. It provides a mechanism to assure continuity of care.

Components of the Plan of Care

For each plan of care presented, the *client assessment data base* is established from information obtained from the *history, physical examination,* and *diagnostic studies. Nursing priorities* are then determined and ranked. The priorities in this book represent a general ranking system for the nursing diagnoses in the plan of care, and may be reworded and reorganized with time lines, according to the individual client and situation, to create short- and long-term goals. The *nursing diagnosis* then follows, with *possible related factors (etiology)* and corresponding *signs and symptoms* when present. *Desired client outcomes* for each problem/need area are followed by appropriate independent and collaborative interventions with accompanying rationales.

ASSESSMENT

As noted, construction of the plan of care begins with the collection of data (assessment). The *assessment data base* consists of subjective and objective information encompassing the various nursing concerns identified in the 1992 list of nursing diagnoses developed by NANDA. Subjective data are those reported by the client and significant others. This information includes the individual's perceptions; that is, what the person wants to share. It is important to accept what is reported, because the client/significant other is the "expert" in this regard. However, the nurse needs to note incongruencies or dissonances, which may indicate the presence of other factors such as lack of knowledge, myths, misconceptions, or fear.

Objective data are those that are observed (quantitatively or qualitatively) and may be verified by others. They include findings from the *physical examination* and *diagnostic testing.* Evaluation of both subjective and objective collected data leads to the identification of problems or areas of concern or need. These problems or needs are expressed as nursing diagnoses (Table 2 – 1).

PROBLEM IDENTIFICATION/ANALYSIS

Analysis involves examining assessment findings, grouping related findings, and comparing the findings against established normal parameters. The key, then, to accurate nursing diagnosis is problem identification, which focuses attention on a current or high-risk physical or behavioral response that interferes with the quality of life the client desires or to which she is accustomed. The nursing diagnosis addresses the concerns of the client, significant others, and/or the nurse that require nursing intervention and management. In this text, the choice of an individual nursing diagnosis is validated by the *related/risk factors and signs and symptoms* most consistently associated with a specific situation or medical condition.

Nurses may feel at risk in committing themselves to documenting a nursing diagnosis; however, many references are currently available to aid in identifying and formulating the diagnostic statement. In addition, unlike medical diagnoses, nursing diagnoses change as the client progresses through various stages of ill-

TABLE 2-1. Nursing Diagnoses Accepted Through the Tenth NANDA Conference, 1992

Activity Intolerance
Activity Intolerance, high risk for
Adjustment, impaired
Airway Clearance, ineffective
Anxiety [specify level]*
Aspiration, high risk for

Body Image disturbance
Body Temperature, altered, high risk for
Bowel Incontinence
Breastfeeding, effective
Breastfeeding, ineffective
Breastfeeding, interrupted
Breathing Pattern, ineffective

Cardiac Output, decreased
Cardiac Output, high risk for decompensation
Caregiver Role Strain
Caregiver Role Strain, high risk for
Communication, impaired verbal
Constipation
Constipation, colonic
Constipation, perceived
Coping, defensive
Coping, Individual, ineffective

Decisional Conflict (specify)
Denial, ineffective
Diarrhea
Disuse Syndrome, high risk for
Diversional Activity deficit
Dysreflexia

Family Coping, ineffective: compromised
Family Coping, ineffective: disabling
Family Coping: potential for growth
Family Processes, altered
Fatigue
Fear
Fluid Volume deficit [active loss]*
Fluid Volume deficit [regulatory failure]*
Fluid Volume deficit, high risk for
Fluid Volume excess

Gas Exchange, impaired
Grieving, anticipatory
Grieving, dysfunctional
Growth and Development, altered

Health Maintenance, altered
Health-Seeking Behaviors (specify)
Home Maintenance Management, impaired
Hopelessness
Hyperthermia
Hypothermia

Incontinence, functional

Incontinence, reflex
Incontinence, stress
Incontinence, total
Incontinence, urge
Infant Feeding Pattern, ineffective
Infection, high risk for
Injury, high risk for

Knowledge Deficit [Learning need]* (specify)
Noncompliance [Compliance, altered]* (specify)
Nutrition, altered, less than body requirements
Nutrition, altered, more than body requirements
Nutrition, altered, high risk for more than body requirements

Oral Mucous Membrane, altered

Pain [acute]
Pain, chronic
Parental Role Conflict
Parenting, altered
Parenting, altered, high risk for
Peripheral Neurovascular Dysfunction, high risk for
Personal Identity disturbance
Physical Mobility, impaired
Poisoning, high risk for
Post-Trauma Response
Powerlessness
Protection, altered

Rape-Trauma Syndrome
Rape-Trauma Syndrome: compound reaction
Rape-Trauma Syndrome: silent reaction
Relocation Stress Syndrome
Role Performance, altered

Self Care deficit (specify): feeding, bathing/hygiene, dressing/grooming, toileting
Self Esteem, chronic low
Self Esteem, disturbance
Self Esteem, situational low
Self-Mutilation, high risk for
Sensory-Perceptual Alterations (specify): visual, auditory, kinesthetic, gustatory, tactile, olfactory
Sexual Dysfunction
Sexuality Patterns, altered
Skin Integrity, impaired
Skin Integrity, impaired, high risk for
Sleep Pattern disturbance
Social Interaction, impaired
Social Isolation
Spiritual Distress (distress of the human spirit)
Spontaneous Ventilation, inability to sustain
Suffocation, high risk for
Swallowing, impaired

Therapeutic Regimen (Individual), ineffective management of

(continued)

TABLE 2–1. Nursing Diagnoses Accepted Through the Tenth NANDA Conference, 1992 (continued)

Thermoregulation, ineffective	Unilateral Neglect
Thought Processes, altered	Urinary Elimination, altered
Tissue Integrity, impaired	Urinary Retention [acute/chronic]*
Tissue Perfusion, altered (specify): cerebral, cardiopulmonary, renal, gastrointestinal, peripheral	
	Ventilatory Weaning Response, dysfunctional (DVWR)
Trauma, high risk for	Violence, high risk for, directed at self/others

*Author recommendations.

ness or maladaptation to problem resolution. From the specific information obtained in the *client assessment data base,* the related factors, signs, and symptoms can be identified, and an individualized statement of the client's problem/need and diagnosis can be formulated. For example, a client may report fatigue and inability to rest adequately while caring for children. This leads to a choice of the nursing diagnosis: Fatigue related to increased energy requirements, altered body chemistry, inadequate support system as evidenced by client reports of lack of energy, inability to maintain usual routines, and emotional irritability.

PLANNING

Goals are established, and outcome statements are formulated, to give direction to nursing care. *Desired client outcomes* emerge from the diagnostic statement and are defined as the results of nursing interventions and patient responses that are achievable, desired by the client and/or nurse, and attainable within a defined period, given the present situation and resources. They have been stated in general terms in this book to permit the practitioner to individualize them by adding time lines, considerations of client circumstances and needs, and other specifics. The terminology must be concise, realistic, measurable, and stated in words that the client can understand. Beginning the outcome statement with an action verb provides direction that is measurable (e.g., "client will: Verbalize"). It is important that multidisciplinary goals do not conflict.

ACTIONS/INTERVENTIONS

Interventions communicate nursing actions to be taken to achieve desired client outcomes. The rationale for interventions needs to be sound and feasible, with the intention of providing individualized care. Actions may be independent or collaborative and encompass orders from nursing, medicine, and other disciplines. Again, using an action verb (e.g., "instruct," "demonstrate") provides direction for the nurse.

The nurse should plan care *with* the client, because both individuals are accountable for that care and for achieving the desired outcomes. The written interventions that guide client care need to be dated and signed to identify the person who is initiating and coordinating the care.

EVALUATION

Evaluation of the client's response to the care delivered and achievement of the desired outcomes (which were developed in the planning phase and documented in the plan of care) are the final step of the nursing process. The evaluation phase is necessary for the determination of how well the plan of care is working, and is an ongoing process. The revision of the plan of care is an essential component of the evaluation phase.

Reassessment is an ongoing evaluation process that occurs not just when a desired client outcome is due to be reviewed or when a determination is needed as to whether or not the client is ready for discharge. Instead, it is a constant "monitoring" of the client's status.

RATIONALES

Although rationales do not appear on agency plans of care, they are included in this book to assist the student and practicing nurse in associating the pathophysiologic and/or psychologic principles with the selected nursing intervention.

Documenting the Nursing Process

In general, the goals of the documentation system are to:

- facilitate the quality of client care.
- ensure documentation of progress with regard to client-focused outcomes.
- facilitate interdisciplinary consistency and the communication of treatment goals and progress.

Two recent publications provide the nurse with guidelines for documenting the nursing process and support the need for a written (or computer-generated) plan of care. The *ANA Standards of Clinical Nursing Practice* ". . . delineate care that is provided to all clients of nursing services," and each standard includes a measurement criterion addressing documentation. In addition, the Nursing Care Standards (Joint Commission on Accreditation of Health Care Organizations [JCAHO], 1992) also focus our attention on documentation, as presented in Table 2 – 2. These revised standards delineate the professional responsibilities of all registered nurses and provide criteria to assist in measuring achievement of identified standards.

From a nursing focus, documentation provides a record of the use of the nursing process for the delivery of individualized client care. The initial *assessment* is recorded in the client history or data base. The *diagnosis* of client problems/needs and the *planning* of client care are recorded in the plan of care. The *implementation* of the plan is recorded in progress notes and/or flow sheets. Finally, the evaluation of care is documented in progress notes and/or the plan of care.

The maintenance of a medical record is one of the most essential requirements for accreditation of healthcare facilities by JCAHO and/or other credentialing and licensing agencies. JCAHO standards state that the medical record must be documented accurately and in a timely manner. Therefore, we emphasize the importance of completing notes on schedule and in a manner that facilitates retrieval of data.

Documentation is not only a requirement for accreditation, but is also a permanent record of what happens with each client and is a legal requirement in any healthcare setting. In our society, with its many lawsuits and aggressive malpractice emphasis, all aspects of the medical record may be important legal documents. The plan of care that has been developed for a particular client serves as a framework or outline for the charting of administered care. Progress notes and flow sheets therefore reflect implementation of the treatment plan by documenting that appropriate actions have been carried out, precautions taken, and so forth. Both implementation of interventions and progress toward measurable outcomes need to be documented in the progress notes. They should be written in a clear and objective fashion and in a manner that reflects progress toward desired measurable outcomes with the use of planned staff interventions. These notations also need to be date and time specific and be signed by the person making the entry. Any

TABLE 2–2. A Sample Portion of One Nursing Care Standard from the Joint Commission on Accreditation of Healthcare Organizations

NC.1. Patients receive nursing care based on a documented assessment of their needs.
    NC.1.3.4. The patient's medical record includes documentation of
        NC.1.3.4.1 The initial assessments and reassessments
        NC.1.3.4.2 The nursing diagnosis and/or patient care needs
        NC.1.3.4.3 The interventions identified to meet the patient's nursing care needs
        NC.1.3.4.4 The nursing care provided
        NC.1.3.4.5 The patient's response to, and the outcomes of, the care provided
        NC.1.3.4.6 The abilities of the patient and/or, as appropriate, his/her significant other(s) to manage continuing care needs after discharge.

TABLE 2–3. Contents of a Progress Note

Unsettled or unclear problems or issues that need to be dealt with, including attempts to contact other client care providers.

Noteworthy incidents or interviews involving the client that would benefit from a more detailed recording.

Other pertinent data, such as notes on phone calls, home visits, and family interactions.

Additional critical incident data, such as seemingly significant or revealing statements made by the client, an insight the nurse has into a client's patterns of behavior, client injuries, the use of any special treatment procedure, or other major events such as episodes of pain, respiratory distress, panic attacks, medication reactions, or suicidal comments.

Administered care, activities, or observations if not recorded elsewhere on flow sheets (physician visits, completion of ordered tests, required medications).

error in the document must be crossed out with one line so that it is still legible, identified by the author as "error," and then initialed. "White-outs" or "cross-outs," which make the information unreadable, are not acceptable, because they could be construed to mean that the individual or facility is trying to alter facts.

The medical record is always the primary source of providing proof of services, which is necessary to maintain revenues. Third-party payors insist that the *why, when, where, how, what,* and *who* of services be clearly documented. Absence of such documentation may result in termination of funding for individual clients and therefore termination of treatment. Therefore, progress notes must document what is happening to the client during all phases of pregnancy, intervention, and recovery. It is important to record information and observations that will assist the oncoming nurse and other healthcare providers to maintain continuity of planned care. Table 2–3 provides examples of information to be documented in the client record.

There are several charting formats currently used for documentation (e.g., problem-oriented medical record, or POMR; Focus® charting). Regardless of the form used, entries should be concise and consistent in style and format to avoid confusion and to comply with existing agency policies and procedures. Examples of documentation formats are included in Chapter 3.

Summary

This book is intended to facilitate the application of the nursing process and the use of nursing diagnosis for the maternity client, newborn, and family. Each plan of care is intended to be an informational guide, designed to provide generalized information on the associated medical condition. The guides can be modified by either using portions of the information provided or adding additional client-care information to the existing guides. The plan of care guidelines were developed using NANDA recommendations except in a few examples where we felt more clarification and enhancement were required. The ongoing controversy on the validity of the NANDA-approved nursing diagnosis *Knowledge Deficit* is one example where further clarification was added; we added the term *Learning Need* to that nursing diagnosis. For example, for the client with severe hypertension, a nursing diagnosis was developed with the following label: Knowledge Deficit [Learning Need] regarding condition, prognosis, and treatment plan.

We recognize that not all of the NANDA-approved nursing diagnoses have been used in these guides but we hope that the guides will assist the nurse in determining the client's needs, outcomes, and nursing interventions. Some diagnoses have been combined for convenience, indicating that two or more factors may be involved; for example, Anxiety/Fear.

We anticipate that the nurse will choose what is applicable. Nurses can be creative as they work with the standardized format, redefining and sharing interventions as they are used with individual clients. We appreciate that not all diagnoses presented in these plans of care will be appropriate for a particular client or locale, in which case alternatives should be chosen to meet the individual client's needs. We support the belief that practicing nurses and researchers need to study, use, and evaluate the diagnoses as presented. As new nursing diagnoses are developed, the information they encompass must be reflected in the data base. The nurse is encouraged to share insights and ideas with the Task Force of the National Group for Nursing Diagnoses, NANDA, 1211 Locust St., Philadelphia, PA 19107; 1-800-647-9002.

The next chapter will assist the nurse in applying and adapting theory to practice.

CHAPTER 3

ADAPTATION OF THEORY TO PRACTICE

Client assessment is the foundation on which identification of individual needs, responses, and problems is based. To facilitate the steps of assessment and diagnosis in the nursing process, assessment data bases have been constructed using a nursing focus instead of the traditional medical approach of "review of systems."

Sample prenatal, intrapartal, and postpartal assessment tools will be presented in the appropriate chapters. These assessment tools are suggested guides for development by an individual or facility to create data bases reflecting a nursing focus.

To achieve this nursing focus, we have grouped the NANDA nursing diagnoses into related categories titled "Diagnostic Divisions" (Table 3–1), which reflect a blending of theories, primarily Maslow's hierarchy of needs and a self-care philosophy. These divisions serve as the framework or outline for collection of data, directing the nurse to the appropriate corresponding nursing diagnoses as the client information is recorded in the *client assessment data base* (Table 3–2).

Because the divisions are based on human responses and needs, and not on specific "systems," information may be recorded in more than one area. For this reason, the nurse is encouraged to keep an open mind, to pursue all leads, and to collect as much data as possible before choosing the nursing diagnosis label that best reflects the client's situation. For example, when the nurse identifies the cue of restlessness in a client, the nurse may infer that the client is anxious. The nurse may believe that the restlessness is psychologically based, overlooking the possibility that it is physiologically based.

From the specific data recorded in the data base, the related/risk factors (etiology) and signs and symptoms can be identified, and an individualized client diagnostic statement can be formulated using the problem, etiology, signs/symptoms (PES) format to accurately represent the client's situation. For example, the diagnostic statement may read: "Knowledge Deficit [Learning Need], regarding preterm labor, related to lack of information/misinterpretation, evidenced by questions and expression of concerns."

Desired client outcomes are identified to facilitate choosing appropriate interventions and to serve as evaluators of both nursing care and client response. These outcomes also form the framework for documentation.

Interventions are designed to specify the action of the nurse, the client, and/or significant other(s). Interventions need to promote movement toward independence, in addition to achieving physiologic stability. This requires involvement of the client in her own care, including participation in decisions about the care and projected outcomes. In addition, although the pregnant woman is the primary client, significant other(s)/family members will also need consideration and inclusion in care.

To assist in visualizing this process, a client situation and sample plan of care (Preterm Labor/Prevention of Delivery) provides an example of data collection and construction of the plan of care. As the *client assessment data base* is reviewed, the nurse can identify the related or risk factors and defining characteristics (signs/symptoms) that were used to formulate the client diagnostic statements. The addition of time lines to specific client outcomes and goals reflects anticipated length of stay and individual client and nurse expectations. Interventions have been chosen based on concerns/needs identified by the client and

TABLE 3-1. Nursing Diagnoses Organized According to Diagnostic Divisions*

ACTIVITY/REST— Ability to engage in necessary/desired activities of life (work and leisure) and to obtain sleep/rest
- Activity Intolerance
- Activity Intolerance, high risk for
- Disuse Syndrome, high risk for
- Diversional Activity deficit
- Fatigue
- Sleep Pattern disturbance

CIRCULATION— Ability to transport oxygen and nutrients necessary to meet cellular needs
- Cardiac Output, decreased
- Dysreflexia
- Tissue Perfusion, altered (specify): cerebral, cardiopulmonary, renal, gastrointestinal, peripheral

EGO INTEGRITY— Ability to develop and use skills and behaviors to integrate and manage life experiences
- Adjustment, impaired
- Anxiety [specify level]
- Body Image disturbance
- Coping, defensive
- Coping, Individual, ineffective
- Decisional Conflict (specify)
- Denial, ineffective
- Fear
- Grieving, anticipatory
- Grieving, dysfunctional
- Hopelessness
- Personal Identity disturbance
- Post-Trauma Response
- Powerlessness
- Rape-Trauma Syndrome
- Rape-Trauma Syndrome: compound reaction
- Rape-Trauma Syndrome: silent reaction
- Relocation Stress Syndrome
- Self Esteem, chronic low
- Self Esteem, disturbance
- Self Esteem, situational low
- Spiritual Distress (distress of the human spirit)

ELIMINATION— Ability to excrete waste products
- Bowel Incontinence
- Constipation
- Constipation, colonic
- Constipation, perceived
- Diarrhea
- Incontinence, functional
- Incontinence, reflex
- Incontinence, stress
- Incontinence, total
- Incontinence, urge

- Urinary Elimination, altered
- Urinary Retention [acute/chronic]

FOOD/FLUID— Ability to maintain intake of and utilize nutrients and liquids to meet physiologic needs
- Breastfeeding, effective
- Breastfeeding, ineffective
- Breastfeeding, interrupted
- Fluid Volume deficit [active loss]
- Fluid Volume deficit [regulatory failure]
- Fluid Volume deficit, high risk for
- Fluid Volume excess
- Infant Feeding Pattern, ineffective
- Nutrition, altered, less than body requirements
- Nutrition, altered, more than body requirements
- Nutrition, altered, high risk for more than body requirements
- Oral Mucous Membrane, altered
- Swallowing, impaired

HYGIENE— Ability to perform activities of daily living
- Self Care deficit (specify): feeding, bathing/hygiene, dressing/grooming, toileting

NEUROSENSORY— Ability to perceive, integrate, and respond to internal and external cues
- Peripheral Neurovascular dysfunction, high risk for
- Sensory-Perceptual alterations (specify): visual, auditory, kinesthetic, gustatory, tactile, olfactory
- Thought Processes, altered
- Unilateral Neglect

PAIN/DISCOMFORT— Ability to control internal/external environment to maintain comfort
- Pain [acute]
- Pain, chronic

RESPIRATION— Ability to provide and use oxygen to meet physiologic needs
- Airway Clearance, ineffective
- Aspiration, high risk for
- Breathing Pattern, ineffective
- Gas Exchange, impaired
- Spontaneous Ventilation, inability to sustain
- Ventilatory Weaning Response, dysfunctional (DVWR)

SAFETY— Ability to provide safe, growth-promoting environment
- Body Temperature, altered, high risk for
- Health Maintenance, altered
- Home Maintenance Management, impaired

(continued)

TABLE 3–1. Nursing Diagnoses Organized According to Diagnostic Divisions* (continued)

Hyperthermia
Hypothermia
Infection, high risk for
Injury, high risk for
Physical Mobility, impaired
Poisoning, high risk for
Protection, altered
Self-Mutilation, high risk for
Skin Integrity, impaired
Skin Integrity, impaired, high risk for
Suffocation, high risk for
Thermoregulation, ineffective
Tissue Integrity, impaired
Trauma, high risk for
Violence, high risk for, directed at self/others

SEXUALITY — [Component of Ego Integrity and Social Interaction] — Ability to meet requirements/characteristics of male or female role
Sexual dysfunction
Sexuality Patterns, altered

SOCIAL INTERACTION — Ability to establish and maintain relationships
Caregiver Role Strain
Caregiver Role Strain, high risk for
Communication, impaired verbal
Family Coping, ineffective: compromised
Family Coping, ineffective: disabling
Family Coping: potential for growth
Family Processes, altered
Parenteral Role Conflict
Parenting, altered
Parenting, altered, high risk for
Role Performance, altered
Social Interaction, impaired
Social Isolation

TEACHING/LEARNING — Ability to incorporate and use information to achieve healthy lifestyle/optimal wellness
Growth and Development, altered
Health-Seeking Behaviors (specify)
Knowledge Deficit [Learning Need] (specify)
Noncompliance [Compliance, altered] (specify)
Therapeutic Regimen (Individual), ineffective management of

*After data are collected, and areas of concern/need identified, the nurse is directed to the *diagnostic divisions* to review the list of nursing diagnoses that fall within the individual categories. This will assist the nurse in choosing the specific diagnostic label to describe the data accurately. Then with the addition of etiology or related/risk factors (when known) and signs and symptoms (defining characteristics), the client diagnostic statement emerges.

nurse during data collection, as well as physician orders. Although not normally included in a plan of care, rationales are included in this sample for the purpose of explaining or clarifying the choice of interventions and enhancing the nurse's learning. Finally, to complete the learning experience, samples of documentation based on the client situation are presented.

TABLE 3-2. Prenatal Assessment Tool

General information:
Name _____ Age ____ DOB _____ Race _____ Visit/Admission date _____
Health care provider: maternal _____ infant _____
Father of child: Age: ____ Race: _____
Source of information: reliability _____ (1–4 with 4 very reliable)

ACTIVITY/REST:

Subjective:

Occupation: _____
Usual activities/hobbies: _____
Leisure time activities: _____
Usual exercise: _____
Limitations imposed by pregnancy/condition: ____
Physical requirements of:
Employment: _____ Home: _____
Sleep: Number of hours: _____ Naps: _____
    Aids: _____ Insomnia: _____
    Reason: _____

Objective:

Observed response to activity:
    Cardiovascular: _____ Respiratory: _____
Mental status (e.g., withdrawn/lethargic): _____
Neuromuscular assessment:
    Muscle mass/tone: _____ Posture: _____
    Tremors: _____ ROM: _____ Strength: _____
    Deformity: _____ Other: _____

CIRCULATION:

Subjective:

History of: Elevated BP: _____
    Heart trouble: _____ Rheumatic fever: _____
    Ankle/leg edema: _____ Phlebitis: _____
    Slow healing: _____
Extremities: Numbness: _____ Tingling: _____
Cough/hemoptysis: _____
Change in frequency/amount of urine: _____

Objective:

BP: R and L: Standing: _____ Sitting: _____
    Lying: _____
Peripheral pulses: Radial: _____
    Dorsalis pedis: _____
    Jugular vein distention: _____
Heart sounds: Rate: _____ Rhythm: _____
    Quality: _____ Rub/murmur: _____
Breath sounds: _____
Extremities: Temperature: _____ Color: _____
    Capillary refill: _____ Homan's sign: _____
    Varicosities: _____
    Nails (abnormalities): _____
Color/cyanosis: Overall: _____
    Mucous membranes: _____ Lips: _____
    Nailbeds: _____ Conjunctiva: _____
    Sclera: _____ Diaphoresis: _____

EGO INTEGRITY:

Subjective:

Pregnancy planned (Y/N): _____
Client/father feelings about pregnancy: _____
Relationship status: _____
Report of stress factors: Financial concerns: ____
    Lifestyle: _____ Recent changes: _____
Ways of handling stress: _____
Religion (practicing): _____
Cultural factors: _____
Feelings of: Helplessness: _____
    Hopelessness: _____ Powerlessness: _____
History of emotional problems: _____
    Psychologic abuse/neglect: _____

Objective:

Emotional status: _____
Observed physiologic response(s): _____

(continued)

TABLE 3-2. Prenatal Assessment Tool (continued)

ELIMINATION:

Subjective:

Usual bowel pattern: _____ Laxative use: _____
  Character of stool: _____ Last BM: _____
  Bleeding: _____ Hemorrhoids: _____
  Diarrhea: _____ Constipation: _____
Usual voiding pattern: _____
  Incontinence/when: _____ Urgency: _____
  Frequency: _____ Retention: _____
  Character of urine: _____
  Pain/burning/difficulty voiding: _____
  History of kidney/bladder disease: _____
  Diuretic use: _____

Objective:

Abdomen tender: _____ Soft/firm: _____
  Palpable mass: _____ Size/girth: _____
  Bowel sounds: _____ Hemorrhoids: _____
  Bladder palpable: _____
  Overflow voiding: _____
Urinalysis: _____ Albuminuria: _____
  Glycosuria: _____ Occult blood: _____
Stool for occult blood: _____

FOOD/FLUID:

Subjective:

Usual diet (type): _____ Number of meals
  daily: _____
  Last meal/intake: _____ Dietary pattern: _____
  Loss of appetite: _____
  Nausea/vomiting: _____
  Heartburn/indigestion: _____
  Related to/relieved by: _____
  Allergy/food intolerance: _____
Mastication/swallowing problems: _____
  Dentures: _____
Average non-pregnant weight: _____
  Current weight: _____ Pattern of weight: gain/
  loss: _____
Diuretic use: _____

Objective:

Current weight: _____ Height: _____
  Body build: _____ Skin turgor: _____
  Mucous membranes moist/dry: _____
Hernia/masses: _____
Edema: _____ General: _____
  Dependent: _____
  Periorbital: _____ Sacral: _____
  Digital: _____
  Jugular vein distention: _____
Thyroid enlarged: _____
Halitosis: _____ Condition of teeth/gums: _____
  Appearance of tongue: _____;
  Mucous membranes: _____
Bowel sounds: _____
Breath sounds: _____
Diabetic screening: GTT: _____
  Thyroid studies: _____
Hb/Hct (anemia): _____

HYGIENE:

Subjective:

Activities of daily living: Independent/dependent
  (specify): _____
Equipment/prosthetic devices required: _____
  Assistance provided by: _____

Objective:

General appearance: _____ Manner of
  dress: _____ Personal habits: _____ Body
  odor: _____ Condition of scalp: _____
  Presence of vermin: _____

NEUROSENSORY:

Subjective:

Fainting spells/dizziness: _____
Headaches: _____ Location: _____
  Frequency: _____ Tingling/numbness/
  weakness (location): _____
Stroke (residual effects): _____
Seizures: _____ Aura: _____
  How controlled: _____

Objective:

Mental status: Oriented/disoriented
  (specify): _____
Glasses: _____ Contacts: _____ Hearing
  aids: _____
Usual speech pattern/impairment: _____

(continued)

TABLE 3–2. Prenatal Assessment Tool (continued)

Eyes: Vision loss: _____ Last examination: _____
  Glaucoma: _____ Cataract: _____
Ears: Hearing loss: _____ Last
  examination: _____
Epistaxis: _____ Sense of smell: _____

PAIN/DISCOMFORT:

Subjective:

Location: _____ Intensity (0–10 with 10 most
  severe): _____ Frequency: _____
  Quality: _____ Duration: _____ Precipitating
  factors: _____
  How relieved: _____ Associated
  symptoms _____

Objective:

Facial grimacing: _____ Guarding affected
  area: _____ Emotional response: _____
  Narrowed focus: _____

RESPIRATION:

Subjective:

Dyspnea (related to): _____ Cough/sputum: _____
History of bronchitis: _____ Asthma: _____
  Tuberculosis: _____ Emphysema: _____
  Recurrent pneumonia: _____
Smoker _____ Pk/day: _____ Number of
  years: _____ Use of respiratory aids: _____
  Oxygen _____

Objective:

Respiratory: Rate: _____ Depth: _____
  Quality: _____
Breath sounds: _____
Sputum characteristics: _____
Chest x-ray results: _____

SAFETY:

Subjective:

Allergies/sensitivity: _____ Reaction: _____
Previous alteration of immune system: _____
  Cause: _____
History of sexually transmitted diseases/
  gynecologic infections (date/type): _____
  High-risk behaviors: _____ Testing: _____
Blood transfusion/number: _____ When: _____
  Reaction: _____ Describe: _____
Childhood diseases: _____ Immunization
  history: _____
Recent exposure to German measles: _____
  Other viral infections: _____
  x-ray/radiation: _____ house pets: _____
Previous obstetrical problems: PIH: _____
  Kidney: _____ Hemorrhage: _____
  Cardiac: _____ Diabetes: _____
  Infection/UTI: _____ ABO/Rh sensitivity: _____
  Uterine surgery: _____ Anemia: _____
Length of time since last pregnancy: _____
  Type of previous delivery: _____
History of accidental injuries: Fractures/
  dislocations: _____ Physical abuse: _____
  Arthritis/unstable joints: _____ Back
  problems: _____
Changes in moles: _____ Enlarged nodes: _____
Impaired vision: _____ Hearing: _____
Prosthesis: _____ Ambulatory devices: _____

Objective:

Temperature: _____ Diaphoresis: _____
  Skin integrity: _____ Scars: _____
  Rashes: _____ Ecchymosis: _____
  Vaginal warts/lesions: _____
General strength: _____ Muscle tone: _____
  Gait: _____ ROM: _____ Paresthesia/
  paralysis: _____
Fetal: Heart rate: _____ Location: _____
  Method of auscultation: _____
  Fundal height: _____ Estimated
  gestation: _____
  Movement: _____ Ballottement: _____
Results of fetal testing: _____ AFT: _____
Results of cultures, cervical/rectal: _____
  Immune system testing: _____ Blood type:
  Maternal: _____ Paternal: _____ Screenings:
  Serology: _____ Syphilis: _____
  Sickle cell: _____ Rubella: _____
  Hepatitis: _____ HIV: _____

(continued)

TABLE 3–2. Prenatal Assessment Tool (continued)

SEXUALITY (Component of Social Interactions)

Subjective:

Sexual concerns: _____
Menarche: _____ Length of cycle: _____
    Duration: _____
First day of last menstrual period: _____
    Amount: _____ Bleeding/cramping since
    LMP: _____
Vaginal discharge: _____
Client's belief of when conception occurred: _____
Estimated date of delivery: _____
Practices breast self exam (Y/N): _____
Last PAP smear: _____ Results: _____
Recent contraceptive method: _____
Ob history: (GPTPAL) gravida: _____ Para: _____
    Term: _____ Preterm: _____ Abortions: _____
    Living: _____ Multiple births: _____
Delivery history: Year: _____ Place of
    delivery: _____ Length of gestation: _____
    Length of labor: _____ Type of delivery: _____
    Born (alive or dead): _____ Weight: _____
    Apgar scores: _____
Complications (maternal/fetal): _____

Objective:

Pelvic: Vulva: _____ Perineum: _____
    Vagina: _____ Cervix: _____ Uterus: _____
    Adnexal: _____ Diagonal conjugate: _____
    Transverse diameter: _____ Outlet (cm): _____
    Shape of sacrum: _____ Arch: _____
    Coccyx: _____ SS Notch: _____ Ischial
    spines:
    _____ Adequacy of inlet: _____ Mid: _____
    Outlet: _____
Prognosis for delivery: _____
Breast exam: _____ Nipples: _____
Pregnancy test: _____
    Serology test (date): _____

SOCIAL INTERACTIONS:

Subjective:

Relationship status: _____ Years in relationship:
    _____ Living with: _____ Role within family
    structure: _____
Extended family: _____ Other support person(s):
    _____ Frequency of social contacts: _____
Concerns/stresses: _____ Coping behaviors:
    _____
Plans for intra/postpartal period: _____

Objective:

Verbal/nonverbal communication with significant
    other/family: _____
Family interaction (behavioral) pattern: _____

TEACHING/LEARNING:

Subjective:

Dominant language (specify): _____
    Literate: _____ Cognitive limitations: _____
Maternal/paternal education levels: _____
    Occupations: _____
Ethnic/cultural background: _____ Health beliefs/
    special practices (including religious factors):
    _____
Familial risk factors (indicate relationship):
    Diabetes: _____ Tuberculosis: _____
    High BP: _____ Epilepsy: _____
    Heart disease: _____
    Strokes: _____ Kidney disease: _____

Discharge Plan Considerations (when hospitalized)

Date information obtained: _____
Anticipated date of discharge: _____
Availability of maternity leave: _____
Resources available: Persons: _____
    Financial: _____
Anticipated needs/assistance required: _____

TABLE 3–2. Prenatal Assessment Tool (continued)

Cancer: _____ Blood disorders: _____
Mental illness: _____ Genetic (congenital)
problems: _____ Cesarean births: _____
Multiple births: _____
Prescribed medications: Drug: _____
   Dose: _____ Times: _____
   Take regularly: _____ Purpose: _____
Non-prescription drugs: Over-the-counter (OTC):
   _____ Street drugs: _____ Use of alcohol
   (amount/frequency): _____ Tobacco: _____
Current complaints/symptoms of
   pregnancy: _____ Effect on lifestyle: _____
   Adaptations made: _____
Relevant illnesses and/or hospitalizations/
   surgeries: _____
Expectations of this pregnancy/hospitalization:
   _____
Last physical exam (date and doctor): _____
Type of delivery: _____ Anesthesia: _____,
   Infant feeding planned: _____
Education classes/resources: _____

SAMPLE MATERNAL CLIENT SITUATION:
Preterm Labor/Prevention of Delivery _____

Mrs. R.F.M., a 30-yr-old gravida 1, para 0, with expected/estimated date of delivery (EDD) of 6/26/90 (24½ weeks' gestation), and ultrasound confirmation of 2 fetuses present (office visit 2/5/90) called physician's office today (3/14/90) at 1400. R.F.M. had experienced a contraction beginning at 1340; at 1400 her abdomen remained firm to touch even after she had attempted to diminish the contraction by: 1) drinking two large glasses of water, 2) voiding a moderate amount, and 3) lying on her left side. She was directed to the hospital for evaluation of labor, and was admitted with an initial diagnosis of possible preterm labor.

ADMITTING PHYSICIAN'S ORDERS

Have patient drink 480 to 720 ml of fluid now.
Apply external fetal monitor (EFM), document uterine activity and fetal status.
Check cervix for dilatation and effacement.
Nitrazine test, vaginal culture now.
Stat CBC, K+, UA.
Fasting blood glucose per fingerstick in AM.
Terbutaline 0.25 mg SC and 5 mg PO now; if contractions do not cease, start 500 ml lactated Ringer's infusion and begin terbutaline drip per protocol.
Betamethasone 12.5 mg (2 ml) IM now and repeat in 12 hours.
VS q4hr.
Complete bedrest.
Regular diet.

NURSING HISTORY AND ASSESSMENT

Name: R.F.M.
Age: 30. DOB: 5/6/62. Sex: F. Race: Caucasian.
Admission date: 3/14/93. Time: 1520. From: Home.
Source of information: Client.
Father of Child: R.L.M. Age: 38. Race: Caucasian.
Health care provider: Maternal: Dr. C.R.
                                    Infant: Has not chosen yet

ACTIVITY/REST

Reports (Subjective):
Sleep: Hours: 8–10 h/night Naps: 2/day Aids: None.

Usual activities/hobbies: Needlework and reading.

Limitations imposed by pregnancy: Bedrest, ordered by physician 2/5/93.

Occupation: RN, worked part time until 2/5/93.

Exhibits (Objective):
Observed response to activity: Cardiovascular: Slight increase in rate (110 bpm). Respiratory: Slight increase in rate (26/min).

Mental status: Outgoing, alert; responds appropriately.

Neuromuscular assessment: Quality of extremities: Moves all four extremities well/equal. Posture: Erect. ROM: Full. Tremors: -0-. Strength: Good/equal in all extremities.

CIRCULATION

Reports (Subjective):
History of: Elevated B/P: -0-. Heart trouble: -0-. Rheumatic fever: -0-. Ankle/leg edema: -0-. Phlebitis: -0-. Slow healing: -0-.

Extremities: Numbness: -0-. Tingling: -0-.

BP: R: Standing: 122/70. Sitting: 120/66. Lying: 120/62. L: Stand: 124/72. Sitting: 122/68. Lying: 120/62.

Peripheral pulses: Radials 3+, Pedals 2+.

Heart sounds: No murmurs or rubs. Apical rate: 100 bpm. Rhythm: Regular. Quality: Strong.

Jugular vein distention: -0-.

Extremities: Temperature: Warm to touch. Color: Pink.

Capillary refill: Rapid, under 3 seconds.

Homans' sign: -0-. Varicosities: -0-.

Nails: Normal; pink nail beds; nail base firm.

Color/cyanosis: Mucous membranes: Pink; intact. Conjunctiva: salmon-colored. Sclera: white.

EGO INTEGRITY

Reports (Subjective):

Pregnancy planned: Yes.

Client feelings about pregnancy: "We waited several years so I'm really happy."

Father's feelings about pregnancy: Excited and relieved as conception had been a difficult process.

Relationship status: Married.

Financial concerns: Has health insurance coverage and sick leave.

Religion: Maternal/Paternal: Both Protestant. Practicing: Yes.

Cultural factors: Urban white-collar workers, middle-class, Western European descent.

Report of stress factors: "It has been frustrating to lie around the house and not be able to do things that need to be done. Now I am very concerned about our babies' health."

Ways of handling stress: Previously walking, now relaxation skills and reading.

Lifestyle: Married, dual-income family. Recent changes: Off work and unable to care for husband and self.

Feelings of helplessness: "Sometimes." Hopelessness: No. Powerlessness: "Some right now."

Exhibits (Objective):

Emotional status: Calm, fearful.

Observed physiologic response(s): Remains calm, yet demonstrates appropriate concern; facial expression tense; body tense guarded.

ELIMINATION

Reports (Subjective):

Usual bowel pattern: Once a day. Laxative use: -0-.

Character of stool: Soft, brown, formed. Last bowel movement: Yesterday.

Bleeding: -0- Hemorrhoids: -0-.

Usual voiding pattern: Moderate amount every 2–4 hours around the clock.

Incontinence: -0-. Urgency: -0-.

Frequency: Since 3rd week of pregnancy. Retention: -0-.

Character of urine: Clear, pale yellow.

Pain/burning/difficulty voiding: -0-. History of kidney/bladder disease: -0-.

Exhibits (Objective):

Abdomen: Slightly tender since 12/92. Soft/firm: Firm. Palpable mass: No abnormalities. Size/girth: 22 cm.

Bowel sounds: Present all quadrants.

Hemorrhoids: None present.

Bladder palpable: -0-. Overflow voiding: -0-.

Urinalysis report: To be done.

Albuminuria/glycosuria: Negative per dipstick.

FOOD/FLUID

**Reports
(Subjective):**

Loss of appetite: -0-.

Nausea: -0-. Vomiting: Severe vomiting during 1st 15 weeks of pregnancy.

Heartburn/food intolerance: -0-.

Normal weight: 140 lb.

Use of diuretics: -0-.

Dietary pattern: eats 3 meals/d.

Last ate/what: Lunch/tomato soup and tuna sandwich, milk, cookie, half an apple.

**Exhibits
(Objective):**

Current weight: 159 lb. Height: 5'5". Body build: Stocky/endomorphic. Skin turgor: Good, elastic.

Edema: Dependent/periorbital: -0-. Thyroid enlarged: No.

Halitosis: -0-.

Condition of teeth/gums: All teeth present and in good condition; gums pink, no bleeding.

Appearance of tongue: Pink; fully mobile within mouth.

Breath sounds: Clear bilateral.

Hb/Hct (anemia): Hb 12.6, Hct 37.8.

Diabetic screening: GTT. N/A. Thyroid studies: N/A.

HYGIENE

**Reports
(Subjective):**

Activities of daily living: Independent: In all areas until 2/5/93; since then has maintained bedrest with bathroom privileges.

Dependent (specify): Husband has done all household tasks and assisted client with self-care activities since client was placed on bedrest.

**Exhibits
(Objective):**

General appearance: Clean and neat, light makeup, hair groomed.

Manner of dress: Maternity dress, low-heeled shoes.

Condition of scalp: Clean, slightly dry.

NEUROSENSORY

**Reports
(Subjective):**

Fainting spells/dizziness: Dizziness during 1st trimester.

Headaches: Location: Right temporal area. Frequency: Occasional, "especially when I am under stress." Has right temporal-mandibular joint (TMJ) disease.

Eyes/vision loss: Near-sighted R/L corrected with glasses.

Ears/hearing loss: None. Nose/epistaxis: Occasional "especially when humidity is very low."

Sense of smell: Reports no problems/not tested.

**Exhibits
(Objective):**

Mental status: Alert, oriented to time, person, place.

Pupils: PERLA.

Glasses: Yes Contacts: -0-. Hearing aid: -0-.

Unusual speech pattern/impairment: -0-.

PAIN/DISCOMFORT

Reports
(Subjective):

Location: Suprapubic.

Intensity (0–10): 3–4. Quality: Dull pain; increases when symphysis pubis is touched. Duration: 1 week.

Precipitating factors: Twin "A" became engaged; experienced a contraction to-day with abdomen remaining tense since.

How relieved: Is not relieved; tried drinking 2 large glasses of water, voiding, and lying on left side.

Exhibits
(Objective):

Facial grimacing: When area is palpated. Narrowed focus: No.

Guarding affected area: Asks medical staff to use light touch when taking uterine measurements.

RESPIRATION

Reports
(Subjective):

Dyspnea/caused by: -0-. Cough/productive: -0-.

History: Bronchitis: -0-. Asthma: -0- Tuberculosis: -0-.

Smoker: -0-/nonsmoking household.

Exhibits
(Objective):

Respiratory: Rate: 20/min. Depth: Shallow. Quality: Equal; bilateral.

Breath sounds: Vesicular, clear bilateral.

SAFETY

Reports
(Subjective):

Allergies/sensitivity: Penicillin. Reaction: Generalized red rash. Occurred when client was a child, has not taken penicillin since.

History of STD (date/type): -0-.

German measles: Immune. Exposure to radiation: Not during pregnancy.

Previous obstetrical problems: N/A. ABO/Rh sensitivity: N/A.

Blood transfusion: -0-.

Fractures/dislocations: Nose was fractured at age 4. Arthritis/unstable joints: -0- Back problems: -0-.

Impaired: Vision: Wears glasses "except to sleep."

Exhibits
(Objective):

Temperature: 98.6, oral.

Skin integrity: Intact/Scars: Inner right forearm, old injury from childhood.

Strength (general): Good; equal in all 4 extremities.

Muscle tone: Firm/Gait: Wide spaced secondary to pregnancy. ROM: Good.

Fetal: Heart rate: Twin "A" 150 bpm, Twin "B" 154 bpm. Location: Twin "A" LLQ (2 fingers above pubic bone), Twin "B" RUQ (4 fingers breadth to R of umbilicus). Method of auscultation: EFM. Fundal height: 22 cm. Estimated gestation: $24^{1}/_{7}$ weeks. Movement: Frequent; active. Ballotment: Absent; Twin "A" engaged.

Blood Type/Rh: Maternal: A+ Paternal: A+.

Screens: Sickle cell: N/A. Rubella: Immune. Hepatitis: -0-.

AFP: -0-.

Serology syphilis: Negative 11/18/92.

Cervical/rectal culture: Pending (done 3/14/93; 1600).

Vaginal warts/lesions: -0-.

SEXUALITY

**Reports
(Subjective):**

Menarche: 10 years old. Length of cycle: 28 days. Duration: 3–5 days.

Last menstrual period: 9/19/92. Amount: Moderate. EDD: 6/26/93.

Vaginal discharge: Odorless, clear, thick.

Bleeding since LMP: Once a month, first trimester: spotting.

Practices breast self-exam: Yes. Last PAP smear: 11/18/92.

Recent contraceptive method: Diaphragm.

Ob history (GPTPAL): (Gravida: 1. Para: 0. Abortions: 0.

**Exhibits
(Objective):**

Pelvic: Vulva: Pink; moist. Perineum: no abnormalities; pink; intact.

Vagina: Dark, pink. Cervix: Closed; Chadwick's sign present.

Uterus: Distended, pear-shaped. Adnexal: Normal.

Diagonal conjugate: 12.5 cm. Transverse diameter: Outlet: 10.5 cm.

Shape of sacrum: Normal, average inclination. Coccyx: Movable.

Ischial spines: >8 cm.

Inlet: Adequate. Mid: Adequate. Outlet: Adequate.

Prognosis for delivery: Good for vaginal delivery.

Breast exam: Supple, symmetric; no abnormalities.

Nipples: Erect/dark in color; no cracks or fissures; no abnormalities.

Serology test: Negative 10/25/92.

SOCIAL INTERACTIONS

**Reports
(Subjective):**

Relationship status: Married. Years in relationship: 8. Living with: Husband.

Role within family structure: Housewife; secondary breadwinner.

Extended family: Married younger brother/nephew in town; all other relatives live out-of-town.

Other support person(s): Many close friends in town; mother available to come if client goes home on bedrest.

Frequency of social contacts: Family/friends in 2–3 times/wk.

Concerns/stresses: Husband has had to carry all responsibilities for both of them.

Coping behaviors: Maintains open communication, acceptance of situation.

Plans for intra/postpartal period: Mother will be available.

**Exhibits
(Objective):**

Verbal/nonverbal communication with family/SO(s): Husband sitting beside bed, speaks quietly and holds client's hand.

TEACHING/LEARNING

**Reports
(Subjective):**

Language dominant: English. Literate: Yes.

Ethnic/cultural background: Anglo-Saxon. Health beliefs/special practices: -0-.

Education: Client: BSN. Cognitive limitations: 0.

Husband: MS degree. Occupation: Respiratory therapist.

Familial risk factors (maternal/paternal; indicate relationship): Tuberculosis: Maternal grandfather. Diabetes: -0-. High BP: maternal aunt. Epilepsy: -0-. Heart disease: -0-. Stroke: -0-. Kidney disease: -0-. Cancer: Maternal grandmother had colon cancer.

Multiple births: Maternal: aunt had twins; father of these babies is a twin.

Genetic conditions: -0-.

Prescribed medications: Drugs: Maternal prenatal vitamin/mineral supplement: Takes 1 tablet daily at 2200, regularly.

Nonprescription drugs: OTC: -0-. Illicit: -0-.

Use of alcohol (amount/frequency): -0-.

Current complaints/symptoms of pregnancy: Called OB at 1400, reported having a contraction that didn't seem to go away and abdomen remained very firm.

Relevant illnesses and/or hospitalization/surgery: 12/10/92: Short stay hospitalization for IV therapy; R.M. experienced 7-lb weight loss in 48 h due to severe prenatal vomiting.

Last physical exam: Last OB appt., 3/7/93; uterine measurement, FHT, and ultrasound done by Dr. C.R.

Ultrasound report: Twin "A" was shown to be engaged and both babies were growing at the same rate. R.M. complained of frequent regular contractions and the day after the appointment, called to report loss of mucus plug.

Expectations of this pregnancy: Full-term, healthy babies.

Type of delivery planned: Vaginal, although twin "B" is breech so realizes cesarean birth is possible.

Type of anesthesia planned: Local, if episiotomy is done; otherwise, none.

Type of infant feeding planned: Breast.

Preparation: Prenatal/intrapartal classes: Prematurity Prevention 2/18/93.

Infant care/feeding: No formal class yet, was to begin childbirth classes 3/31/93.

Books: Several medical books dealing with obstetrics and bonding.

Other (specify): Contacted local chapters of La Leche League and the Twins Club.

Discharge Plan Considerations:

On 3/14/93
If delivery delayed: Will require periodic home health monitoring/visitation; homemaker assistance.

Anticipated discharge: Within 5 days—by 3/19/93.

Resources available: Husband, mother.

SAMPLE MATERNAL CLIENT PLAN OF CARE: Preterm Labor/Prevention of Delivery

CLIENT DIAGNOSTIC STATEMENT (NURSING DIAGNOSIS):	ANXIETY [MODERATE], related to the possibility of premature delivery, perceived or actual threat to fetuses and self, evidenced by expressions of concern regarding current events, increased tension, apprehension, narrowed focus.
DESIRED OUTCOMES— CLIENT WILL:	Verbalize awareness of feelings of anxiety within 24 hours (3/15 1600).
	Appear relaxed and report anxiety is reduced to a manageable level within 24 hours (3/15 1600).
	Identify three ways she is dealing with anxieties within 48 hours (3/16 1600).

ACTIONS/INTERVENTIONS	RATIONALE
Introduce self to R.F.M. and family. Maintain "primary caregiver."	Important for couple to feel "connected" to the caregiver to promote a sense of trust.
Explain procedures, nursing interventions, and treatments.	Knowledge of the reasons for these activities can decrease fear of the unknown.
Orient couple to labor suite environment.	Helps client/husband to feel at ease and more comfortable in their surroundings.
Keep communication open; discuss the possible side effects and outcomes, maintaining an optimistic attitude.	Knowing information will be given freely and questions will be answered can help to reduce anxiety and promote hope and strengthen "working" relationship between client and staff.
Control external stimulation. Review restrictions/rationale (e.g., TV, radio, visitors, phone).	Quiet atmosphere promotes rest and relaxation, which can assist in decreasing muscle tension and may enhance uterine and fetal blood flow. In turn, this may reduce the perceived/actual threat to fetuses.
Encourage use of relaxation techniques (e.g., deep breathing exercises, visualization, guided imagery).	Enables the client to obtain maximum benefit from rest periods; prevents muscle fatigue and may improve uterine blood flow. Provides opportunity for active participation and enhances sense of control.
Encourage verbalization of fears and concerns.	Helps client to define and become aware of specific problems, providing opportunity for problem solving and thereby reducing anxiety.
Monitor maternal/fetal vital signs.	Vital signs of client and fetuses may be altered by anxiety. Stabilization may reflect reduction of anxiety level.
Assess support systems available to R.F.M./couple.	Availability of the assistance and caring of significant others, including caregivers, is extremely important during this time of stress and uncertainty to decrease anxiety and enhance coping.

CLIENT DIAGNOSTIC STATEMENT (NURSING DIAGNOSIS):	**ACTIVITY INTOLERANCE, related to muscle/cellular hypersensitivity, evidenced by increased uterine irritability and cervical dilatation; and adverse effect on uteroplacental perfusion evidenced by change in fetal heart rate (FHR).**
DESIRED OUTCOMES— CLIENT WILL:	Report/display cessation of uterine contractions within 12–36 hours (3/14–15 0400).

ACTIONS/INTERVENTIONS

Expedite the admissions process and institute bed rest using left lateral position.

Explain the reasons for requiring bedrest, lying on left side, and decreasing activity.

Demonstrate/encourage use of relaxation techniques.

Provide comfort measures such as changes of position/linen, back rub, and Therapeutic Touch. Decrease stimuli in room (e.g., lighting).

Offer diversional activities, such as reading, television, or visits with selected friends or family as appropriate.

Monitor maternal and fetal vital signs per protocol.

RATIONALE

Facilitating reduction of activity and psychologic stressors may help decrease tension and relieve uterine contractions. Left lateral position improves uterine flow and may decrease uterine irritability.

These measures are intended to keep the pressure of the fetus off the cervix and to enhance placental perfusion. Bedrest may decrease uterine irritability.

Helps reduce muscle tension and client's perception of discomfort.

Relieves muscle fatigue and promotes sense of well-being.

Refocuses attention, reduces boredom, and may enhance coping ability.

Reflects effectiveness of and determines need for further interventions.

CLIENT DIAGNOSTIC STATEMENT (NURSING DIAGNOSIS):	**POISONING, HIGH RISK FOR, related to possibility of toxic side effects (cardiovascular) of treatments and medications used to stop labor.**
DESIRED OUTCOMES— CLIENT WILL:	Verbalize understanding of potential dangers, maternal/fetal side effects within 4 hours (3/14 2000).
	Display no untoward effects/complications (ongoing).

ACTIONS/INTERVENTIONS

Place in left lateral position. Elevate head of bed slightly.

Have R.F.M. drink 480–720 ml of fluid now.

RATIONALE

Decreases uterine irritability, increases placental perfusion, and prevents supine hypotension.

Helps rule out preterm labor related to dehydration.

ACTIONS/INTERVENTIONS	RATIONALE
Assist as needed with sterile vaginal examination. Obtain vaginal culture on admission.	Necessary to assess cervical status; however, vaginal examinations are kept to a minimum, because they may contribute to uterine irritability. Safety of tocolytic agents when cervix is greater than 4 cm dilated or more than 80% effaced is not documented. Culture is done to rule out infection, STD.
Apply EFM and assess uterine contractions and FHR electronically on admission and continuously until stable, then b.i.d. (0900, 2000).	Tactile and electronic monitoring of uterine contractions and fetal heart rate provides ongoing fetal/uterine assessment and basis for altering or maintaining drug administration. Note: External monitors may increase contractions in some clients.
Provide information about the actions and side effects of drug therapy. Obtain release for administration of terbutaline sulfate.	Important for the client/couple to know the purpose of the drug(s) being administered. Terbutaline sulfate is still considered an experimental drug and may cause fetal tachycardia, hyperglycemia, acidosis, and hypoxia.
Administer terbutaline 0.25 mg SC and 5 mg PO now. Document response.	Promotes relaxation of uterine muscle and vessel walls.
Monitor vital signs q4h, noting cardiac rhythm. Auscultate lung sounds. Record intake and output.	Terbutaline sulfate, which stimulates beta$_2$ receptors, may cause complications such as tachycardia/cardiac dysrhythmias and an increase in plasma volume.
Observe for development of side effects (e.g., palpitations, increased respiratory rate, chest pain, dyspnea, agitation). If present, discontinue drug, give oxygen by mask, start lactated Ringer's infusion (fluid expander), administer mild sedation (Secobarbital [Seconal] 100 mg, flurazepam [Dalmane] 15 mg, or hydroxyzine [Vistaril] 25 mg) per protocol, and notify physician.	Prompt action can reverse untoward or toxic effects.
Maintain fluid intake between 2000 and 3000 ml per day.	Amniotic fluid exchange occurs every 3 to 4 hours so it is advisable for client to drink something every 2 hours and maintain high daily intake.
Weigh daily.	Detects fluid shifts/retention, possible alteration in urinary functioning, and adequacy of nutritional intake.
Obtain urine sample for routine urinalysis.	Urinary tract infection may cause/enhance uterine irritability.
Review/monitor laboratory findings: CBC, UA, cultures, serum glucose and potassium.	Check for anemia, presence of infection. Terbutaline sulfate causes movement of potassium ions into cells, decreasing plasma K$^+$ levels, increasing blood glucose and plasma insulin levels, and stimulating release of glycogen from muscle and liver.

CLIENT DIAGNOSTIC STATEMENT (NURSING DIAGNOSIS):	INJURY, HIGH RISK FOR, FETAL, related to insufficient development to maintain physiologic self outside of uterine environment if delivered prematurely.
DESIRED OUTCOMES — CLIENT WILL:	Maintain pregnancy until fetal viability is reached (at least 25 weeks, or longer if possible).

ACTIONS/INTERVENTIONS	RATIONALE
Perform nitrazine test now.	Verifies ruptured membranes (PROM), which presents increased risk of infection and affects choice of interventions and timing of delivery.
Assess for maternal conditions that would contraindicate steroid therapy.	In pregnancy-induced hypertension (PIH) and chorioamnionitis, steroid therapy may aggravate-hypertension and mask signs of infection. Steroids may increase blood glucose levels in the client with diabetes.
Assess FHR; note presence of uterine activity or cervical dilation.	Tocolytics can increase FHR. Delivery may be extremely rapid with small infant if persistent uterine contractions are unresponsive to tocolytics, or if cervical changes continue.
Review pros and cons of steriod therapy with R.F.M./couple.	Steroid therapy is most effective between 28 and 34 weeks' gestation to stimulate lung maturity. Long-term effects on the development of the child cannot be known until longitudinal studies have been completed.
Administer betamethasone 12.5 mg (2 ml) IM 1800, repeat at 0600.	Although steroid therapy is still controversial, research indicates that it prevents or decreases the severity of respiratory distress syndrome (RDS) by stimulating fetal surfactant production.
Stress necessity of follow-up care if discharged without delivering.	If fetuses are not delivered within 7 days of administration of steroids, dose should be repeated weekly.

CLIENT DIAGNOSTIC STATEMENT (NURSING DIAGNOSIS):	KNOWLEDGE DEFICIT [LEARNING NEED], regarding condition, prognosis, and treatment related to lack of information/misinterpretation evidenced by questions and expressions of concerns.
DESIRED OUTCOMES — CLIENT WILL:	Verbalize awareness of implications and possible outcomes of condition and preterm labor within 16 hours (3/15 0800).
	Ask questions appropriately within 24 hours (3/15 1600).
	Assume responsibility for own learning and participate in learning process within 48 hours of admission (3/16 1600).

ACTIONS/INTERVENTIONS	RATIONALE
Ascertain knowledge about preterm labor and possible outcomes.	Establishes data base and identifies individual client learning needs.
Determine readiness to learn.	Factors such as anxiety or lack of awareness of need for information (denial) can interfere with readiness to learn.
Include husband in the teaching process.	Support from significant other(s) can help allay anxiety as well as reinforce learning.
Review signs and symptoms of "early" labor.	Helps client to recognize preterm labor so that therapy to suppress this labor can be initiated or reinstituted promptly.
Discuss need for bedrest, limitation of activity, restriction of sexual and nipple activity.	Activity, orgasm, and stimulation of the nipples (which releases oxytocin) may stimulate uterine activity.
Stress avoidance of use of OTC drugs while tocolytic agents are administered, unless approved by physician.	Concurrent use of OTC drugs may cause deleterious effects, especially if drug has side effects similar to those of tocolytic agent (e.g., antihistamines or inhalers with bronchodilating effects, such as epinephrine [Primatene Mist]).
Recommend taking oral tocolytic agents with food if drug is continued.	Food improves tolerance to drug and reduces GI side effects.
Provide information about follow-up care, including home monitoring programs.	Cooperation is enhanced when client understands need of regular monitoring/treatment.
Arrange for visit to neonatal intensive care unit.	Helps alleviate fears and facilitates adjustment to the potential realities of the situation.
Refer to community health nurse, childbirth education class, another couple who have experienced a similar episode with a successful outcome.	Additional help may assist client/couple to cope with situation, especially if she returns home to await delivery.

Evaluation

As nursing care is provided, ongoing assessments determine the client's response to therapy and progress toward accomplishing the desired outcomes. This activity serves as the feedback and control part of the nursing process, through which the status of the individual client diagnostic statement is judged to be resolved, continuing, or requires revision.

This process is visualized in Figure 3–1. Discussion with Mrs. R.F.M. verifies she is aware of her feelings of anxiety and is gathering information she needs to deal more effectively with her concerns. She appears relaxed and states she feels more in control of her immediate situation. Therefore, she is progressing toward resolving and managing her anxiety, and this problem will continue to be addressed, although no revision in the treatment plan is required at this time.

Documentation

There are several charting formats that have been used for documentation. These include block notes, with a single entry covering an entire shift (e.g., 7–3 PM); narrative timed notes (e.g., 8:30 AM, ate all of break-

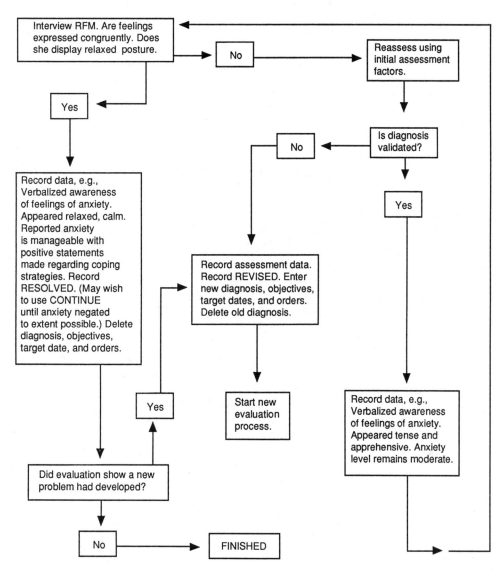

Figure 3–1. Outcome-based evaluation of the client's response to therapy related to nursing diagnosis, Anxiety. (Adapted from Cox, HC, et al: Clinical Applications of Nursing Diagnosis. FA Davis, Philadelphia, 1993, p 616.)

fast); and the problem-oriented medical record system (POMR or PORS) using the SOAP/SOAPIER approach, to name a few. The latter can provide thorough documentation, but it was designed by physicians for episodic care and requires that the entries be tied to a client problem identified from a problem list.

A new system format created by nurses for documentation of frequent/repetitive care is FOCUS® Charting. It was designed to encourage looking at the client from a positive rather than a negative (or problem-oriented) perspective by using precise documentation to record the nursing process. Recording of assessment, interventions, and evaluation information in a Data, Action, and Response (DAR) format facilitates tracking and following what is happening to the client at any given moment. Charting focuses on client and nursing concerns. The focal point is client status and the associated nursing care. The Focus is always stated in a way that reflects the *client's* concern/need rather than reflecting a nursing task or medical diagnosis.

Thus, the focus can be a client problem/concern or nursing diagnosis, signs/symptoms of potential importance (e.g., fever, blood pressure fluctuations, edema), a significant event or change in status, or specific standards of care/hospital policy. Based on the client situation of Mrs. R.F.M., the following examples of documentation are provided:

SOAP/SOAPIER Format

Date	Time	Number/Problem	Progress Notes
3/14/93	1600	1 Anxiety	S: "I feel so helpless. what's going to happen to me and the babies?" O: Crying, hands trembling, voice quivering, pulse 110. A: Moderate anxiety with concern regarding changes in life events and fear of unspecific consequences. P: Demonstrate and encourage use of relaxation techniques. Encourage verbalization of fears/concerns. Provide information as indicated. Signed: M. Sickus, RN
3/15/93	0800	5 Knowledge	S: "The signs of early labor include uterine contractions every 10 minutes or sooner, pelvic pressure, abdominal cramping, low back ache, and/or increase in vaginal discharge. Without prompt intervention, labor could progress to point that my babies will be born prematurely, increasing their risk of complications and threatening their survival. If any of these symptoms occur, I should empty my bladder, lie down on my left side, drink 3 to 4 glasses of water, palpate for uterine contractions, and notify the clinic nurse if symptoms continue." O: Displays relaxed posture, thoughtful expression. A: Has achieved outcome #1. P: Continue teaching plan as outlined. Signed: M. Sickus, RN

Other examples of documentation:

DAR Format

Date	Time	Focus	Progress Notes
3/15/93	0800	Learning Needs	D: Identified implications/signs of labor, and appropriate responses. Listed available resources/support groups. Verbalized benefits of activity limitations. Appeared relaxed; thoughtful expression as she recounted information. A: Provided positive feedback regarding client's understanding and awareness. R: Demonstrated learning and achievement of outcome 1. Signed: M. Sickus, RN
3/15/93	1600	Anxiety	D: Verbalizes awareness of feelings of anxiety. Reports she is gathering information to deal more effectively with her concerns and feels more in control of situation. A: Continued open communication and optimistic attitude. Provided information regarding usual home monitoring program. R: Identified additional supports available to self/husband and reported anxiety is manageable. Appeared relaxed and calm. Resting quietly. B. Briner, RN

The following is an example of documentation of a client need/concern that currently does not require identification as a client problem (nursing diagnosis) or inclusion in the plan of care and therefore is not easily documented in the SOAP format:

DAR Format

Date	Time	Focus	Progress Notes
3/15/93	1920	Gastric distress	D: Reports "indigestion/burning sensation" with hand over epigastric area. Skin warm/dry, color pink, vital signs unchanged. A: Given Mylanta 30 ml PO. Head of bed elevated approximately 15 degrees. R: Reports pain relieved. Appears relaxed, resting quietly. B. Briner, RN

CHAPTER 4
PRENATAL CONCEPTS

The Trimesters: Prenatal Assessment _____

CLIENT ASSESSMENT DATA BASE

ACTIVITY/REST

Blood pressure slightly lower than normal (8 to 12 wks), returning to prepregnancy levels during the last half of pregnancy.

Pulse rate may increase 10–15 bpm.

Short systolic murmur may develop related to increased volume.

Syncopal episodes.

Varicosities.

Slight edema of lower extremities/hands may be present (particularly in last trimester).

EGO INTEGRITY

Expresses changes in perception of self.

ELIMINATION

Changes in stool consistency/frequency.

Increased frequency of urination.

Urinalysis: increased specific gravity.

Hemorrhoids.

FOOD/FLUID

Nausea and vomiting, primarily first trimester; heartburn is common.

Weight gain: 2 to 4 lb first trimester; second and third trimesters, 11 to 12 lb each.

Dry mucous membranes; hypertrophy of gingival tissue may occur, may bleed easily.

Low Hb and Hct may be present (physiologic anemia).

Slight dependent edema.

Slight glycosuria may be present.

Diastasis recti (separation of the rectus muscle) may occur late in pregnancy.

PAIN/DISCOMFORT

Leg cramps, breast tenderness and swelling; Braxton Hicks contractions noted after 28 weeks; back pain.

RESPIRATION

Nasal stuffiness; mucosa redder than normal.

Respiratory rate may increase relative to size/height of uterus; thoracic breathing.

SAFETY

Temperature 98–99.6° F (36.1–37.6° C)

Fetal heart tones (FHT) audible with Doptone (beginning 10–12 wk) or fetoscope (17–20 wk).

Fetal movement noted on exam after 20 weeks, quickening (sensation of fetal movement in the abdomen) between 16 and 20 weeks.

Ballottement present 4th and 5th month.

SEXUALITY

Cessation of menses.

Change in sexual response/activity.

Leukorrhea may be present.

Progressive increase in uterine size; e.g., fundus slightly above symphysis pubis (at 10–12 wk), at umbilicus (at 20–22 wk), slightly below ensiform cartilage (at 36 wk).

Breast changes: Enlargement of adipose tissue, increased vascularity, tenderness on palpation, increase in diameter and pigmentation of areolar tissue, hypertrophy of Montgomery tubercles; tingling sensation (first and third trimester), possible striae gravidarum; colostrum may appear after 12 wk.

Pigmentation changes: Chloasma, linea nigra, palmar erythema, spider nevi, striae gravidarum.

Positive Goodell's, Hegar's, Chadwick's, Ladin's signs.

SOCIAL INTERACTION

Confusion/questioning of anticipated role changes.

Maturational/development stage varies and may regress with stressor of pregnancy.

Responses of other family members can vary from positive and supportive to dysfunctional.

TEACHING/LEARNING

Individual expectations of pregnancy, labor/delivery dependent on age, level of knowledge, experiences, parity, desire for child, economic stability.

DIAGNOSTIC STUDIES

CBC: Denotes anemia, hemoglobinopathies (e.g., sickle cell).

Blood type: ABO and Rh to identify risk of incompatibility.

Vaginal/rectal smear: Tests for *Neisseria gonorrhea*, *Chlamydia*.

Serologic tests: Determine presence of syphilis (RPR), other sexually transmitted diseases (STDs) (as indicated by vaginal warts, lesions, abnormal discharge).

Screening: For HIV, hepatitis, tuberculosis.

Rubella titer: > a:a0 denotes immunity.

Papanicolaou smear: Identifies neoplasia, herpes simplex type 2.

Urinalysis: Screen for medical conditions (e.g., verification of pregnancy; infection, diabetes, renal disease).

Serum/urine testing for human chorionic gonadotrophin (HCG): Positive.

Sonography: Evidence of fetus after 8 weeks' gestation.

Serum glucose screen/1 hr glucose test: <140 mg/dl (usually done between 24 and 28 wk).

Subsequent evaluations and focused assessments are done at each prenatal visit.

Genetic Counseling _____

Genetic counseling is a communication process that deals with human problems associated with the occurrence or risk of a genetic disorder in a family. The process can be prospective (counseling delivered to a client/couple of reproductive age before conception or the birth of an affected child), or it can be retrospective (counseling delivered after the birth of an affected child). In many cases, however, the need for genetic counseling first becomes apparent during the first trimester.

Counseling also involves genetic screening, whereby a high-risk or general population is analyzed to detect the presence of disease, and case-finding for couples at potential risk based on medical/family histories.

CLIENT ASSESSMENT DATA BASE

CIRCULATION

Hypertension.

Bleeding.

EGO/INTEGRITY

May express feelings of inadequacy.

FOOD/FLUID

Weight gain may be inappropriate for gestational stage (smaller gain may negatively affect fetus).

Maternal insulin-dependent diabetes.

Presence of eating disorders (e.g., anorexia nervosa, bulimia, or obesity).

SAFETY

Infection (e.g., sexually transmitted diseases [STDs], pelvic inflammatory disease).

Presence of seizure disorder, degree/method of control.

Significant exposure to radiation, toxic chemicals, or infectious teratogens (e.g., rubella, toxoplasmosis, cytomegolovirus, human immunodeficiency virus/AIDS and other STDs), postnatal infections (e.g., meningitis, encephalitis); postnatal nutritional/stimulatory deprivation.

Breech presentation (especially with anencephaly).

SEXUALITY

History of two or more first-trimester abortions, fetal demise, or previous child with chromosomal abnormality.

Birth trauma or identifiable genetically transmitted disorder.

Use of ovulation stimulant such as clomiphene or menotropins (Pergonal).

SOCIAL INTERACTION

Interfamily marriage (consanguinity).

Guilt/blame toward self and/or partner who carries defective gene.

TEACHING/LEARNING

Positive family history/pedigree of known genetic or inherited disorders (e.g., sickle cell, cystic fibrosis, hemophilia, phenylketonuria, craniospinal defects, renal malformations, thalassemia, Huntington chorea), familial disorders (cancer, heart disease, diabetes, allergies), congenital abnormalities (Down syndrome, mental retardation, neural tube defects), or inborn metabolic disorder (e.g., maple syrup urine disease, Tay-Sachs disease).

Ethnic background at risk for specific disorder (e.g., black African, Mediterranean, Ashkenazi Jewish).

Drug usage (alcohol; over-the-counter [OTC], prescribed, or street drugs; anticonvulsant medication).

DIAGNOSTIC STUDIES

Chromosomal analysis: Using buccal smear/serum.

Prenatal diagnosis:

Amniocentesis (at 14–16 weeks): Determines sex chromatin (rules out sex-linked disorders), karyotype (rules out chromosomal disorders), biochemical studies (rules out inborn errors of metabolism), elevation of alpha-fetoprotein (AFP) levels reflecting neural tube defects (NTD).

Ultrasonography (using real time) preceding/during amniocentesis: Rules out missed abortion, visualizes term pregnancies, and identifies gross anomalies/problems.

Serum AFP levels (16–18 weeks): Identifies NTD; if abnormality high/low, test is repeated.

Amniography/fetography: Identifies gross problems such as major soft-tissue abnormalities, esophageal/duodenal atresia, and bone abnormalities using special x-ray technique (may be potentially teratogenic).

Fetoscopy (considered experimental, of limited availability): Permits direct visual examination of the fetus and sampling of fetal blood/tissue samples to diagnose hereditary blood disorders (e.g., sickle cell anemia, hemophilia).

Chorionic villi sampling (CVS) (at 8 weeks): May replace amniocentesis as a genetic diagnostic tool.

NURSING PRIORITIES

1. Assist client/couple/family to recognize and understand specific situation.
2. Facilitate therapeutic use of informational resources.
3. Provide ongoing emotional support.

DISCHARGE GOALS

1. Coping effectively with situation.
2. Completes counseling process.
3. Understands information specific to individual situation.

NURSING DIAGNOSIS:	ANXIETY [SPECIFY LEVEL]
May be related to:	Presence of specific risk factors (e.g., history of genetic problem, exposure to teratogens), situational crisis, threat to self-concept (perceived/actual), conscious or unconscious conflict about essential values (beliefs) and goals of life.
Possibly evidence by:	Increased tension, apprehension, uncertainty, feelings of inadequacy, or expressed concern regarding changes in life events, insomnia.

DESIRED OUTCOMES— CLIENT/COUPLE WILL:	Acknowledge awareness of feelings of anxiety.
	Verbalize realistic concerns related to process of genetic counseling/prenatal diagnosis.
	Appear relaxed and report that anxiety is reduced to a manageable level.
	Identify and use resources/support systems effectively.

ACTIONS/INTERVENTIONS	RATIONALE
Independent	
Assess nature, source, and manifestations of anxiety.	Identifies specific areas of concern and determines direction for and possible options/interventions.
Provide information about specific genetic disorder, risks involved in reproduction, and available prenatal diagnostic measures/options. (Refer to ND: Knowledge Deficit [Learning Need].)	May relieve anxiety associated with the unknown and assist family to cope with stress, make decisions, and adapt positively to choices. (Note: A large number of clients at risk of producing a child with a genetic abnormality do not receive prospective counseling/diagnostic services due to ineffective case-finding/lack of awareness and enter counseling retrospectively [often during the first trimester]. New genetic research at the gene level will have future implications for diagnosis, carrier status, or prenatal detection of genetic disease. Such techniques include restriction endonuclease, DNA probes, polymerase chain reaction [PCR], Southern blot, restriction fragment length polymorphisms [RFLPs].)
Promote ongoing sharing of concerns/feelings.	Opportunity for client/couple to begin resolution of situation. Level of anxiety is usually higher in the couple who have already given birth to a child with a chromosomal disorder.
Review procedure and what to expect in terms of discomfort, if fetus is affected and couple elects to terminate pregnancy and so on. (Refer to CP: Elective Termination.)	Client/couple may be extremely anxious, guilt-ridden during uncomfortable procedure, information can reduce anxiety.
Visit couple after procedure. Provide anticipatory guidance in terms of physical/psychologic changes.	Follow-up visit by the primary nurse may relieve anxiety/depression in couple following abortion for genetic indications.
Provide opportunity for discussion of test results on fetus and assist with interpretation of information, especially following abortion. Listen to expressions of concern/feelings about situation.	Helps to confirm the diagnosis; reduces anxiety associated with uncertainty of whether fetus was really affected and whether couple made the "right" choice. When concerns and feelings are expressed/listened to, client needs can be identified more readily.
Collaborative	
Refer for further counseling (e.g., psychiatric, group).	Anxiety may not be resolved sufficiently, necessitating additional professional assistance.

43

ACTIONS/INTERVENTIONS

Collaborative

Assist couple in identifying community agencies to aid in care of their newborn in the event that they elect to continue the pregnancy after fetus is found to be affected, or when diagnosis is made after delivery. (Refer to CP: The Parents of a Child with Special Needs.)

RATIONALE

Helps to reduce anxieties regarding how the couple will meet their baby's special needs.

NURSING DIAGNOSIS:	KNOWLEDGE DEFICIT [LEARNING NEED], regarding purpose/process of genetic counseling
May be related to:	Lack of awareness of the purpose/ramifications of genetic counseling, its applicability to their situation, components of the decision-making process necessary for analyzing available options, and available methods of prenatal diagnosis.
Possibly evidenced by:	Verbalization of the problem, statement of misconceptions, request for information.
DESIRED OUTCOMES— CLIENT/COUPLE WILL:	Describe the disorder in question.
	Identify available options.
	Discuss, in own words, purpose and findings of specific prenatal detection methods.
	Estimate risks associated with reproduction.

ACTIONS/INTERVENTIONS

Independent

Discuss the purpose/goals of genetic counseling.

Obtain pertinent family history; create pedigree chart from information. Include both parents in interview.

Identify risk factors in obstetric history, such as three or more miscarriages, fetal demise, hypertension, bleeding, infection, significant exposure to radiation, low-level exposure to environmental pollutants (e.g., lead, formaldehyde, anesthetic gases), drug use (over-the-counter, prescribed, street), birth trauma, or identifiable genetically transmitted disorder.

RATIONALE

Serves to educate parents about the risks in their situation and ultimately to help them make educated/informed decisions. Misconceptions may interfere with the decision-making process.

Provides accurate picture of the proband (afflicted person/index case) in relation to other family members and serves to identify other persons similarly affected. Ensures both parents are provided the same information.

These factors may produce a phenocopy, an imitation of a genetic disorder.

ACTIONS/INTERVENTIONS	RATIONALE

Independent

Distinguish between environmental causes of mental retardation and those with a genetic component (e.g., Down syndrome).

Environmental causes include birth trauma, chemical teratogens, infectious teratogens (e.g., rubella, toxoplasmosis, cytomegalovirus), postnatal infections (e.g., meningitis, encephalitis), and postnatal nutritional/stimulatory deprivation.

Define specific genetic disorder in question. Provide prognosis/estimate of risks and probable consequences. Clarify/interpret data; avoid making recommendations/decisions for the client/couple.

Determines the probability of risk and recurrence of risk, allows client/couple to make informed choices incorporating values/goals/personal circumstances, free of biases or recommendations from the nurse.

Carry out ongoing family assessment for available support systems. Note signs of inappropriate coping/maladaptation. Offer information as family is ready to hear it.

Negative coping may interfere with cognitive functioning and hinder educational process. Some families are not ready to listen immediately after a diagnosis is made, and many do not listen effectively the first time information is presented.

Arrange for follow-up, telephone calls, visits to home/counseling service.

Provides opportunity to reinforce information when family is "ready" to hear it.

Provide information about readily available/individually appropriate diagnostic procedures/screenings, such as amniocentesis, serum testing for AFP, and ultrasonography, as well as newer methods such as CVS, fetoscopy, amniography, percutaneous umbilical blood sampling (PUBS, or cordocentesis), computed tomography scanning, and magnetic resonance imaging.

Prenatal diagnosis permits preparation for or offers an alternative to having children with genetic disorders.

Permit couple to arrive at own decision regarding their participation in or refusal of prenatal testing procedures.

Allows couple to make informed choices based on understanding of long-term problems associated with the disorder in question, at their own pace. May assist in determining whether the fetus at risk for a genetic disorder is actually affected.

Review anticipated follow-up evaluative procedures, especially if client is currently pregnant.

May include regular assessment of fetal heart tones, obtaining 20-minute tracing on electronic monitoring, and so forth.

Discuss time element associated with receiving test results.

Test results may take up to 4 weeks to analyze. Although CVS is currently limited in its availability, it has advantages over amniocentesis because it can be performed earlier in the pregnancy (first versus second trimester) and results are available quickly (in 1 to 2 wk versus 2 to 4 wk). PUBS, or cordocentesis, provides a rapid fetal karyotype. Prior knowledge of length of time required to obtain results can lessen client's anxiety.

Encourage participation in community programs; i.e., education/support groups and groups concerned with specific genetic disorders as indicated (Tay-Sachs disease, Down syndrome, and so forth).

Helps client identify with others who have dealt with genetic disorders. Provides role models and information about the identified disorder.

ACTIONS/INTERVENTIONS

Independent

Obtain/coordinate referrals with support groups, specialty clinics, and adoptive agencies that deal with specific genetic disorders (e.g., cystic fibrosis, hemophilia).

Obtain informed consent/surgical permit for procedures/tests. Review risks associated with procedure.

RATIONALE

May be needed to answer questions/concerns that are presented in genetic counseling, especially if genetic component is involved.

Client needs to be aware of any risks involved to herself or the fetus, especially if the procedure is invasive, such as amniocentesis, CVS, fetoscopy, or PUBS.

NURSING DIAGNOSIS:	FAMILY PROCESSES, ALTERED, HIGH RISK FOR
Risk factors may include:	Situational crisis, individual/family vulnerability, difficulty reaching agreement regarding decision.
Possibly evidenced by:	[Not applicable; presence of signs/symptoms establishes an **actual** diagnosis.]
DESIRED OUTCOMES— CLIENT/COUPLE WILL:	Discuss available options.
	Participate in the decision-making process.
	Verbalize comfort with final decision.

ACTIONS/INTERVENTIONS

Independent

Determine couple's relationship to one another, strength of intrafamily bonds, and support systems.

Assess couple's perception of disorder as well as their attitudes/religious beliefs. (Refer to ND: Spiritual Distress [distress of the human spirit].)

Provide information about risk estimates for disorder. Assess meaning of "carrier" status to client/couple, especially if couple desires male child and diagnosis is X-linked.

Provide opportunity to verbalize concerns. Be truthful and straightforward about genetic transmission.

RATIONALE

Establishes baseline. The threat of a hereditary disorder often results in intrafamily strife as well as marital disharmony, and family disintegration (separation and divorce).

The way family members respond depends on the nature of the condition and on their perception of the "burden" (total amount of distress created by the diagnosis/birth of an affected child). Reactions may be more negative in dominant, X-linked disorders where only one member of the couple is to "blame" or is identified as the carrier.

Allows couple to deal with the reality of the situation. For instance, if both parents are carriers of an autosomal recessive disorder for a deleterious gene, the risk is 1 in 4, or 25%, that an offspring will be affected. The nature of the condition influences the family's responses. If female is carrier for X-linked disorder such as hemophilia, male fetuses have a 50% risk of being affected.

Helps absolve feelings of guilt by exploring random nature of genetic transmission. Knowledge that everyone has 6–10 defective genes and that it is just chance that spouses have the same recessive deleterious gene may be reassuring/limit "blame".

ACTIONS/INTERVENTIONS	RATIONALE
Independent	
Review all options available to the client/couple, e.g., adoption, postponing childbearing, artificial insemination by donor sperm, electing to reproduce using prenatal diagnosis, or surrogate parenting. If client is carrying an affected child, options include terminating the pregnancy, treating the fetus in utero (if possible), carrying the pregnancy to term and keeping the neonate, and placing the child for adoption/foster care or institutionalization. (Refer to CP: The Parents of a Child with Special Needs.)	Promotes communication between client and partner. Provides opportunity to begin decision-making process based on factual information.
Assist in problem-solving and exploring alternative solutions, weighing impact on family members.	Helps to arrive at a decision, bringing family out of crisis, and facilitates growth of individual members and family as a unit.
Provide emotional support individually and to the couple as a unit.	Sometimes it is helpful to talk to members of the couple individually as well as together to assess individual perceptions of situation. Separate meetings are particularly critical if the couple are not in agreement about possible solutions.
Collaborative	
Refer to community support groups, counseling, or social service worker.	May be necessary to help problem-solve and prevent family disintegration. Situations may arise whereby the couple are unable to agree on a decision when aware of risks/potential outcomes.
Refer to early intervention programs, community groups, or specialists after birth of an affected child.	Assists in management of short- and long-term medical/psychologic problems.

NURSING DIAGNOSIS:	**SPIRITUAL DISTRESS (DISTRESS OF THE HUMAN SPIRIT)**
May be related to:	Intense inner conflict about the outcome, normal grieving for the loss of a perfect child, anger that is often directed at God, religious beliefs/moral convictions.
Possibly evidenced by:	Verbalization of inner conflict about beliefs, questioning of the moral and ethical implications of therapeutic choices, questioning the meaning of this event, regarding condition as punishment, the development of anger, hostility, and crying.
DESIRED OUTCOMES— CLIENT/COUPLE WILL:	Make informed choice regarding childbearing/childrearing within their religious/moral framework.
	Verbalize acceptance/resolution of stress if prenatal diagnosis is positive.

ACTIONS/INTERVENTIONS

Independent

Assist in identifying/discussing concerns and analyzing options based on religious beliefs and value system.

Analyze client's/couple's emotional state. Assess for normal or abnormal states of grieving.

Collaborative

Refer to pastor/rabbi/priest or counselor as appropriate, especially if client/couple has religious affiliations that might affect decisions regarding conditions such as Tay-Sachs disease or Down syndrome.

RATIONALE

Helps couple to recognize their dilemma. The decision regarding the pregnancy outcome and participation in prenatal diagnosis is ultimately the right/responsibility of the prospective parents, with informed decision making dependent on ethical/religious/moral convictions.

Grieving is anticipated, but excessive denial may interfere with progression/resolution of grief work.

May assist in or be necessary for resolution of ethical issues. In many religions, such as Catholicism and Orthodox Judaism, abortion is viewed as an attack on the sanctity of life, with the mother's endangerment being the only generally permissible reason, in which case permission from a higher church authority is required.

NURSING DIAGNOSIS:	SELF ESTEEM, DISTURBANCE
May be related to:	Perceived failure at a life event.
Possibly evidenced by:	Denial; self-negating verbalization; feelings of guilt, powerlessness, anger; expressions of the unfairness of the situation; projection of blame/responsibility for problem.
DESIRED OUTCOMES— CLIENT/COUPLE WILL:	Verbalize lessened sense of guilt and restored feelings of self-worth.
	Set realistic goals.
	Participate actively in conflict resolution process.

ACTIONS/INTERVENTIONS

Independent

Determine self-perception of client/couple. Identify and reinforce individual/mutual strengths.

Provide or reinforce information regarding risk estimate, to discuss with client and couple together and separately. Reaffirm inability to control outcome of conception; affirm ability to control decision to reproduce, adopt, or remain childless.

RATIONALE

Provides opportunity for nurse to learn about client's/couple's expectations/perceptions of genetic disorder. Helps put feelings/opinions into perspective. When the diagnosis of genetic inheritance is involved, and one or both parents are found to be carriers of the defect, guilt, powerlessness, anger, and feelings of unfairness are normal/universal reactions and to be anticipated.

Helps reduce guilt feelings; promotes recognition by couple that some control over outcome is possible.

ACTIONS/INTERVENTIONS	RATIONALE

Independent

Arrange for follow-up visit in clinic or office to assess status after abortion.

Feelings of loss/depression/negativism often occur following discharge from the hospital, resulting in alteration in ego functioning.

Assess for recurring unresolved conflicts.

Professional help may be required to resolve low self-esteem.

Collaborative

Refer for counseling/psychiatric care as needed.

May be necessary to assist in working through the grief process in a healthy manner so that a positive sense of self emerges. Provides opportunity to establish or reestablish family integrity.

NURSING DIAGNOSIS:	INJURY, HIGH RISK FOR, complications of testing procedures
Risk factors may include:	Invasive procedure, tissue hypoxia/changes in circulation, teratogenic effects of radiation.
Possibly evidenced by:	[Not applicable; presence of signs/symptoms establishes an **actual** diagnosis.]
DESIRED OUTCOMES— CLIENT/COUPLE WILL:	Identify individual risks and ways of minimizing them. Be free of preventable complications.

ACTIONS/INTERVENTIONS	RATIONALE

Independent

Identify the necessity of the specific test(s) and associated risks.

Testing involving radiation, CVS, amniocentesis, and so forth carries with it some degree of risk; i.e., spontaneous abortion/preterm labor, bleeding, infection, rupture of membranes, direct fetal injury/loss. Information helps the client/couple make informed decisions.

Review indications for genetic testing.

Some indications for this procedure are the previous birth of a child with a chromosomal disorder or known metabolic defects, any woman identified as a carrier of a sex-linked trait, any woman age 35 or older, paternal age of 45 or older, family history of NTD, or both parents carrying an autosomal recessive disease or a chromosomal abnormality.

Review signs/symptoms of complications such as premature labor, infection, and abruptio placentae.

Client needs to recognize these as being important to report to healthcare provider.

Collaborative

Assist with obtaining blood or tissue, placental or chromosomal analysis/biopsy.

In the event of a stillbirth/neonatal death/birth of an affected child, determines nature of disorder; is helpful in counseling couple regarding future pregnancies.

ACTIONS/INTERVENTIONS	RATIONALE

Independent

Assist with procedures such as amniocentesis, taking necessary measures (e.g., monitor blood pressure, pulse, respiration, and fetal heart rate). Assess fetal/uterine activity; use external fetal monitor for 20 to 30 minutes after procedure.

Testing procedures carry risks to the pregnancy/fetus. Careful monitoring may reduce untoward effects.

Position mother on left side.

Increases placental circulation, dilating blood vessels and reducing risk of supine hypotension and uterine irritability.

Administer medications as indicated:
  Rh immune globulin (Rh-Ig) after amniocentesis and CVS;

Protects Rh-negative client from sensitization. (Note: CVS is contraindicated in an Rh-sensitized woman unless the purpose of the test is to detect an Rh-positive fetus.)

  Antibiotics.

Given prophylactically for 10 days after fetoscopy to prevent amnionitis.

(Refer to CP: The High-Risk Pregnancy.)

NURSING DIAGNOSIS:	HEALTH MAINTENANCE, ALTERED, HIGH RISK FOR
Risk factors may include:	Ineffective coping methods, unresolved grief, disabling distress, lack of material resources.
Possibly evidenced by:	[Not applicable; presence of signs/symptoms establishes an **actual** diagnosis.]
DESIRED OUTCOMES— CLIENT/COUPLE WILL:	Assume responsibility for health care needs.
	Identify factors contributing to condition/situation.
	Verbalize ability to cope adequately with the existing situation.

ACTIONS/INTERVENTIONS	RATIONALE

Independent

Assess level of dependence/independence and ability to make decisions to meet own needs.

May need more help to gain information necessary for problem resolution.

Determine needs (e.g., communication skills, knowledge of resources, motivation).

To determine extent and type of interventions necessary.

Initiate/participate in case-finding/referral of individuals with real or potential genetic concerns.

Helps reduce the number of children born with genetic defects.

Encourage participation in group activities, such as diagnosis-related support groups, March of Dimes, or Easter Seals.

Can assist client/family in dealing with own situation.

First Trimester

NURSING PRIORITIES

1. Encourage client to adopt health-promoting behaviors.
2. Detect actual or potential risk factors.
3. Prevent/treat complications.
4. Foster client's/couple's positive adaptation to pregnancy.

NURSING DIAGNOSIS:	NUTRITION, ALTERED, LESS THAN BODY REQUIREMENTS, HIGH RISK FOR
Risk factors may include:	Changes in appetite, presence of nausea/vomiting, insufficient finances, unfamiliarity with increasing metabolic/nutritional needs.
Possibly evidenced by:	[Not applicable; presence of signs/symptoms establishes an **actual** diagnosis.]
DESIRED OUTCOMES— CLIENT WILL:	Explain the components of a well-balanced prenatal diet, giving food sources of vitamins, minerals, protein, and iron.
	Follow recommended diet.
	Take iron/vitamin supplement as prescribed.
	Demonstrate individually appropriate weight gain (usually a minimum of 3 lb by the end of the first trimester).

ACTIONS/INTERVENTIONS	RATIONALE
Independent	
Determine adequacy of past/present nutritional habits using 24-hour recall. Note condition of hair, nails, and skin.	Fetal/maternal well-being depends on maternal nutrition during pregnancy as well as during the 2 years preceding pregnancy.
Obtain health history; note age (especially less than 17 years, more than 35 years).	Adolescents may be prone to malnutrition/anemia, and older clients may be prone to obesity/gestational diabetes. (Refer to CPs: The Pregnant Adolescent; Diabetes Mellitus: Prepregnancy/Gestational.)
Ascertain knowledge level of dietary needs.	Determines specific learning needs. In the prenatal period, the basal metabolic rate increases by 20%–25% (especially in late pregnancy), owing to increased thyroid activity associated with the growth of fetal and maternal tissues, creating a potential risk for the client with poor nutrition. An additional 800 mg of iron is necessary during pregnancy for developing maternal/fetal tissue and fetal storage. During the first trimester, the demand for iron is minimal, and a balanced diet meeting increased caloric needs is usually adequate. (Note: Iron preparations are not commonly prescribed in the first trimester because they may potentiate nausea.)

ACTIONS/INTERVENTIONS	RATIONALE
Independent	
Provide appropriate oral/written information about prenatal diet and daily vitamin/iron supplements.	Reference material can be reviewed at home, increasing the likelihood that the client will select a well-balanced diet.
Evaluate motivation/attitude by listening to client's comments and asking for feedback about information given.	If client is not motivated to improve diet, further evaluation or other interventions may be indicated.
Elicit beliefs regarding culturally proscribed diet and taboos during pregnancy.	May affect motivation to follow recommendations of healthcare provider. For example, some cultures refuse iron, believing that it hardens maternal bones and makes delivery difficult.
Note presence of pica. Assess choices of nonfood substances and degree of motivation for eating them.	The ingestion of nonfood substances in pregnancy may be based on a psychologic need, cultural phenomenon, response to hunger, and/or a bodily response to the need for nutrients (e.g., chewing on ice may indicate anemia). Note: Ingestion of laundry starch may potentiate iron-deficiency anemia; and the ingestion of clay may lead to fecal impaction.
Weigh client; ascertain usual pregravid weight. Provide information about optimal prenatal gain.	Inadequate prenatal weight gain and/or below normal prepregnancy weight increases the risk of intrauterine growth retardation (IUGR) in the fetus and delivery of low-birth-weight infant. Research studies have found a positive correlation between pregravid maternal obesity and increased perinatal morbidity rates associated with preterm births.
Review frequency and severity of nausea/vomiting. Rule out pernicious vomiting (hyperemesis gravidarum). (Refer to CP: The High-Risk Pregnancy, ND: Nutrition, altered, less than body requirements, high risk for.)	First-trimester nausea/vomiting can have a negative impact on prenatal nutritional status, especially at critical periods in fetal development.
Monitor hemoglobin (Hb)/hematocrit (Hct) levels.	Identifies presence of anemia and potential for reduced maternal oxygen-carrying capacity. Clients with Hb levels less than 12 g/dL or Hct levels less than or equal to 37% are considered anemic in the first trimester.
Test urine for acetone, albumin, and glucose.	Establishes baseline; is performed routinely to detect potential high-risk situations such as inadequate carbohydrate ingestion, diabetic ketoacidosis, and pregnancy-induced hypertension (PIH).
Measure uterine growth.	Maternal malnutrition may negatively affect fetal growth and contribute to reduced complement of brain cells in the fetus, which results in developmental lags in infancy and possibly beyond.
Collaborative	
Make necessary referrals as indicated (e.g., dietitian, social services).	May need additional assistance with nutritional choices; may have budget/financial constraints.

ACTIONS/INTERVENTIONS

Collaborative

Refer to Women, Infant, Children (WIC) food program as appropriate.

RATIONALE

Supplemental federally funded food program helps promote optimal maternal/fetal nutrition.

NURSING DIAGNOSIS:	DISCOMFORT*
May be related to:	Physical changes and hormonal influences.
Possibly evidenced by:	Verbalizations, restlessness, alteration in muscle tone.
DESIRED OUTCOMES— CLIENT WILL:	Identify measures that provide relief.
	Assume responsibility for alleviation of discomforts.
	Report absence/successful management of discomforts.

*Authors' note: Currently there is no NANDA diagnostic label that addresses issues of comfort below the level of Pain [acute] or chronic. Although the label of **Discomfort** is not approved, we believe it speaks more directly to the identified problem.

ACTIONS/INTERVENTIONS

Independent

Note presence/degree of minor discomforts.

Evaluate degree of discomfort during internal examination. Use extreme gentleness/pictures/models especially for the client with infibulation or female circumcision.

Recommend wearing of supportive bra. Review nipple care (e.g., expose to air for 20 minutes daily; avoid soaps).

Stress importance of avoiding excessive nipple manipulation.

Instruct in use of Hoffman technique for flat/inverted nipples, or recommend wearing of hard plastic cup (such as Confi-Dry) in bra.

RATIONALE

Provides information for selection of interventions; is clue to client's response to discomfort and pain.

Discomfort during internal examination may occur, especially in the foreign client who has had a female circumcision or infibulation (whereby, after removal of the clitoris, labia minora, and medial aspect of the labia majora, the raw areas are drawn over the vagina to heal closed). Although many women are intimidated by the American healthcare system and male physicians, it is important to anticipate the discomfort experienced by foreign clients because they may not ask questions or express discomfort/pain, especially when the husband is present at the procedure. Adolescents may be self-conscious during an examination, which may further increase discomfort.

Provides proper support for enlarging breast tissues; toughens areolar tissue.

Excessive nipple stimulation may contribute to preterm labor through the release of oxytocin.

Hoffman technique and use of plastic cups help break adhesions and cause flat/inverted nipple to evert and to become more erect.

ACTIONS/INTERVENTIONS	RATIONALE

Independent

Assess for hemorrhoids: note complaints of itching, swelling, bleeding.

Reduced gastrointestinal (GI) motility and displacement of bowel and pressure on vasculature by enlarging uterus can predispose client to the development of hemorrhoids.

Instruct in use of ice packs, heat, or topical anesthetics; teach how to reinsert hemorrhoid with lubricated finger; encourage diet high in fiber, fruits, and vegetables; suggest periodically elevating buttocks on pillow. (Refer to ND: Constipation.)

Reduces discomfort and swelling; promotes GI motility.

Leg cramps: instruct client to dorsiflex foot with leg extended and to reduce amount of cheese and milk ingested.

Increases blood supply to the leg. Excess intake of dairy products results in greater levels of phosphorus than calcium, creating an imbalance that may result in muscle cramping.

Leukorrhea: encourage frequent bathing and perineal care, use of cotton underwear, and a dusting of cornstarch to absorb discharge. Tell client to avoid the use of talcum powder.

Promotes hygiene by removing/absorbing excess vaginal secretions. Application of talcum powder in the genital area is believed to contribute to development of cervical cancers.

Nausea/vomiting: recommend increasing carbohydrate intake on arising (e.g., eating dry toast), eating small and frequent meals, and avoiding strong odors. (Refer to ND: Fluid Volume deficit, high risk for.)

Reduces likelihood of gastric disturbances that may be caused by the effects of hydrochloric acid on the empty stomach or by increased sensitivity/aversion to odors, spices, or certain foods.

Stuffiness: encourage humidification of air and avoidance of nasal sprays and decongestants.

Increased estrogen levels contribute to nasal congestion. Although humidification of air may be of limited benefit, sprays/decongestants absorbed systemically can be harmful to the fetus.

Review physiologic changes resulting in urinary frequency. Recommend avoidance of caffeinated beverages.

Urinary frequency caused by pressure of the enlarging uterus on the bladder although normal, can be a cause of irritation. Caffeine has diuretic properties that can further aggravate the problem of frequency.

Assess fatigue level and nature of family/work commitments. (Refer to NDs: Coping, Individual, ineffective; Family Coping, ineffective: compromised; and Fatigue.)

Encourages client to set priorities and include time for rest.

Collaborative

Substitute daily calcium supplements if intake of dairy products is reduced.

Assists in restoring calcium/phosphorus balance and reducing muscle cramping.

NURSING DIAGNOSIS:	FLUID VOLUME DEFICIT, HIGH RISK FOR
Risk factors may include:	Impaired intake and/or excessive losses (vomiting), increased fluid needs.
Possibly evidenced by:	[Not applicable; presence of signs/symptoms establishes an **actual** diagnosis.]

<table>
<tr>
<td>DESIRED OUTCOMES—
CLIENT WILL:</td>
<td>Identify and practice measures to reduce frequency and severity of episodes of nausea/vomiting.

Ingest individually appropriate amounts of fluid daily.

Identify signs and symptoms of dehydration necessitating treatment.</td>
</tr>
</table>

ACTIONS/INTERVENTIONS	RATIONALE
Independent	
Auscultate fetal heart tones (FHT).	Presence of a fetal heart confirms presence of a fetus and rules out a hydatidiform mole.
Determine frequency/severity of nausea/vomiting.	Provides data regarding extent of condition. Increased levels of human chorionic gonadotropin (HCG), changes in carbohydrate metabolism, and reduced gastric motility contribute to first-trimester nausea and vomiting.
Review history for other possible medical problems (e.g., peptic ulcer, gastritis, cholecystitis).	Assists in ruling out other causes and in identifying interventions to address specific problems.
Recommend client maintain diary of intake/output, urine testing, and weight loss. (Refer to CP: The High-Risk Pregnancy, ND: Nutrition, altered, less than body requirements.)	Helpful in determining presence of pernicious vomiting (hyperemesis gravidarum). Initially, vomiting may result in alkalosis, dehydration, and electrolyte imbalance. Untreated or severe vomiting may lead to acidosis, necessitating further intervention.
Assess skin temperature and turgor, mucous membranes, blood pressure (BP), temperature, intake/output, and urine specific gravity. Obtain client weight and compare with baseline weight.	Indicators assisting in evaluation of hydration level/needs.
Encourage increased intake of carbonated beverages, six small meals per day, and foods high in carbohydrates (e.g., plain popcorn, dry toast before arising).	Helpful in minimizing nausea/vomiting by reducing gastric acidity.

<table>
<tr>
<td>NURSING DIAGNOSIS:</td>
<td>KNOWLEDGE DEFICIT [LEARNING NEED], regarding natural progression of pregnancy</td>
</tr>
<tr>
<td>May be related to:</td>
<td>Lack of understanding of normal physiologic/psychologic changes and their impact on the client/family.</td>
</tr>
<tr>
<td>Possibly evidenced by:</td>
<td>Request for information, statement of misconceptions.</td>
</tr>
<tr>
<td>DESIRED OUTCOMES—
CLIENT WILL:</td>
<td>Explain normal physiologic/psychologic changes associated with the first trimester.

Display self-care behaviors that promote wellness.

Identify danger signs of pregnancy.</td>
</tr>
</table>

ACTIONS/INTERVENTIONS	RATIONALE
Independent	
Establish an ongoing and supportive nurse–client relationship.	The role of teacher/counselor can provide anticipatory guidance and promote individual responsibility for wellness.
Evaluate current knowledge and cultural beliefs regarding normal physical/psychologic changes of pregnancy, as well as beliefs about activities, self-care and so forth.	Provides information to assist in identifying needs and creating a plan of care.
Clarify misconceptions.	Fears usually arise out of misinformation and may interfere with further learning.
Determine degree of motivation for learning.	Client may have difficulty learning unless the need for it is clear.
Identify who provides support/instruction within the client's culture (e.g., grandmother/other family member, cuerandero, other healer). Work with support person(s) when possible, using interpreter as needed.	Helps ensure quality/continuity of care because support person(s) may be more successful than the physician/nurse/midwife in presenting information.
Maintain open attitude toward beliefs of client/couple.	Acceptance is important to developing and maintaining relationship.
Determine attitude of client toward care given by male provider versus midwife or female practitioner.	Some cultures view the medical doctor as someone seen for illness and use midwives/cueranderos for healthy state of childbirth. Modesty or cultural demands may prohibit care by males and/or may require that husband remain in room when care is being given.
Explain office visit routine and rationale for interventions (e.g., urine testing, BP monitoring, weight). Reinforce importance of keeping regular appointments.	Reinforces relationship between health assessment and positive outcome for mother/baby. Different cultures put emphasis on different phases of pregnancy (e.g., prenatal, delivery, or postnatal), and the client's cultural group may not consider prenatal visits as important.
Provide anticipatory guidance, including discussion of nutrition, exercise, comfort measures, rest, employment, breast care, sexual activity, and health habits/lifestyle.	Information encourages acceptance of responsibility and promotes willingness to assume self-care.
Review need for prenatal vitamins, ferrous sulfate, and folic acid.	Helps maintain normal Hb levels. Folic acid deficiency contributes to megablastic anemia, possible abruptio placentae, abortion, and fetal malformation. Research indicates that iron supplements may not be necessary until the second and third trimester, when fetal demand is great. (Note: Iron may be contraindicated in the presence of sickle cell anemia because of the possibility of overload; however, client may require increased folic acid during and following sickle cell crisis.)
Discuss fetal development, using pictures.	Visualization enhances reality of child and strengthens learning process.
Answer questions about infant care and feeding.	Provides information that can be useful for making choices.

ACTIONS/INTERVENTIONS

Independent

Identify danger signals of pregnancy, such as bleeding, cramping, acute abdominal pain, backache, edema, visual disturbance, headaches, and pelvic pressure.

Identify agents harmful to the fetus. Assess client's use of drugs (nicotine, alcohol, cocaine, marijuana, and so forth). Stress the need to avoid all medications until the health team member is consulted.

Refer client/couple to childbirth preparation class. Provide list of suggested readings.

RATIONALE

Helps client to distinguish normal from abnormal findings, thus assisting her in seeking timely, appropriate health care. (Adverse signs and symptoms may be viewed as "normal" occurrences for pregnancy and assistance may not be sought.)

The fetus is most vulnerable in the first trimester during critical periods of organ development.

Knowledge gained helps reduce fear of unknown and increases confidence that couple can manage their preparation for the birth of their child.

NURSING DIAGNOSIS:	INJURY, HIGH RISK FOR, fetal
Risk factors may include:	Maternal malnutrition, exposure to teratogens/infectious agents, presence of genetic disorders.
Possibly evidenced by:	[Not applicable; presence of signs/symptoms establishes an **actual** diagnosis.]
DESIRED OUTCOMES— CLIENT WILL:	Initiate behaviors that promote health for self and fetus.
	Refrain from self-medication without first contacting the obstetrical health practitioner.
	Abstain from smoking and use of alcohol or illicit drugs.

ACTIONS/INTERVENTIONS

Independent

Discuss importance of maternal well-being.

Discuss normal activity level and exercise practices. Encourage client to engage in moderate, non-weight-bearing exercise (e.g., swimming, bicycling).

Encourage client to engage in safer sex activities, proper use of condoms. (Refer to CP: Prenatal Infection.)

RATIONALE

Fetal well-being is directly related to maternal well-being, especially during the first trimester, when developing organ systems are most vulnerable to injury from environmental/hereditary factors.

Blood flow to the uterus can decrease by 70% with strenuous exercises, producing transient bradycardia, possible fetal hyperthermia, and IUGR. Yet, nonendurance antepartal exercise regimens tend to shorten labor, increase likelihood of a spontaneous vaginal delivery, and decrease need for oxytocin augmentation.

Failure to use condoms during intercourse may increase risk of transmission of sexually transmitted diseases (STDs), especially human immunodeficiency virus (HIV), if client does not know sexual history/contacts of partner.

ACTIONS/INTERVENTIONS	RATIONALE

Independent

Review dietary habits and cultural practices. Weigh client. Discuss normal weight gain curve for each trimester.	Malnutrition in the mother is associated with IUGR in fetus and low-birth-weight infants. Pregravid maternal obesity has been linked to preterm births.
Note protein intake. Monitor Hb and Hct. (Refer to ND: Nutrition, altered, less than body requirements, high risk for.)	Protein intake is essential to development of fetal brain tissue; Hb is essential for oxygen transport.
Review obstetrical/medical history for high-risk factors (e.g., lifestyle, altitude, culture, emotional stressors, use of medications, potential teratogens such as alcohol or nicotine or environmental toxins, or exposure to STDs, including HIV and other viruses).	Identifies physical and psychologic risk factors and need for additional evaluation and/or intervention.
Assess for possible high-risk situation associated with genetic disorders (e.g., advancing maternal age for Down syndrome, Jewish background for Tay-Sachs disease). Discuss options, including chorionic villus sampling (CVS) in first trimester or amniocentesis in second trimester. (Refer to CP: Genetic Counseling.)	Clients at risk for certain genetic disorders may desire testing to determine whether fetus is affected.
Provide information about potential teratogens, such as x-rays, alcohol, nicotine, live attenuated viruses, STORCH group of viruses (syphilis, toxoplasmosis, other, rubella, cytomegalovirus, herpes simplex), and HIV.	Helps client make decisions/choices about behaviors/environment that can promote healthy offspring.
Discuss mode of transmission of certain infections. Stress need to wash hands after animal contact. Advise against changing cat's litter box or eating improperly cooked meat. Recommend wearing gloves while gardening. Determine history of *Listeria monocytogenes* infection. (Refer to CP: Prenatal Infection.)	In the United States, *Toxoplasma gondii* is most frequently transmitted in cat feces; other cultures may acquire it through ingestion of raw or improperly cooked meat. Therapeutic abortion may be considered if disease is diagnosed prior to 20 week's gestation. *Listeria monocytogenes* is thought to be transmitted via animal contact. Vaginal culture should be obtained from client with fever of nonspecific origin or with history of *Listeria* infection.
Provide information about avoiding contact with persons known to have rubella infection if client is not immune, and about the need to be immunized following delivery. (Refer to CP: Prenatal Infection.)	Approximately 5%–15% of women of childbearing age are still susceptible to rubella, which is spread by droplet infection. Exposure may have negative effects on fetal development, especially in first trimester. Immunization after delivery results in immunity during subsequent pregnancies.
Encourage cessation of tobacco usage.	Smoking negatively affects placental circulation. Low Apgar scores at birth (below 7 at 5 minutes) are associated with smoking.

ACTIONS/INTERVENTIONS	RATIONALE
Collaborative	

Assess uterine growth through internal examination.

Provides information about gestation of fetus; screens for IUGR; identifies multiple pregnancies.

Obtain vaginal/rectal culture to rule out STDs and *Listeria*; serum should be obtained for HIV testing.

Appropriate treatment may be instituted based on culture report.

Do serologic testing.

Positive diagnosis of conditions such as toxoplasmosis can be made.

Treat client appropriately when herpes culture is positive; i.e., for active infection, medication such as acyclovir may be ordered; if inactive, information for self-care is provided.

In cases of herpes simplex virus type II, the client should have at least two consecutive negative cultures, the most recent within 4 days of delivery, to allow a vaginal delivery.

Evaluate rubella titer for immunity (>1:10). Note need for postpartum immunization.

Screening for susceptibility allows client to take appropriate precautions, thereby reducing likelihood of prenatal exposure.

Refer to appropriate resources if substance abuse exists.

More help may be needed to deal with resolution of problem and ensure well-being of pregnancy and fetus.

Refer for CVS if client is over age 35 or is at risk for a specific genetic disorder (Refer to CP: Genetic Counseling.)

CVS can detect abnormalities or genetic defects between 9 and 12 weeks' gestation. CVS is an earlier alternative to amniocentesis, which cannot be performed until 14–16 weeks' gestation.

Refer for genetic counseling if appropriate.

Additional information may be necessary.

Prepare for/discuss transvaginal sonography.

Can be carried out as early as $4\frac{1}{2}$ weeks' gestation as a diagnostic tool for suspected fetal abnormalities or for prompt detection of tubal gestation.

Discuss possible treatment options, such as abortion.

Therapeutic abortion may be considered if disease is diagnosed prior to 20 weeks' gestation.

NURSING DIAGNOSIS:	**FATIGUE, HIGH RISK FOR**
Risk factors may include:	Increased carbohydrate metabolism, altered body chemistry, increased energy requirements to perform activities of daily living.
Possibly evidenced by:	[Not applicable; presence of signs/symptoms establishes an **actual** diagnosis.]
DESIRED OUTCOMES— CLIENT WILL:	Identify basis of fatigue and individual areas of control.
	Modify lifestyle to meet changing needs/energy level.
	Report improved sense of energy.

ACTIONS/INTERVENTIONS	RATIONALE

Independent

Determine normal sleep-wake cycle and commitments to work, family, community, and self.	Helps in setting realistic priorities and examining time commitments. Client may need to make adjustments, such as changing work shift to accommodate early-morning nausea (changing to a later morning shift) or provide more rest (changing from night shift to day shift), shifting of household chores/responsibilities, and so forth.
Encourage a 1- to 2-hr nap each day, 8 hr of sleep each night.	Provides rest to meet metabolic needs associated with growth of maternal/fetal tissues.
Monitor Hb level. Explain role of iron in the body; encourage daily iron supplement to be taken between meals, as indicated.	Low Hb levels result in greater fatigue due to decreased oxygen-carrying capacity. (Note: Iron may need to be restricted in the presence of sickle cell anemia.)

NURSING DIAGNOSIS:	CONSTIPATION, HIGH RISK FOR
Risk factors may include:	Smooth muscle relaxation, increased absorption of water from GI tract, presence of hemorrhoids, ingestion of iron supplements.
Possibly evidenced by:	[Not applicable; presence of signs/symptoms establishes an **actual** diagnosis.]
DESIRED OUTCOMES— CLIENT WILL:	Maintain normal pattern of bowel functioning.
	Identify individual contributing factors/risk behaviors.
	Report adoption of individually appropriate behaviors to promote elimination.

ACTIONS/INTERVENTIONS	RATIONALE

Independent

Determine prepregnancy elimination habits, noting alteration with pregnancy.	Usual elimination patterns need to be maintained, when possible. Increasing progesterone levels relax smooth muscle within the GI tract, resulting in reduced peristalsis and increased reabsorption of water and electrolytes. Iron supplements also contribute to problems of constipation.
Assess for hemorrhoids. (Refer to ND: Discomfort.)	Varicosities of the rectum frequently develop with prolonged constipation, increased efforts at bearing down, or as a result of increased circulating volume and hormonal relaxation of blood vessels. The presence of hemorrhoids can cause pain with defecation, resulting in reluctance of the client to evacuate her bowels.
Provide dietary information about fresh fruits, vegetables, grains, fiber, roughage, and adequate fluid intake.	Bulk and consistency in diet choices help promote effective bowel pattern.

ACTIONS/INTERVENTIONS	RATIONALE

Independent

Encourage regular nonstrenuous exercise program, such as walking. Tell client to avoid strenuous, prolonged exercise. Note cultural beliefs about exercise.

Promotes peristalsis and assists in prevention of constipation. Strenuous exercise is thought to reduce uteroplacental circulation, possibly resulting in fetal bradycardia, hyperthermia, or growth retardation. In some cultures, inactivity may be viewed as a protection for mother/child.

Collaborative

Discuss cautious use of stool softener or bulk-producing agent if diet/exercise is not effective.

May be necessary to assist in combatting constipation and establishing a regular routine.

NURSING DIAGNOSIS:	INFECTION, HIGH RISK FOR, urinary tract infection (UTI)
Risk factors may include:	Urinary stasis, poor hygienic practices, insufficient knowledge to avoid exposure to pathogens.
Possibly evidenced by:	[Not applicable; presence of signs/symptoms establishes an **actual** diagnosis.]
DESIRED OUTCOMES— CLIENT WILL:	Identify behaviors to reduce urinary stasis/risk of infection.
	List signs and symptoms requiring evaluation/interventions.
	Be free of signs and symptoms of infection.

ACTIONS/INTERVENTIONS	RATIONALE

Independent

Provide information about signs/symptoms of UTI. Stress need to report signs of infection to healthcare provider and to avoid self-medication until after such notification.

Maternal UTI responds well to treatment and may not be serious; however, it is associated with preterm labor/birth.

Stress need for frequent/thorough handwashing before meals and food handling, and after toileting.

Many viruses, such as cytomegalovirus (CMV), can be excreted in the urine for up to 4 years after exposure and possibly transmitted through poor hygienic practices.

Provide information about other hygiene measures, including wiping vulva from front to back after urinating and voiding after intercourse.

Helps prevent rectal *E. coli* contaminants from reaching the vagina. May help to prevent transmission of STDs, especially CMV and nongonococcal urethritis.

Recommend client drink 6 to 8 glasses of liquid daily. Discuss role of acid residue in diet and addition of cranberry/orange juice.

Helps prevent stasis in the urinary tract; may acidify urine and help prevent UTI.

Encourage practice of Kegel exercise (tightening of the perineum) throughout the day.

Improves support to the pelvic organs, strengthening and increasing elasticity of the pubococcygeus muscle; provides more control over urination.

ACTIONS/INTERVENTIONS	RATIONALE

Independent

Suggest use of cotton underwear and avoidance of baths if client has a history of UTI.

Urinary stasis and glycosuria can predispose the prenatal client to UTI, especially if history includes urinary/kidney problems. Contributory factors such as wearing man-made fabrics and sitting in bathwater can add to potential for exposure to infection.

Collaborative

Obtain routine urine sample for microscopic examination, pH, presence of white blood cells, and culture and sensitivity, as indicated. Report colony counts of greater than 100,000/ml.

Alkaline urine predisposes client to a possible *Proteus vulgaris* infection. As many as 2%–10% of pregnant women have asymptomatic bacteriuria (colony count greater than 100,000/ml), which increases risk of premature rupture of membranes, preterm labor, and chorioamnionitis.

Administer antibiotics (e.g., ampicillin, erythromycin) as appropriate.

Treats infection as indicated. Care must be taken in prescribing antibiotics prenatally, owing to potentially negative effects on the fetus.

NURSING DIAGNOSIS:	CARDIAC OUTPUT [maximally compensated]
May be related to:	Increased fluid volume (preload), ventricular hypertrophy, changes in peripheral resistance (afterload).
Possibly evidenced by:	Variations in blood pressure and pulse, syncopal episodes, presence of pathologic edema.
DESIRED OUTCOMES— CLIENT WILL:	Differentiate normal and abnormal changes.
	Remain normotensive.
	Be free of pathologic edema.
	Display no more than 1+ albumin in urinalysis.

ACTIONS/INTERVENTIONS	RATIONALE

Independent

Review physiologic process and normal or abnormal changes and signs/symptoms.

Prenatally, circulating blood volume in the form of plasma and red blood cells increases 30%–50% to meet maternal/fetal nutritional and oxygen needs and to act as a safeguard against blood loss during delivery. The body compensates for the increase in fluid volume by increasing cardiac output through ventricular hypertrophy. Hormonal effects of progesterone and relaxin reduce resistance to cardiac output by relaxing smooth muscle within the blood vessel walls. Although this is a normal process, the client is maximally compensated and could be at risk for hypertension and/or circulatory failure as the pregnancy progresses. Prompt recognition and intervention reduces risk of adverse outcome.

ACTIONS/INTERVENTIONS	RATIONALE

Independent

Obtain baseline BP and pulse measurement. Report systolic increase of greater than 30 mm Hg or diastolic increase greater than 15 mm Hg.

An increase in BP may indicate PIH. Pulse increase above 10 to 15 bpm may indicate cardiac stress.

Auscultate heart sounds; note any murmurs. Review contributory history of cardiac problems or rheumatic fever.

Cardiac ventricles undergo slight hypertrophy to compensate for increase in circulating volume and to maximize output. Systolic murmur may be created by decreased blood viscosity, displacement of the heart, or torsion of great vessels.

Assess for location/degree of edema. Distinguish between physiologic and potentially harmful edema. (Refer to CP: Pregnancy-Induced Hypertension, ND: Fluid Volume deficit, high risk for.)

Dependent edema of the lower extremities (physiologic edema) often occurs, owing to venous stasis caused by uterine pressure and hormonal effects of progesterone and relaxin, which relax blood vessel walls. Edema of facies and/or upper extremities may indicate PIH.

Assess for varicosities of legs, vulva, rectum.

Increased fluid load and hormonal relaxation of blood vessel walls increases risk for vascular engorgement and venous stasis, especially in client whose lifestyle requires prolonged sitting/standing.

Discuss the need to avoid rapid position changes from sitting or lying to standing.

Client may be prone to postural hypotension due to reduced venous return.

Collaborative

Monitor Hb and Hct levels.

Low Hb may indicate anemia, which can increase heart rate and cardiac workload; elevated Hct may indicate dehydration with PIH fluid shifts.

Test urine for albumin as indicated.

Proteinuria with elevation of albumin above 1+ suggests glomerular edema or spasm (developing PIH), requiring prompt intervention.

NURSING DIAGNOSIS:	BODY IMAGE DISTURBANCE, HIGH RISK FOR
Risk factors may include:	Perception of biophysical changes; psychosocial, cultural, and spiritual beliefs.
Possibly evidenced by:	[Not applicable; presence of signs/symptoms establishes an **actual** diagnosis.]
DESIRED OUTCOMES— CLIENT WILL:	Verbalize understanding/acceptance of body changes.
	Verbalize acceptance of self in situation.
	Demonstrate a positive self-image by maintaining an overall satisfactory appearance.

ACTIONS/INTERVENTIONS	RATIONALE

Independent

Determine attitude toward pregnancy, changing body image, and job situation, and how these issues are viewed by significant other(s).

The client's feelings toward the pregnancy affect her ability to develop positive feelings about her changing body contours, as well as her ability to adapt positively to her parenting roles.

Identify basic sense of client's self-esteem in relation to the changes of pregnancy and responsibilities related to this new role.

Alterations in body image occur normally in pregnancy due to a changing body shape and may create a crisis situation negatively impacting both the pregnancy and parenting abilities in clients with poor self-esteem and a weak ego identity.

Assess support systems such as aunt, grandmother, cultural healer, and so on.

Adequate support can help client to cope positively with her changing body shape and maintain positive self-esteem.

Review physiologic changes of pregnancy; assure client that mixed feelings are normal. Provide environment in which couple can discuss feelings.

Helps decrease stress associated with pregnancy. Verbalizing helps sort out feelings, attitudes, and past experiences.

Collaborative

Refer to other resources as indicated (e.g., counseling/therapy).

Client may require more intensive intervention to facilitate acceptance of self/pregnancy.

NURSING DIAGNOSIS:	ROLE PERFORMANCE, ALTERED, HIGH RISK FOR
Risk factors may include:	Maturational crisis, developmental level (immaturity on the part of the client and/or significant other), history of maladaptive coping, absence of support systems.
Possibly evidenced by:	[Not applicable; presence of signs/symptoms establishes an **actual** diagnosis.]
DESIRED OUTCOMES— CLIENT WILL:	Identify perceived stressors.
	Verbalize realistic perception and acceptance of self in changing role.
	Talk with family/significant other about situation and changes that have occurred or may occur.
	Develop realistic plans for adapting to new role/role changes.

ACTIONS/INTERVENTIONS	RATIONALE

Independent

Evaluate the client's/couple's response to pregnancy, individual and family stressors, and cultural implications of pregnancy/childbirth.

Identifies needs to assist in planning interventions. The client's/couple's ability to adapt positively to this "crisis" depends on support systems, cultural beliefs, resources, and effective coping mechanisms developed in dealing with past stressors. Initially, even if the pregnancy is planned, the expectant mother may feel ambivalent toward the pregnancy due to personal/professional goals, fi-

ACTIONS/INTERVENTIONS	RATIONALE
Independent	
	nancial concerns, and possible role changes a child will necessitate.
Ascertain from client/couple how stressors have been dealt with in the past.	Provides information regarding client's/couple's ability to deal positively with stress. Learned coping methods, either positive or negative, tend to be used in subsequent crises.
Assess economic situation and financial needs. Make necessary referrals.	Impact of pregnancy on family without adequate resources can create added stress. Members of some cultures may view healthcare as unaffordable and, as a result, may seek abortion or may not seek prenatal care.
Elicit information about preparations or lack of preparations being made for this infant.	May have fears that visible preparations may result in child's death or that planning ahead has the potential of "defying God's will."
Explain emotional lability as characteristic of pregnancy. Discuss normalcy of ambivalence.	Helps client/couple understand mood swings. Partner realizes the need to offer support/affection at these times.
Provide information about and encourage attendance at childbirth classes.	Provides an opportunity for formal/informal sharing of problems, feelings, and peer support.
Assess for maladaptive behaviors (e.g., withdrawal, inappropriate anger/reactions, lack of or inappropriate self-care).	Provides information about client's ability to deal with stress and the need for intervention.
Collaborative	
Refer for psychologic counseling, if necessary.	Further assistance in developing problem-solving skills may be helpful. By the end of the first trimester, the client/couple should have successfully achieved the task of accepting the pregnancy.

NURSING DIAGNOSIS:	FAMILY COPING: POTENTIAL FOR GROWTH
May be related to:	Client and family needs are sufficiently met, adaptive tasks are effectively addressed to enable goals of self-actualization to surface.
Possibly evidenced by:	Family member/individual makes realistic appraisal of growth impact of pregnancy on own values, priorities, goals or relationships; moving in direction of health-promoting and enriching lifestyle; chooses experiences that optimize wellness.
DESIRED OUTCOMES— CLIENT/COUPLE WILL:	Explore anticipated role changes.
	Undertake appropriate tasks in preparation for the birth.
	Report feelings of self-confidence and satisfaction with progress being made.

ACTIONS/INTERVENTIONS	RATIONALE

Independent

Identify relationship of family members to one another. Note strengths/stressors (e.g., communication styles, interactions between members).

Pregnancy is a crisis situation for client/couple and family members, resulting in a disequilibrium that necessitates adaptation to new roles and responsibilities.

Assess relationship of client/couple to parents.

May provide insight for assisting couple in assuming parenting role. New parents tend to use their own parents as role models and may thus adopt positive or negative parenting behaviors.

Evaluate sibling responses to pregnancy and upcoming change in family structure.

In the first trimester, young siblings may not be aware of the reality and long-term consequences of pregnancy. Older children may not manifest negative feelings outwardly, yet internally they may begin to fear a change in the security of their relationship with their parent(s). Family members may be concerned about anticipated changes and may express a desire to prepare themselves and siblings for role/life change(s).

Provide information about father/sibling attendance at childbirth classes and participation in delivery, as desired.

Helps family members to realize they are an integral part of the pregnancy and delivery.

Encourage father/siblings to attend prenatal office visits and listen to FHT.

Promotes a sense of involvement; helps to make baby a reality for family members.

Provide list of appropriate reading materials for client/couple/siblings regarding adjusting to newborn.

Information helps individual to realistically analyze changes in family structure, roles, and behaviors.

Collaborative

Provide information/referral about community resources if client/couple is having concerns about parenting abilities. (Refer to ND: Role Performance, altered, high risk for.)

Reducing stressors in the home allows the expectant couple to devote emotional energy to the pregnancy.

NURSING DIAGNOSIS:	SEXUALITY PATTERNS, ALTERED
May be related to:	Knowledge/skill deficit about altered body function/structure, changes in comfort level.
Possibly evidenced by:	Reported difficulties, limitations, or changes in sexual response/activities.
DESIRED OUTCOMES— CLIENT/PARTNER WILL:	Share feelings related to changes in sexual desire.
	Take desired steps to remedy situation.
	Report satisfaction with/acceptance of changes or modifications required by pregnancy.

ACTIONS/INTERVENTIONS	RATIONALE
Independent	
Determine the couple's usual pattern of sexual activity using a sexual assessment tool. Assess the impact of pregnancy on the pattern and the couple's response to the changes.	How the couple copes with changes in sexuality and sexual patterns during pregnancy may affect the relationship. Client/couple may be helped when they know that desire may be diminished because the woman isn't feeling well, owing to breast tenderness, fatigue, nausea, vomiting, and a changing body image. However, they should know it is alright to continue sexual activity/alternatives as the couple desires.
Review information about the normalcy of these changes; correct misconceptions.	Helps the couple understand the changes from a physiologic viewpoint. Reduced libidinal urges in the first trimester are common for the prenatal client. This decreased desire may be difficult for the couple, and especially for the male partner, to understand.
Assess couple's relationship to one another and ability to cope with decrease in frequency of sexual intercourse.	The nature of the relationship prior to pregnancy affects how well the couple copes during pregnancy.
Assess client/couple response to changing body shape. Create a teaching plan to discuss sexual changes for prenatal client in the second and third trimester. (Refer to ND: Body Image disturbance, high risk for.)	Acceptance of sexuality issues is directly related to a positive self-concept and individual's sense of identity.
Review obstetrical history with couple. Assess for vaginal bleeding/spotting.	Intercourse is not usually contraindicated in the first trimester unless the client has experienced complications such as bleeding during this pregnancy or in past pregnancies.
Collaborative	
Refer the couple for counseling if sexual concerns are not resolved.	Professional counseling may be necessary to help couples to cope positively with sexuality issues in pregnancy.

NURSING DIAGNOSIS:	BODY IMAGE DISTURBANCE, HIGH RISK FOR
Risk factors may include:	Perception of biophysical changes, responses of others.
Possibly evidenced by:	[Not applicable; presence of signs/symptoms establishes an **actual** diagnosis.]
DESIRED OUTCOMES— CLIENT WILL:	Verbalize gradual acceptance/adaptation to changing self-concept/body image.
	Demonstrate a positive self-image by maintaining an overall satisfactory appearance; dress in appropriately fitting clothes, and low-heeled shoes.

ACTIONS/INTERVENTIONS	RATIONALE
Independent	
Review/assess attitude toward pregnancy, changing body shape, and so forth. (Refer to CP: First Trimester, ND: Body Image disturbance.)	In the second trimester, the changing body contours are readily visible. Negative responses to such changes may occur in the client/couple whose fragile self-concept is based on physical appearance. Other visible effects from prenatal hormones such as chloasma, striae gravidarum, telangiectasia (vascular spiders), palmar erythema, acne, and hirsutism can contribute to the client's emotional changes. These changes may affect how she deals with the changes that are occurring.
Discuss physiologic aspects of, and client's response to, changes. Provide information about normalcy of changes.	Individuals react differently to the changes that occur, and information can help the client understand/accept what is happening.
Suggest styles and available sources of maternity clothing.	Individual circumstances indicate needs for clothing that will enhance the client's appearance for work and leisure activities.
Discuss methods of skin care and makeup (to minimize/hide darkened areas of the skin), the use of support hose, maintenance of posture, and a moderate exercise program.	Learning about and being involved in ways to look and feel better may be helpful for maintaining positive feelings about the self. A nonendurance perinatal exercise regimen tends to shorten labor, increase the likelihood of a spontaneous vaginal delivery, and decrease the need for oxytocin augmentation. (Note: Strenuous exercise may result in reduced uterine blood flow/fetal bradycardia.)
Collaborative	
Refer to other resources such as counseling and/or classes in childbirth education and parenting.	May be helpful in providing additional support during this period of change; identifies role models.

NURSING DIAGNOSIS:	BREATHING PATTERN, INEFFECTIVE
May be related to:	Impingement of the diaphragm by the enlarging uterus.
Possibly evidenced by:	Complaints of shortness of breath, dyspnea, changes in respiratory depth.
DESIRED OUTCOMES— CLIENT WILL:	Report decrease in frequency/severity of complaints.
	Demonstrate behaviors that optimize respiratory functioning.

ACTIONS/INTERVENTIONS	RATIONALE
Independent	
Assess respiratory status (e.g. shortness of breath on exertion, fatigue).	Determines existence/severity of problem, which occurs in approximately 60% of prenatal clients. Even though vital capacity increases, respiratory function is modified as the diaphragm's ability to descend on inspiration is reduced by the enlarging uterus.
Obtain history of and monitor preexisting/developing medical problems (e.g., allergic rhinitis, asthma, sinus problems, tuberculosis). (Refer to CP: The High-Risk Pregnancy, ND: Injury, High Risk For, fetal.)	Other problems may further alter breathing patterns and may compromise maternal/fetal tissue oxygenation.
Assess hemoglobin (Hb) and hematocrit (Hct) levels. Stress importance of daily prenatal vitamins/ferrous sulfate intake (except in client with sickle cell anemia).	Increased plasma levels at 24–32 weeks' gestation further dilute Hb levels, resulting in possible anemia and decreased oxygen-carrying capacity. (Note: Iron may be contraindicated for client with sickle cell anemia.)
Provide information about rationale for respiratory difficulties and realistic activity/exercise program. Encourage frequent rest periods, providing extra time for certain activities, and participation in mild exercise, such as walking.	Reduces the likelihood of respiratory symptoms caused by overexertion.
Review measures client can take to ease problems; e.g., good posture, avoiding smoking, eating smaller more frequent meals, using modified semi-Fowler's position for sitting/sleeping if symptoms are severe.	Good posture and small meals help to maximize diaphragmatic descent, increasing space available for lung expansion. Smoking reduces oxygen available for maternal-fetal exchange. Upright positioning may increase lung expansion as the gravid uterus descends.

NURSING DIAGNOSIS:	KNOWLEDGE DEFICIT [LEARNING NEED], regarding natural progression of pregnancy
May be related to:	Continued need for information as the changes of the second trimester are experienced.
Possibly evidenced by:	Request for information, statement of concerns or misconceptions.

ACTIONS/INTERVENTIONS	RATIONALE
Independent	
Review changes to be expected during the second trimester.	Questions continue to arise as new changes occur, regardless of whether changes are expected or unexpected.
Institute/continue a learning program as outlined in CP: First Trimester, ND: Knowledge Deficit [Learning Need].	Repetition reinforces learning, and if client has not been seen previously, information is useful at this point.
Provide information about need for ferrous sulfate and folic acid.	Ferrous sulfate and folic acid help maintain normal Hb levels. Folic acid deficiency contributes to megaloblastic anemia, possible abruptio placentae, abortion, and fetal malformation. (Note: Clients with sickle cell anemia require increased folic acid during and following crisis episode.)
Identify possible individual health risks (e.g., spontaneous abortion, hypoxia related to asthma or tuberculosis, heart disease, pregnancy-induced hypertension [PIH], kidney disorders, anemia, gestational diabetes mellitus [GDM], sexually transmitted diseases [STDs]). Review danger signs and appropriate actions.	Helpful reminder/information for client about potential high-risk situation requiring closer monitoring and/or intervention.
Discuss any medications that may be needed to control or treat medical problem.	Helpful in choosing treatment options because need must be weighed against possible harmful effects to the fetus.
Discuss need for specific laboratory studies, screening, and close monitoring as indicated.	More frequent prenatal visits may be needed to promote maternal well-being. Monitoring Hb and Hct using electrophoresis detects specific anemias and is helpful in determining cause. Screening for GDM at 24–26 weeks' gestation or at 12, 18, and 32 weeks' gestation in high-risk client can detect developing hyperglycemia, which may need treatment with insulin and/or the American Diabetes Association diet. (Refer to CPs: Diabetes Mellitus: Prepregnancy/Gestational; The High-Risk Pregnancy.)

Possibly evidenced by:	[Not applicable; presence of signs/symptoms establishes an **actual** diagnosis.]
DESIRED OUTCOMES— CLIENT WILL:	Verbalize awareness of individual risk factors.
	Avoid factors and/or refrain from behaviors that may contribute to fetal injury.

ACTIONS/INTERVENTIONS	RATIONALE
Independent	
Determine understanding of information previously provided. (Refer to CP: First Trimester, ND: Injury, high risk for, fetal.)	Identifies individual needs/concerns and provides opportunity to clarify misconceptions, especially for clients whose initial prenatal visit occurs at this time.
Review maternal health status; e.g., malnutrition, substance use/abuse. (Refer to CP: First Trimester, ND: Nutrition, altered, less than body requirements.)	These factors can have great impact on developing fetal tissues and organs, and early identification and intervention may prevent untoward results.
Assess for other factors existing in the individual situation that may be harmful to the fetus (e.g., exposure to viruses/other STDs, environmental factors). (Refer to CP: Prenatal Infection.)	Identification enables client and nurse to discuss ways to minimize/prevent injury. STDs or other viruses may be only mildly problematic for the client, but often have a great negative impact on fetal well-being.
Note quickening (maternal perception of fetal movements) and fetal heart tones (FHT). Refer to physician if problem is detected.	Perceivable fetal movements first occur between 16 and 20 weeks' gestation as fetal size increases; lack of movement may indicate an existing problem. Failure to detect FHT may indicate fetal demise or absence of fetus/presence of hydatidiform mole.
Assess uterine growth and fundal height at each visit.	Screens for multiple gestation, normal or abnormal fetal growth; may detect problems related to polyhydramnios or oligohydramnios.
Provide information about diagnostic tests or procedure(s). Review risks and potential side effects.	Having information helps client/couple to deal with situation and make informed decisions. Certain genetic problems such as neural tube defects (NTD) may be detected at this stage.
Collaborative	
Assist with ultrasonographic procedure, and explain its purpose.	Detects presence of fetus as early as 5–6 weeks' gestation and provides information about fetal growth using measurements of crown to rump, length of femur, and biparietal diameter, to confirm gestational age and rule out intrauterine growth retardation. Also determines placental size and location and may detect some fetal abnormalities.
Obtain maternal serum sample for alpha-fetoprotein (AFP) level between 14 and 16 weeks.	With an open NTD (most commonly, spina bifida and anencephaly), AFP, a protein produced by the yolk sac and fetal liver, is present in maternal serum at a level 8 times higher than normal at 15 weeks' gestation. Thereafter, it decreases until term.

ACTIONS/INTERVENTIONS

Collaborative

Assist with amniocentesis when AFP level is abnormal, especially in high-risk population (e.g., clients with possible genetic disorders/previous child having a chromosomal abnormality, older gravidas over age 35 years), if client has not already had chorionic villus sampling (CVS).

Follow with genetic counseling, as appropriate. (Refer to CP: Genetic Counseling.)

Screen client for GDM with glucose tolerance test (GTT) at 24–26 weeks' gestation, as indicated. (Refer to CP: Diabetes Mellitus; Prepregnancy/Gestational.)

RATIONALE

Analysis of amniotic fluid detects genetic/chromosomal disorders and NTD.

Client/couple will need information to make informed decisions about course of action in this pregnancy as well as future pregnancies.

GDM is associated with macrosomia and problems of dystocia.

NURSING DIAGNOSIS:	CARDIAC OUTPUT, high risk for decompensation
Risk factors may include:	Increased circulatory demand, changes in preload (decreased venous return) and afterload (increased peripheral vascular resistance), ventricular hypertrophy.
Possibly evidenced by:	[Not applicable; presence of signs/symptoms establishes an **actual** diagnosis.]
DESIRED OUTCOMES— CLIENT WILL:	Remain normotensive during the prenatal course.
	Be free of pathologic edema and signs of PIH.
	Identify ways to control and reduce cardiovascular problems.

ACTIONS/INTERVENTIONS

Independent

Review physiologic process and normal and abnormal changes, signs, and symptoms. (Refer to CP: Cardiac Conditions.)

Note history of preexisting or potential cardiac/kidney/diabetic problems.

RATIONALE

During the second trimester, hypertrophy of the cardiac ventricles ensures increased cardiac output, which peaks at 25–27 weeks' gestation to meet maternal/fetal oxygen and nutrient needs. Normally, the cardiovascular system compensates for increased cardiac output with dilation of blood vessels, which reduces resistance to cardiac output. This lowers the systolic pressure readings approximately 8 mm Hg while the diastolic pressure decrease averages 12 mm Hg. Increases in fluid, stress, and/or preexisting cardiac problems, however, can compromise the system.

These clients face the greatest risk for cardiac involvement during the second trimester, when cardiac output peaks.

ACTIONS/INTERVENTIONS	RATIONALE

Independent

Obtain blood pressure (BP) and pulse measurement. Report systolic increase greater than 30 mm Hg and diastolic increase greater than 15 mm Hg.

An increase in BP may indicate PIH, especially in clients with preexisting cardiac or kidney disease, diabetes, or in the presence of multiple pregnancies or hydatidiform mole.

Auscultate heart sounds; note presence of murmurs.

Systolic murmurs are often benign and may be created by increased volume, decreased blood viscosity, displacement of the heart, or torsion of great vessels. However, a murmur may indicate developing failure.

Assess for presence of ankle edema and varicosities of legs, vulva, and rectum. Distinguish between physiologic and potentially harmful edema. (Refer to CP: Pregnancy-Induced Hypertension, ND: Fluid Volume deficit [active loss].)

Dependent edema of the lower extremities (physiologic edema) often occurs because of venous stasis due to vasodilation from progesterone activity, heredity, excess fluid retention, and uterine pressure on pelvic blood vessels. This increases the risk of venous thrombus formation. Edema of facies and/or upper extremities may indicate PIH.

Encourage client to avoid crossing legs, sitting, and standing for long periods; to put on support hose before arising in the morning; to wear loose, nonconstricting clothing; to elevate legs when sitting; to elevate legs, hips, and vulva vertical to the wall three times a day for 20 minutes; and to turn feet upward in dorsiflexion if sitting or standing for long periods.

Promotes venous return and reduces risk of developing edema, varicosities, or venous thrombosis.

Dorsiflex foot to test for Homans' sign. If present, refer to physician.

A positive Homans' sign may indicate thrombophlebitis.

Assess for faintness. Encourage client to avoid changing position rapidly.

Sudden position changes may result in dizziness as blood pools in lower extremities, reducing circulating volume.

NURSING DIAGNOSIS:	FLUID VOLUME EXCESS, HIGH RISK FOR
Risk factors may include:	Changes in regulatory mechanisms, sodium/water retention.
Possibly evidenced by:	[Not applicable; presence of signs/symptoms establishes an **actual** diagnosis.]
DESIRED OUTCOMES— CLIENT WILL:	List ways to minimize problem.
	Identify signs/symptoms requiring medical evaluation/intervention.
	Be free of hypertension, albuminuria, excessive fluid retention, and edema of facies.

ACTIONS/INTERVENTIONS	RATIONALE
Independent	
Monitor weight regularly.	Detects excessive weight gain and invisible fluid retention, which may be potentially pathologic. During the second trimester, total body water (plasma and red blood cells) increases by 1,000 ml, owing in part to estrogen levels stimulating the adrenal gland to secrete aldosterone, which retains sodium and water. Although up to 5 lb of fluid can be retained with no visible edema, this increase can contribute to cardiac decompensation.
Assess for signs of PIH, noting blood pressure. Monitor location/extent of edema, and fluid intake and output. Note reports of visual disturbances, headache, epigastric pain, or presence of hyperreflexia.	Indicators of pathologic edema. Although PIH due to excessive fluid retention is not usually seen until the last 10 weeks of pregnancy, it may develop earlier, especially in the client with predisposing factors such as diabetes, renal disease, hypertension, multiple gestation, malnutrition (overweight or underweight), hydatidiform mole.
Test urine for albumin.	Detects vascular involvement associated with glomerular spasms of the kidney, which reduce resorption of albumin.
Provide information about diet (e.g., increased protein, no added table salt, avoidance of foods and beverages high in sodium).	Adequate nutrition, especially increased protein, reduces likelihood of PIH. Excess sodium may contribute to water retention (too little sodium may result in dehydration.)
Recommend elevating extremities periodically during the day.	Physiologic edema of the lower extremities occurring at the end of the day is normal, but it should resolve with simple corrective measures. If it does not resolve, the healthcare provider should be notified.
Review Hct levels. (Note effects of variables, such as altitude and race.)	In general, levels >41% (Caucasian) or >38% (African heritage) indicate intravascular fluid shifts resulting in tissue edema.
Collaborative	
Schedule more frequent prenatal visits and institute treatment if PIH exists. (Refer to CP: Pregnancy-Induced Hypertension.)	Treatment helps promote positive maternal/fetal outcomes.

NURSING DIAGNOSIS:	**DISCOMFORT***
May be related to:	Changes in body mechanics, effects of hormones, electrolyte imbalances.
Possibly evidenced by:	Reports of back strain, leg cramps, heartburn.

DESIRED OUTCOMES— CLIENT WILL:	Identify and demonstrate appropriate self-care measures.
	Report discomfort is prevented or minimized.
	*Author's note: Currently there is no NANDA diagnostic label that addresses issues of comfort below the level of Pain [acute] or chronic. Although the label of **Discomfort** is not approved, we believe it speaks more directly to the identified problem.

ACTIONS/INTERVENTIONS

Independent

Note presence of problems related to cardiac output or breathing difficulties, and refer to appropriate nursing diagnoses.

Reassess for changes in bowel elimination and hemorrhoids.

Discuss dietary intake, exercise, and use of stool softener as presented in CP: First Trimester, ND: Constipation, high risk for.

Note presence of heartburn (pyrosis); review dietary history. Explain physiology of problem. Suggest client avoid fried/fatty foods, eat six small meals per day, assume semi-Fowler's position after meals, decrease fluid intake with meals, and avoid very cold food.

Note presence of backache and lower back pressure. Demonstrate exercises (e.g., pelvic tilt, lying flat on back and pressing back to floor). Review proper dress (e.g., low-heeled shoes; loose, comfortable clothing).

Reassess for leg cramps; teach client to extend leg and dorsiflex foot.

Recommend reducing intake of milk products and taking aluminum lactate, or continuing with 1 quart of milk daily and taking aluminum hydroxide, if leg cramps are severe or persist.

RATIONALE

Although these conditions are often sources of discomfort, the client usually experiences a sense of physical well-being free of the typical discomforts of the first trimester.

Reduced gastrointestinal motility, the effect of iron supplements, and increasing pressure/displacement from enlarging uterus interfere with normal functioning.

Aids in the prevention/management of constipation.

Fatty foods increase gastric acidity; small, frequent meals neutralize acidity. Semi-Fowler's position, decreased fluid intake, and avoidance of cold food help to prevent gastric reflux.

Relieves strain on lower back caused by increased curvature of the lumbosacral vertebrae and strengthens back muscles.

Pressure on nerves in the pelvis, as well as low tissue calcium levels, potentiate leg cramps. Extension of the leg and dorsiflexion of the foot increase perfusion/oxygenation of tissue and helps relieve pressure on nerves of lower extremities.

Continued intake of calcium-containing foods/products elevates ionized plasma levels. Aluminum hydroxide traps dietary phosphorus in intestinal tract, offsetting calcium-phosphorus imbalances.

ACTIONS/INTERVENTIONS

RATIONALE

Independent

Provide information about appropriate choices of over-the-counter antacids. Avoid use of bicarbonate as a neutralizer or calcium products, as appropriate.

May be constipating and/or may contain substances, such as sodium, that may be contraindicated in certain situations owing to its water-retaining properties. Frequent use of calcium-containing antacids in addition to intake of high-calcium foods may contribute to calcium-phosphorus imbalance and development of muscle cramps.

Collaborative

Administer low-sodium antacid.

Neutralizes gastric acidity; decreases phosphorus levels.

Give calcium supplements and aluminum gel as appropriate.

Substitutes for milk products in presence of dietary intolerance. Can reduce phosphorus levels.

NURSING DIAGNOSIS:	**COPING, INDIVIDUAL, INEFFECTIVE, HIGH RISK FOR**
Risk factors may include:	Situational/maturational crisis, personal vulnerability, unrealistic perceptions.
Possibly evidenced by:	[Not applicable; presence of signs/symptoms establishes an **actual** diagnosis.]
DESIRED OUTCOMES— CLIENT WILL:	Express feelings freely.
	Identify individual strengths.
	Display effective problem-solving and coping skills.

ACTIONS/INTERVENTIONS

RATIONALE

Independent

Identify fears/fantasies client/partner may have. Discuss meaning of these thoughts.

Common female/male fears and fantasies may arise at this time. Women may fear the death of the spouse, and the male partner may fantasize about himself being pregnant.

Reinforce the normalcy of these fears and fantasies.

May result in difficulties for the individual who does not see the normalcy of this experience.

Evaluate degree of dysfunction client/partner is experiencing in relation to changes that are occurring and those that are anticipated.

Clients experiencing difficulty adjusting to the overwhelming tasks associated with pregnancy/parenting may manifest inappropriate follow-through with prenatal healthcare or greater than normal states of emotional lability. The male partner may demonstrate negative coping in preoccupation with work or a new hobby, lack of interest in the pregnancy, or involvement in extramarital activity.

Encourage client/partner to express feelings about pregnancy and parenting.

Acknowledging and expressing feelings can help the individual begin to identify problems and begin the problem-solving process.

ACTIONS/INTERVENTIONS

Collaborative

Refer to counseling and classes as needed. (Refer to CP: First Trimester, ND: Role Performance, altered, high risk for.)

RATIONALE

May need additional help to solve underlying issues.

NURSING DIAGNOSIS:	SEXUALITY PATTERNS, ALTERED
May be related to:	Conflict regarding changes in sexual desire and expectations, fear of physical injury.
Possibly evidenced by:	Reported difficulties, limitations or changes in sexual behaviors/activities.
DESIRED OUTCOMES— CLIENT/COUPLE WILL:	Discuss sexual concerns.
	Verbalize understanding of possible reasons for changes noted.
	Identify acceptable alternatives to meet individual needs.
	Verbalize mutual satisfaction or seek counseling, if appropriate.

ACTIONS/INTERVENTIONS

Independent

Discuss impact of pregnancy on normal patterns of sexual intercourse. (Refer to CP: First Trimester, ND: Sexuality Patterns, altered.)

Review normalcy of feelings and discuss possible choice of increasing physical contact through hugging and fondling rather than actually engaging in intercourse.

Review possible alterations in position for sexual activity.

Be alert to indications of possible sexual difficulties or inappropriate behaviors by the man.

Collaborative

Refer to clinical nurse specialist/counseling as indicated.

RATIONALE

Optimal sexual satisfaction for the prenatal client occurs in the second trimester due to pelvic/perineal vasocongestion increasing orgasmic pleasure. The man may experience mixed feelings in response to his partner's increased arousal and be confused by his own reduced or increased sexual desire in response to his partner's changing body.

Fear of injuring the fetus during intercourse is another common concern. Reinforcement of the normalcy of these feelings and concerns can help allay anxiety. Other choices are perfectly acceptable if both parties are satisfied.

Assists couple in considering alternatives/making choices.

There appears to be a higher rate of deviations (such as rape, incest, violent crimes, and extramarital affairs) when mate is pregnant.

May need additional help to solve underlying problems, which may develop as pregnancy progresses or which may be preexisting.

NURSING DIAGNOSIS:	DISCOMFORT*
May be related to:	Physical changes, hormonal influences.
Possibly evidenced by:	Reports of back strain/pain, leg cramps, paresthesia, pruritus, uterine contractions.
DESIRED OUTCOMES—CLIENT WILL:	Use appropriate self-care activities to reduce discomforts.
	Report discomfort minimized/controlled.
	Seek medical attention appropriately.
	*Authors' note: Currently there is no NANDA diagnostic label that addresses issues of comfort below the level of Pain [acute] or chronic. Although the label of **Discomfort** is not approved, we believe it speaks more directly to the identified problem.

ACTIONS/INTERVENTIONS	RATIONALE
Independent	
Continue ongoing assessment of client's discomforts and her methods of dealing with problems. (Refer to CP: Second Trimester, ND: Discomfort.)	Updates data base for planning care.
Assess client's respiratory status. (Refer to CP: Second Trimester, ND: Breathing Pattern, ineffective.)	Reduced respiratory capacity as the uterus presses on the diaphragm results in dyspnea, especially for the multigravida who may not experience relief with engagement (lightening) until the onset of labor.
Note reports of back strain and altered gait. Suggest use of low-heeled shoes, pelvic-rock exercise, maternity girdle, heat application, Therapeutic Touch, or transcutaneous electrical nerve stimulation (TENS), as appropriate.	Lordosis and muscle strain are caused by the influence of hormones (relaxin, progesterone) on pelvic articulations and a shift in the center of gravity as the uterus enlarges. Multiple interventions are usually more helpful to alleviate discomfort.
Note presence of leg cramps. Encourage client to extend leg and turn foot upward in dorsiflexion, to reduce milk intake, to change position frequently; and to avoid prolonged standing/sitting.	Reduces discomfort associated with altered calcium levels/calcium-phosphorus imbalance, or with pressure from enlarging uterus compressing nerves supplying the lower extremities.
Assess for presence/frequency of Braxton-Hicks contractions. Provide information regarding physiology of uterine activity.	These contractions may create discomfort for the multigravida in both second and third trimesters. The primigravida usually does not experience this discomfort until the last trimester, when progesterone's protective effect on uterine activity is decreasing and oxytocin levels are increasing.
Note paresthesia of toes and fingers. Suggest that client remove constrictive jewelry, maintain adequate intake of prenatal vitamins (take vitamin B_6 supplement with orange juice or banana), use correct posture, exercise limbs regularly throughout the day, and avoid extremes of temperatures.	Reduces effects of extreme lordotic posture (which strains brachial nerves and compresses nerve roots and femoral veins), edema, pressure of carpal tunnel nerves/ligaments, and vitamin B_6 deficiency. (Note: some sources report controversy over the use of vitamin B_6.)

ACTIONS/INTERVENTIONS

Independent

Note reports of urinary frequency and bladder pressure. (Refer to ND: Urinary Elimination, altered.)

Assess for constipation and hemorrhoids.

Discuss dangers of using cathartics during the ninth month, and suggest other means of resolving constipation, such as a high-fiber diet. Note cultural practices that might influence behaviors. (Refer to CP: First Trimester, NDs: Discomfort; Constipation, high risk for.)

Assess for pyrosis (heartburn). Review dietary limitations.

Note presence of leukorrhea and pruritus. Encourage client to bathe frequently, use cotton underwear, wear loose clothing, and to avoid long periods of sitting.

Assess for problems related to diaphoresis; suggest use of lightweight clothing, frequent bathing, and cool environment.

Collaborative

Give calcium supplements as appropriate. Recommend use of aluminum hydroxide gel as needed.

RATIONALE

Third-trimester uterine enlargement reduces bladder capacity, resulting in urinary frequency.

Increasing displacement of the bowel contributes to problems of elimination.

The use of cathartics may stimulate the onset of early labor. Some cultures, such as Hispanic, believe such use of cathartics ensures good delivery of a healthy boy.

Problem often occurs in second trimester and may continue, especially when diet is not modified.

As estrogen levels increase, secretions of the cervical glands create an acid medium that encourages proliferation of organisms.

Increased metabolism and body temperature, caused by progesterone activity and excess weight gain, may create a constant feeling of being overheated and may increase diaphoresis.

Substitutes for milk products when intolerance is a problem. Gel can reduce phosphorus levels, correcting calcium-phosphorus imbalance.

NURSING DIAGNOSIS:	KNOWLEDGE DEFICIT [LEARNING NEED], regarding preparation for labor/delivery; infant care
May be related to:	Lack of exposure/experience, misinterpretation of information.
Possibly evidenced by:	Request for information, statement of concerns or misconceptions.
DESIRED OUTCOMES— CLIENT/COUPLE WILL:	Discuss physical/psychologic changes associated with labor/delivery.
	Identify appropriate resources to obtain information about infant care.
	Verbalize preparedness for labor/delivery and infant.

ACTIONS/INTERVENTIONS

Independent

Continue/institute learning program as outlined in CP: First Trimester.

RATIONALE

Reinforces previous learning and/or provides new information. Of greatest concern for the couple in

ACTIONS/INTERVENTIONS

Independent

Provide information about normal physical/physiologic changes associated with third trimester. (Refer to ND: Self Esteem, situational low, high risk for.)

Provide oral/written information about signs of labor onset; distinguish between false and true labor. Discuss when to notify physician or healthcare provider and when to leave for hospital or alternative birth center (ABC). Discuss stages of labor/delivery.

Provide oral/written information about infant care, development, and feeding; offer appropriate references. Assess cultural beliefs.

Encourage enrollment in childbirth classes (if not already attending) and tour of hospital or ABC.

RATIONALE

this trimester is how to prepare physiologically and psychologically for the event of labor/delivery and issues surrounding infant care.

Understanding the normalcy of such changes can reduce anxiety and foster adoption of self-care activities.

Helps client to recognize onset of labor, to ensure timely arrival at hospital or ABC, and to cope with labor/delivery.

Helps prepare for new caretaking role, acquiring necessary items of furniture, clothing, and supplies; helps prepare for breastfeeding and/or bottle feeding. Lack of preparation may be culturally linked, indicating belief that preparation may be associated with increased risk of infant's death because they are "defying God's will."

Reduces anxiety associated with the unknown; enhances coping mechanisms for labor/delivery.

NURSING DIAGNOSIS:	**SELF ESTEEM, SITUATIONAL LOW, HIGH RISK FOR**
Risk factors may include:	Concern about ability to accomplish tasks of pregnancy/childrearing.
Possibly evidenced by:	[Not applicable; presence of signs/symptoms establishes an **actual** diagnosis.]
DESIRED OUTCOMES— CLIENT WILL:	Discuss reactions to altered body image, dreams.
	Seek positive role models in preparation for parenting.
	Verbalize feelings of confidence in self regarding new role.

ACTIONS/INTERVENTIONS

Independent

Note client's/couple's verbal and nonverbal cues in discussion of issues related to body change and role expectations. (Refer to CP: First Trimester, ND: Family Coping: potential for growth.)

Discuss nature/frequency of dreams.

RATIONALE

A crisis situation may result in this last trimester as the client feels anxious, ambivalent, and depressed about her body and the effects of pregnancy on her abilities/activities. She may also fear injury to herself and the fetus and may feel vulnerable to rejection, loss, or insult.

At this time, dreams and fantasies related to the birth experience, possible abnormalities of the newborn, and role changes intensify.

ACTIONS/INTERVENTIONS	RATIONALE
Independent	
Evaluate client's/couple's psychologic adaptation to pregnancy.	Normal third-trimester tasks focus on preparation for motherhood/fatherhood. If the client and/or her partner have weak egos and do not accomplish the tasks of pregnancy, difficulties coping with the stresses of labor and delivery as well as parenting are possible.
Determine cultural background, including values regarding family.	Society and culture influence the couple's response to pregnancy and to role changes necessitated by the birth of the baby.
Provide information to couple regarding normalcy of introspection, mood swings, and fears.	Turning inward (self-preoccupation) may confuse the man, but allows the client to adjust, adapt, and gain inner strength needed for childbirth, parenting, and role changes. Dreams/fears about labor are common.
Provide/review information about normal physical changes in the third trimester.	Education/communication about how normal body changes can positively affect attitudes and perceptions facilitates understanding and appreciation of the pregnancy by both members of the couple.
Encourage participation in childbirth classes, if not already enrolled.	Allows opportunity for development of peer support group to share emotional reactions to pregnancy and prepare for successful delivery.
Assess availability and nature of support systems, role models, and cultural beliefs.	Availability of sufficient supports can foster positive adjustment to pregnancy and parenting.

NURSING DIAGNOSIS:	**INJURY, HIGH RISK FOR, maternal**
Risk factors may include:	Presence of hypertension, infection, substance use/abuse, altered immune system, abnormal blood profile, tissue hypoxia, premature rupture of membranes (PROM).
Possibly evidenced by:	[Not applicable; presence of signs/symptoms establishes an **actual** diagnosis.]
DESIRED OUTCOMES— CLIENT WILL:	Verbalize understanding of potential individual risk factors. Be free of complications.

ACTIONS/INTERVENTIONS	RATIONALE
Independent	
Screen/evaluate preexisting/newly developed high-risk factors (e.g., heart, kidney, or lung conditions; genetic disorders). Monitor blood pressure, (BP), pulse, and heart sounds. Screen for signs of pregnancy-induced hypertension (PIH) such as edema, albuminuria and hypertension.	Potential high-risk situations often become problematic and necessitate intervention at this time, when circulatory and metabolic demands are greatest. Varying degrees of cardiovascular involvement (vasoconstriction, vasospasm) occur, with sodium/water retention negatively affecting kidney, uterine circulation, and CNS functioning.

ACTIONS/INTERVENTIONS	RATIONALE

Independent

Obtain vaginal culture. Assess for infections and sexually transmitted diseases (STDs) (e.g., *Monilia*, *Trichomonas*, gonorrhea, herpes simplex virus type II, *Chlamydia*, pruritus, and visible warts/lesions). If present, refer for appropriate treatment.

Untreated vaginal infections or STDs create intense discomfort for the client, and pose risk for the fetus, either through placental transmission or at the time of delivery.

Review need for cesarean birth and schedule the procedure, if within 4 days of delivery and vaginal culture is positive for herpes simplex virus. (Refer to CP: Prenatal Infection.)

Prevents infection of neonate during birth process.

Obtain hemoglobin (Hb) and hematocrit (Hct) at 28 weeks' gestation. Verify that client is following prescribed daily iron intake and prenatal vitamins. Screen for genetic problems (e.g., sickle cell, thalassemia) if not previously done. (Refer to CP: The High-Risk Pregnancy.)

Detects anemia with potential hypoxemia/anoxia problems for client and fetus.

Provide close, ongoing supervision of diabetic client. At 28 weeks' gestation, obtain results of glucose tolerance test. (Refer to CP: Diabetes Mellitus; Prepregnancy/Gestational.)

Diabetic women are most prone to third-trimester problems related to abruptio placentae, urinary tract infections (UTI), PIH, stillbirths, placental aging, and ketoacidosis.

Provide information about signs of labor onset; review history for PROM or preterm labor.

Positive history increases likelihood of similar problems in subsequent pregnancies.

Determine use of alcohol/other drugs.

Substance use/abuse places client at increased risk of premature labor and the fetus at risk for difficulties following delivery.

Collaborative

Assess for vaginal bleeding, presence of ecchymotic areas, and signs of disseminated intravascular coagulation; refer for appropriate treatment. (Refer to CP: Prenatal Hemorrhage.)

Presents an obstetrical emergency, with reduction in fluid volume and decreased oxygen-carrying capacity posing a threat to maternal organs, placental circulation, and fetal systems.

NURSING DIAGNOSIS:	URINARY ELIMINATION, ALTERED
May be related to:	Uterine enlargement, increasing abdominal pressure, fluctuation of renal blood flow and glomerular filtration rate (GFR).
Possibly evidenced by:	Urinary frequency, urgency; dependent edema.
DESIRED OUTCOMES— CLIENT WILL:	Verbalize understanding of condition.
	Identify ways to prevent urinary stasis and/or tissue edema.

ACTIONS/INTERVENTIONS	RATIONALE

Independent

Provide information about urinary changes associated with third trimester.

Helps client understand the physiologic reason for urinary frequency and nocturia. Third-trimester

ACTIONS/INTERVENTIONS	RATIONALE
Independent	
	uterine enlargement reduces bladder capacity, resulting in frequency. Positioning affects kidney functioning so that a supine, upright position decreases renal blood flow by 50%, and a left lateral recumbent position increases GFR and renal blood flow.
Encourage client to assume left lateral position while sleeping. Note reports of nocturia.	Increases kidney perfusion; mobilizes dependent edema. Edema is reduced by morning in cases of physiologic edema.
Advise client to avoid long periods in upright or supine position.	These positions potentiate vena caval syndrome and reduce venous return.
Provide information regarding need for fluid intake of 6 to 8 glasses/day, reduction of intake 2–3 hr before retiring, and moderate use of salt- or sodium-containing foods or products.	Maintains adequate fluid levels and kidney perfusion, which relies on dietary sodium to maintain an isotonic state.
Provide information regarding danger of taking diuretics and of eliminating sodium from diet.	Sodium losses/restrictions may overstress renin-angiotensin-aldosterone regulators of fluid levels, resulting in severe dehydration/hypovolemia.
Test midstream urine for presence of albumin. Note location and extent of tissue edema and urine output.	May indicate glomerular spasms or decreased kidney perfusion associated with PIH.
Collaborative	
Reassess contributory preexisting medical problems (e.g., kidney disease, hypertension, heart disease).	Problems affecting kidney function combined with increased fluid volume and stasis increase the client's risk for circulatory problems affecting the placenta/fetus.
Assess for signs and symptoms of UTI; obtain urine for colony count, and for culture and sensitivity if count is greater than 100,000/ml.	The prenatal client is susceptible to urinary stasis/UTI due to progesterone's vasodilating effect on ureters and to compression of the ureters by the enlarging uterus. Women with bacteriuria are also at high risk for preterm labor, PROM, and chorioamnionitis.

NURSING DIAGNOSIS:	**SEXUALITY PATTERNS, ALTERED**
May be related to:	Changes in sexual desire, discomfort (shortness of breath, fatigue, abdominal enlargement), misconceptions/fears.
Possibly evidenced by:	Reported difficulties, limitations or changes in sexual behavior, concerns about fetal safety.
DESIRED OUTCOMES—CLIENT/COUPLE WILL:	Discuss concerns related to sexual issues in the third trimester.
	Express mutual satisfaction with sexual relationship.

ACTIONS/INTERVENTIONS	RATIONALE

Independent

Continue/initiate sexual assessment, looking for changes in patterns from first and second trimesters.

Diminished interest in sexual activity/intercourse often occurs in the third trimester, owing to physical changes/discomforts.

Assess couple's perception of sexual relationship.

The couple's ability to identify/verbalize/accept changes in sexuality during the third trimester may influence the relationship and their ability to support each other emotionally.

Encourage couple to discuss, separately and with one another, feelings and concerns related to changes in sexual relationship. Provide information as to the normalcy of changes.

Communication between the couple is critical to constructive resolution of problems. The client may feel less sexually attractive as her body enlarges, and the man's responses to the client's changing shape may vary from increased desire to disinterest or repulsion. In addition, the client often notes changes in orgasmic experience with a single prolonged contraction rather than rhythmic contractions.

Provide information about alternative methods of achieving sexual satisfaction to meet needs for intimacy/closeness.

Sexual needs can be met through masturbation, fondling, stroking, and so forth, if mutually desired/acceptable. Client may find masturbation creates a more intense orgasm than does intercourse.

Recommend alternative positions for intercourse other than traditional male superior position (e.g., side lying or female superior position).

The client's enlarging abdomen requires change of positioning for comfort and safety.

Discuss importance of not blowing air into the vagina.

Maternal deaths due to air embolism have been reported.

Encourage client/couple to verbalize fears that may reduce desire for intercourse.

Misconceptions and fears that intercourse may result in fetal injury, infection, and initiation of labor may also influence sexual desires. Intercourse has not been found to cause fetal injury, PROM, onset of labor, or infections in most women.

Collaborative

Instruct client to discuss the safety of intercourse in the last 6 to 8 weeks with her healthcare provider.

Specific instructions may be needed if there is a history of complications or if complications are anticipated.

Refer for sexual counseling if concerns are not resolved.

May be needed to promote positive adaptation to sexual changes.

NURSING DIAGNOSIS:	**CARDIAC OUTPUT, high risk for decompensation**
Risk factors may include:	Increased fluid volume/altered venous return, changes in capillary permeability.
Possibly evidenced by:	[Not applicable; presence of signs/symptoms establishes an **actual** diagnosis.]

DESIRED OUTCOMES— CLIENT WILL:	Remain normotensive, free of pathologic edema.
	Display albuminuria not greater than 1+.
	Identify abnormal signs requiring further evaluation.

ACTIONS/INTERVENTIONS	RATIONALE
Independent	
Review normal physiologic changes. Identify signs/symptoms requiring medical evaluation or intervention.	Near term, fluid volume continues to increase by an additional 700 ml, necessitating an accompanying increase in cardiac output. Increased capillary permeability and hydrostatic pressure favors filtration from the vascular bed. Excess fluid retention and initiation of the renin-angiotensin II-aldosterone stress response may cause fluid to leave the cardiovascular system, resulting in dehydration that negatively affects cardiac output.
Monitor pulse/heart rate.	Resting heart rate increases normally at this time by as much as 15 bpm to facilitate circulation of the additional fluid volume.
Note signs of PIH; i.e., generalized edema, albuminuria 2+, and hypertension with systolic increases greater than 30 mm Hg or diastolic increases greater than 15 mm Hg.	Differentiates between physiologically normal edema and potential for developing problems. (Refer to CPs: Second Trimester, Pregnancy-Induced Hypertension; ND: Cardiac Output, high risk for decompensation.)
Determine client's knowledge about the effect positioning has on cardiac functioning.	Supine/recumbent positions and prolonged upright positions severely reduce venous return and cardiac output in the third trimester, negatively affecting flow to the uterus and kidneys. A lateral Sims'/semi-Fowler's position optimizes placental/kidney perfusion.
Recommend frequent position changes.	Promotes venous return, thereby reducing edema.

NURSING DIAGNOSIS:	**SLEEP PATTERN DISTURBANCE**
May be related to:	Changes in level of activity, psychologic stress, inability to maintain comfort.
Possibly evidenced by:	Interrupted sleep, awakening earlier/later than desired, difficulty in falling asleep, not feeling well rested, dark circles under eyes.
DESIRED OUTCOMES— CLIENT WILL:	Report improvement in sleep/rest.
	Report increased sense of well-being and feeling rested.

ACTIONS/INTERVENTIONS

Independent

Review normal sleep requirement changes associated with pregnancy. Determine current sleep pattern.

Evaluate level of fatigue; encourage client to rest 1–2 hr daily and obtain 8 hr sleep per night. Give information about normalcy of moderate fatigue. Reassess commitments to work and family. (Refer to CP: First Trimester, ND: Fatigue.)

Assess for occurrence of insomnia and for client's response to sleep loss. Suggest aids to sleep, such as relaxation techniques, reading, warm baths, and reduced activity just before retiring.

Note reports of positional breathing difficulties. Suggest sleeping in a semi-Fowler's position.

Collaborative

Obtain red blood cell (RBC) count and Hb level; rule out organic problems such as anemia.

Refer client for counseling if sleep deprivation/fatigue is interfering with activities of daily living.

RATIONALE

Helps identify need for establishing different sleep patterns (e.g., earlier bedtime and naps).

Increased fluid retention, weight gain, and fetal growth all contribute to feelings of fatigue, especially in the multipara with other children and/or demands.

Excess anxiety, excitement, physical discomforts, nocturia, and fetal activity all may contribute to sleeping difficulties.

In a recumbent position, the enlarging uterus as well as abdominal organs compress the diaphragm, thereby restricting lung expansion. Use of semi-Fowler's position allows the diaphragm to descend, fostering optimal lung expansion.

Anemia and reduced Hb/RBC levels, resulting in reduced oxygenation of tissues may contribute to feeling of excessive fatigue.

May be necessary for client to cope with alterations in sleep-wake cycle, identify appropriate priorities, and modify commitments.

NURSING DIAGNOSIS:	GAS EXCHANGE, IMPAIRED, HIGH RISK FOR, fetal
Risk factors may include:	Altered blood flow within decidua, altered oxygen supply/altered oxygen-carrying capacity of blood (anemia, cigarette smoking).
Possibly evidenced by:	[Not applicable; presence of signs/symptoms establishes an **actual** diagnosis.]
DESIRED OUTCOMES— CLIENT WILL:	Identify individual risk factors.
	Demonstrate techniques to control/alleviate risk factors.
	Display normal fetal heart rate (FHR), appropriate daily fetal movements and progressive fundal growth.

ACTIONS/INTERVENTIONS

Independent

Evaluate normal growth progression using fundal height measurement and fetal outline size. Investigate measurements greater than or less than expected levels.

RATIONALE

Approximate fundal height at 28 weeks' gestation is 28 cm, and it increases approximately 1 cm/week until lightening occurs from 38 weeks' gestation on. At term, the fetus obtains oxygen from the maternal portion of the placenta at a rate

ACTIONS/INTERVENTIONS

Independent

RATIONALE

of 20 to 30 L/min. Because the fetus has such critical needs at that time, any maternal condition that affects cardiac functioning within the decidua basalis, such as placental aging, diabetes, hypertension, or a kidney disorder, as well as high altitude, reduces fetal oxygen levels and nutrient transfers.

Help client/couple assess fetal movement. Demonstrate method and review rationale for daily count. Instruct client/couple to notify healthcare provider if less than 10 fetal movements are felt for 2 consecutive days.

Placental insufficiency can be detected by a reduction in fetal movement, usually before any perceivable alteration in FHR occurs. The fetus with adequate placental perfusion demonstrates peak movement between 29 and 38 weeks' gestation.

Continue ongoing assessment, and encourage cessation of tobacco use.

Tobacco may negatively affect placental circulation. Low Apgar scores (below 7 at 5 minutes) are associated with cigarette smoking.

Assess client's prenatal exercise program. Encourage client to engage in moderate, non-weight- bearing exercise (e.g., swimming, bicycling).

Blood flow to the uterus can decrease by 70% with strenuous exercise, producing transient fetal bradycardia, possible fetal hyperthermia, and intrauterine growth retardation.

Evaluate for other risk factors (e.g., maternal anemia).

May indicate potential incompatibility problems and decreased placental perfusion.

Collaborative

Prepare for and assist with ultrasonography, if indicated.

Comparative biparietal diameter measurements, estimated fetal weight, and femur length obtained by ultrasonography can accurately assess growth.

Test serum for Rh incompatibility in Rh-negative client. Repeat test every 4 wk until term, or until high titer (greater than 1:8 or 1:16) indicates a need for further intervention, such as amniocentesis or intrauterine transfusion.

Determines level of anti-D antibodies in serum of Rh-negative client with an Rh-positive partner, permitting early intervention.

Administer Rh-immune globulin at 28 weeks' gestation. (Refer to CP: The High-Risk Pregnancy.)

In the unsensitized client, may decrease possibility of transplacental bleeding.

NURSING DIAGNOSIS:	INJURY, HIGH RISK FOR, fetal
Risk factors may include:	Maternal health problems, exposure to teratogens/infectious agents.
Possibly evidenced by:	[Not applicable; presence of signs/symptoms establishes an **actual** diagnosis.]
DESIRED OUTCOMES— CLIENT WILL:	Identify individual risk factors.
	Alter lifestyle/behaviors to reduce risks.

ACTIONS/INTERVENTIONS	RATIONALE

Independent

Continue ongoing assessment of maternal nutrition. (Refer to CP: First Trimester, ND: Nutrition, altered, less than body requirements, high risk for.)

Alterations in maternal nutrition can reduce fetal iron stores, limit fat reserves, delay neurologic development in the neonate/child, and reduce protein available for brain growth, thereby reducing head circumference in offspring.

Discourage use of tobacco.

May limit maternal weight gain, reduce intrauterine/placental growth, and result in low Apgar scores at birth.

Provide information about risks of drug therapy (e.g., sulfonamide, tetracycline, streptomycin) in the event of maternal infection.

In the third trimester, sulfonamides increase the risk of hyperbilirubinemia by interfering with albumin-bilirubin bond. Tetracycline causes staining of deciduous teeth and inhibits bone growth in premature infants. Streptomycin may cause damage to auditory nerve, resulting in possible hearing losses.

Collaborative

Monitor fetal biophysical profile.

Determine uteroplacental/fetal well-being. (Refer to CP: The High-Risk Pregnancy, ND: Injury, high risk for, fetal.)

Note condition of membranes; hospitalize client if ruptured.

Rupture of membranes places fetus and client at risk for sepsis.

NURSING DIAGNOSIS:	COPING, INDIVIDUAL/FAMILY, INEFFECTIVE, HIGH RISK FOR
Risk factors may include:	Situational/maturational crises, personal vulnerability, unrealistic perceptions, inadequate coping methods, absent/insufficient support systems.
Possibly evidenced by:	[Not applicable; presence of signs/symptoms establishes an **actual** diagnosis.]
DESIRED OUTCOMES— CLIENT/COUPLE WILL:	Discuss emotional reaction to third trimester.
	Prepare for birth of baby, in accordance with cultural beliefs, through education/acquisition of supplies.
	Identify with appropriate role models.
	Ascribe personality characteristics to fetus.

ACTIONS/INTERVENTIONS	RATIONALE

Independent

Assess preparation for labor, delivery, and arrival of newborn.

Enrollment in childbirth classes and acquisition of nursery equipment and supplies may indicate psychologic preparedness. Lack of preparation may be based on cultural belief, or may indicate financial or psychologic problems.

ACTIONS/INTERVENTIONS	RATIONALE
Independent	
Determine client's/couple's perception of fetus as a separate entity.	Such perceptions indicate completion of psychologic tasks of pregnancy.
Determine how the man is handling the pregnancy as labor and delivery approaches.	The man with strong dependency needs himself may have difficulty meeting the client's increasing need for dependence, which may create conflict. In addition, negative coping may be manifested in lack of preparation for labor and/or for the newborn. The man may resort to work, hobbies, or an extramarital affair if he is not accomplishing the tasks of pregnancy.
Note any previous pregnancy loss, genetic factors, or history of stillbirth, and discuss meaning of the incident to the client/couple. (Refer to CPs: Genetic Counseling; Perinatal Loss.)	The high-risk couple may choose not to undergo appropriate preparation as a means of protecting themselves from possible loss/injury in the event that the fetus does not survive.
Evaluate support systems available to client/couple.	Availability of family and friends can help client/couple to manage tasks of upcoming labor and delivery.

The High-Risk Pregnancy _____

This plan of care provides a general framework for assessing and caring for the client and fetus in a high-risk situation during the prenatal period. Specific high-risk problems that occur in 6% or more of the prenatal population are discussed in the individual plans of care that follow. Less common problems can occur, placing both the client and the fetus in a potentially compromised situation. This plan of care focuses on these less common problems, as well as on general psychosocial considerations for all high-risk clients.

CLIENT ASSESSMENT DATA BASE

ACTIVITY/REST

May be pale, listless, fatigued.

CIRCULATION

Blood pressure (BP), pulse may be elevated.

EGO INTEGRITY

May express concern about own self-esteem regarding problems of pregnancy.

Pregnancy may not be planned/desired.

ELIMINATION

May practice colonic therapy (diminishes normal colon bacteria).

FOOD/FLUID

May be malnourished/obese or underweight (weight less than 100 lb/greater than 200 lb).

History of anemia (differentiate iron deficiency, sickle cell trait/disease, hemorrhage).

Edema may be confined to lower extremities, include both upper/lower extremities, or be generalized.

NEUROSENSORY

May have difficulty with muscle function (i.e., multiple sclerosis, myasthenia gravis, paralysis/spinal cord trauma).

RESPIRATION

Breath sounds: crackles, ronchi, expiratory wheeze.

SAFETY

History of previous obstetrical complications, such as premature rupture of membranes (PROM), placenta previa, abruptio placentae, miscarriage, 2 or more episodes of preterm labor/deliveries, Rh incompatibility, previous birth defects, hydatidiform mole, hyperemesis gravidarum, one or more pregnancy losses due to premature dilation of the cervix, pregnancy-induced hypertension (PIH), or postpartal hemorrhage, infection, or phlebitis.

History of sexually-transmitted diseases (STDs), a virus of the TORCH group, or _Listeria_; repeated urinary tract/vaginal infections; bowel problems; diarrhea; or recent flu.

May have history of intrapartal complications (e.g., hemorrhage, dystocia, PIH, meconium staining, fetal distress).

May be jaundiced, screening positive for active hepatitis.

Vaginal discharge may have foul odor.

SEXUALITY

Fundal height may be inappropriate for gestation.

Perineum may have visible lesions.

May be adolescent (age 17 years or younger); nullipara, age 35 years or older; multipara age 40 years or older; pregnant less than 3 months after last delivery, or have interval of 8 or more years between pregnancies.

May have history of large for gestational age infant (macrosomia).

May have had a previous cesarean birth, now opting for attempted vaginal birth after cesarean (AVBAC) or planning a repeat cesarean birth if the primary intervention was based on cephalopelvic disproportion.

Pelvic diameter may be smaller than normal.

Vaginal bleeding or spotting may be present.

History of menstrual problems,such as cramping, or irritable uterus.

SOCIAL INTERACTION

May have history of abusive relationship.

Lack of support systems.

TEACHING/LEARNING

History of preexisting medical complications (e.g., diabetes, kidney disease, acquired/congenital cardiac problems, asthma, tuberculosis).

History of substance dependency/abuse.

(Refer to Prenatal Assessment Data Base; First Trimester; specific plans of care related to The Pregnant Adolescent; Diabetes; Pregnancy-Induced Hypertension; Cardiac Conditions; Prenatal Hemorrhage; Prenatal Infection; Preterm Labor/Prevention of Delivery.)

DIAGNOSTIC STUDIES

Ultrasonography (using real time): Assesses gestational age of fetus and presence of multiple gestations; detects fetal abnormalities; locates placenta and amniotic fluid pockets prior to amniocentesis.

Amniocentesis for lecithin to sphingomyelin (L/S) ratio: Detects presence of phosphatidylglycerol (pg); measures optical density of fluid for detection of hemolysis in Rh incompatibility or infection in fluid.

Glucose tolerance test: Screens for gestational diabetes mellitus (GDM).

Platelet count: Drop may be associated with PIH and HELLP syndrome (hemolysis, elevated liver enzymes, and/or low platelet count).

Blood type, Rh group, and screen for antibodies in Rh-negative/Du-negative client: Identifies incompatibility risks.

Coagulation studies (activated partial thromboplastin time (APPT), partial thromboplastin time (PTT), prothrombin time (PT)), fibrin split degradation products (FSP/FDP): Identify clotting disorders in presence of hemorrhage.

Bilirubin, liver function studies (AST, ALT, and LDH levels): Assess hypertensive liver involvement.

Urinalysis, culture/sensitivity: Detects bacteriuria. *Dipstick:* Determines glucose/protein levels.

Vaginal, cervical, or rectal smear: Identifies STDs (e.g., genital herpes, gonorrhea, *Chlamydia*, or *Listeria*).

Serologic studies, VDRL: Screen for hepatitis, human immunodeficiency virus, AIDS, syphilis.

Biophysical profile (BPP) criteria: Assesses fetal well-being.

NURSING PRIORITIES

1. Identify high-risk situations.
2. Minimize risk factors for client and/or fetus.
3. Create ongoing program of education and support.
4. Prevent/minimize deterioration of maternal/fetal status.
5. Counsel client regarding present and/or future pregnancies.

NURSING DIAGNOSIS:	GAS EXCHANGE, IMPAIRED, HIGH RISK FOR, maternal
Risk factors may include:	Altered blood flow, alveolar-capillary changes, reduced oxygen-carrying capacity of blood.
Possibly evidenced by:	[Not applicable, presence of signs/symptoms establishes an **actual** diagnosis.]
DESIRED OUTCOMES— CLIENT WILL:	Verbalize understanding of individual risk factors.
	Identify and use interventions to reduce risks.
	Display BP, pulse, respiratory rate, and hemoglobin (Hb) and hematocrit (Hct) within normal limits.

Refer to discussion of circulatory considerations in CPs: Pregnancy-Induced Hypertension; Cardiac Conditions.

ACTIONS/INTERVENTIONS	RATIONALE

Independent

Assess for respiratory disorders that may interfere with lung function, such as asthma or tuberculosis. Note maternal respiratory rate or effort and adventitious lung sounds.

Any condition, either preexisting or developing during the pregnancy, that reduces or interferes with oxygen-carrying capacity impairs normal gas exchange. Such conditions may be due to problems related to respiration, circulation, or cellular components.

Note conditions potentiating vascular changes/reduced placental circulation (e.g., diabetes, PIH, cardiac problems) or those that alter oxygen-carrying capacity (e.g., anemias, hemorrhage). (Refer to specific plans of care as needed).

Extent of maternal vascular involvement and reduction of oxygen-carrying capacity have a direct influence on uteroplacental circulation and gas exchange. Intrauterine growth retardation (IUGR) and birth of a low-birth-weight (LBW) or small for gestational age infant are associated with maternal vascular changes.

Monitor BP and pulse.

Elevated BP may indicate PIH; reduced BP and increased pulse may accompany hemorrhage.

Promote bed/chair rest. Position in upright or semi-Fowler's position when respiratory effort is compromised; otherwise, encourage client to assume left lateral position.

Reduces respiratory effort and increases oxygen consumption as diaphragm falls, increasing vertical chest diameter. Left lateral position increases renal/placental perfusion; either position is effective in preventing supine hypotensive syndrome.

Monitor maternal kidney function, noting overall intake/output, and measure specific gravity as indicated.

Kidney function may deteriorate during pregnancy, negatively affecting cardiovascular function, elevating BP, and reducing placental circulation.

ACTIONS/INTERVENTIONS	RATIONALE

Independent

Encourage increased fluid intake as appropriate/tolerated.

Prevents dehydration, enhances organ perfusion/function, and liquefies respiratory secretions to facilitate expectoration.

Review dietary sources of vitamin C, iron, and protein. Discuss individual need for sufficient calories. Identify substances that foster iron absorption (acid medium, vitamin C) and those that reduce absorption (alkaline medium, milk).

Inadequate nutrition results in iron deficiency anemia and may lead to problems of oxygen transport.

Reduce stressors precipitating allergic/asthmatic response in susceptible client.

Decreases incidence of attacks. Impact of asthma on pregnancy is questionable, although it may be associated with increased incidence of abortion and preterm labor.

Encourage maternal avoidance of potential stressors that may precipitate sickle cell crisis (e.g., hypoxia, dehydration, acidosis, exposure to cold).

Maternal acidosis/hypoxia, especially in third trimester, can result in fetal CNS disorders. Repeat crises predispose the client/fetus to increased mortality/morbidity.

Collaborative

Monitor maternal laboratory studies as indicated:
Hb/Hct using electrophoresis.

Any reduction in Hb levels or circulating blood volume reduces oxygen available for maternal tissues. Treatment depends on the cause of the anemia as diagnosed by electrophoresis.

Blood urea nitrogen (BUN), creatinine clearance, 24-hour protein, and uric acid levels.

Evaluates adequacy of renal function.

Arterial blood gases (ABGs).

Determines oxygenation and therapy needs.

Administer medications, as indicated:
Theophylline.

Assists in bronchial dilation but may be associated with side effects of tachycardia in client/fetus.

Iron dextran (Imferon).

Parenteral administration may be necessary in presence of severe iron deficiency anemia to increase maternal oxygen-carrying capacity.

Isoniazid/ethambutol/rifampin.

Active tuberculosis requires treatment. Isoniazid crosses the placenta but does not appear to have teratogenic effects. Rifampin also crosses the placenta, but studies of fetal effects are still in progress. Streptomycin is avoided owing to association with vestibular/auditory defects. (Note: Isoniazid therapy requires supplementation of pyridoxine [vitamin B_6].)

Provide supplemental oxygen.

May be indicated in presence of severe anemias or during sickle cell crisis.

Assist with prophylactic exchange transfusion or crisis/anemia transfusion as indicated.

Helps maintain maternal hemoglobin S (HbS, abnormal sickle cell) level at less than 50%–60% of total Hb, or Hct at 30%, to improve oxygen-carrying capacity.

ACTIONS/INTERVENTIONS	RATIONALE
Independent	
Note maternal conditions that impact fetal circulation, such as PIH, diabetes, cardiac or kidney disease, anemia, Rh incompatibility, or hemorrhage (Refer to appropriate plans of care.)	Any factor that interferes with or reduces maternal circulation/oxygenation has a similar impact on placental/fetal oxygen levels. The fetus who is unable to obtain sufficient oxygen for metabolic needs from maternal circulation resorts to anaerobic metabolism, which produces lactic acid leading to an acidotic state.
Assess for excessive nausea/vomiting.	Exposes developing fetus to acidotic state and malnutrition and may contribute to IUGR and poor brain growth. Development of hyperemesis gravidarum may require hospitalization.
Determine abuse of substances such as tobacco, alcohol, and other drugs. Provide information about negative effects on fetal growth.	Depending on its extent, use/abuse may result in varying degrees of involvement, ranging from an identifiable syndrome such as fetal alcohol syndrome to less specific developmental disorders/delays.
Note estimated date of delivery (EDD).	Placental function is characterized by intense metabolic activity and oxygen consumption, which increases until term and then begins to fall. A post-term placenta becomes calcified and degenerates, thereby reducing surface available for oxygen and nutrient transfer, increasing perinatal mortality.
Assist in screening for and identifying genetic/chromosomal disorders. (Refer to CP: Genetic Counseling.)	Disorders such as phenylketonuria (PKU) or sickle cell anemia necessitate special treatment to prevent negative effects on fetal growth.
Discuss potential negative effects of genetic/chromosomal disorders (e.g., PKU) on fetus, and review options available to client. (Refer to ND: Nutrition, altered, less/more than body requirements and CP: Genetic Counseling.)	Intrauterine/postnatal growth retardation, malformation, or mental retardation may occur in PKU if pregnant woman does not resume diet low in phenylalanine for the duration of the pregnancy.
Assess fetal heart rate (FHR), noting rate and regularity. Have client monitor fetal movement daily as indicated. Note presence of maternal conditions that may also impact FHR (e.g., maternal hyperthyroidism or Graves' disease).	Tachycardia in a term infant may indicate a compensatory mechanism to reduced oxygen levels and/or sepsis. A reduction in fetal activity occurs prior to bradycardia. Although fetal thyrotoxicosis is rare, IUGR or tachycardia may result if maternal

ACTIONS/INTERVENTIONS	RATIONALE
Independent	condition is untreated. (Note: Fetal hypothyroidism may result from low-dose antithyroid drug therapy; higher doses may produce a goiter or mental retardation.)
Assess or screen for preterm uterine contractions, which may or may not be accompanied by cervical dilatation. (Refer to CP: Preterm Labor/Prevention of Delivery.)	Occurs in 6%–7% of all pregnancies and may result in delivery of a preterm infant if tocolytic management is not successful in reducing uterine contractility and irritability.
Monitor FHR during sickle cell crisis.	Maternal acidosis/hypoxia, especially in third trimester, can result in fetal CNS disorders. Repeat crises predispose the client and fetus to increased mortality and morbidity rates.
Collaborative	
Monitor maternal laboratory studies: Serology tests.	Assess for presence of TORCH group of viruses and active/carrier state of hepatitis. (Refer to CP: Prenatal Infection.)
Blood type/group.	Identifies fetus at risk for isoimmunization.
Serum human placental lactogen (HPL), and serum/urinary estriol levels (Note: Recent studies suggest use of BPP/nonstress test (NST) rather than estriol/HPL levels.)	Alterations in placental secretion of HPL/estriol may indicate fetal/placental problems. Low levels occur in toxemia, IUGR, and postmaturity; elevated levels accompany Rh sensitization, diabetes, maternal sickle cell anemia, and liver diseases.
Serum alpha-fetoprotein (AFP) levels at 14 to 16 weeks' gestation and amniocentesis if levels are abnormal.	With a neural tube defect (NTD), most commonly spina bifida and anencephaly, AFP (a protein produced by the yolk sac and fetal liver) is present in maternal serum at a level 8 times higher than normal at 15 weeks' gestation. The AFP level then decreases until term.
Administer Rh-immune globulin (Rh IgG) to client at 28 weeks' gestation, then again 72 hours post partum if indicated.	In Rh-negative clients with Rh-positive partners, Rh IgG helps reduce incidence of maternal isoimmunization in nonsensitized mothers and helps prevent erythroblastosis fetalis and fetal red blood cell (RBC) hemolysis.
Prepare client for/review serial testing: Ultrasonography. (Refer to ND: Gas Exchange, impaired, maternal and CPs: Diabetes Mellitus: Prepregnancy/Gestational; Pregnancy-Induced Hypertension; Cardiac Conditions.)	Monitors clients at risk for reduced/inadequate placental perfusion, such as adolescents, clients older than age 35 years, or those clients with diabetes, PIH, cardiac/kidney disease, anemia, or respiratory disorders. Inadequate placental perfusion with reduced transfer of oxygen/nutrients may result in fetal IUGR.
BPP and contraction stress test (CST) (if result of NST nonreactive or unequivocable).	Assess uteroplacental/fetal well-being. Chronic intrauterine hypoxia due to vascular changes or postmaturity results in reduced fetal activity, tachycardia, reduced beat-to-beat variability, possibly nonreactive stress test, positive CST, falling estriol levels, and decreased fetal muscle tone

95

ACTIONS/INTERVENTIONS	RATIONALE
Collaborative	
	and breathing movements. (Note: A reactive NST indicates integrity of placental circulation and fetal CNS. A positive CST with late decelerations indicates a high-risk client/fetus with possible reduced uteroplacental reserves; a negative CST indicates adequate fetal oxygen reserve/placental functioning.)
Provide supplemental oxygen as appropriate.	Increases the oxygen available for fetal uptake, especially in presence of severe anemias or sickle cell crisis, or when maternal/fetal circulation is compromised.
Provide information and assist with procedures as indicated: Amniocentesis;	Amniocentesis may be performed for genetic purposes or to assess fetal lung maturity. Spectrophotometric fluid analysis may be done to detect bilirubin after 26 weeks' gestation.
Administer Rh IgG after amniocentesis based on results from Betke-Kleihauer test;	If serum titer is greater than 1:16, sensitization occurs when maternal/fetal cells mix, creating an antigen–antibody response with hemolysis of fetal RBCs and release of bilirubin. Betke-Kleihauer test detects presence of fetal blood in maternal system. Rh IgG may prevent procedural isoimmunization.
Observe external fetal monitor for 20–30 min after amniocentesis. Position client on left side;	Helps detect negative fetal/uterine response to procedure. Left lateral position increases uteroplacental perfusion.
Assist with intrauterine fetal exchange transfusion. Repeat transfusion every 2 wk as indicated by titers (Betke-Kleihauer test) followed by administration of Rh IgG;	If excess fetal RBC hemolysis occurs, transfusion into fetal peritoneal cavity with Rh_O-negative blood replaces hemolyzed RBCs when fetus is determined at risk of dying before 32 weeks' gestation.
Fetoscopy.	Although it is not widely used, fetoscopy permits fetal blood/skin sampling and direct visualization of the fetus with identification of genetic or developmental problems such as sickle cell anemia, hemophilia, thalassemia major; immunologic problems, Rh isoimmunization; and NTD.
Assess fetal maturity when early delivery is anticipated, using results from amniotic fluid analysis for surfactant pg, creatinine, bilirubin, and cytologic analysis.	Fetal lung maturity is indicated by an L/S ratio of 2:1 or greater, except in an infant of a diabetic mother. Presence of pg and creatinine levels of 2.0 mg/100 ml reflects kidney maturity. Cornified cells are present at 36 weeks' gestation. Bilirubin levels of 0 in mothers having no Rh isoimmunization indicate fetal maturity.
Prepare for and assist with termination of pregnancy by induction or cesarean delivery as indicated.	Pregnancy may be terminated if desired for such conditions as toxoplasmosis occurring prior to 20 weeks' gestation, rubella during the first trimester, or elevated AFP levels indicating NTD. Labor may be induced in event of post-term placental calcification of deterioration of maternal condition.

NURSING DIAGNOSIS:	FLUID VOLUME DEFICIT, HIGH RISK FOR
Risk factors may include:	Inability to ingest and retain fluids.
Possibly evidenced by:	[Not applicable, presence of signs/symptoms establishes an **actual** diagnosis.]
DESIRED OUTCOMES— CLIENT WILL:	Maintain adequate circulating volume as evidenced by vital signs WNL and urine output greater than 30 ml/hr.

ACTIONS/INTERVENTIONS	RATIONALE
Independent	
Determine presence/frequency of excessive or persistent nausea and vomiting/retching.	Pernicious vomiting (hyperemesis gravidarum) results in dehydration, hypovolemia, and metabolic changes, exposing the developing fetus to acidotic state and malnutrition, which may contribute to IUGR and poor brain growth or possibly death.
Note client reports of nervousness or heat intolerance, and presence of fine tremors, temperature elevation, excessive diaphoresis, or tachycardia.	Signs suggestive of hyperthyroid state may cause excessive vomiting.
Monitor BP and pulse.	Dehydration/hypovolemia may cause hypotension or tachycardia.
Encourage bedrest.	Conserves energy; allows for closer monitoring of physical status.
Record intake/output; measure urine specific gravity.	Provides information regarding hydration and effectiveness of fluid replacement.
Provide frequent oral care.	Dehydration and acid emesis may cause drying and irritation of mucous membranes.
Note signs of mucosal bleeding or hemorrhage. Recommend use of soft toothbrush and/or alcohol-free mouthwash and ingestion of soft foods.	Severe vitamin deficiencies and hypothrombinemia may alter coagulating ability. Preventing trauma to mucous membranes reduces likelihood of bleeding.
Review need for and/or use of antithyroid drugs, such as propylthiouracil (PTU) or methimazole.	Interferes with synthesis of thyroid hormone and helps overcome intractable vomiting (hyperemesis) caused by hyperthyroid state. However, fetal consequences may include hypothyroidism, goiter, or mental retardation.
Collaborative	
Monitor laboratory studies as indicated:	
Electrolytes.	Electrolyte/acid-base imbalances are common and may be life-threatening.
Hct.	Elevated in dehydration. May be useful in assessing fluid needs.
BUN.	Hypovolemia reduces renal perfusion and function, elevating BUN.
Thyroid studies and serum thyroxine levels.	Elevated in client with hyperthyroidism/Graves' disease.

ACTIONS/INTERVENTIONS

Collaborative

Administer prochlorperazine (Compazine) or hydroxyzine (Vistaril) as indicated, or monitor low-dose promethazine (Phenergan) infusion.

Administer parenteral fluids, electrolytes, glucose, or vitamins, as indicated.

Provide diet as tolerated (may be NPO for 24–48 hr) starting with small/dry feedings followed by clear liquids and progressing to low-fat, soft then regular foods.

Refer to psychologic counseling if no improvement occurs.

Prepare for therapeutic abortion if warranted by patient's condition.

RATIONALE

Provides sedative action and prevents vomiting. (Note: May have teratogenic effects.)

Helps reverse or prevent possible hypokalemia, severe protein/vitamin deficiencies, or acidosis, which may negatively affect maternal/fetal well-being.

Allows the gastrointestinal tract an initial period of rest. Gradually increasing oral feedings may improve food tolerance.

There may be a psychologic component to problem of vomiting.

Early recognition and treatment should prevent such a severe situation from developing, but it may be indicated when mother's life is threatened, as evidenced by jaundice, prolonged fever greater than 101°F, tachycardia, retinal hemorrhage, and delirium.

NURSING DIAGNOSIS:	NUTRITION, ALTERED, LESS/MORE THAN BODY REQUIREMENTS, HIGH RISK FOR
Risk factors may include:	Extremes of weight (less than 100 lb/greater than 200 lb), inability to ingest/digest food, excessive/inappropriate intake, limited financial resources.
Possibly evidenced by:	[Not applicable, presence of signs/symptoms establishes an **actual** diagnosis.]
DESIRED OUTCOMES— CLIENT WILL:	Gain 24–28 lb during the pregnancy.
	Follow a well-balanced diet.
	Be free of ketones in urine.

ACTIONS/INTERVENTIONS

Independent

Ascertain current/past dietary patterns and practices.

Weigh client. Compare current weight with pre-pregnancy weight.

RATIONALE

Ascertaining the nutritional state prior to conception is critical to ensuring proper organ development, especially brain tissue, in the early weeks of pregnancy.

Underweight clients are at risk for anemia, inadequate protein/calorie intake, vitamin/mineral deficiencies, and PIH. Overweight women are at risk for possible changes in the cardiovascular system that create risks for development of PIH, for GDM,

ACTIONS/INTERVENTIONS	RATIONALE
Independent	
	and for excess glucose intake with hyperinsulinemia of the fetus, resulting in macrosomia. Sudden weight gain of 2.5 lb or more in a week may indicate PIH; a weight loss of 3 lb or more near term suggests postmaturity.
Provide information about risks of weight reduction during pregnancy and about nourishment needs of client and fetus.	Prenatal calorie restriction and resultant weight loss may result in nutrient deficiency or ketonemia, with negative effects on fetal CNS and possible IUGR.
Test urine for presence of ketones.	Indicates inadequate glucose utilization and breakdown of fats for metabolic processes.
Develop plan with client that provides necessary nutrients, including adequate fluid intake. Recommend 2 quarts of fluid per day.	Prevents malnutrition and dehydration, which appear to compromise optimal uterine and placental functioning and increase uterine irritability, which could potentiate premature labor.
Discuss importance of staying on low-phenylalanine diet for the woman with PKU.	To prevent elevated phenylpyruvic acid levels and reduce the risk of mental retardation, microcephaly, congenital heart defects, and growth retardation, this client should have begun the diet before becoming pregnant and should continue the diet throughout the pregnancy.

(Refer to CPs: First Trimester, Diabetes Mellitus: Prepregnancy/Gestational; ND: Nutrition, altered, less than body requirements, high risk for.)

NURSING DIAGNOSIS:	**INJURY, HIGH RISK FOR, maternal**
Risk factors may include:	Preexisting medical conditions, complications of pregnancy.
Possibly evidenced by:	[Not applicable, presence of signs/symptoms establishes an **actual** diagnosis.]
DESIRED OUTCOMES— CLIENT WILL:	Identify signs/symptoms requiring medical evaluation/intervention.
	Verbalize understanding of individual risk factors.
	Be free of maternal injury.

ACTIONS/INTERVENTIONS	RATIONALE
Independent	
Review obstetrical/medical history.	Helps identify individual risk factors.
Discuss the option of AVBAC in client with incision into the lower uterine segment and potential risks associated with previous classical incision into uterus.	Potential for uterine rupture in subsequent pregnancies exists when incision is a classical (vertical) incision or gestational age is not accurately determined, resulting in overdistention and stimulating onset of labor.

ACTIONS/INTERVENTIONS	RATIONALE

Independent

Refer client/couple for AVBAC or cesarean classes, as appropriate.

Provides information/opportunity for asking questions to prepare client for AVBAC or cesarean delivery.

Discuss unpredictable effect of pregnancy on epileptic/seizure disorders. Review information regarding medical control with diazepam (Valium), chlordiazepoxide hydrochloride (Librium), and phenytoin (Dilantin).

Pregnancy may cause an increase in seizure activity, especially if complications occur. (Note: Dilantin has been associated with cleft lip or cleft palate in the newborn. Other anticonvulsants may impair clotting, requiring prophylactic use of vitamin K during the last month of pregnancy to prevent neonatal hemorrhage.)

Assess renal/cardiac involvement in client with systemic lupus erythematosus (SLE). Provide information about the need to continue with corticosteroid intake throughout pregnancy.

Increased rates of spontaneous abortion, cardiac problems, preterm labor, stillbirth, PIH, and even maternal death occur in the client with SLE-related kidney involvement.

Discuss safety concerns related to presence of spinal cord injury/paralysis.

For clients at risk for autonomic dysreflexia, episode may be relieved or prevented by appropriate emptying of the bladder. Other concerns, such as altered mobility/transfer and increased attention to skin care needs, generally can be managed with preventive planning.

Monitor for temperature elevation. Note diaphoresis, tachycardia, fine tremors, weight loss, and altered bowel function.

May indicate onset of hyperthyroidism/thyrotoxicosis, which in addition to deleterious fetal effects (increased mortality and LBW infants), may result in pernicious vomiting and cardiac stress.

Investigate reports of excessive nausea/vomiting in conjunction with elevated BP, pathologic edema, and proteinuria.

Hyperemesis gravidarum and PIH prior to 24 weeks' gestation may develop in association with hydatidiform mole.

Collaborative

Assist with ultrasonography; note absence of fetal heart outline or fetal heart tones. Monitor elevation of human chorionic gonadotropin (HCG) titers.

Diagnostic for hydatidiform mole, which is most likely to occur in older women or women treated with clomiphene citrate. Sequelae of choriocarcinoma may develop if HCG titers remain high after evacuation.

Assist in uterine evacuation by induced abortion, dilatation and curettage (D and C), or hysterectomy, as indicated.

Surgery ensures complete removal of all placental fragments. In the presence of excessive bleeding, or with older clients who have increased risk of malignant sequelae, hysterectomy may be the treatment of choice.

Stress need to follow up HCG titers for at least 1 year.

Pregnancy should be delayed for 1 full year after negative HCG titers are achieved. Chemotherapy is recommended if titers rise/remain high and D and C reveals malignant cells.

Review thyroid profile studies and serum thyroxine values.

Help to confirm hypothyroid or hyperthyroid state and identify treatment needs. (Note: Untreated hypothyroidism markedly increases the risk of fetal loss, congenital goiter, and true cretinism; untreated hyperthyroidism potentiates risk of abortion or fetal demise.)

ACTIONS/INTERVENTIONS

Collaborative

Administer propylthiouracil (PTU) or methimazole.

RATIONALE

Helps reduce effects of Graves' disease and thyrotoxicosis by interfering with synthesis of thyroid hormones. Radioisotope treatment is contraindicated in pregnancy.

NURSING DIAGNOSIS:	KNOWLEDGE DEFICIT [LEARNING NEED], regarding high-risk situation/preterm labor
May be related to:	Lack of exposure to and/or misinterpretation of information, unfamiliarity with individual risks/own role in risk prevention/management.
Possibly evidenced by:	Request for information, statement of concerns or misconceptions, inaccurate follow-through of instructions.
DESIRED OUTCOMES— CLIENT WILL:	Verbalize awareness of condition(s) placing her at risk.
	Identify signs/symptoms of preterm labor.
	List possible preventive measures.
	Participate in achieving the best possible pregnancy outcome.

ACTIONS/INTERVENTIONS

Independent

Provide information related to specific high-risk situation, including clear, simple explanations of pathophysiologic changes and maternal and fetal implications.

Provide appropriate information related to screening and testing methods and procedures.

Emphasize the *normalcy* of pregnancy.

Assist client to identify individually appropriate adaptations/self-care techniques: maintaining fluid volume (2 to 3 L/day), voiding every 2 hr during the day, scheduling rest periods 2 to 3 times a day using left lateral position, avoiding overexertion or heavy lifting, and maintaining contact with family/daily life when bedrest is required.

Identify danger signals requiring immediate notification of healthcare provider (e.g., PROM, preterm labor, vaginal bleeding).

RATIONALE

Increases understanding of the impact of pregnancy on the disease process. Client's/significant other(s)' level of knowledge of and involvement in preventive measures appears to have a direct impact on the outcome of an at-risk pregnancy.

Understanding of tests can reduce anxiety and may increase client cooperation.

Avoids/limits perception of "sick role" and provides support to client/couple to deal with their specific situation.

Preventive problem solving promotes participation in own care and enhances self-confidence, sense of control, and client/couple satisfaction.

Recognizing risk situations encourages prompt evaluation/intervention, which may prevent or limit untoward outcomes.

ACTIONS/INTERVENTIONS	RATIONALE

Independent

Define labor, and review possible symptoms of preterm labor: painless or painful uterine contractions or rhythmic pressure, occurring 10 or less min apart; contractions lasting 30 sec or longer for 1 hr (unrelieved by rest, drinking fluids, or emptying bladder); cramps resembling those of menstruation; abdominal cramping with or without diarrhea; and pressure or aching of the low back and/or vulva unrelieved by resting on left side (though may sometimes be relieved by sacral massage).

May help clarify misconceptions regarding "false labor," and aid client in distinguishing between preterm labor and Braxton-Hicks contractions. Symptoms of preterm labor may be overlooked by confusing them with normal "aches and pains" of pregnancy.

Describe potential implications of premature birth.

Increases understanding of need for prevention and motivation to follow therapeutic regimen.

Encourage client to assess uterine tone/contractions for 1 hr, once or twice a day.

Although uterine contractions occur occasionally, cervical dilation can occur with contractions occurring every 10 min or less for a period of 1 hr.

Stress importance of reporting increased or altered vaginal discharge.

May reflect cervical changes; indicates need to screen for vaginal infections, which may precipitate preterm labor or may indicate PROM.

Discuss implications of unknown progression of degenerative neurologic conditions for client/infant.

Conditions such as multiple sclerosis may occasionally complicate pregnancy or develop afterward; however, exacerbations or remissions seem unrelated to pregnancy. If severely affected, client may elect to interrupt pregnancy or undergo sterilization. (Note: Decreased sensation may alter client's ability to sense uterine contractions/presence of labor.)

Review significance of symptoms of respiratory difficulty, fatigue, and upper eyelid drooping in client with myasthenia gravis. Discuss implications for care of self and infant after birth.

Peak prevalence of this motor endplate disorder occurs at age 25 years, and pregnancy may increase severity of symptoms. Myasthenia gravis is not an indication for therapeutic abortion, but adjustments may be required to care for infant and self.

Discuss impact of rheumatoid arthritis on pregnancy/postpartal period, as well as need to avoid nonsteroidal anti-inflammatory drugs such as aspirin.

Severity of symptoms often subside during pregnancy, yet severe exacerbations may occur 1 month after delivery, making infant care difficult. Aspirin is contraindicated owing to its effect on maternal/fetal platelets, coagulation, and corresponding anemia related to blood loss. (Note: Extra rest is important to protect weight-bearing joints.)

NURSING DIAGNOSIS:	ANXIETY [SPECIFY LEVEL]
May be related to:	Situational crises, threat of maternal/fetal death (perceived/actual), interpersonal transmission/contagion.
Possibly evidenced by:	Increased tension, apprehension, feelings of inadequacy, somatic complaints, difficulty sleeping.

DESIRED OUTCOMES— CLIENT WILL:	Verbalize fears and concerns related to complication and/or pregnancy.
	Identify healthy ways to deal with anxiety.
	Demonstrate problem-solving skills.
	Use resources/support systems effectively.

ACTIONS/INTERVENTIONS	RATIONALE

Independent

Note level of anxiety and degree of interference with ability to function/make decisions.	Unresolved stress may interfere with accomplishment of the tasks of pregnancy, with normal acceptance of the pregnancy/fetus, and with decisions regarding future pregnancies versus sterilization.
Provide emotionally warm and supportive atmosphere; accept client/couple as they present themselves.	Facilitates development of trusting relationship. Nonjudgmental acceptance promotes sense of trust.
Assume an unhurried attitude whenever dealing with the client/family.	Fear of the unknown and fear of becoming a burden are incompatible with psychologic and emotional rest.
Provide 24-hour access to healthcare team.	Decreases sense of being alone. Anxiety can be reduced when information or help is readily available.
Review possible sources of anxiety (e.g., prior high-risk pregnancy or premature birth, alterations in family life or role performance, financial concerns related to pregnancy, possible delivery of preterm infant, or employment restrictions).	An uncomplicated pregnancy is associated with some anxiety for the client/couple; a medical complication further intensifies feelings of uncertainty concerning the outcome of the pregnancy. Acknowledgment of the realities of what is happening can provide support.
Assess stress level of client/couple associated with the medical complication, couple's relationship, the relationship of the client/couple to family members, and the availability of a support network.	Poor family relationships and unavailability of support systems may increase stress level. Client may become dependent on other family members, which may affect her self-esteem and increase her feelings of anxiety, as well as adding to the family's level of stress.
Encourage client/couple to express feelings of frustration related to therapy regimen and/or lifestyle changes. Explain to client that verbalization is acceptable and important. (Be alert to expressions of concern regarding children at home and "wanting to deliver and get it over with.")	Client/couple needs frequent opportunities to vent anger/frustration about changes in family life in order to minimize anxiety levels. Allowing such expression assures client that these feelings are normal and expressing them is helpful. Anxiety/frustration may interfere with making realistic decisions.
Observe for signs of emotional changes, imbalance, or conflict with family/significant other(s).	Provides opportunity for early intervention. Anxiety is "contagious" and may be transmitted between family, client, and staff members.
Assess physiologic response to anxiety (e.g., BP, pulse).	Anxiety/stress may be accompanied by the release of catecholamines, creating physical responses that affect the client's sense of well-being and thus increasing anxiety.

103

ACTIONS/INTERVENTIONS	RATIONALE

Independent

Provide individually appropriate information regarding interventions or treatments (inpatient or outpatient basis) and the potential impact of condition on client and fetus.

Helps to reduce anxiety associated with the unknown. May enhance cooperation with treatment regimen, promoting optimal pregnancy outcome.

Reinforce positive aspects of maternal/fetal condition, if present, such as fetal growth and activity.

Increases confidence and hope for client and significant other(s).

Collaborative

Coordinate team conference including client/couple. Create ongoing plan of care.

Promotes continuity of care and team approach to situation. If hospitalization is necessary, stress levels tend to increase further after 2 wks and remain elevated for the remainder of the hospitalization.

Refer to community support group, such as the American Diabetes Association, or to couples who have successfully completed a high-risk pregnancy.

Decreases sense of being alone and can help couple develop a positive outlook on pregnancy.

Refer to other resources/counseling, as indicated. (Refer to NDs: Family Processes, altered, high risk for; Family Coping: potential for growth).

May need help with child care and housekeeping. Counseling or therapy may be necessary to help client/couple verbalize more freely and examine unmanageable anxiety.

NURSING DIAGNOSIS:	ACTIVITY INTOLERANCE, HIGH RISK FOR
Risk factors may include:	Presence of circulatory/respiratory problems, uterine irritability.
Possibly evidenced by:	[Not applicable; presence of signs/symptoms establishes an **actual** diagnosis.]
DESIRED OUTCOMES— CLIENT WILL:	Report an awareness of activity tolerance.
	Plan necessary alterations in lifestyle/daily activities.
	Be free of excessive fatigue or uterine irritability/sustained contractions.

ACTIONS/INTERVENTIONS	RATIONALE

Independent

Encourage client to pace activities and allow for sufficient rest.

Conserves energy and avoids overexertion to minimize fatigue/uterine irritability.

Review home/employment situation, noting activity levels and individual responses.

Modifications may be required, depending on symptoms and previous history.

Encourage adequate rest and use of left lateral position.

Increases uterine blood flow and may decrease uterine irritability/activity.

Instruct client to avoid heavy lifting, strenuous activity/housework, sports, and motor trips longer than 1–2 hr. (Note: Client with cardiac condition may face more severe restrictions.)

Previously tolerated activity may not be indicated for women at risk. Aerobic exercise/abdominal muscle strain may decrease uterine blood flow and increase uterine irritability.

ACTIONS/INTERVENTIONS	RATIONALE

Independent

Instruct client to modify or eliminate any type of sexual activity in the presence of symptoms of preterm labor, cervical changes, or bleeding.

Sexual activity, including orgasms and breast stimulation, appears to increase uterine irritability, owing to release of oxytocin.

Recommend avoiding travel and altitude changes in the third trimester.

Motion of travel, prolonged sitting position, and decreased oxygen appear to increase uterine irritability.

Stress importance of quiet diversional activities.

Prevents boredom and enhances cooperation with activity restrictions.

Collaborative

Encourage modified/complete bedrest as indicated.

Activity level may need modification depending on symptoms of uterine activity, cervical changes, or bleeding.

NURSING DIAGNOSIS:	SELF ESTEEM, SITUATIONAL LOW, HIGH RISK FOR
Risk factors may include:	Perceived failure at a life event.
Possibly evidenced by:	[Not applicable; presence of signs/symptoms establishes an **actual** diagnosis.]
DESIRED OUTCOMES— CLIENT/COUPLE WILL:	Verbalize thoughts/feelings about situation.
	Express positive self-appraisal.
	Seek appropriate referral as needed.

ACTIONS/INTERVENTIONS	RATIONALE

Independent

Encourage verbalization of feelings. Assess perception of self in nonpregnant state and alteration in perception with pregnancy.

Helps detect problems and determine their severity. Because pregnancy is thought to be a normal physiologic process, a high-risk situation can lead to alterations in self-concept, a lowered self-esteem, and ego disintegration, especially if one or both members of the couple associate childrearing with success as a man or woman.

Facilitate positive adaptation to altered self-concept through "Active Listening," acceptance, and problem solving.

Helps in successful accomplishment of the psychologic tasks of pregnancy, although the high-risk couple may remain ambivalent as a self-protective mechanism against possible loss of the pregnancy or fetal death.

Encourage involvement in decisions about care when possible.

Enhances sense of control and increased self-esteem.

Promote attendance at classes/support groups as appropriate.

Provides information for client/couple and reinforces that they are not alone.

Collaborative

Refer for individual/group counseling, if indicated.

May be necessary for positive ego integration.

105

NURSING DIAGNOSIS:	FAMILY COPING: POTENTIAL FOR GROWTH
May be related to:	Needs sufficiently gratified and adaptive tasks effectively addressed to enable goals of self-actualization to surface.
Possibly evidenced by:	Attempts to describe growth impact of this crisis on own values, priorities, and goals; moving in direction of health-promoting and enriching lifestyle that supports and monitors maturational process; generally chooses experiences that optimize wellness.
DESIRED OUTCOMES— FAMILY WILL:	Verbalize fears/perceived disruptions in family life caused by high-risk pregnancy.
	Seek assistance/counseling, as needed.

ACTIONS/INTERVENTIONS	RATIONALE

Independent

Assess perceived impact of complication on client and family members. Encourage verbalization of concerns.	Family stress often occurs in an uncomplicated pregnancy, and it is amplified in a high-risk pregnancy, where concerns focus on the health of both the client and fetus. Family is strengthened if all members have a chance to express fears openly and work cooperatively.
Provide primary caregiver and thorough documentation.	Ensures continuity of care, enhances ongoing identification and prevention of additional problems, and ensures appropriate follow-up to assist during postpregnancy readjustment.
Help client/couple plan restructuring of roles/activities necessitated by complication of pregnancy.	Education, support, and assistance in maintenance of family integrity help foster growth of its individual members and reduce stress that the client may feel from her dependent role.
Include partner/siblings in prenatal office visits or hospital visits if client is hospitalized. Arrange place for family to stay overnight.	Helps family members to view the outcome of the pregnancy as a cooperative effort. Proper management of stress at this time may promote growth within the family and individual members.
Listen for expressions of helplessness and concern about how current situation is affecting the family and home. Problem-solve solutions.	Medical problems necessitating special therapy/restrictions at home or hospitalization significantly disrupt normal routines and cause stress and guilt feelings in the client, partner, and/or siblings. Creative solutions enhance self-esteem, may increase cooperation, and can promote family involvement.

Collaborative

Refer to community service agencies (e.g., Visiting Nurse Association, social service).	Community supports may be needed for ongoing assessment of medical problem, family status, coping behaviors, and financial stressors.
Refer for counseling if family does not sustain positive coping and growth. (Refer to ND: Family Processes, altered, high risk for.)	May be necessary to promote growth and to prevent family disintegration.

NURSING DIAGNOSIS:	FAMILY PROCESSES, ALTERED, HIGH RISK FOR
Risk factors may include:	Situational crisis.
Possibly evidenced by:	[Not applicable; presence of signs/symptoms establishes an **actual** diagnosis.]
DESIRED OUTCOMES— FAMILY WILL:	Express feelings freely and appropriately.
	Direct energies in a purposeful manner to plan for resolution of crisis.
	Seek appropriate help.

ACTIONS/INTERVENTIONS	RATIONALE

Independent

Determine degree of lifestyle change and extent of financial burden of pregnancy.	Provides information to identify needs and create plan of care.
Encourage verbalization and sharing of feelings.	Helps promote integrity of mutual support system.
Assess verbal/nonverbal cues and negative behaviors, such as inappropriate diet, eating improperly; excessive use of alcohol, tobacco, or tranquilizers; and avoidance of discussion of concerns.	The client who does not appropriately verbalize negative feelings or hostility about the complicated pregnancy may express such feelings with nonverbal cues or behaviors.
Assess partner for behaviors that negatively affect family process.	Expectant fathers may begin working longer hours, spending increased amounts of time away from home, abusing alcohol, which are signs of negative coping.
Assess siblings for negative, attention-getting behaviors toward parents or authority figures, such as difficulty in school, truancy, or failure to carry out responsibilities.	Such behaviors may signal anger, jealousy, or resentment of changes in lifestyle necessitated by the complicated pregnancy.
Involve in procedures and decisions regarding therapeutic regimen, when possible.	Provides client/family with some degree of control in what is often viewed as an uncontrollable situation.
Acknowledge strengths, such as client's effective monitoring for diabetes.	Provides positive reinforcement and helps client/couple to view efforts as worthwhile.
Provide anticipatory guidance.	Knowing what is ahead may decrease stress and allow time for adaptation.
Encourage family to verbalize significance of situation if hospitalization is required.	Separation necessitated by hospitalization of the client may place stress on family members, who may also experience relief or guilt because the healthcare system has relieved them of the burden of care.

Collaborative

Refer to social worker, hospital chaplain, other families in similar situation, and/or community agencies.	May assist in providing sources of financial/emotional assistance.

107

ACTIONS/INTERVENTIONS	RATIONALE

Collaborative

Refer for professional counseling, if necessary.

May be needed to maintain family integrity. Family members who are not positively adjusting to a complicated pregnancy may experience a high level of stress and/or negative coping. Such negative coping may result in family disintegration, separation, or divorce.

NURSING DIAGNOSIS:	COPING, INDIVIDUAL/FAMILY, INEFFECTIVE: COMPROMISED, HIGH RISK FOR
Risk factors may include:	Situational crisis, personal vulnerability, inadequate support systems.
Possibly evidenced by:	[Not applicable; presence of signs/symptoms establishes an **actual** diagnosis.]
DESIRED OUTCOMES— CLIENT/FAMILY WILL:	Identify ineffective coping behaviors and consequences.
	Verbalize awareness of own strengths/coping abilities.
	Demonstrate coping by discussing fears and dealing positively with the situation.
	Seek help appropriately.

ACTIONS/INTERVENTIONS	RATIONALE

Independent

Assess past and present coping strategies and emotional response to event/diagnosis.

In coping with a high-risk pregnancy, the client/couple/family often uses denial, then guilt, blame, or feelings of ambivalence, as emotional protection from possible loss of the pregnancy and fetus/newborn.

Evaluate client's/couple's support systems, including ability to comfort one another. Note negative coping, and discuss consequences.

Often, as a protective mechanism, the client and her partner do not form positive emotional attachment ("give of themselves") to the fetus. Lack of adequate support systems and failure to achieve the normal developmental tasks of pregnancy may result in continuation of high-risk situation into the childrearing phase and may create potential problems associated with physical or emotional child abuse and high-risk parenting.

Discuss normalcy of feelings; encourage couple to verbalize (separately and together) their feelings and concerns.

Helps assure client/couple that feelings are appropriate in high-risk situation; promotes open lines of communication. (Note: One member of the couple may be reluctant to discuss fears openly in front of partner; may require additional support to facilitate interaction with one another.)

Note client reports of increasing fatigue and inability to manage daily household activities.

Lack of family's assistance may indicate a need for help to resolve situation. Significant other(s) may be preoccupied with own emotional con-

ACTIONS/INTERVENTIONS

Independent

Encourage family to restructure daily activities to meet client's needs without negating their own needs.

Obtain/review history of increasing severity of symptoms, especially if hospitalization is necessary.

Collaborative

Identify available community support groups.

Refer family for homemaker/child care and financial assistance as necessary.

Refer for counseling as appropriate.

RATIONALE

flicts/personal suffering and express lack of understanding/knowledge about how to be helpful.

Family may need assistance in recognition of the importance of time planning to meet such needs as increased rest during pregnancy. However, family needs to work as a group to problem-solve solutions that meet individual needs and prevent negative feelings and "sabotage behaviors."

Problems may require a reduction in activity level and/or hospitalization, necessitating changes in family life.

Discussion of situation with others who share the same problem can be helpful and can enhance problem-solving.

Additional outside assistance with everyday activities, sibling care, and/or financial help may be required for client to cope positively with daily needs/therapy regimen.

May be needed in presence of negative coping to assure attachment to pregnancy/fetus/newborn. Helps to resolve concerns and/or develop effective coping skills; may prevent high-risk parenting.

NURSING DIAGNOSIS:	NONCOMPLIANCE [COMPLIANCE, ALTERED], HIGH RISK FOR
Risk factors may include:	Patient value system, health beliefs/cultural influences, issues of control, presence of anxiety.
Possibly evidenced by:	[Not applicable; presence of signs/symptoms establishes an **actual** diagnosis.]
DESIRED OUTCOMES— CLIENT WILL:	Participate in the prescribed regimen during pregnancy.
	Use appropriate self-care behaviors.

ACTIONS/INTERVENTIONS

Independent

Identify cause of/contributing factors to perceived lack of cooperation.

RATIONALE

The client/couple may find it difficult to follow a prescribed health regimen that significantly alters their lifestyle and requires a great deal of time and energy. In addition, loss of control and anxiety contribute to feelings of helplessness/hopelessness, which increase the possibility of rejection of a specific health regimen. Furthermore, misunderstandings can result in client not following prescribed regimen.

ACTIONS/INTERVENTIONS	RATIONALE
Independent	
Determine goals that client wants to achieve and the motivating factors.	Full cooperation and commitment are needed to obtain or maintain control of condition.
Assist client in reducing/modifying causative factors of medical complication. Avoid being judgmental. Encourage an objective problem-solving approach using a cooperative decision-making model.	Gives a sense of control. Pointing out failure only leads to despair.
Discuss and have client demonstrate behaviors/techniques in question.	During pregnancy, control of condition may require many specific modified or new behaviors. Demonstration allows accurate assessment of learning.
Collaborative	
Refer to community resources or to a peer who has had a positive outcome with a complicated pregnancy.	Decreases overwhelming feelings of aloneness; provides role model and opportunity for sharing common experiences. Reinforces idea that efforts can have a positive outcome.

Prenatal Substance Dependence/Abuse _____

This disorder is a continuum of phases incorporating a cluster of cognitive, behavioral, and physiologic symptoms that include loss of control over use of the substance and a continued use of the substance despite adverse maternal/fetal consequences (e.g., poor nutrition/weight gain, anemia, predisposition to infection, pregnancy-induced hypertension [PIH], fetal defects/intrauterine growth retardation [IUGR], fetal alcohol syndrome [FAS]). The drugs most often abused are alcohol, cocaine (crack), heroin, methamphetamine, barbiturates, marijuana, and phencyclidine (PCP). Care depends on the degree of abuse and whether the client is intoxicated or is in the withdrawal phase. The client who is addicted may not seek care during the prenatal period, compounding any existing or developing problems. In addition, negative attitudes on the part of society and often from caregivers affect the pregnant woman and her care.

This plan of care is to be used in conjunction with the CP: The High-Risk Pregnancy.

CLIENT ASSESSMENT DATA BASE

ACTIVITY/REST

Lack of energy/fatigue, malaise.

Incoordination, unsteady gait.

Sleeplessness/insomnia.

Yawning.

CIRCULATION

Systemic hypertension; orthostatic hypotension.

Tachycardia, palpitations.

Ventricular arrhythmias.

History of endocarditis, sudden coronary artery spasm, myocardial infarction.

EGO INTEGRITY

Pregnancy usually not planned.

May express indecision about pregnancy (i.e., issues of abortion, adoption), concern regarding involvement of social/legal agencies.

Labile mood, irritability, lack of motivation, denial of problem.

Low self-esteem; feelings of guilt regarding substance use.

Presence of stressors (financial, changes in lifestyle).

Increased dependency needs.

Inadequate coping skills/support systems.

ELIMINATION

Diarrhea or constipation.

FOOD/FLUID

Appetite changes, anorexia, nausea, vomiting.

Inadequate nutritional/fluid intake.

Low weight gain.

Pathologic edema.

HYGIENE

Poor oral/body hygiene.

NEUROSENSORY

Dizziness.

Slurred speech.

Hyperactivity; tremors of hands, tongue, eyelids.

Pupillary dilation or constriction, nystagmus, diplopia.

Decreased attention span, impaired memory.

Irritability, depression, confusion, hallucinations, delirium, coma.

History of seizure activity.

PAIN/DISCOMFORT

Low threshold for pain or decreased response to pain.

Muscle pain, headache.

Early uterine contractions.

RESPIRATION

Nasal sinus drainage, inflamed mucosa, nosebleeds, septal defect.

Tachypnea.

Frequent sore throats.

Cigarette smoker/exposure to secondhand smoke.

History of recurrent pneumonia.

SAFETY

Hyperthermia, diaphoresis.

Evidence of needle tracks on extremities.

Presence of cellulitis, superficial abscesses, septic phlebitis.

History of traumatic injuries; physical/emotional abuse.

Inadequate maintenance of home environment.

History of jaundice.

Positive screen for hepatitis, sexually transmitted disease, or human immunodeficiency virus.

Previous obstetrical problems (e.g., PIH, abruptio placenta, premature rupture of membranes).

Fetal hyperactivity, bradycardia.

SEXUALITY

Decreased libido.

History of multiple sexual partners.

Fundal height inappropriate for length of gestation.

Vaginal spotting/bleeding.

GPTPAL may reveal spontaneous abortion, premature birth/fetal death, meconium staining, low-birth-weight infant, fetal withdrawal/alcohol syndrome, infant death/(SIDS).

SOCIAL INTERACTIONS

Lack of support systems.

Loss of job; financial problems.

Relationship/family discord (manipulative behavior).

TEACHING/LEARNING

Use of alcohol, prescription, over-the-counter, and/or illicit drugs.

Difficulty maintaining self drug-free; ineffective recovery attempts; drug hunger.

Absence of/limited prenatal care or preparation.

Lack of cooperation with therapeutic regimen.

DIAGNOSTIC STUDIES

Toxicology screen: Identifies drug(s) used and current status.
Various blood studies (e.g., complete blood count (CBC), serum glucose, electrolytes): Determine presence of anemia and nutritional status.
Liver studies: Detect presence and degree of involvement/damage.
Ultrasonography: Locates placental implantation; assesses fetal size in relation to length of gestation.
Chest x-ray: Reveals presence of pneumonia, foreign body, emboli, or pulmonary edema.
Screening tests/cultures: Determine presence of infectious diseases.
Addiction Severity Index: Produces a "problem severity profile" of the client, including chemical, medical, psychologic, legal, family/social, and employment/support aspects, indicating areas of treatment needs.

NURSING PRIORITIES

1. Promote physiologic stability and well-being of client and fetus.
2. Support client's acceptance of reality of situation.
3. Facilitate learning of new ways to reduce anxiety; strengthen individual coping skills.
4. Promote family involvement in treatment process.
5. Provide information about condition, prognosis, and treatment needs.

DISCHARGE GOALS

1. Free of injury/complications to self and fetus/newborn.
2. Responsibility for own life and behavior assumed.
3. Abstinence from drug(s) maintained on a day-to-day basis.
4. Support systems identified and used; attending group rehabilitation program, as appropriate.
5. Dependence condition and its impact on pregnancy, prognosis, and therapeutic regimen understood.

NURSING DIAGNOSIS:	NUTRITION, ALTERED, LESS THAN BODY REQUIREMENTS
May be related to:	Insufficient dietary intake to meet metabolic needs for psychologic, physiologic, or economic reasons.
Possibly evidenced by:	Low weight gain, prepregnant weight below norm for height/body build, decreased subcutaneous fat/muscle mass, poor muscle tone, reported altered taste sensation, lack of interest in food; sore, inflamed buccal cavity; laboratory evidence of protein/vitamin deficiencies.
DESIRED OUTCOMES— CLIENT WILL:	Demonstrate progressive weight gain toward goal, with normalization of laboratory values and absence of signs of malnutrition.
	Verbalize understanding of effects of substance abuse and reduced dietary intake on nutritional status and pregnancy.
	Demonstrate behaviors and lifestyle changes to regain/maintain appropriate weight for pregnancy.

ACTIONS/INTERVENTIONS	RATIONALE
Independent	
Determine age, height/weight, body build, strength, and activity/rest pattern. Note condition of oral cavity.	Provides information on which to base caloric needs/dietary plan. Type of diet/foods may be affected by condition of mucous membranes and teeth.
Obtain anthropometric measurements, e.g., triceps skinfold.	Calculates subcutaneous fat and muscle mass to aid in determining dietary needs.
Note total daily calorie intake. Encourage client to maintain a diary of intake, times, and patterns of eating.	Information about patient's dietary pattern will identify nutritional strengths/needs/deficiencies.
Evaluate energy expenditure (e.g., pregnancy needs, pacing or sedentary activities), and establish an individualized exercise program.	Pregnant state and activity level affect nutritional needs. Exercise enhances muscle tone, may stimulate appetite, and promotes sense of well-being.
Provide opportunity to choose foods or snacks to meet dietary plan.	Enhances participation/sense of control and may promote resolution of nutritional deficiencies.
Weigh client weekly and record.	Provides information regarding current status/effectiveness of dietary plan.
Collaborative	
Consult with dietitian.	Useful in establishing individual dietary needs/ plan. Provides additional resource for learning about the importance of nutrition in nonpregnant and pregnant states.
Review laboratory work as indicated; e.g., glucose, serum albumin, and electrolytes.	Identifies anemias, electrolyte imbalances, and other abnormalities that may be present, requiring specific therapy. (Note: Toxic vapor abuse of toluene-based solvents [such as spray paint or

ACTIONS/INTERVENTIONS

Collaborative

Refer for dental consultation as necessary.

RATIONALE

glue] may cause a distal renal tubular acidosis with resultant hypokalemia, hypophosphatemia, hypomagnesemia, and hypocalcemia as well as rhabdomyolysis.)

Teeth are essential to good nutritional intake, and dental hygiene/care is often neglected in this population.

NURSING DIAGNOSIS:	**DENIAL, INEFFECTIVE; COPING, INDIVIDUAL, INEFFECTIVE**
May be related to:	Personal vulnerability, difficulty handling new situations, previous ineffective/inadequate coping skills with substitution of drug(s), inadequate support systems, anxiety/fear.
Possibly evidenced by:	Denial (one of the strongest and most resistant symptoms of substance abuse), lack of acceptance that drug use is causing the present situation, use of manipulation to avoid responsibility for self, altered social patterns/participation, impaired adaptive behavior and problem-solving skills, decreased ability to handle stress of illness/hospitalization, financial affairs in disarray, employment difficulties (e.g., losing time on job/not maintaining steady employment, poor work performance, on-the-job injuries).
DESIRED OUTCOMES— CLIENT WILL:	Verbalize awareness of relationship of substance abuse to current situation.
	Identify ineffective coping behaviors and their consequences.
	Use effective coping skills/problem solving.
	Initiate necessary lifestyle changes.
	Attend support group (e.g., Cocaine/Narcotics/Alcoholics Anonymous) regularly.

ACTIONS/INTERVENTIONS

Independent

Determine client's understanding of pregnancy and current situation and previous methods of coping with life's problems.

Remain nonjudgmental. Be alert to changes in behavior; e.g., restlessness, increased tension.

Provide positive feedback when client expresses awareness of denial in self and recognizes it in others.

RATIONALE

Provides information about degree of denial; identifies coping skills that may be used in present plan of care.

Confrontation can lead to increased agitation, which may compromise safety of client/staff.

Denial is the major defense mechanism in addictive disease, and may block progress of therapy until client accepts reality of the problem. Positive feedback is necessary to enhance self-esteem and to reinforce insight into behavior.

ACTIONS/INTERVENTIONS	RATIONALE
Independent	
Maintain firm expectation that client will attend recovery support/therapy groups regularly.	Attending is related to admitting need for help, to working with denial and for an optimal outcome of the pregnancy, as well as maintenance of a long-term drug-free existence.
Provide information about addictive use versus experimental, occasional use of drugs; biochemical/genetic disorder theory (genetic predisposition); and use activated by environment, pharmacology of stimulant, or compulsive desire as a lifelong occurrence.	Progression of use continuum in the addict is from experimental/recreational to addictive use. Comprehending this process is important in combatting denial. Education may relieve client of guilt and blame, and may help awareness of recurring addictive characteristics.
Discuss ways to use diversional activities that relate to recovery (e.g., social activities within support group) wherein issues of being chemically free are examined.	Discovery of alternative methods of recreation and methods for coping with drug hunger can remind client that addiction is a lifelong process and that opportunity for changing patterns is available.
Encourage and support client's taking responsibility for own recovery (e.g., development of alternative behaviors to drug use).	Denial can be replaced with responsible action when client accepts the reality of own responsibility.
Set limits and confront efforts to get caregiver to grant special privileges, making excuses for not following through on behaviors agreed on, and attempting to continue drug use.	Client has learned manipulative behavior throughout life and needs to learn a new way of getting needs met. Following through on consequences of failure to maintain limits can help the client to change ineffective behaviors.
Assist client to learn relaxation skills, guided imagery, or visualizations; encourage her to use them.	Helps client to relax and develop new ways to deal with stress and problem-solve.
Be aware of family/staff enabling behaviors and feelings.	Lack of understanding of enabling and codependence can result in nontherapeutic approaches to addicts.
Collaborative	
Administer medications as indicated, noting restrictions on use in pregnancy: Disulfiram (Antabuse).	This drug can be helpful in maintaining abstinence from alcohol while other therapy is undertaken; however, safety in pregnancy has not been established.
Methadone.	This drug is thought to blunt the craving for and/or diminish the effects of heroin and is used to assist in withdrawal and long-term maintenance programs. It has fewer side effects than heroin and allows the client to maintain daily activities and ultimately withdraw from drug use.
Encourage involvement with self-help associations; e.g., Alcoholics/Narcotics Anonymous.	Puts client in direct contact with support systems necessary for managing sobriety/drug-free life. Self-help groups are valuable for learning and promoting abstinence in each member with understanding and support as well as peer pressure.

NURSING DIAGNOSIS:	POWERLESSNESS
May be related to:	Substance addiction with or without periods of abstinence, episodic compulsive indulgence, failed attempts at recovery, lifestyle of helplessness.
Possibly evidenced by:	Ineffective recovery attempts, statements of inability to stop behavior (even with awareness of effects on pregnancy) and/or requests for help, continuous/constant thinking about drug and/or obtaining drug; alterations in personal, occupational, and social life.
DESIRED OUTCOMES— CLIENT WILL:	Admit inability to control drug habit, surrender to powerlessness over addiction.
	Verbalize acceptance of need for treatment and awareness that willpower alone cannot maintain abstinence.
	Engage in peer support.
	Demonstrate active participation in program.
	Maintain healthy state during pregnancy with an optimal outcome.

ACTIONS/INTERVENTIONS	RATIONALE
Independent	
Use crisis intervention techniques:	Client is more amenable to acceptance of need for treatment in the crisis presented by the pregnancy. (Note: Typical binging pattern of cocaine use may promote or inhibit client's responsiveness to intervention.)
Assist client to recognize that a problem exists.	While client is hurting and recognizing that substance abuse is harmful to her fetus, it is easier to admit drug use is a problem.
Identify goals for change.	Helpful in planning direction for care and promoting belief that change can occur.
Discuss alternative solutions.	Brainstorming helps creatively identify possibilities and provides sense of control.
Assist in selecting most appropriate alternative.	As possibilities are discussed, the most useful solution becomes clear.
Support decision and implementation of selected alternative(s).	Helps the client to persevere in process of change.
Discuss need for help in a caring, nonjudgmental way.	A caring nonconfrontive manner is more therapeutic, because the client may respond defensively to a moralistic attitude, blocking recovery.

ACTIONS/INTERVENTIONS	RATIONALE

Independent

Discuss ways in which drug use has interfered with life, occupation, and personal/interpersonal relationships.

Awareness of how the drug has controlled life is important in combatting denial/sense of powerlessness.

Assist client to learn ways to enhance health, meet pregnancy needs, and structure healthy diversion from drug use (e.g., a balanced diet, adequate rest, acupuncture, biofeedback, deep meditative techniques, and exercise, such as walking, swimming, or other activity tailored to pregnant state).

Learning to empower self in constructive areas can strengthen ability to continue recovery. These activities help restore natural biochemical balance, aid detoxification, and manage stress, anxiety, and use of free time as well as promote positive pregnancy outcomes. These diversions can increase self-confidence, thereby improving self-esteem. (Note: Release of endorphins from sustained exercise can create a feeling of well-being.)

Assist client in self-examination of spirituality and faith.

Surrendering to a power greater than oneself and faith in that power have been found to be effective in substance recovery; may decrease sense of powerlessness.

Assist client to learn assertive communication.

Effective in assisting in ability to refuse use, to stop relationships with users and dealers, to build healthy relationships, and to regain control of own life.

Collaborative

Refer to/assist with making appointment to treatment program, e.g., partial hospitalization drug treatment programs, Narcotics/Alcoholics Anonymous.

Follow-through on appointments may be easier than making the initial contact, and continuing treatment is essential to positive outcome of both substance abuse problem and pregnancy. (Note: To date, treatment programs admitting pregnant clients have been very limited in number, reducing treatment options and jeopardizing client/fetal outcomes.)

NURSING DIAGNOSIS:	SELF ESTEEM, DISTURBANCE; SELF ESTEEM, SITUATIONAL LOW
May be related to:	Social stigma attached to substance abuse, social expectation that one control behavior (e.g., abuse of drugs, sexual activity, and use of birth control), biochemical body change (e.g., withdrawal from alcohol/drugs), situational crisis of pregnancy with loss of control over life events.

Possibly evidenced by:	Not taking responsibility for self/self-care, lack of follow-through, self-destructive behavior, change in usual role patterns or responsibility (family, job, legal); confusion about self, purpose, or direction in life; denial that substance use is a problem.
DESIRED OUTCOMES— CLIENT WILL:	Identify feelings and methods for coping with negative perception of self.
	Verbalize acceptance of self as is and an increased sense of self-esteem.
	Set goals and participate in realistic planning for lifestyle changes necessary to live without drugs and bring pregnancy to the desired outcome.

ACTIONS/INTERVENTIONS	RATIONALE
Independent	
Provide opportunity for and encourage verbalization/discussion of individual situation.	Client often has difficulty expressing self and even more difficulty accepting the degree of importance substance has assumed in life and its relationship to present situation/pregnancy. (Note: pregnancy may not have been planned, and client may feel indecisive about plans for the future.)
Assess mental status. Note presence of other psychiatric disorders (dual diagnosis).	May affect decisions regarding pregnancy. Many clients use substances (alcohol and other drugs) to seek relief from depression or anxiety. (Note: approximately 60% of substance-dependent individuals also have mental illness problems, and there is an increasing awareness that treatment for both is imperative.)
Spend time with client. Discuss client's behavior/substance use in a nonjudgmental way.	Presence of the nurse conveys acceptance of the individual as a worthwhile person. Discussion provides opportunity for insight into the problems substance abuse has created for the client.
Provide reinforcement for positive actions, and encourage client to accept this input.	Failure and lack of self-esteem have been problems for this client, who needs to learn to accept self as an individual with positive attributes.
Observe family/significant other interactions; note dynamics and presence/effectiveness of support.	Substance abuse is a family disease, and how the members act and react to the client's pregnancy and her behavior affects the course of the disease and how client sees herself. Many unconsciously become "enablers," helping the individual to cover up the consequences of the abuse. (Refer to NDs: Family Coping, ineffective: compromised/disabling; Caregiver Role Strain.)

ACTIONS/INTERVENTIONS	RATIONALE

Independent

Encourage expression of feelings of guilt, shame, and anger.

The client often has lost respect for self and believes that the situation is hopeless. Expression of these feelings helps the client begin to accept responsibility for self and take steps to make changes.

Help the client to acknowledge that substance use is the problem and that problems can be dealt with without the use of drugs. Confront the use of defenses (e.g., denial, projection, rationalization).

When drugs can no longer be blamed for the problems that exist, the client can begin to deal with them and live without substance use. Confrontation helps the client accept the reality of the problems as they exist.

Ask the client to list and review past accomplishments and positive happenings, including previous pregnancy experiences.

There are things in everyone's life that have been successful. Often when self-esteem is low, it is difficult to remember these successes or to view them as successes.

Use techniques of role rehearsal.

Assists client to practice the development of skills to cope with new role as a person who no longer uses or needs drugs to handle life's problems.

Collaborative

Involve client in group therapy.

Group sharing helps encourage verbalization because other members of group are in various stages of abstinence from drugs and can address the client's concerns/denial. The client can gain new skills, hope, and a sense of family/community from group participation.

Refer to other resources, such as Narcotics/Alcoholics Anonymous.

One of the oldest and most popular forms of group treatment uses a basic strategy known as the Twelve Steps. The client admits powerlessness over drug, and, although not necessary, may seek help from a "higher power." Members help one another, and meetings are available at many different times and places in most communities. The philosophy of "one day at a time" helps attain the goal of abstinence.

Formulate plan to treat other mental illness problems.

Clients who seek relief for other mental health problems through drugs will continue to do so. Both the substance use and the mental health problems need to be treated together to maximize abstinence potential.

Administer antipsychotic medications as necessary, noting precautions of use in pregnancy.

Prolonged/profound psychosis following LSD or PCP use can be treated with antipsychotic drugs because it is probably the result of an underlying functional psychosis that has now emerged. (Note: avoid the use of phenothiazines because they may decrease seizure threshold and cause hypotension in the presence of LSD/PCP.)

NURSING DIAGNOSIS:	FAMILY COPING, INEFFECTIVE: COMPROMISED/DIS-ABLING; CAREGIVER ROLE STRAIN
May be related to:	Personal vulnerability of individual family members, codependency issues, situational crises of drug abuse and pregnancy, compromised social systems, family disorganization/role changes, prolonged disease progression that exhausts supportive capability of family members; significant person(s) with chronically unexpressed feelings of guilt, anger, hostility, or despair.
Possibly evidenced by:	Denial, or belief that all problems are due to substance use; severely dysfunctional family (family violence, spouse/child abuse, separation/divorce, children displaying acting-out behaviors); financial affairs in disarray; employment difficulties; altered social patterns/participation; significant other demonstrating enabling or codependent behaviors (avoiding and shielding, attempting to control, taking over responsibilities, rationalizing and accepting, cooperating and collaborating, rescuing and self-serving).
DESIRED OUTCOMES— FAMILY WILL:	Verbalize understanding of dynamics of codependence and participate in individual and family programs. Identify ineffective coping behaviors/consequences. Demonstrate/plan for necessary lifestyle changes. Take action to change self-destructive behaviors and/or alter behavior that contributes to client's addiction.

ACTIONS/INTERVENTIONS	RATIONALE

Independent

ACTIONS/INTERVENTIONS	RATIONALE
Assess family history; explore roles of family members and circumstances involving drug use, strengths, and areas for growth. Note attitudes/beliefs regarding pregnancy and parenting.	Determines areas for focus and potential for change.
Explore how the family/significant other has coped with the client's habit (e.g., denial, repression, rationalization, hurt, loneliness, projection).	The codependent person suffers from the same feelings as the client (e.g., anxiety, self-hatred, helplessness, low self-worth, guilt) and needs help in learning new/effective coping skills.
Determine understanding of current situation/pregnancy and previous methods of coping with life's problems.	Identifies misconceptions/areas of need on which to base present plan of care.
Assess current level of functioning of family members.	Affects individual's ability to cope with situation.
Determine extent of enabling behaviors being evidenced by family members; explore with individual and client.	*Enabling* is doing for the client what she needs to do for herself. People want to be helpful and do not want to feel powerless to help their loved one to stop drinking and change the behavior that is so destructive. However, in many cases the substance abuser relies on others to cover up own inability to cope with daily responsibilities.

121

ACTIONS/INTERVENTIONS	RATIONALE
Independent	
Provide information about enabling behavior and addictive disease characteristics for both user and nonuser person who is codependent.	Awareness and knowledge provide opportunity for individuals to begin the process of change.
Provide factual information to client and family about the effects of addictive behaviors on the family and what to expect regarding abstinence from drugs and course of pregnancy.	Many individuals are not aware of the nature of addiction, the involvement of the family, and the effects on pregnancy/fetus. (Note: if client is using legally obtained drugs, family members may believe this does not constitute abuse.)
Encourage family members to be aware of their own feelings and to look at the situation with perspective and objectivity. They can ask themselves, "Am I being conned? Am I acting out of fear, shame, guilt, or anger? Do I have a need to control?"	When the codependent family members become aware of their own actions that perpetuate the addict's problems, they can decide to change themselves. If they change, the client can then face the consequences of her own actions and may choose to get well.
Involve significant other in referral plans.	Drug abuse is a family illness. Because the family has been so involved in dealing with the substance abuse behavior, they need help adjusting to the new behavior of sobriety/abstinence. Incidence of recovery is almost doubled when the family is treated along with the client.
Be aware of staff's enabling behaviors and feelings about client, pregnancy, and partners who are codependent.	Lack of understanding of enabling and codependence can result in nontherapeutic approaches to addicts and their families. Staff may feel angry toward client who uses or continues to use drug(s) even though she has been given information regarding possibility of damage to the developing fetus.
Collaborative	
Encourage involvement with self-help associations (e.g., Alcoholics/Narcotics Anonymous, Al-Anon, Al-Ateen) and professional family therapy.	Puts client/family in direct contact with support systems necessary for continued sobriety and assistance with learning problem resolution.

NURSING DIAGNOSIS:	**KNOWLEDGE DEFICIT [LEARNING NEED], regarding condition/pregnancy, prognosis, and treatment needs**
May be related to:	Lack/misinterpretation of information, lack of recall, cognitive limitations/interference with learning (other mental illness problems/organic brain syndrome).
Possibly evidenced by:	Statements of concern, questions/misconceptions, inaccurate follow-through of instructions, development of preventable complications, continued use in spite of complications/bad trips.
DESIRED OUTCOMES— CLIENT WILL:	Verbalize understanding of own condition/pregnancy/disease process, prognosis, and treatment plan.
	Identify/initiate necessary lifestyle changes to remain drug-free with optimal pregnancy outcome.
	Participate in treatment program.

ACTIONS/INTERVENTIONS	RATIONALE
Independent	
Provide information about effects of drugs on the reproductive system/fetus (e.g., increased risk of premature birth, brain damage, and fetal malformation). Review drinking/drug history of client/partner.	Awareness of the negative effects of alcohol/other drugs on reproduction may motivate client to stop using drug(s). When client is pregnant, identification of potential problems aids in planning for future fetal needs/concerns.
Review results of sonogram.	Assesses fetal growth and development to identify possibility of IUGR or FAS and future needs.
Be aware of and deal with anxiety of client and family members.	Anxiety can interfere with ability to hear and assimilate information.
Provide an active role for the client/partner in the learning process through discussions, group participation, and role-playing.	Learning is enhanced when people are actively involved.
Provide written and verbal information as indicated. Include list of articles and books related to client/family needs, and encourage reading and discussing what they learn.	Helps individuals to make informed choices about future. Bibliotherapy can be a useful addition to other therapy approaches if materials chosen consider the individual's educational and cognitive abilities.
Assess client's knowledge of own situation; i.e., pregnancy, complications, and needed changes in lifestyle.	Assists in planning for long-range changes necessary for maintaining sobriety/drug-free status. Client may have street knowledge of the drug but be ignorant of medical facts and relationship to pregnancy.
Review condition and prognosis/future expectations.	Provides knowledge base on which client can make informed choices.
Time activities to individual needs.	Facilitates learning because information is more readily assimilated when individual learning pace is considered.
Discuss relationship of drug use to current situation/pregnancy.	In many cases, client has misperception (denial) of real reason for admission to the medical/psychiatric setting/when hospitalized.
Discuss variety of helpful organizations and programs that are available for assistance/referral.	Long-term support is necessary to maintain optimal recovery and/or assist with pregnancy needs. Psychosocial needs may require addressing as well as other issues.

The Pregnant Adolescent _____

Pregnant adolescents are at risk physically, emotionally, and socially. The impact of adolescent pregnancy on the individual has far-reaching consequences, which may restrict or limit future opportunities for the adolescent and the child(ren). Educational goals may be altered or eliminated, thus limiting potential for a productive life. The client frequently may be of lower socioeconomic status, with the pregnancy perpetuating financial dependence and lowered self-esteem. Statistically, the obstetrical hazards for adolescents and their infants include increased mortality and morbidity. Therefore, individualized prenatal nursing care for the adolescent client/family/partner that incorporates developmental needs and health education with prenatal needs has the potential to contribute positively to prenatal, intrapartal, and postpartal outcomes. Additionally, neonatal outcomes associated with better Apgar scores, lower incidence of resuscitation, and fewer low-birth-weight (LBW) infants can also be expected. (Refer to CPs: First Trimester; Second Trimester; Third Trimester, for discussion of usual/expected pregnancy needs.)

CLIENT ASSESSMENT DATA BASE

(In addition to Prenatal Client Assessment Data Base.)

CIRCULATION

Elevated blood pressure (BP), a risk indicator of pregnancy-induced hypertension (PIH).

EGO INTEGRITY

Pregnancy may or may not be wanted by client; may be result of abuse.

Varied cultural/religious response to pregnancy out of wedlock; or as a stressor on teen marriage (note whether client's mother was a teenage mother).

Expressions of worthlessness, discounting self.

Decision making varies from abdicating all responsibility to extreme independence.

May or may not be involved with father of child by own/partner's choice, family demands, or question of paternity.

May feel helpless, hopeless; fear family/peer response.

Emotional status varies; e.g., calm, accepting, denial, hysteria.

History of limited/no financial resources.

History of encounters with judicial system.

ELIMINATION

Proteinuria (risk indicator of PIH).

FOOD/FLUID

Weight gain may be less than optimal.

Dietary choices may not include all food groups.

Edema (risk indicator of PIH).

Hemoglobin (Hb) and/or hematocrit (Hct) may reveal anemia and hemoconcentration, suggesting PIH.

HYGIENE

Dress may be inappropriate for stage of gestation (e.g., wearing restrictive or bulky clothing to conceal pregnancy).

RESPIRATORY

May be a cigarette smoker.

SAFETY

History/presence of sexually transmitted diseases (STD).

Fundal height may be less than normal for gestation (indicating intrauterine growth retardation [IUGR] of fetus).

Ultrasonography may reveal inappropriate fetal growth, low-lying placental implantation.

SEXUALITY

Lack of/incorrect use of contraception.

Pelvic measurements may be borderline/contracted.

SOCIAL INTERACTIONS

May report problems with family dynamics, lack of available resources/support.

Little or no concept of reality of situation; future expectations, potential responsibilities.

TEACHING/LEARNING

Level of maturity varies/may regress; barriers of age and developmental stage.

Experimentation with substance use or abuse.

Lack of achievement in school.

Lack of awareness of own health/pregnancy needs.

Fantasies/fears about childbirth.

NURSING PRIORITIES

1. Promote optimal physical/emotional well-being of client.
2. Monitor fetal well-being.
3. Provide information and review the options available.
4. Facilitate positive adaptation to new and changing roles.
5. Encourage family/partner participation in problem-solving.

NURSING DIAGNOSIS:	NUTRITION, ALTERED, LESS THAN BODY REQUIREMENTS
May be related to:	Intake insufficient to meet metabolic demands.
Possibly evidenced by:	Lack of information, misconceptions, body weight below (or possibly above) ideal, inappropriate uterine/fetal growth; reported intake that does not meet recommended daily allowance (RDA); anemia, pregnancy-induced hypertension.
DESIRED OUTCOMES— CLIENT WILL:	Ingest nutritionally adequate diet.
	Gain prescribed weight.
	Take daily iron/vitamin supplement as appropriate.
	Maintain normal Hb and Hct levels, free of anemia and without signs of PIH.

ACTIONS/INTERVENTIONS	RATIONALE

Independent

Assess dietary intake using 24-hour recall.	Information about current intake is helpful/necessary to planning changes or additions for adequate diet. Adolescents, especially age 17 or younger, are at risk for malnutrition, because their normally increased bodily requirements for growth are stressed by the metabolic demands associated with pregnancy.
Weigh client and determine prepregnancy weight. Provide information about risk of dieting in pregnancy.	Weight gain needed during pregnancy is calculated according to normal growth demands and prepregnancy weight. Food idiosyncrasies, which are related to the adolescent's developmental stage, and delayed prenatal care contribute to poor or inadequate intake, possible fetal IUGR and resultant LBW infant, and maternal complications, such as PIH and associated uterine ischemia. Weight loss places client and fetus at risk for acidosis.
Provide individual prescription for weight gain based on growth needs and prepregnancy weight, recognizing adolescent lifestyle and preferences for "fast foods."	Adequate calories are necessary to spare proteins and ensure iron intake. An underweight client needs an additional 500 calories daily; an overweight client needs 17 calories per pound of pregnancy weight.
Stress importance of daily vitamin/iron intake. (Refer to CP: First Trimester, ND: Nutrition, altered, less than body requirements, high risk for.)	Pregnant adolescents are prone to problems of malnutrition and anemia, owing to incomplete growth and/or dietary habits, which necessitate increased dietary protein, iron, and calories.
Identify individual protein requirement.	Requirements in pregnancy for the client age 15–18 years are equal to 1.5 g/kg of pregnant body weight; for clients younger than age 15, requirements equal 1.7 g/kg of pregnant body weight.
Provide information about role of protein in terms of maternal/fetal development.	Low/inadequate protein intake during pregnancy, especially in the first trimester, places fetus at risk for IUGR and lack of brain cell hyperplasia and hypertrophy, and may contribute to development of maternal PIH. (Refer to CP: Pregnancy-Induced Hypertension.)
Assess client's situation, and determine who is responsible for food purchasing and meal preparation. Provide information about ways of improving nutritional intake.	Socioeconomic status, financial concerns, or lack of experience with grocery shopping and meal preparation may interfere with proper nutrition.

Collaborative

Refer to Women, Infants, and Children (WIC) program through local public health department.	When client qualifies, programs such as this enable the adolescent to manage a better nutritional program.
Assess Hb/Hct initially and again at 7 months' gestation.	Iron deficiency anemia, which is common in the adolescent, places the fetus at risk for lowered Hb/Hct levels and for continuation of low iron stores/iron deficiency anemia in the infant after delivery.

NURSING DIAGNOSIS:	KNOWLEDGE DEFICIT [LEARNING NEED], regarding pregnancy process, individual needs, future expectations
May be related to:	Lack of information, unfamiliarity with resources, information misinterpretation, lack of interest in learning, developmental stage/cognitive deficit, psychologic stressors/absence of support systems.
Possibly evidenced by:	Request for information, statement of misconception, inaccurate follow-through of instructions, development of complications.
DESIRED OUTCOMES— CLIENT WILL:	Participate in learning process.
	Verbalize understanding of condition.
	Discuss and adhere to components of adequate prenatal diet.
	Identify potential teratogens, physiologic/psychologic aspects of reproduction, pregnancy, labor and delivery.

ACTIONS/INTERVENTIONS	RATIONALE

Independent

Evaluate client's age and stage of adolescent development.	The age and stage of the adolescent will influence the approach to teaching because the late adolescent (aged 17–20 years) may be better able to conceptualize, process, and synthesize information than the client in early (aged 11–14 years) or middle (aged 14–17 years) adolescence.
Note readiness to learn.	Depending on the stage of development, the adolescent is self-focusing. The client may not be motivated because of difficulty recognizing the need or importance of learning.
Encourage client to explore options regarding outcomes of pregnancy, including termination of pregnancy (dependent on stage of gestation), keeping the baby, or giving the baby up for adoption. (Note implications of culture on decisions.)	Although currently many adolescents elect to keep their babies, the client must be given freedom of choice based on available options. In some situations and/or cultures (e.g., Cambodian), the family makes decisions about the pregnancy for the adolescent rather than allowing her to make her own decisions.
Assess client's understanding of male/female anatomy and physiology. Provide appropriate information; correct misconceptions.	For the pregnant client in early adolescence, pregnancy and parenthood are often not recognized as possible outcomes of sexual activity.
Assess factors related to high rate of recidivism. Identify community resources and potential support systems.	If pregnancy is not accompanied by emotional maturation, a high rate of recidivism may be anticipated, especially if the teenager uses sexual activity to demonstrate independence or enhance her self-concept. A comprehensive assessment of the adolescent mother and early intervention are helpful in preventing second and subsequent unplanned pregnancies.

127

ACTIONS/INTERVENTIONS	RATIONALE

Independent

Obtain drug use/abuse history; screen for STDs and for human immunodeficiency virus (HIV) risk behaviors. Provide information about possible negative effects on fetus. (Refer to ND: Injury, high risk for, fetal (following) and in CP: First Trimester; and CPs: The High-Risk Pregnancy, Prenatal Infection.)

Helps prevent fetal complications. Adolescents, however, frequently do not enter the healthcare system until the second trimester, by which time fetal injury may have already occurred. Reasons for this delay include shame, fear of parental reaction, denial, and failure to recognize pregnancy.

Provide information about nutrition, meal planning, and need to avoid empty calories. (Refer to ND: Nutrition, altered, less than body requirements.)

Adolescents, in desiring to achieve independence, may repeat poor nutritional habits practiced by parents/peers, thereby risking malnutrition, IUGR, and birth of LBW infant.

Refer client to adolescent clinic for peer support and informational services such as prenatal, parenting, and infant care classes.

Adolescent clinics, which are responsive to the unique needs of the teenager, provide information in concrete terms, which is appropriate for the client unable to cope with abstractions or to solve problems based on inference.

Provide information about importance of establishing individual long-range personal and educational goals for client and her offspring. Refer to appropriate social agencies.

Two out of three pregnant adolescents drop out of school, which often results in their being economically dependent on the welfare system, creating a perpetual cycle for the offspring. Establishing realistic educational goals may interrupt or prevent the development of this cycle.

Discuss signs of labor. Identify factors that place the adolescent at risk for preterm labor/delivery.

Client needs to know when to call the physician or caregiver and how to differentiate between true and false labor.

Present/discuss available methods of birth control, giving advantages and disadvantages of each. Be realistic and nonjudgmental. Present information appropriate for the adolescent's particular developmental stage.

Information presented prenatally assists client in selection of contraception following delivery. Rates of recidivism tend to decrease if effective contraception material and methods are provided immediately after the pregnancy.

(Refer to CP: The High-Risk Pregnancy, ND: Knowledge Deficit [Learning Need].)

NURSING DIAGNOSIS:	**INJURY, HIGH RISK FOR, fetal**
May be related to:	Maternal malnutrition, preexisting health problems and/or maternal complications/susceptibility, inadequate prenatal care and screening.
Possibly evidenced by:	[Not applicable; presence of signs/symptoms establishes an **actual** diagnosis.]
DESIRED OUTCOMES— CLIENT WILL:	Verbalize understanding of individual risk factors.
	Demonstrate behaviors/lifestyle changes to reduce risk factors and protect self and fetus.
	Display fetal growth within normal limits.
	Carry pregnancy to term, with delivery of full-term infant of size appropriate for gestational age.

ACTIONS/INTERVENTIONS	RATIONALE

Independent

Assess for potential risks to fetus.

Infants born to adolescent mothers are at risk for prematurity, low birth weight, birth trauma, and resultant sequelae of mental retardation, cerebral palsy, and epilepsy.

Weigh client. Provide individual prescription for weight gain based on body structure, prepregnancy weight, and normal growth (anabolic) needs.

Clients who give birth to LBW infants weigh less before pregnancy and gain less prenatally. Statistics reveal that birth weight of babies born to adolescent mothers averages 94 g less than in those born to nonadolescent mothers.

Provide oral/written information about dietary requirements, sources of vitamins/minerals, and food groups. Rule out anorexia nervosa. (Refer to CP: The High-Risk Pregnancy, ND: Nutrition, altered, less/more than body requirements, high risk for.)

Malnutrition contributes to inadequate development of neonatal/fetal brain cells during the prenatal hyperplasia phase and the combined hyperplasia/hypertrophy phase of the first 6 months of life, resulting in fewer total brain cells and smaller individual cell size.

Discuss negative aspects of dieting on fetus.

One in 10 adolescents who become pregnant is obese and, in many cases, is dieting during pregnancy, which results in weight loss, maternal/fetal acidosis, and possible CNS damage to fetus, especially in third trimester.

Stress importance of ongoing prenatal care.

Adolescents often feel well and do not follow up with prenatal protocols of care, especially if they do not understand the importance of frequent checkups and health promotion. This could result in inadequate screening or early intervention, which might otherwise ensure normal fetal growth and development.

Discuss role and food sources of iron, and need to supplement food intake with daily iron/folic acid.

Low maternal iron stores reduce available oxygen-carrying capacity and fetal oxygen uptake, decrease fetal iron stores during third trimester, and result in iron deficiency anemia of the infant.

Obtain sexual history, including STD exposure or episodes and high-risk behaviors for HIV. Note presence of active herpetic lesions or warts, and review culture reports. (Refer to CPs: The High-Risk Pregnancy, Prenatal Infection; ND: Injury, high risk for, fetal.)

STDs can contribute to fetal developmental problems as well as neonatal infections. STDs (including HIV) can either be transmitted to the fetus transplacentally or contracted during the delivery. Hepatitis and HIV are transmitted in blood products, so infant could contract either disease through vaginal or cesarean birth.

Provide information related to condom use/safer sexual practices if client is engaging in sexual activity outside of a monogamous relationship or with an at-risk partner. Discuss sexual abstinence.

Use of condoms/safer sexual behaviors in adolescents who are not in a monogamous sexual relationship tend to reduce risk of STD, including HIV infection. Although abstinence may be preferred, once an individual becomes sexually active, it is often difficult to make the decision to abstain.

Obtain history of use of tobacco, alcohol, or other substances; provide information about potentially harmful effects on fetal development. (Refer to CP: Prenatal Substance Dependence/Abuse.)

Adolescents typically have a higher substance abuse rate than nonadolescents, and in many cases, substance abuse occurs during critical periods of fetal development before client suspects she is pregnant. Substance abuse places the client at higher risk for complications of pregnancy and preterm labor.

129

ACTIONS/INTERVENTIONS	RATIONALE
Independent	
Screen for PIH at each prenatal visit. (Refer to CP: Pregnancy-Induced Hypertension.)	Adolescents are at risk for developing PIH, possibly due to malnutrition and inadequate protein intake, which may cause placental inadequacies and placental separation (abruptio placentae).
Collaborative	
Obtain pelvic measurements; determine prognosis for eutocia. Discuss possibility of cesarean birth if measurements are small.	Inadequate pelvic measurements due to physiologic immaturity place the client/fetus at risk for cephalopelvic disproportion and potential fetal injury intrapartally.
Review results of diagnostic/screening studies: Hb and Hct.	Reflect level of oxygen-carrying capacity and potential iron stores.
Rapid plasma reagin (RPR); cultures for herpes virus (HV) and gonorrhea/chlamydia.	If HV cultures are positive just prior to labor/delivery, a cesarean section may need to be scheduled.
Assist with appropriate treatment as needed. Serial ultrasonography.	Determines fetal growth. IUGR, possibly due to malnutrition or vascular changes with PIH, is reflected in biparietal diameter, femur length, estimated fetal weight, and abdominal circumference that are below normal limits for gestational age.
Biophysical Profile, nonstress test (NST), or contraction stress test (CST) if more than two NSTs are nonreactive. (Refer to CP: The High-Risk Pregnancy, ND: Injury, high risk for, fetal.)	Assess placental/fetal well-being. A compromised placenta is reflected in a nonreactive NST, necessitating confirmation by CST.
Refer to appropriate resources/drug program if client needs assistance with withdrawal from substance use/abuse.	Physiologic drug addiction/withdrawal increase risks to both client and fetus and thereby require specialized support and monitoring.

NURSING DIAGNOSIS:	**BODY IMAGE DISTURBANCE; ROLE PERFORMANCE, ALTERED; PERSONAL IDENTITY DISTURBANCE; SELF ESTEEM (specify)**
May be related to:	Situational and maturational crises, fear of failure at life events, biophysical changes, absence of support systems.
Possibly evidenced by:	Self-negating verbalizations, expressions of shame/guilt, hypersensitivity to criticism, fear of rejection, lack of follow-through and/or nonparticipation in care.
DESIRED OUTCOMES— CLIENT WILL:	Identify feelings and methods for coping with negative perception of self/abilities.
	Verbalize increased sense of self-esteem in relation to current situation.
	Demonstrate adaptation to changes/events as evidenced by setting of realistic goals and active participation in meeting own needs.

ACTIONS/INTERVENTIONS	RATIONALE

Independent

Establish a therapeutic nurse-client relationship.	Adolescent client needs a caring, nonjudgmental adult with whom to talk. Important to establish trust and cooperation so that the client is free to hear the information available.
Assess use of terms/language used by the client/ significant other(s).	Terminology may be specific to the adolescent culture, and words may have different meanings for client and nurse.
Determine developmental level and needs relative to age as early, middle, or late adolescence.	Cognitive development during this period moves from concrete to abstract thinking (formal operations). The younger client may see control of the situation as external and beyond her grasp, and have little ability to understand the consequences of her behavior. With maturity, the abilities to understand possible consequences and to accept individual responsibility develop.
Identify client's self-perception as positive or negative.	Helps client to become aware of how she views herself and to begin to increase her self-esteem. Until late adolescence, body image is still formative. The client is dealing with adolescent developmental tasks, establishing an adult identity. Low self-worth may lead to feelings of hopelessness about the future and inability to visualize a successful outcome.
Elicit the client's feelings about sexual identity/ roles.	May have difficulty seeing herself as a mother. The adolescent must make a role transition from child/daughter to adult/mother, which can create conflicts for the client and significant other(s).
Discuss concerns and fears about body image and transitory changes associated with pregnancy; discuss personal value system.	Establishes a basis for future learning. Conflicts may exist regarding how client has previously seen herself, what her expectations of pregnancy had been, and what the realities of pregnancy are. By mid-pregnancy, the enlarging abdomen and the increasing size of breasts and buttocks may prompt the teenager to try to control her appearance by dieting, with adverse consequences for fetal health and her own growth needs.
Discuss ways to promote positive self-image (e.g., clothing style, makeup) and recognition of positive aspects of the situation.	Assists in coping with changes in appearance and presenting a positive image.
Discuss appropriate adaptation techniques and the communication skills to implement these techniques.	Role-playing and active listening can be used to learn skills of communication and adaptation. Helps client learn information necessary to development of improved self-esteem.

NURSING DIAGNOSIS:	SOCIAL ISOLATION
May be related to:	Alterations in physical appearance, perceived unacceptable social behavior, inadequate personal resources, difficulty in engaging in satisfying personal relationships (developmental or situational).
Possibly evidenced by:	Expressed feelings of rejection or aloneness imposed by others, seeks solitude, inability to meet expectations of others, absence of effective support system.
DESIRED OUTCOMES— CLIENT WILL:	Remain involved in school and activities at the level of desire and ability.
	Participate in established social, community, and educational programs.

ACTIONS/INTERVENTIONS

Independent

Ascertain changes in client's relationships with others that have occurred with the pregnancy.

Discuss resources available for assistance and ways to use them.

Involve client with others who have shared interests.

Provide positive reinforcement as appropriate.

Encourage enrollment in childbirth and parent-education classes.

Collaborative

Arrange and assist with placement in foster or group home, if necessary.

RATIONALE

Initial reactions of parents and boyfriend may include shock, anger, guilt, and shame. The pregnant adolescent often finds herself isolated from her peer group. She may be isolated from school and the normal contacts it affords. Her social sphere may be restricted to other pregnant teenagers, her boyfriend (if he remains involved and if circumstances do not force separation), and perhaps her relatives, who may or may not include an extended family. Extent of isolation may depend on whether client is in early, middle, or late adolescence.

Acquaints the client with potential avenues for help. Client in late adolescence (aged 17–19) may be more resourceful financially.

Establishes peer/support group.

Helps adolescent develop sense of self-esteem in a situation in which criticism may be overwhelming.

Provides a learning environment for client with others who share similar circumstances and physical constraints.

May provide more positive environment if family is nonsupportive; may also be beneficial in enhancing self-esteem.

NURSING DIAGNOSIS:	FAMILY PROCESSES, ALTERED
May be related to:	Situational and developmental crises, faulty family relationships, impaired patterns of communication.
Possibly evidenced by:	Family fails to adapt to or deal with situation, verbalizes difficulty coping with situation, expresses confusion about what to do, displays unhealthy decision-making process and inability to express/accept own feelings or feelings of other family members.
DESIRED OUTCOMES— FAMILY WILL:	Express feelings freely, honestly, and appropriately.
	Participate in efforts directed toward establishing and/or reestablishing healthy communication and interaction.
	Provide adequate support for the pregnant adolescent/ partner.
	Seek professional counseling as appropriate.

ACTIONS/INTERVENTIONS	RATIONALE

Independent

Assess family life stressors and involved members within the client's family of origin. (Refer to ND: Family Coping, ineffective: compromised/disabling, high risk for.)	The reasons adolescents give for becoming pregnant may be directly related to the family unit. For some clients, there may be faulty relationships within the family. The pregnancy may be an act of rebellion toward parental constraints, or it may represent a search for outside nurturance if parents have not satisfied this need appropriately. At the same time, parents of the adolescent may be experiencing their own mid-life crisis. Even more destructive to the family, the pregnancy may be the result of incest/abuse.
Assess client's relationship with mother. Note cultural impact of pregnancy out of wedlock.	Mother may feel guilty, see daughter as too young to assume responsibility, and take over inappropriately. If client does not assume her new role as mother effectively, the mother may have difficulty assuming her new role as grandmother.
Identify the mode of communication and interaction within the family. Assess role expectations of family members.	Understanding the dynamics of the family and the roles of individual members can assist with change. Family disruption can best be resolved by assessing reasons for role changes and ways to facilitate them.
Treat family members in a warm caring way; encourage establishment of support systems.	Acceptance of the situation can strengthen the family and encourage members to extend their support to each other.
Encourage discussion of plans for the future of client, infant, and family.	At this time of crisis, members are apt to respond with anger, blaming each other, and may need help in focusing energies on practical solutions. The relationships with the baby's father and with family members in relation to future personal or

ACTIONS/INTERVENTIONS

Independent

Encourage supportive association with father of the child if agreeable to both parties.

Provide information about risks of marriage precipitated by the pregnancy alone.

Refer client to counseling and parenting classes.

RATIONALE

educational goals may be unclear. Furthermore, the decision whether client will relinquish or keep the infant will add to the uncertainties.

Father of the child may or may not be known; reaction of various family members may strain/prohibit involvement. However, with some understanding and assistance, in many cases the teen father would like to be involved in this event and can provide support for the client. (Note: When the pregnancy is the result of incest/abuse, personal and legal constraints will likely preclude inclusion of the father and will have an impact on the support provided by other family members.)

Although 50%–75% of adolescent marriages end in divorce, some teenage couples have a strong love relationship and may eventually marry or maintain a relationship.

Additional information and assistance with resolution of conflicts and/or coping with stressors may aid family in developing new and positive relationships.

NURSING DIAGNOSIS:	PARENTING, ALTERED, HIGH RISK FOR
Risk factors may include:	Chronologic age/developmental stage, lack of knowledge, lack of support between/from significant other(s), ineffective role models, unrealistic expectations for self, lack of role identity, presence of stressors.
Possibly evidenced by:	[Not applicable; presence of signs/symptoms establishes an **actual** diagnosis.]
DESIRED OUTCOMES— CLIENT WILL:	Participate in activities/classes to promote growth.
	Identify appropriate parenting role.
	Demonstrate behavior/lifestyle changes to reduce risk of short- and long-term problems.
	Use appropriate individual, family, and community resources to support the new family unit.

ACTIONS/INTERVENTIONS

Independent

Assess client's ego development, educational level, stressors, and understanding of infant capabilities.

RATIONALE

Helps identify needs for establishing educational program if client has decided to keep infant. May identify potentially abusive parent(s). Often, ability to master parenting skills effectively is directly related to educational level, socioeconomic factors, stress level, ego development, and social support.

ACTIONS/INTERVENTIONS	RATIONALE

Independent

Assess potential parenting capabilities of both teenage mother and father, if present.

Adolescent mothers and fathers, because of their own developmental needs, are less likely to be accepting, cooperative, accessible, and sensitive to their child's needs than are more mature parents.

Use visual data, audiovisual aids, film, lecture, and hands-on instruction to give information on bathing and other aspects of caring for a new baby.

Provides information about skills needed by the new parent(s).

Provide opportunity for the adolescent parent to ask questions and communicate freely.

Offers opportunity to clarify misunderstandings and allows for expressions of frustrations, disappointments, and concerns without judgment; can help both mother and father begin to cope with situation.

Make opportunities for client and involved father to interact with infants/toddlers and appropriate role models. Encourage discussion about full-time responsibility associated with children.

Helps adolescent parents to internalize/adopt appropriate parenting behaviors and gain realistic perceptions of infant capabilities/behaviors. The adolescent mother/father is a high-risk parent known to be less responsive to infant cues, more likely to use punishment and to be unrealistic in expectations of infant behavior.

Assist to develop support systems within the family and/or community.

Making contacts that allow freedom to discuss situation, fears, and confusion can help client make decisions appropriate for her and the infant. Social/extended family supports assist the client in her ability to parent effectively.

Provide information about ongoing prenatal/postnatal classes that focus on learning parenting skill and on infant capabilities, caretaking, and stimulation.

Will help to promote positive parenting. Children born to adolescent mothers are at greater risk for behavioral, social, and intellectual retardation and possible physical retardation than those children born to older mothers.

Assist client with learning methods of relaxation and ways of conserving energy.

Will help the client learn skills for keeping energy level up after the baby is born in order to care adequately for the infant. She may not be aware of her need for time out and fail to care for her own needs.

NURSING DIAGNOSIS:	FAMILY COPING, INEFFECTIVE: COMPROMISED/DISABLING, HIGH RISK FOR
Risk factors may include:	Temporary disorganization of the client's family of origin, family having difficulty providing support for the client/couple, situational and/or developmental crises the father may be facing, insufficient reciprocity of support between client and father of the baby.
Possibly evidenced by:	[Not applicable; presence of signs/symptoms establishes an **actual** diagnosis.]

ACTIONS/INTERVENTIONS	RATIONALE
Independent	
Assess family constellation/organization and nature of individual relationships to one another.	Family may consist of the client alone or may encompass an extended family, including the adolescent father and his family. The extended family may have a negative impact on the maturity and development of the young couple by either withdrawing its support or by overcompensating and interfering.
Assess individual and family response to pregnancy.	Response to pregnancy depends on culture, value systems, socioeconomic status, circumstances of pregnancy, and educational level. In some cultures, teenage parenting is common, and the girl's mother may have been a teenage mother.
Assess client's ability to achieve tasks of pregnancy concurrently with developmental tasks.	In many cases, adolescent is unable to achieve pregnancy tasks as well as normal developmental tasks. This may result in long-term psychologic effects associated with impaired adult identity formation.
Determine the client's/couple's perception of individual and collective strengths and weaknesses.	Provides information for developing an individualized plan of care.
Assess father's developmental, educational, and socioeconomic status.	Developmental tasks are disrupted for the male partner as well as for the client. His level of maturation and education may influence his decision to remain in or leave the situation/relationship.
Provide opportunities for the father to talk about his feelings and perceptions. Listen in a nonjudgmental manner.	Helps him to identify and clarify what is happening. The adolescent father needs an opportunity to verbalize his concerns, have his feelings validated, and assume an active role in all aspects of the pregnancy. (Note: In order to provide nonjudgmental listening and care, nurses need to be aware of their own moral and ethical conflicts.)
Help father, and couple as a unit, to identify stressors and ways of dealing positively with them.	Awareness of stressors can facilitate growth; effective coping promotes positive outcomes. (Note: Father/couple may already possess effective coping skills, especially if in late adolescence.)

ACTIONS/INTERVENTIONS	RATIONALE

Independent

Identify available support systems.

The adolescent father may find himself bearing the brunt of family anger and shame.

Involve father in activities related to pregnancy and childbirth.

Helps him to know that he is an integral part of the process and that his support is important to the client.

Discuss with client/couple individual expectations/plans for the future and the perception of each regarding the response of both families.

The pregnant adolescent may receive appropriate physical/emotional care while the needs of the father/couple go unidentified and/or unmet. The family may have moral/ethical conflict about providing support to a couple who may not be married or may not intend to get married. Although the relationship may not survive the stress of the pregnancy and accompanying decisions, the couple may see it as important at the moment.

Collaborative

Refer for appropriate assistance: counseling, financial, educational, and/or social services.

The father/couple/family may need help for a prolonged period, depending on how stressors are handled and whether client chooses to keep or relinquish infant.

NURSING DIAGNOSIS:	FAMILY COPING: POTENTIAL FOR GROWTH
May be related to:	Client and family achieving the developmental tasks of the pregnancy, demonstrating readiness to address goals of self-actualization.
Possibly evidenced by:	Participation in prenatal classes, physical preparation for infant, establishment of realistic goals for the future.
DESIRED OUTCOMES— FAMILY WILL:	Participate in activities related to childbearing and child-rearing.
	Seek information designed to enhance growth.
	Report feelings of confidence and satisfaction with progress being made.

ACTIONS/INTERVENTIONS	RATIONALE

Independent

Assess stage of family development and potential for growth.

Determines necessary steps to assist in further growth. A supportive family is critical to fostering growth and appropriate parenting behaviors.

Ascertain impact of cultural and maturational factors.

These factors may hinder a family from expressing or recognizing their readiness to progress. Sensitivity to these issues can facilitate growth.

Listen to client's/family's expressions of hope and plans for the future. Support continuation of formal education as appropriate.

Can build on awareness of possibilities for the situation. Early termination of education has a severe impact on the client's earning capacity throughout life.

ACTIONS/INTERVENTIONS

Independent

Assist client/family with communication skills, and provide experiences in which they can learn ways of supporting one another.

Discuss feelings about and plans for the future with client who has decided to give infant up for adoption. Include family in discussion as possible.

Collaborative

Refer to other resources as appropriate (e.g., support group or psychiatric counseling).

RATIONALE

Learning effective communication skills enhances potential for growth.

Helping this client deal with issues of loss and grieving will enable her to go on with her life in a positive manner. Family understanding of client's feelings/needs can facilitate this process.

May need additional assistance in learning to express feelings, manage crisis situations, and so forth.

NURSING DIAGNOSIS:	HOME MAINTENANCE MANAGEMENT, IMPAIRED, HIGH RISK FOR
Risk factors may include:	Chronologic age/developmental stage, lack of knowledge, inadequate support systems, insufficient finances.
Possibly evidenced by:	[Not applicable; presence of signs/symptoms establishes an **actual** diagnosis.]
DESIRED OUTCOMES— CLIENT/COUPLE OR FAMILY WILL:	Develop a plan for maintaining a clean, safe, growth-promoting environment.
	Demonstrate appropriate/effective use of resources.

ACTIONS/INTERVENTIONS

Independent

Assess developmental level; cognitive, emotional, and physical functioning; and financial situation.

Identify support systems available to the client/couple.

Assist client/significant other(s) to develop a plan for maintaining a clean, healthful environment.

Collaborative

Identify resources available for appropriate assistance.

RATIONALE

These factors may impair functioning and, therefore, influence creation of the plan of care and available options.

Availability of a good supportive network fosters positive adaptation to caretaking roles. Many teenage clients have few resources and depend on either parents and/or social agencies for assistance.

Helps develop responsibility for having an environment conducive to health and growth of mother and child.

May need help with budget counseling, financial and living arrangements, social work services, and so forth.

Cardiac Conditions _____

Blood volume increases about 45% above the nonpregnant level during pregnancy, necessitating a drop in systemic and pulmonary vascular resistance. The client with heart disease may not be able to readily accommodate for the higher workload of pregnancy due to decreased cardiac reserves.

CLIENT ASSESSMENT DATA BASE

ACTIVITY/REST

Inability to carry on normal activities.

Nocturnal/exertion-related dyspnea.

CIRCULATION

Tachycardia, palpitations.

History of congenital/organic heart disease, rheumatic fever.

Upward displacement of the diaphragm and heart proportionate to uterine size.

May have a continuous diastolic or presystolic murmur; cardiac enlargement; loud systolic murmur, associated with a thrill; severe dysrhythmia.

Blood pressure (BP) and pulse may be elevated, or BP may be decreased with decreased vascular resistance.

Clubbing of toes and fingers may be present with symmetric cyanosis in surgically untreated tetralogy of Fallot.

ELIMINATION

Urine output may be decreased.

FOOD/FLUID

Obesity.

May have edema of the lower extremities.

PAIN/COMFORT

May report chest pain with/without activity.

RESPIRATION

Cough; may or may not be productive.

Hemoptysis.

Respiratory rate may be increased.

Dyspnea/shortness of breath, orthopnea may be reported.

Rales may be present.

SAFETY

Repeated streptococcal infections.

TEACHING/LEARNING

Possible history of valve replacement/prosthetic device, Marfan's syndrome, surgically treated/untreated (rare) tetralogy of Fallot.

DIAGNOSTIC STUDIES

White blood cell (WBC) count: Leukocytosis indicative of generalized infection, primarily streptococcal.

Hemoglobin (Hb)/hematocrit (Hct): Reveals actual versus physiologic anemia; polycythemia.

Maternal arterial blood gases (ABGs): Provide secondary assessment of potential fetal compromise due to maternal respiratory involvement.

Sedimentation rate: Elevated in the presence of cardiac inflammation.

Maternal electrocardiogram (ECG): Demonstrates patterns associated with specific cardiac disorders, dysrhythmias.

Echocardiography: Diagnoses mitral valve prolapse or Marfan's syndrome.

Radionuclide cardiac imaging: Evaluates suspected atrial or ventricular septal defects, patent ductus arteriosus, or intracardiac shunts.

Amniocentesis: Determines fetal maturity.

Serial ultrasonography: Detects gestational age of fetus and possible intrauterine growth retardation (IUGR).

Biophysical profile (BPP) criteria, nonstress test (NST), contraction stress test (CST), amniotic fluid volume, fetal tone, fetal movements (FM), fetal breathing movements: Determine fetal well-being.

NURSING PRIORITIES

1. Monitor degree/progression of symptoms.
2. Promote client involvement in control of condition and self-care.
3. Monitor fetal well-being.
4. Support client/couple toward culmination of a safe delivery.

NURSING DIAGNOSIS:	CARDIAC OUTPUT, high risk for decompensation
Risk factors may include:	Increased circulating volume, dysrhythmias, altered myocardial contractility, inotropic changes in the heart.
Possibly evidenced by:	[Not applicable; presence of signs/symptoms establishes an **actual** diagnosis.]
DESIRED OUTCOMES— CLIENT WILL:	Identify/adopt behaviors to minimize stressors and maximize cardiac function.
	Tolerate the stress of increasing blood volume as indicated by BP and pulse within individually appropriate limits.
	Demonstrate adequate placental circulation, kidney function with fetal heart rate (FHR) and fetal movement within normal limits (WNL), and individually appropriate urine output.

ACTIONS/INTERVENTIONS	RATIONALE
Independent	
Determine/monitor client's functional classification (as outlined by the New York Heart Association):	Useful for identifying client needs and progression/remission of condition.

ACTIONS/INTERVENTIONS	RATIONALE
Independent	
Class I: No limitation of physical activity, no discomfort during exertion. Class II: Ordinary activity may cause symptoms of palpitation, dyspnea, and angina. Class III: Less than ordinary activity causes cardiac symptoms, such as fatigue, dyspnea, and angina. Class IV: Symptoms of cardiac insufficiency occur in the absence of physical activity.	
Monitor client's vital signs.	Beginning stage of decompensation due to intolerance of circulatory load, infection, or anxiety may first be noted by an insidious change in the vital sign pattern, associated with increased temperature, pulse (110 bpm or greater), respiration (greater than 20–34/minute), and BP.
Auscultate client's breath sounds.	Congestive heart failure (CHF) may develop, especially in clients whose functional classification is Class III or IV. Conversely, clients with mitral valve prolapse may be symptom-free during pregnancy, owing to the increase in left ventricular volume, yet are at high risk for involvement related to chest pain, palpitations, and possibly death after delivery.
Evaluate FHR, daily fetal movement count, and NST results as indicated. (Refer to CP: The High-Risk Pregnancy.)	Fetal hypoxia caused by beginning stage of maternal cardiac decompensation may be noted in the form of tachycardia, bradycardia, or reduction in fetal activity.
Provide information about the necessity of adequate rest (e.g., 8–10 hr at night and 1/2 hr after each meal).	Minimizes cardiac stress and conserves energy. Class IV clients may require bed rest for the duration of the pregnancy.
Investigative reports of chest pain and palpitations. Recommend limiting caffeine as appropriate.	Clients with mitral valve prolapse may develop arrhythmias resulting in chest pain and palpitations. Limiting caffeine may reduce frequency of episodes.
Assess for evidence of venostasis with resulting dependent edema of extremities or generalized edema. Instruct client to elevate legs when sitting down and periodically during the day.	Prolonged positioning of legs and ankles below the level of the heart further impairs venous return in an already stressed circulatory system and places the client at risk for pregnancy-induced hypertension (PIH).
Assess amount and concentration of urine output; assess urine specific gravity. Instruct client to monitor fluid intake.	Cardiovascular involvement may negatively affect kidney function, resulting in oliguria/anuria or increased specific gravity. Intake and output should be approximately the same.
Provide information regarding use of left lateral position.	The occurrence of supine hypotension to the point of loss of consciousness can be prevented if the client avoids the supine position and adopts the lateral recumbent resting position.

141

ACTIONS/INTERVENTIONS	RATIONALE

Collaborative

Administer medications such as digitalis glycosides (digoxin or digitoxin) or propranolol (Inderal) as indicated. Monitor for early labor.

Cardiac stress due to increased demand for output is greatest between 28 and 32 weeks' gestation, then levels off until delivery. Digitalis glycosides maximize ventricular contractions, but increased plasma volume may lower circulating levels of the drug, necessitating increased or more frequent doses. Digitalis has a direct effect on the myometrium, often causing early labor as well as shortening the length of labor. Propranolol may be used to control dysrhythmias associated with mitral valve prolapse. (Note: Although these drugs cross the placenta and have no reported teratogenic effects, studies have not clearly established their safety in pregnancy.)

Treat underlying respiratory infections as necessary.

Cardiac decompensation is worsened by superimposed upper respiratory infection, which is usually associated with coughing and increased secretions, and which may mask deterioration of cardiac function.

Assess placental functioning, using sequential serum/urine estriol levels and CST/NST. (Refer to CP: The High-Risk Pregnancy, ND: Injury, high risk for, fetal.)

Reduced cardiac function may negatively affect placental functioning.

Obtain/review sequential ECGs.

May demonstrate pathologic pattern if decompensation is present; identify type of dysrhythmia.

Encourage use of antithrombotic stockings.

Promotes venous return; limits venous stasis.

Prepare client for hospitalization as warranted by her condition.

Clients with a functional classification of Class II through Class IV are usually hospitalized 2 weeks before expected delivery, because likelihood of decompensation is greatest during the latter part of the third trimester. Clients with Class IV function may be hospitalized earlier in the pregnancy, depending on fetal status/developing complications.

Monitor hemodynamic pressures using arterial and central venous pressure (CVP) lines or Swan-Ganz catheter to monitor pulmonary artery wedge pressure.

CVP lines measure venous return/circulating volume; the Swan-Ganz catheter may be required to monitor pulmonary pressures and, indirectly, left-sided heart function.

NURSING DIAGNOSIS:	FLUID VOLUME EXCESS, HIGH RISK FOR
Risk factors may include:	Increasing circulating volume, changes in renal function, dietary indiscretion.
Possibly evidenced by:	[Not applicable; presence of signs/symptoms establishes an **actual** diagnosis.]

DESIRED OUTCOMES—CLIENT WILL:	Demonstrate stable fluid balance with vital signs WNL, appropriate weight gain, absence of edema.
	Verbalize understanding of restrictions/therapy needs.
	List signs that require notification of care provider.

ACTIONS/INTERVENTIONS	RATIONALE
Independent	
Obtain baseline weight. Instruct client to monitor her weight at home daily.	Weight gain exceeding the normal 2–2$\frac{1}{2}$ lb/wk may indicate accumulating fluid and potential CHF. Rule out toxemia if weight gain is sudden.
Assess dietary factors that may contribute to excessive fluid retention; provide information as needed.	Improper diet, specifically deficiency of protein and excess of sodium, contributes to fluid retention.
Assess for/review signs of CHF (e.g., dyspnea, distended neck veins, crackles, hemoptysis, and so forth).	Indicates developing failure and need for immediate treatment. The normal increase of 1,300 ml in circulatory volume that occurs in pregnancy can put stress on the cardiac system. Further increase of fluid can be especially dangerous for the client with existing cardiac problems.
Investigate unexplained cough.	Cough unrelated to respiratory problems may indicate developing CHF.
Collaborative	
Restrict fluids and sodium in presence of CHF.	Minimizes risk of fluid retention/overload.
Administer diuretics (e.g., chlorothiazide, hydrochlorothiazide).	Helps rid body of excess fluid resistant to conservative treatment of rest and decreased sodium intake.

NURSING DIAGNOSIS:	**TISSUE PERFUSION, ALTERED, HIGH RISK FOR: uteroplacental**
Risk factors may include:	Changes in circulating volume, right to left shunt.
Possibly evidenced by:	[Not applicable; presence of signs/symptoms establishes an **actual** diagnosis.]
DESIRED OUTCOMES—CLIENT WILL:	Display BP, pulse, ABGs, and WBC count WNL.
	Demonstrate adequate placental perfusion as indicated by reactive fetus with heart rate ranging from 120 to 160 bpm and size appropriate for gestational age.

ACTIONS/INTERVENTIONS	RATIONALE

Independent

Note individual risk factors and prepregnancy state.

Any preexisting cardiac problems complicated by increased circulatory needs during pregnancy may result in impaired tissue oxygenation. (Note: Such problems are greater in the older client with obesity and long-standing cardiac involvement.)

Assess BP and pulse. Note behavior changes, cyanosis of mucous membranes and nail beds, activity intolerance, and signs of decompensation (i.e., excessive weight gain, unexplained cough, crackles, wheezes, hemoptysis, and increased pulse and respiratory rate).

Tachycardia (heart rate greater than 110 bpm) at rest, increasing BP, and behavior changes may indicate early cardiac failure or hypoxia. A fall in peripheral vascular resistance may result in a worsening of right-to-left shunting and cyanosis. Presence of cyanosis, a late sign of hypoxia, reflects severe problems and indicates severity of tissue damage and cardiac compromise.

Provide information about use of modified upright position for sleeping and resting.

Eases respiratory rate by reducing pressure of the enlarging uterus on the diaphragm and helps increase vertical diameter for lung expansion. Helps prevent venous stasis in lower extremities.

Collaborative

Monitor laboratory studies as indicated:
    ABGs.

Reflects adequacy of ventilation and oxygenation.

    Hb/Hct

Anemia further reduces oxygen-carrying capacity of blood and may require treatment.

    WBC count, culture of upper/lower respiratory secretions.

Any respiratory involvement reduces intake of oxygen. Infection increases metabolic rates and oxygen needs and may have a negative impact on tissue oxygenation.

Administer antibiotics (e.g., ampicillin) as needed.

Prophylactic antibiotics help prevent bacterial endocarditis in client with diseased heart valves.

Assess uterine/fetal blood flow using NST/CST; check estriol levels and FHR. (Refer to CP: The High-Risk Pregnancy, ND: Injury, high risk for, fetal.)

Uterine/placental hypoxia reduces fetal activity and FHR, and presents as late decelerations on CST. Hypoxia may result in placental deterioration and falling estriol levels.

NURSING DIAGNOSIS:	INFECTION, HIGH RISK FOR, maternal
Risk factors may include:	Inadequate primary/secondary defenses, chronic disease/condition, insufficient information to avoid exposure to pathogens.
Possibly evidenced by:	[Not applicable; presence of signs/symptoms establishes an **actual** diagnosis.]
DESIRED OUTCOMES— CLIENT WILL:	Identify/adopt behaviors to reduce individual risk.
	Remain free of bacterial infection.
	Demonstrate appropriate use of antimicrobial agents as indicated.

ACTIONS/INTERVENTIONS	RATIONALE
Independent	
Assess for individual risk factors and history of rheumatic fever.	There is increased risk of bacterial endocarditis in the prenatal client with underlying heart disease, such as valvular damage caused by rheumatic or congenital processes, mitral valve prolapse, ventricular septal defect, tetralogy of Fallot, pulmonic stenosis, coarctation of the aorta, or prosthetic valve.
Provide information about risk of bacterial endocarditis during specific medical-surgical procedures.	Transient bacteremia may occur following medical-surgical procedures. About 60%–90% of clients develop bacteremia after dental extraction; the risk of bacteremia during parturition is 0%–5%. (Note: The client with a prosthetic valve is at high risk for bacterial endocarditis and emboli even in an uncomplicated vaginal delivery.)
Review medication needs and reason for conversion to heparin by warfarin (Coumadin) users.	Because of its large molecular size, heparin sodium does not cross the placenta as does warfarin, and it may prevent clot formation in the client with valve prosthesis.
Assist client in learning administration of medication such as heparin. Observe return demonstration of procedure by client.	Involves client in therapeutic process, and promotes self-care.
Assess for/review signs of ecchymosis, epistaxis, and so forth during anticoagulant therapy.	Signs of bleeding may indicate a need to reduce heparin levels.
Collaborative	
Administer penicillin intramuscularly or by mouth.	Prophylactic antibiotics may be recommended for prevention of streptococcal infection during pregnancy, especially in the client with previous rheumatic fever.
Administer loading dose of heparin.	Warfarin users should have their anticoagulant converted to heparin. Initial dose may be administered intravenously by healthcare provider.
Monitor blood studies, such as clotting times and electrolyte levels.	Prolonged clotting times may indicate need to adjust heparin dosage. Hyponatremia/hypokalemia may occur, owing to reduced sodium intake or diuretic therapy.

NURSING DIAGNOSIS:	**ACTIVITY INTOLERANCE, HIGH RISK FOR**
Risk factors may include:	Presence of circulatory problems, previous episodes of intolerance, deconditioned status.
Possibly evidenced by:	[Not applicable; presence of signs/symptoms establishes an **actual** diagnosis.]
DESIRED OUTCOMES— CLIENT WILL:	Demonstrate self-responsibility for monitoring activity tolerance/intolerance.
	Adopt behaviors to maximize tolerance.
	Take appropriate actions if cardiac/respiratory symptoms arise.

ACTIONS/INTERVENTIONS

Independent

Assess for development of subjective/objective symptoms (e.g., lessening of tolerance to ordinary physical activity, fatigue, cyanosis, inability to carry on normal daily activities, increasing dyspnea with or without physical activity, nocturnal dyspnea, change in pulse rate, development of respiratory symptoms).

Review signs/symptoms with the client and significant other(s).

Assist client in restructuring daily routine to reduce physical activity; include needed rest/sleep periods.

Identify need for household assistance and any available resources.

RATIONALE

Indicates a worsening of the cardiac condition evidenced by a decrease in the client's functional capacity.

Promotes self-care and timely medical interventions.

Circulatory/respiratory impairment may interfere with ability to perform and may result in fatigue. Activity is limited in relation to the extent of cardiac impairment. Clients with Class I or II limitation may only need to include midmorning and midafternoon rest periods, whereas Class III or Class IV clients may need bedrest for much or all of the day.

May be needed to maximize rest, limit fatigue, and preserve cardiac function.

NURSING DIAGNOSIS:	KNOWLEDGE DEFICIT [LEARNING NEED], regarding condition, prognosis, and treatment needs
May be related to:	Lack of exposure to and/or misinterpretation of information.
Possibly evidenced by:	Request for information, statement of misconception, inaccurate follow-through of instructions.
DESIRED OUTCOMES— CLIENT WILL:	Verbalize understanding of individual condition and treatment needs.
	Identify symptoms indicating deterioration of cardiac functioning.
	Intervene and/or notify healthcare provider appropriately.

ACTIONS/INTERVENTIONS

Independent

Assess understanding of pathology/complications regarding pregnancy. Review history, incidence of complications, and so forth.

Discuss necessity for frequent monitoring; i.e., every 2 wk during first 20 weeks, then every week until delivery.

RATIONALE

Establishes data base for health teaching. Increasingly severe cardiac symptoms may indicate client's need for more information and/or assistance to manage necessary self-care.

Provides for early detection of problems and prompt intervention.

ACTIONS/INTERVENTIONS	RATIONALE
Independent	
Provide information about symptoms indicative of cardiac involvement, such as shortness of breath, cough, palpitations, unusual or rapid weight gain (i.e., 2.2–4.4 lb or 1–2 kg in a 2-day period), edema, or anorexia.	Symptoms associated with decompensation should be differentiated from symptoms associated with PIH. (Refer to CP: Pregnancy-Induced Hypertension, ND: Fluid Volume deficit.)
Provide information as appropriate regarding diet, rest/sleep, exercise, and relaxation.	Allows client to feel some control in decision-making process; helps reduce likelihood of complications. The impact of pregnancy superimposed on an existing cardiac problem may necessitate changes in lifestyle. An understanding of techniques designed to lessen cardiac stress may require the acquisition of new knowledge.
Review need to avoid infection.	Resistance may be lowered because of general condition.
Review drug side effects (e.g., hemorrhage).	Determines client's level of knowledge and provides current information.
Discuss special considerations, such as need to avoid foods high in vitamin K (raw, deep green leafy vegetables) when on anticoagulants.	Such foods may counteract/alter anticoagulant drug effect.
Collaborative	
Include healthcare team in teaching/planning.	Provides continuity and completeness of care.
Provide appropriate information for protocol of care in community/hospital setting, as well as at home.	May foster self-responsibility and reduce anxiety.
Identify support groups for high-risk clients.	May serve as role model for necessary adaptations, enhance coping ability, and provide encouragement for a successful outcome.
(Refer to CP: Pregnancy-Induced Hypertension.)	

Pregnancy-Induced Hypertension _____

This is a disorder of unknown etiology occurring in pregnancy, manifested by hypertension (systolic pressure of 30 mm Hg and/or diastolic pressure of 15 mm Hg above baseline), edema, and proteinuria (preeclampsia) that may progress to seizures/coma (eclampsia).

CLIENT ASSESSMENT DATA BASE

CIRCULATION

Persistent increase in blood pressure (BP) over baseline readings after 20 weeks of pregnancy.

History of chronic hypertension.

Pulse may be decreased.

May have spontaneous bruising, prolonged bleeding, or epistaxis (thrombocytopenia).

ELIMINATION

Renal function may be reduced (less than 400 ml/24 hr) or absent.

FOOD/FLUID

Nausea/vomiting.

Weight gain of 2+ lb or more in 1 wk, 6 lb or more per month (depending on length of gestation).

Malnourished (overweight or underweight by 20% or greater); poor protein/caloric intake.

Edema may be present, ranging from mild to severe/generalized and may involve facies, extremities, and organ systems (i.e., liver, brain).

Diabetes mellitus.

NEUROSENSORY

Dizziness, frontal headaches.

Diplopia, blurred vision.

Hyperreflexia.

Convulsions—tonic, then tonic-clonic phases, followed by a period of loss of consciousness.

Funduscopic examination may reveal edema or vascular spasm.

PAIN/DISCOMFORT

Pain in epigastric (right upper quadrant [RUQ]) region.

RESPIRATION

Respirations may be less than 14/minute.

Crackles may be present.

SAFETY

Rh incompatibility may be present.

SEXUALITY

Primigravida, multiple gestation, hydramnios, hydatidiform mole, hydrops fetalis (Rh antigen–antibody).

Fetal movement may be diminished.

Signs of abruptio placentae may be present.

TEACHING/LEARNING

Adolescent (under age 15 years) and elderly primigravida (age 35 years or older) are at greatest risk.

Family history of pregnancy-induced hypertension (PIH).

DIAGNOSTIC STUDIES

Supine pressor test ("rollover test"): May be used to screen for clients at risk for PIH, between 28–32 weeks' gestation, although accuracy is questionable; an increase of 20–30 mm Hg in systolic pressure or 15–20 mm Hg in diastolic pressure indicates a positive test.

Mean arterial pressure (MAP): 90 mm Hg at second trimester indicates PIH.

Hematocrit (Hct): Elevated with fluid shifts, or decreased in HELLP syndrome (hemolysis, elevated liver enzymes, low platelet count).

Hemoglobin (Hb): Low when hemolysis occurs (HELLP syndrome).

Peripheral smear: Distended blood cells or schistocytes in HELLP syndrome or intravascular hemolysis.

Serum platelet counts: Less than 100,000/mm^3 in disseminated intravascular coagulation (DIC) or in HELLP syndrome, as platelets adhere to collagen released from damaged blood vessels.

Serum creatinine level: Elevated.

AST (SGOT), lactic dehydrogenase (LDH), and serum bilirubin levels (indirect particularly): Elevated in HELLP syndrome with liver involvement.

Uric acid level: As high as 7 mg/100 ml, if renal involvement is severe.

Prothrombin time (PT), partial thromboplastin time (PTT), clotting time: Prolonged; fibrinogen decreased; fibrin split products (FSP) and fibrin degradation products (FDP) positive when coagulopathy occurs.

Urine specific gravity: Elevated, reflecting fluid shifts/vascular dehydration.

Proteinuria: By dipstick may be 1+ to 2+ (moderate), 3+ to 4+ (severe), or greater than 5 g/L in 24 hours.

Urinary/plasma estriol levels: Decline indicates reduced placental functioning. (Estriols are not as useful a predictor as biophysical profile [BPP] due to the lag time between fetal problem and test results.)

Human placental lactogen levels: Less than 4 mEq/ml suggests abnormal placental functioning (not frequently done in PIH screening).

Ultrasonography: At 20 to 26 weeks' gestation and repeated 6–10 wk later, establishes gestational age and detects intrauterine growth retardation (IUGR).

Tests of amniotic fluid (lecithin to sphingomyelin [L/S] ratio, phosphatidylglycerol (pg), saturated phosphatidylcholine levels): Determine fetal lung maturity.

BPP, including amniotic fluid volume, fetal tone, fetal breathing movements (FBM), fetal movements, and fetal heart rate reactivity/nonstress test: Determines fetal risk/well-being.

Contraction stress test (CST): Assesses the response of the fetus to the stress of uterine contractions.

NURSING PRIORITIES

1. Monitor maternal, fetal, and placental status.
2. Prevent or reduce progressive fluid accumulation or complications.
3. Promote positive maternal/fetal outcome.
4. Provide information to enhance self-care.

<table>
<tr><td>NURSING DIAGNOSIS:</td><td>FLUID VOLUME DEFICIT [REGULATORY FAILURE]</td></tr>
<tr><td>May be related to:</td><td>Plasma protein loss, decreasing plasma colloid osmotic pressure allowing fluid shifts out of the vascular compartment.</td></tr>
<tr><td>Possibly evidenced by:</td><td>Edema formation, sudden weight gain, hemoconcentration, nausea/vomiting, epigastric pain, headaches, visual changes, decreased urine output.</td></tr>
<tr><td rowspan="4">DESIRED OUTCOMES—CLIENT WILL:</td><td>Verbalize understanding of need for close monitoring of weight, BP, urine protein, and edema.</td></tr>
<tr><td>Participate in therapeutic regimen and monitoring as indicated.</td></tr>
<tr><td>Display hematocrit (Hct) within normal limits (WNL) and physiologic edema with no signs of pitting.</td></tr>
<tr><td>Be free of signs of generalized edema (i.e., epigastric pain, cerebral symptoms, dyspnea, nausea/vomiting).</td></tr>
</table>

ACTIONS/INTERVENTIONS	RATIONALE

Independent

Weigh client routinely. Encourage client to monitor weight at home between visits.	Sudden, significant weight gain (e.g., more than 1.5 Kg/month in the second trimester or more than 0.5 Kg/wk in the third trimester) reflects fluid retention. Fluid moves from the vascular to interstitial space, resulting in edema.
Distinguish between physiologic and pathologic edema of pregnancy. Monitor location and degree of pitting.	The presence of pitting edema (mild, 1+ to 2+; severe, 3+ to 4+) of face, hands, legs, sacral area, or abdominal wall, or edema that does not disappear after 12 hr of bedrest, is significant.
Note signs of progressive or excessive edema (i.e., epigastric/RUQ pain, cerebral symptoms, nausea, vomiting). Assess for possible eclampsia. (Refer to ND: Injury, high risk for, maternal.)	Edema and intravascular fibrin deposition (in HELLP syndrome) within the encapsulated liver are manifested by RUQ pain, dyspnea indicating pulmonary involvement, cerebral edema possibly leading to seizures, and nausea and vomiting indicating gastrointestinal (GI) edema.
Note changes in Hct/Hb levels.	Identifies degree of hemoconcentration caused by fluid shift. If Hct is less than 3 times Hb level, hemoconcentration exists.
Reassess dietary intake of proteins and calories. Provide information as needed.	Adequate nutrition reduces incidence of prenatal hypovolemia and hypoperfusion; inadequate protein/calories increases the risk of edema formation and PIH. Intake of 80–100 g of protein may be required daily to replace losses.
Monitor intake and output. Note urine color, and measure specific gravity as indicated.	Urine output is a sensitive indicator of circulatory blood volume. Oliguria and specific gravity of 1.040 indicate severe hypovolemia and kidney involvement. (Note: Administration of magnesium sulfate ($MgSO_4$) may cause transient increase in output.)

ACTIONS/INTERVENTIONS

Independent

Test clean voided urine for protein each visit, or daily/hourly if hospitalized. Report readings of 2+, or greater.

Assess lung sounds and respiratory rate/effort.

Monitor BP and pulse. (Refer to ND: Cardiac Output, decreased.)

Answer questions and review rationale for avoiding use of diuretics to treat edema.

Collaborative

Schedule prenatal visit every 1–2 wk if PIH is mild; weekly if severe.

Review moderate sodium intake of up to 6 g/day. Instruct client to avoid foods high in sodium (e.g., bacon, luncheon meats, hot dogs, and potato chips).

Place client on strict regimen of bedrest; encourage left lateral position.

Replace fluids either orally or parenterally, via infusion pump, as indicated.

When fluid deficit is severe and client is hospitalized:

Insert indwelling catheter if kidney output is reduced or is less than 50 ml/hr.

Assist with insertion of lines and/or monitoring of invasive hemodynamic parameters, such as central venous pressure (CVP) and pulmonary artery wedge pressure (PAWP).

RATIONALE

Aids in determining degree of severity/progression of condition. A 2+ reading suggests glomerular edema or spasm. Proteinuria affects fluid shifts from the vascular tree. (Note: Urine contaminated by vaginal secretions may test positive for protein.)

Dyspnea and crackles may indicate pulmonary edema, which requires immediate treatment.

Elevation in BP may occur in response to catecholamines, vasopressin, prostaglandins, and, as findings suggest, recent decreased levels of prostacyclin.

Diuretics further increase state of dehydration by decreasing intravascular volume and placental perfusion, and they may cause thrombocytopenia, hyperbilirubinemia, or alteration in carbohydrate metabolism in fetus/newborn. (Note: May be useful in presence of pulmonary edema.)

May be necessary to monitor changes more closely.

Some sodium intake is necessary because levels below 2 to 4 g/day result in greater dehydration in some clients.

Left lateral recumbent position decreases pressure on the vena cava, increasing venous return and circulatory volume. This enhances placental and renal perfusion, reduces adrenal activity, and may lower BP and account for weight loss of up to 4 lb in 24-hr period through diuresis.

Fluid replacement corrects hypovolemia, yet must be administered cautiously to prevent overload, especially if interstitial fluid is drawn back into circulation when activity is reduced. With renal involvement, fluid intake is restricted; i.e., if output is reduced (less than 700 ml/24 hr), total fluid intake is restricted to approximate output plus insensible loss.

Allows more accurate monitoring of output/renal perfusion.

Provides a more accurate measurement of fluid volume. In normal pregnancy, plasma volume increases by 30%–50%, yet this increase does not occur in the client with PIH.

ACTIONS/INTERVENTIONS	RATIONALE
Collaborative	
Administer plasma expander or osmotic diuretic, if necessary.	May help to draw fluid back into intravascular compartment. Such treatment is controversial because it may compromise cardiac functioning and placental circulation.
Monitor serum uric acid and creatinine levels, and blood urea nitrogen (BUN).	Elevated levels, especially of uric acid, indicate impaired kidney function, worsening of maternal condition, and poor fetal outcome.

NURSING DIAGNOSIS:	**CARDIAC OUTPUT, DECREASED**
May be related to:	Hypovolemia/decreased venous return, increased systemic vascular resistance.
Possibly evidenced by:	Variations in blood pressure/hemodynamic readings, edema, shortness of breath, change in mental status.
DESIRED OUTCOMES— CLIENT WILL:	Remain normotensive throughout remainder of pregnancy.
	Report absence and/or decreased episodes of dyspnea.
	Alter activity level as condition warrants.

ACTIONS/INTERVENTIONS	RATIONALE
Independent	
Monitor BP and pulse.	The client with PIH does not manifest the normal cardiovascular response to pregnancy (left ventricular hypertrophy, increase in plasma volume, vascular relaxation with decreased peripheral resistance). Hypertension (the second manifestation of PIH after edema) occurs owing to increased sensitization to angiotensin II, which increases BP, promotes aldosterone release to increase sodium/water reabsorption from the renal tubules, and constricts blood vessels.
Assess MAP at 22 weeks' gestation. A pressure of 90 mm Hg is considered predictive of PIH. Assess for crackles, gurgles, and dyspnea; note respiratory rate/effort.	Pulmonary edema may occur, with changes in peripheral vascular resistance and decline in plasma colloid osmotic pressure.
Institute bedrest with client in left lateral position.	Increases venous return, cardiac output, and renal/placental perfusion.
Collaborative	
Monitor invasive hemodynamic parameters.	Provides accurate picture of vascular changes and fluid volume. Prolonged vascular constriction, increased hemoconcentration, and fluid shifts decrease cardiac output.

ACTIONS/INTERVENTIONS

Collaborative

Administer antihypertensive drug such as hydralazine (Apresoline) P.O./I.V., so that diastolic readings are between 90 and 110 mm Hg. Follow with administration of methyldopa (Aldomet) for maintenance therapy as needed.

Monitor BP and side effects of antihypertensive drugs. Administer propranolol as appropriate.

Prepare for birth of fetus by cesarean delivery, if vaginal delivery is not feasible, when severe PIH/eclamptic condition is stabilized.

RATIONALE

If BP does not respond to conservative measures, medication may be necessary. Antihypertensive drugs act directly on arterioles to promote relaxation of cardiovascular smooth muscle and help increase blood supply to cerebrum, kidneys, uterus, and placenta. Hydralazine is the drug of choice because it does not produce effects on the fetus.

Side effects include tachycardia, headache, nausea and vomiting, and palpitations; may be treated with propranolol. Newer drugs, such as ketanserin, and sodium nitroprusside (especially in HELLP syndrome) are being used with some success to lower BP.

Surgical procedure is the only means of halting the hypertensive problems if conservative treatment is ineffective and labor induction is ruled out.

NURSING DIAGNOSIS:	TISSUE PERFUSION, ALTERED, uteroplacental
May be related to:	Maternal hypovolemia, interruption of blood flow (progressive vasospasm of spiral arteries).
Possibly evidenced by:	Intrauterine growth retardation, changes in fetal activity/heart rate, premature delivery, fetal demise.
DESIRED OUTCOMES—FETUS WILL:	Demonstrate normal CNS reactivity on NST (nonstress test); be free of late decelerations; have no decrease in fetal heart rate on CST/OCT (contraction stress test/oxytocin challenge test).
	Be full-term, AGA.

ACTIONS/INTERVENTIONS

Independent

Provide information to client/couple regarding home assessment/recording of daily fetal movements.

Identify factors affecting fetal activity.

RATIONALE

Reduced placental blood flow results in reduced gas exchange and impaired nutritional functioning of the placenta. Potential outcomes of poor placental perfusion include a malnourished, low-birth-weight infant and prematurity associated with early delivery, abruptio placentae, and fetal death. Reduced fetal activity indicates fetal compromise and occurs prior to detectable alteration in fetal heart rate (FHR).

Cigarette smoking, medication/drug use, serum glucose levels, environmental sounds, time of day, and sleep-wake cycle of the fetus can increase or decrease fetal movement.

ACTIONS/INTERVENTIONS	RATIONALE

Independent

Review signs of abruptio placentae (i.e., vaginal bleeding, uterine tenderness, abdominal pain, and decreased fetal activity).

Prompt recognition and intervention increase the likelihood of a positive outcome.

Provide contact number for client to ask questions, report changes in daily fetal movements, and so forth.

Provides opportunity to address concerns/misconceptions and intervene in a timely manner as indicated.

Evaluate fetal growth; measure progressive fundal growth at each visit.

Decreased placental functioning may accompany PIH, resulting in IUGR. Chronic intrauterine stress and uteroplacental insufficiency decrease amount of fetal contribution to amniotic fluid pool.

Note fetal response to medications such as $MgSO_4$, phenobarbital, and diazepam.

Depressant effects of medication reduce fetal respiratory and cardiac function and fetal activity level, even though placental circulation may be adequate.

Monitor FHR manually or electronically, as indicated.

Evaluates fetal well-being. An elevated FHR may indicate a compensatory response to hypoxia, prematurity, or abruptio placentae.

Collaborative

Assess fetal response to BPP criteria or CST, as maternal status indicates. (Refer to ND: Injury, high risk for, maternal.)

BPP helps evaluate fetus and fetal environment on five specific parameters to assess CNS function and fetal contribution to amniotic fluid volume. CST assesses placental functioning and reserves.

Assist with assessment of fetal maturity and well-being using L/S ratio, presence of pg, estriol levels, FBM, and sequential sonography beginning at 20 to 26 weeks' gestation. (Refer to CP: The High-Risk Pregnancy, ND: Injury, high risk for, fetal.)

In the event of deteriorating maternal/fetal condition, risks of delivering a preterm infant are weighed against the risks of continuing the pregnancy, using results from evaluative studies of lung and kidney maturity, fetal growth, and placental functioning. IUGR is associated with reduced maternal volume and vascular changes.

Assist with assessment of maternal plasma volume at 24 to 26 weeks' gestation using Evans blue dye, when indicated.

Identifies fetus at risk for IUGR or intrauterine fetal demise associated with reduced plasma volume and reduced placental perfusion.

Assist with assessment of placental size using ultrasonography.

Decreased placental function and size are associated with PIH.

Administer corticosteroid (dexamethasone, betamethasone) I.M. for at least 24–48 hr but not more than 7 days before delivery when severe PIH necessitates premature delivery between 28 and 34 weeks' gestation.

Corticosteroids are thought to induce fetal pulmonary maturity (surfactant production) and prevent respiratory distress syndrome, at least in fetus delivered prematurely because of condition or inadequate placental functioning. Best results are obtained when fetus is less than 34 weeks' and delivery occurs within a week of corticosteroid administration.

NURSING DIAGNOSIS:	INJURY, HIGH RISK FOR, maternal
May be related to:	Tissue edema/hypoxia, tonic-clonic convulsions, abnormal blood profile and/or clotting factors.
Possibly evidenced by:	[Not applicable: presence of signs/symptoms establishes an **actual** diagnosis.]
DESIRED OUTCOMES— CLIENT WILL:	Participate in treatment and/or environmental modifications to protect self and enhance safety.
	Be free of signs of cerebral ischemia (visual disturbances, headache, changes in mentation).
	Display normal levels of clotting factors and liver enzymes.

ACTIONS/INTERVENTIONS	RATIONALE

Independent

ACTIONS/INTERVENTIONS	RATIONALE
Assess for CNS involvement (i.e., headache, irritability, visual disturbances or changes on funduscopic examination).	Cerebral edema and vasoconstriction can be evaluated in terms of symptoms, behaviors, or retinal changes.
Stress importance of client reporting signs/symptoms of CNS involvement.	Delayed treatment or progressive onset of symptoms may result in tonic-clonic convulsions or eclampsia.
Note changes in level of consciousness.	In progressive PIH, vasoconstriction and vasospasms of cerebral blood vessels reduce oxygen consumption by 20% and result in cerebral ischemia.
Assess for signs of impending eclampsia: hyperactivity (3+ to 4+) of deep tendon reflexes, ankle clonus, decreased pulse and respirations, epigastric pain, and oliguria (less than 50 ml/hr).	Generalized edema/vasoconstriction, manifested by severe CNS, kidney, liver, cardiovascular, and respiratory involvement, precede convulsive state.
Institute measures to reduce likelihood of seizures; i.e., keep room quiet and dimly lit, limit visitors, plan and coordinate care, and promote rest.	Reduces environmental factors that may stimulate irritable cerebrum and cause a convulsive state.
Implement seizure precautions per protocol.	Reduces risk of injury if seizure does occur.
In the event of a seizure, turn client on side; insert airway/bite block if mouth is relaxed; suction nasopharynx, as indicated; administer oxygen; remove restrictive clothing; do not restrict movement; and document motor involvement, duration of seizure, and postseizure behavior.	Maintains airway by reducing risk of aspiration and preventing tongue from occluding airway. Maximizes oxygenation. (Note: Be cautious with use of airway/bite block; do not attempt to insert when jaws are set because injury may occur.)
Palpate for uterine tenderness or rigidity; check for vaginal bleeding. Note history of other medical problems.	These signs may indicate abruptio placentae, especially if there is a preexisting medical problem such as diabetes mellitus or a renal or cardiac disorder causing vascular involvement.
Monitor for signs and symptoms of labor or uterine contractions.	Convulsions increase uterine irritability; labor may ensue.

ACTIONS/INTERVENTIONS	RATIONALE
Independent	
Monitor for signs of DIC: easy/spontaneous bruising, prolonged bleeding, epistaxis, GI bleeding. (Refer to CP: Prenatal Hemorrhage.)	Abruptio placentae with release of thromboplastin predisposes client to DIC.
Collaborative	
Hospitalize if CNS involvement is present.	Prompt initiation of therapy helps to ensure safety and limit complications.
Administer amobarbital or diazepam, as indicated.	Depresses cerebral activity; has sedative effect when convulsions are not controlled by $MgSO_4$.
Administer $MgSO_4$ I.M. (using Z-track technique) or I.V. using infusion pump.	$MgSO_4$, a CNS depressant, decreases acetylcholine release, blocks neuromuscular transmission, and prevents seizures. It has a transient effect of lowering BP and increasing urine output by altering vascular response to pressor substances. Although I.V. administration of $MgSO_4$ is easier to regulate in the event of a toxic reaction, some facilities may still use the I.M. route if continuous surveillance is not possible and/or if appropriate infusion apparatus is not available. (Note: Addition of 1 ml of 2% lidocaine to the I.M. injection may reduce associated discomfort.)
Monitor BP before, during, and after $MgSO_4$ administration. Note serum magnesium levels in conjunction with respiratory rate, patellar reflex, and urine output.	A therapeutic level of $MgSO_4$ is achieved with serum levels of 4.0–7.5 mEq/L or 6 to 8 mg/dl. Adverse/toxic reactions develop above 10–12 mg/dl, with loss of reflexes occurring first, respiratory paralysis between 15 to 17 mg/dl, or heart block occurring at 30 to 35 mg/dl.
Have calcium gluconate available. Administer 10 ml (1 g/10 ml) over 3 minutes as indicated.	Serves as antidote to counteract adverse/toxic effects of $MgSO_4$.
Perform funduscopic examination daily.	Helps to evaluate changes or severity of retinal involvement.
Monitor test results of clotting time, PT, PTT, fibrinogen levels, and FSP/FDP.	Such tests can indicate depletion of coagulation factors and fibrinolysis, which suggest DIC.
Monitor sequential platelet count. Avoid amniocentesis if platelet count is less than 50,000/mm^3. If thrombocytopenia is present during operative procedure, use general anesthesia. Transfuse with platelets, packed red blood cells, fresh frozen plasma, or whole blood as indicated. Rule out HELLP syndrome.	Thrombocytopenia may occur due to platelet adherence to disrupted endothelium or reduced prostacyclin levels (a potent inhibitor of platelet aggregation). Anesthesia requiring needle puncture (such as spinal/epidural) could result in excessive bleeding.
Monitor liver enzymes and bilirubin; note hemolysis and presence of Burr cells on peripheral smear.	Elevated liver enzyme (AST [SGOT], ALT [SGPT]) and bilirubin levels, microangiopathic hemolytic anemia, and thrombocytopenia may indicate presence of HELLP syndrome, signifying a need for immediate cesarean delivery if condition of cervix is unfavorable for induction of labor.
Prepare for cesarean birth, if PIH is severe, placental functioning is compromised, and cervix is not ripe or is not responsive to induction.	When fetal oxygenation is severely reduced owing to vasoconstriction within malfunctioning placenta, immediate delivery may be necessary to save the fetus.

NURSING DIAGNOSIS:	NUTRITION, ALTERED, LESS THAN BODY REQUIRE-MENTS, HIGH RISK FOR
May be related to:	Intake insufficient to meet metabolic demands and replace losses.
Possibly evidenced by:	[Not applicable; presence of signs/symptoms establishes an **actual** diagnosis.]
DESIRED OUTCOMES— CLIENT WILL:	Verbalize understanding of individual dietary needs.
	Demonstrate knowledge of proper diet as evidenced by developing a dietary plan within own financial resources.
	Display appropriate weight gain.

ACTIONS/INTERVENTIONS	RATIONALE
Independent	
Assess client's nutritional status, condition of hair and nails, and prepregnancy weight and height.	Establishes guidelines for determining dietary needs and educating client. Malnutrition may be a contributing factor to the onset of PIH, specifically when client follows a low-protein diet, has insufficient caloric intake, and is overweight or underweight by 20% or more before pregnancy.
Provide information about normal weight gain in pregnancy, modifying it to meet client's needs.	The underweight client may need a diet higher in calories; the obese client should avoid dieting because it places the fetus at risk for ketosis.
Provide oral/written information about action and uses of protein and its role in development of PIH.	Daily intake of 1.5 g/kg is sufficient to replace proteins lost in urine and allow for normal serum oncotic pressure.
Provide information about effect of bedrest and reduced activity on protein requirements.	Reducing metabolic rate through bedrest and limited activity decreases protein needs.

NURSING DIAGNOSIS:	KNOWLEDGE DEFICIT [LEARNING NEED], regarding condition, prognosis, and treatment needs
May be related to:	Lack of exposure/unfamiliarity with information resources, misinterpretation.
Possibly evidenced by:	Request for information, statement of misconceptions, inaccurate follow-through of instructions, development of preventable complications.
DESIRED OUTCOMES— CLIENT/COUPLE WILL:	Verbalize understanding of disease process and appropriate treatment plan.
	Identify signs/symptoms requiring medical evaluation.
	Perform necessary procedures correctly.
	Initiate lifestyle/behavior changes as indicated.

ACTIONS/INTERVENTIONS	RATIONALE
Independent	
Assess client's/couple's knowledge of the disease process. Provide information about pathophysiology of PIH, implications for mother and fetus, and the rationale for interventions, procedures, and tests, as needed.	Establishes data base and provides information about areas in which learning is needed. Receiving information can promote understanding and reduce fear, helping to facilitate the treatment plan for the client. (Note: Current research in progress may provide additional treatment options, such as using low-dose [60 mg/day] aspirin to reduce thromboxane generation by platelets, limiting the severity/incidence of PIH.)
Provide information about signs/symptoms indicating worsening of condition, and instruct client when to notify healthcare provider.	Helps ensure that client seeks timely treatment and may prevent worsening of preeclamptic state or additional complications.
Keep client informed of health status, results of tests, and fetal well-being.	Fears and anxieties can be compounded when client/couple does not have adequate information about the state of the disease process or its impact on client and fetus.
Instruct client in how to monitor her own weight at home, and tell her to notify healthcare provider if gain is in excess of 2 lb per week, or 0.5 lb/day.	Gain of 3 lb or greater per month in second trimester or 1 lb or greater per week in third trimester is suggestive of PIH.
Assist family members in learning the procedure for home monitoring of BP, as indicated. Review techniques for stress management and diet restriction.	BP elevation occurs owing to increased resistance to cardiac output. Review reinforces importance of client's responsibility in treatment.
Provide information about ensuring adequate protein in diet for client with possible or mild preeclampsia.	Protein is necessary for intravascular and extravascular fluid regulation.
Review self-testing of urine for protein. Reinforce rationale for and implications of testing.	A test result of 2+ or greater is significant and needs to be reported to healthcare provider. Urine specimen contaminated by vaginal discharge or RBCs may produce positive test result for protein.
(Refer to CP: The High-Risk Pregnancy.)	

Diabetes Mellitus: Prepregnancy/Gestational _____

This disorder of carbohydrate metabolism of variable severity may be preexisting (pregestational insulin-dependent diabetes mellitus [IDDM] or non-insulin-dependent diabetes mellitus [NIDDM]), or may develop during pregnancy (gestational diabetes mellitus [GDM]).

CLIENT ASSESSMENT DATA BASE

CIRCULATION

Pedal pulse and capillary refill of extremities may be diminished or slowed with diabetes of long duration.

Edema, elevated BP. (Refer to CP: Pregnancy-Induced Hypertension.)

ELIMINATION

May have history of pyelonephritis, recurrent urinary tract infection (UTI), nephropathy.

Polyuria.

FOOD/FLUID

Polydipsia, polyphagia.

Nausea and vomiting.

Obesity; excessive or inadequate weight gain (client with GDM is usually obese; client with IDDM is usually not obese prior to pregnancy).

Abdominal tenderness.

May report episodes of hypoglycemia, glycosuria.

SAFETY

Skin integrity/sensation of arms, thighs, buttocks, and abdomen may be altered from frequent injections of insulin.

Visual impairment/retinopathy may be present.

History of symptoms of infection and/or positive cultures for infection, especially urinary or vaginal.

SEXUALITY

Fundal height may be higher or lower than normal for gestational age (hydramnios, inappropriate fetal growth).

History of large for gestational age (LGA) neonate, hydramnios, congenital anomalies, unexplained still-birth.

SOCIAL INTERACTION

Socioeconomic concerns/factors can increase risk of complications.

Inadequate or lack of committed support system (may adversely affect diabetic control).

TEACHING/LEARNING

Client's own birth weight may have been 9 lb or more.

May report recent problems/change in stability of diabetes.

Family history of diabetes, gestational diabetes, pregnancy-induced hypertension (PIH), infertility problem; LGA infant, history of neonatal death(s), stillbirth, congenital anomalies, spontaneous abortion, hydramnios, macrosomia (greater than 4,000 g or 9 lb at birth).

DIAGNOSTIC STUDIES

Glycosylated hemoglobin (HbA$_{1C}$): Reveals diabetic control (HbA$_{1C}$ greater than 8.5%, especially before pregnancy, puts the fetus at risk for congenital anomalies).
Random serum glucose level: Determines immediate diabetic control.
Urine ketone levels: Determines nutritional state.
Urine culture: Identify asymptomatic UTI.
Protein and creatinine clearance (24 hour): Verify level of kidney function, especially in diabetes of long duration.
Thyroid function tests: Establish baseline and/or identify coexisting hypothyroidism or hyperthyroidism.
Hemoglobin/hematocrit (Hb/Hct): May reveal anemia.
Triglycerides and cholesterol levels: May be elevated.
Estriol level: Indicates level of placental function.
Glucose tolerance test (GTT): Elevated at 20 or 28 weeks' gestation.
Glycosylated albumin: Measures diabetic control; screens for GDM. (If screening result is positive, GTT and glucose challenge test should be done at 24 to 28 weeks' gestation, to screen for gestational diabetes.)
Electrocardiogram (ECG): May reveal altered cardiovascular function in diabetes of long duration.
Vaginal culture: May be positive for *Candida albicans* (monilia infection).
Nonstress test (NST): May demonstrate reduced fetal response to maternal activity.
Serial ultrasonography: Determines presence of macrosomia or intrauterine growth retardation (IUGR).
Contraction stress test (CST), oxytocin challenge test (OCT): Positive results indicate placental insufficiency.
Amniocentesis: Ascertains fetal lung maturity using lecithin to sphingomyelin (L/S) ratio or presence of phosphatidylglycerol (pg).
Biophysical profile (BPP) criteria: Assesses fetal well-being/maturity.

NURSING PRIORITIES

1. Determine immediate and previous 8-week diabetic control.
2. Evaluate ongoing client/fetal well-being.
3. Achieve and maintain normoglycemia (euglycemia).
4. Provide client/couple with appropriate information.

NURSING DIAGNOSIS:	NUTRITION, ALTERED, LESS THAN BODY REQUIREMENTS, HIGH RISK FOR
Risk factors may include:	Inability to ingest/utilize nutrients appropriately.
Possibly evidenced by:	[Not applicable; presence of signs/symptoms establishes an **actual** diagnosis.]
DESIRED OUTCOMES—CLIENT WILL:	Gain 24–30 lb prenatally, or as appropriate for prepregnancy weight.
	Maintain fasting blood glucose (FBS) levels between 60–100 mg/dl, and 1 hour postprandial no higher than 140 mg/dl.
	Verbalize understanding of individual treatment regimen and need for frequent self-monitoring.

ACTIONS/INTERVENTIONS	RATIONALE

Independent

Weigh client each prenatal visit. Encourage client to periodically monitor weight at home between visits.	Weight gain is the key index for deciding caloric adjustments.
Assess caloric intake and dietary pattern using 24-hour recall.	Aids in evaluating client's understanding of and/or adherence to dietary regimen.
Review/provide information regarding required changes in diabetic management; i.e., switch from oral agents to insulin if not done prior to conception, use of Humulin insulin only, self-monitoring of serum glucose levels at least 6 times a day (e.g., before and 1 hour after each meal), and reducing carbohydrates in the diet.	Metabolism and fetal/maternal needs change greatly during gestation, requiring close monitoring and adaptation. Research suggests antibodies against insulin may cross the placenta, causing inappropriate fetal weight gain. The use of human insulin decreases the development of these antibodies. Reducing carbohydrates to less than 40% of the calories ingested decreases the degree of the postprandial glucose peak or hyperglycemia. Because pregnancy produces severe morning carbohydrate intolerance, the first meal of the day should be small, with minimal carbohydrates.
Review importance of regularity of meals and snacks (e.g., 3 meals/4 snacks) when taking insulin.	Small, frequent meals avoid postprandial hyperglycemia and fasting/starvation ketosis.
Note presence of nausea and vomiting, especially in first trimester.	Nausea and vomiting may result in carbohydrate deficiency, which may lead to metabolism of fats and development of ketosis.
Assess understanding of the effect of stress on diabetes. Provide information about stress management and relaxation. (Refer to CP: The High-Risk Pregnancy.)	Stress can elevate glucose levels, creating fluctuations in insulin needs.
Teach client finger-stick method for self-monitoring of glucose using enzyme strips and reflectance meters. Have client demonstrate procedure.	Insulin needs for the day can be adjusted based on periodic serum glucose readings. (Note: Values obtained by reflectance meters are 15% lower than plasma values.)
Recommend monitoring urine for ketones on awakening and when a planned meal or snack is delayed.	Insufficient caloric intake is reflected by ketonuria, indicating need for an increase of carbohydrates or addition of an extra snack in the dietary plan (i.e., recurrent presence of ketonuria on awakening may be eliminated by a 3 A.M. glass of milk).
Review/discuss signs and symptoms and significance of hypoglycemia or hyperglycemia.	Hypoglycemia may be more sudden or severe in first trimester, owing to increased usage of glucose and glycogen by client and developing fetus, as well as low levels of the insulin antagonist human placental lactogen (HPL). Ketoacidosis occurs more frequently in second and third trimesters because of the increased resistance to insulin and elevated HPL levels. Sustained or intermittent pulses of hyperglycemia are mutagenic and teratogenic for the fetus during the first trimester; may also cause fetal hyperinsulinemia, macrosomia, inhibition of lung maturity, cardiac

ACTIONS/INTERVENTIONS	RATIONALE
Independent	
	dysrhythmias, neonatal hypoglycemia, and risk of permanent neurologic damage. Maternal effects of hyperglycemia can include hydramnios, UTI and/or vaginal infections, hypertension, and spontaneous termination of pregnancy.
Instruct client to treat symptomatic hypoglycemia, if it occurs, with an 8-oz glass of milk and to repeat in 15 min if serum glucose level remains below 70 mg/dl.	Using large amounts of simple carbohydrates to treat hypoglycemia causes blood glucose values to overshoot. A combination of complex carbohydrates and protein maintains normoglycemia longer and helps maintain stability of blood glucose throughout the day.
Collaborative	
Discuss dosage, schedule and type of insulin (i.e., usually 4 times/day: 7:30 A.M.—NPH, 10 A.M.—Regular, 4 P.M.—NPH, 6 P.M.—Regular).	Division of insulin dosage considers maternal basal needs and mealtime insulin-to-food ratio, and allows more freedom in meal scheduling. Total daily dosage is based on gestational age, current maternal body weight, and serum glucose levels. A mix of NPH and Regular human insulin helps mimic the normal insulin release pattern of the pancreas minimizing "peak/valley" effect of serum glucose level.
Adjust diet or insulin regimen to meet individual needs.	Prenatal metabolic needs change throughout the trimesters, and adjustment is determined by weight gain and laboratory test results. Insulin needs in the first trimester are 0.7 unit/kg of body weight. Between 18 and 24 weeks' gestation, they increase to 0.8 unit/kg body weight; at 34 weeks' gestation, 0.9 unit/kg body weight, and 1.0 unit/kg body weight by 36 weeks' gestation.
Refer to registered dietitian to individualize diet and counsel regarding dietary questions.	Diet specific to the individual is necessary to maintain normoglycemia and to obtain desired weight gain. In-depth teaching promotes understanding of own needs and clarifies misconceptions, especially for client with GDM. (Note: New recommendations [Peterson, Peterson, 1992] set dietary needs at 25 kcal/kg dependent on the client's current pregnant weight.)
Monitor serum glucose levels (FBS, preprandial, 1 and 2 hours postprandial) on initial visit, then as indicated by client's condition.	Incidence of fetal and newborn abnormalities is decreased when FBS levels range between 60 and 100 mg/dl, preprandial levels between 60 and 105 mg/dl, 1-hour postprandial remains below 140 mg/dl, and 2-hour postprandial is less than 120 mg/dl.
Ascertain results of HbA_{1c} every 2–4 wk.	Provides accurate picture of average serum glucose control during the preceding 60 days. Serum glucose control takes 6 weeks to stabilize.
Prepare for hospitalization if diabetes is not controlled.	Infant morbidity is linked to maternal hyperglycemia-induced fetal hyperinsulinemia.

NURSING DIAGNOSIS:	INJURY, HIGH RISK FOR, fetal
Risk factors may include:	Elevated maternal glucose levels, changes in circulation.
Possibly evidenced by:	[Not applicable; presence of signs/symptoms establishes an **actual** diagnosis.]
DESIRED OUTCOMES— FETUS WILL:	Display normally reactive NST and negative oxytocin challenge test (OCT) and/or contraction stress test (CST).
	Be full-term, with size appropriate for gestational age.

ACTIONS/INTERVENTIONS	RATIONALE

Independent

Determine White's classification for diabetes; explain classification and significance to client/couple.	Fetus is at less risk if White's classification is A, B, or C. The client with classification D or above who develops kidney or acidotic problems or PIH is at high risk. As a means of determining prognosis for perinatal outcome, White's classification has been used in conjunction with (1) evaluation of diabetic control or lack of control and (2) presence or absence of Pederson's prognostically bad signs of pregnancy (PBSP), which include acidosis, mild/severe toxemia, and pyelonephritis. The National Diabetes Data Group Classification of diabetes (type I, insulin-dependent; type II, non-insulin-dependent) has not yet had prognostic significance in predicting perinatal outcomes.
Assess client's diabetic control before conception.	Strict control (normal HbA_{1c} levels) before conception helps reduce the risk of fetal mortality and congenital anomalies.
Assess fetal movement and fetal heart rate (FHR) each visit as indicated. (Refer to CP: Third Trimester, ND: Injury, high risk for, fetal.) Encourage client to periodically count/record fetal movements beginning about 18 weeks' gestation, then daily from 34 weeks' gestation on.	Fetal movement and FHR may be negatively affected when placental insufficiency and maternal ketosis occur.
Monitor fundal height each visit.	Useful in identifying abnormal growth pattern (macrosomia or IUGR, small or large for gestational age [SGA/LGA]).
Monitor urine for ketones.	Irreparable CNS damage or fetal death can occur as result of maternal ketonemia, especially in the third trimester.
Provide information and reinforce procedure for home glucose monitoring and diabetic management. (Refer to NDs: Knowledge Deficit [Learning Need]; Nutrition, altered, less than body requirements, high risk for.)	Decreased fetal/newborn mortality and morbidity complications and congenital anomalies are associated with optimal FBS levels between 70 and 95 mg/dl, and 2-hour postprandial glucose level of less than 120 mg/dl. Frequent monitoring is necessary to maintain this tight range and to reduce incidence of fetal hypoglycemia or hyperglycemia

163

ACTIONS/INTERVENTIONS	RATIONALE

Independent

Monitor for signs of PIH (edema, proteinuria, increased blood pressure).

About 12%–13% of diabetics develop hypertensive disorders owing to cardiovascular changes associated with diabetes. These disorders negatively affect placental perfusion and fetal status.

Provide information about possible effect of diabetes on fetal growth and development.

Knowledge helps client to make decisions about managing regimen and may increase cooperation.

Review procedure and rationale for weekly NST after 30 weeks' gestation, twice-weekly NST after 36 weeks' gestation.

Fetal activity and movement are good predictors of fetal wellness. Activity level decreases before alterations in FHR occur.

Discuss rationale/procedure for carrying out weekly OCT/CST beginning at 30 to 32 weeks' gestation. (Refer to CP: Third Trimester, ND: Injury, high risk for, fetal.)

CST assesses placental perfusion of oxygen and nutrients to fetus. Positive results indicate placental insufficiency, in which case fetus may need to be delivered surgically.

Review procedure and rationale for amniocentesis using L/S ratio and presence of pg. (Refer to CP: Second Trimester, ND: Injury, high risk for, fetal.)

Fetal lung maturity is criterion used to determine whether survival is possible when maternal/placental functioning is impaired before term. Hyperinsulinemia inhibits and interferes with surfactant production; therefore, in the diabetic client, testing for presence of pg is more accurate than using L/S ratio.

Collaborative

Assess HbA$_{1c}$ every 2–4 wk as indicated.

Incidence of congenitally malformed infants is increased in women with high HbA$_{1c}$ level (greater than 8.5%) early in pregnancy or before conception.

Assess glycolysated albumin level at 24 to 28 weeks' gestation, especially for client in high-risk category (history of macrosomic infants, previous GDM, or positive family history of GDM). Follow with GTT if test results are positive.

Serum test for glycolysated albumin reflects glycemia over several days and may gain acceptance as screening tool for GDM because it does not involve potentially harmful glucose loading as does GTT. HbA$_{1c}$ is not sensitive enough as a screening tool for GDM.

Obtain serum for alpha-fetoprotein levels at 14 to 16 weeks' gestation.

Incidence of neural tube defects is greater in diabetic client than in nondiabetic clients, especially if poor control existed prior to pregnancy.

Prepare for ultrasonography at 8, 12, 18, 28, and 36 to 38 weeks' gestation as indicated.

Ultrasonography is useful in confirming gestation date and helps to evaluate IUGR.

Perform NST and OCT/CST, as appropriate.

Assesses fetal well-being and adequacy of placental perfusion.

Review periodic creatinine clearance levels.

There is a slight parallel between renal vascular damage and impaired uterine blood flow.

Obtain sequential serum or 24-hour urinary specimen for estriol levels after 30 weeks' gestation.

Although estriol levels are not used as often now, falling levels may indicate decreased placental functioning, leading to possibility of IUGR and stillbirth.

ACTIONS/INTERVENTIONS	RATIONALE
Collaborative	
Assist as necessary with BPP assessment.	Provides a score to assess fetal well-being/risk. The criteria include NST results, fetal breathing movements, amniotic fluid volume, fetal tone, and fetal body movements. For each criteria met, a score of 2 is given. A total score of 8 to 10 is reassuring, a score of 4 to 7 indicates need for further evaluation and retesting, and a score of 0 to 3 is ominous.
Assist with preparation for delivery of fetus vaginally or surgically if test results indicate placental aging and insufficiency.	Helps ensure positive outcome for neonate. Incidence of stillbirths increases significantly with gestation more than 36 weeks. Macrosomia often causes dystocia with cephalopelvic disproportion (CPD).

NURSING DIAGNOSIS:	INJURY, HIGH RISK FOR, maternal
Risk factors may include:	Changes in diabetic control, abnormal blood profile/anemia, tissue hypoxia, altered immune response.
Possibly evidenced by:	[Not applicable; presence of signs/symptoms establishes an **actual** diagnosis.]
DESIRED OUTCOMES— CLIENT WILL:	Remain normotensive.
	Maintain normoglycemia.
	Be free of complications (e.g., infection, placental separation).

ACTIONS/INTERVENTIONS	RATIONALE
Independent	
Note White's classification for diabetes. Assess degree of diabetic control (Pederson's criteria). (Refer to ND: Injury, high risk for, fetal.)	Client classified as D, E, or F is at higher risk for complications, as is client with PBSP.
Assess client for vaginal bleeding and abdominal tenderness.	Vascular changes associated with diabetes place client at risk for abruptio placentae.
Monitor for signs and symptoms of preterm labor.	Overdistention of uterus due to macrosomia or hydramnios may predispose client to early labor.
Assist client in learning home monitoring of blood glucose, to be done a minimum of 6 times/day. (Refer to NDs: Nutrition, altered, less than body requirements, high risk for; Knowledge Deficit [Learning Need].)	Allows greater accuracy than urine testing because renal threshold for glucose is lowered during pregnancy.
Request that client check urine for ketones daily on awakening and when scheduled food intake is delayed.	Ketonuria indicates presence of starvation state, which may negatively affect the developing fetus.

ACTIONS/INTERVENTIONS	RATIONALE

Independent

Identify for hypoglycemia episodes occurring at home.	Hypoglycemic episodes occur most frequently in the first trimester, owing to continuous fetal drain on blood glucose and amnio acids, and to low levels of HPL. Vomiting may lead to ketosis.
Identify for episodes of hyperglycemia.	Diet/insulin regulation is necessary for normoglycemia, especially in second and third trimesters, when insulin requirements often double (may quadruple in third trimester).
Assess for and/or monitor presence of edema. (Refer to CPs: Pregnancy-Induced Hypertension, ND: Fluid Volume deficit.)	The diabetic client is prone to excess fluid retention and PIH because of vascular changes. The severity of the vascular changes before pregnancy influences the extent and time of onset of PIH.
Determine fundal height; check for edema of extremities and dyspnea.	Hydramnios occurs in 6%–25% of pregnant diabetic clients; may possibly be associated with increased fetal contribution to amniotic fluid, because hyperglycemia increases fetal urine output.
Assess for and review with client signs and symptoms of UTI.	Early detection of UTI may prevent pyelonephritis, which is thought to contribute to premature labor.
Assess nature of vaginal discharge.	If glycosuria is present, client is more likely to develop monilial vulvovaginitis, which is caused by *Candida albicans* and may result in oral thrush in newborn.
Monitor client closely if tocolytic drugs are used to arrest labor.	Tocolytic drugs may elevate blood glucose and plasma insulin.

Collaborative

Monitor serum glucose levels each visit.	Detects impending ketoacidosis; determines times of day in which client is prone to hypoglycemia
Obtain HbA$_{1C}$ every 2–4 wk as indicated.	Allows accurate assessment of glucose control for past 60 days.
Assess Hb/Hct on initial visit, then during second trimester and at term.	Anemia may be present in client with vascular involvement.
Instruct in insulin administration as required. Ensure that client is adept at self-administration, either s.c. or with pump, depending on client's needs or care setting.	Insulin requirements are decreased in first trimester, then double and quadruple in second and third trimesters, respectively. Highly motivated and cooperative clients may do well with a continuous subcutaneous insulin infusion pump to more naturally meet insulin needs.
Obtain urinalysis and urine culture; administer antibiotic as indicated.	Helps prevent or treat pyelonephritis. (Note: Some antibiotics might be contraindicated because of danger of teratogenic effects.)
Obtain culture of vaginal discharge, if present.	Monilial vulvovaginitis can cause oral thrush in the newborn.
Collect specimens for total protein excretion, creatinine clearance, blood urea nitrogen, and uric acid levels.	Progressive vascular changes may impair renal function in client with severe or long-standing diabetes.

ACTIONS/INTERVENTIONS

Collaborative

Schedule ophthalmologic examination during first trimester for all clients, and in second and third trimesters if client is class D or above.

Prepare client for ultrasonography at 8, 12, 18, 26, and 36 to 38 weeks' gestation to determine fetal size using biparietal diameter, femur length, and estimated fetal weight.

Start I.V. therapy with 5% dextrose; administer glucagon S.C. if client is hospitalized with insulin shock and is unconscious. Follow with 8 oz skim milk when client is able to swallow.

RATIONALE

Background retinopathy may progress during pregnancy, owing to severe vascular involvement. Laser coagulation therapy may improve client's condition and reduce optic fibrosis.

Client is at increased risk for CPD and dystocia due to macrosomia.

Glucagon is a naturally occurring substance that acts on liver glycogen and converts it to glucose, which corrects hypoglycemic state. (Note: Hypertonic glucose *(D50) administered I.V. may have negative effects on fetal brain tissue because of its hypertonic action. Protein helps sustain normoglycemia over a longer period of time.)

NURSING DIAGNOSIS:	KNOWLEDGE DEFICIT [LEARNING NEED], regarding diabetic condition, prognosis, and treatment needs
May be related to:	Lack of exposure to information, misinformation, lack of recall, unfamiliarity with information resources.
Possibly evidenced by:	Questions, statement of misconception, inaccurate follow-through of instructions, development of preventable complications.
DESIRED OUTCOMES— CLIENT WILL:	Participate in the management of diabetes during pregnancy.
	Verbalize understanding of the procedures, laboratory tests, and activities involved in controlling diabetes.
	Demonstrate proficiency in self-monitoring and insulin administration.

ACTIONS/INTERVENTIONS

Independent

Assess client's/couple's knowledge of disease process and treatment, including relationships between diet, exercise, illness, stress, and insulin requirements.

RATIONALE

Clients with either preexisting diabetes or GDM are at risk for ineffective glucose uptake within the cells, excess utilization of fats/proteins for energy, and cellular dehydration as water is drawn from the cell by a hypertonic concentration of glucose within the serum. Pregnancy alters insulin requirements drastically and necessitates more intense control. Control of diabetes depends on the client/couple taking an active role. Informed decisions can be made only when there is a clear understanding of both the disease process and the rationale for management.

ACTIONS/INTERVENTIONS	RATIONALE

Independent

Review importance of home serum glucose monitoring using reflectance meter and enzyme strips, and the need for frequent readings (at least 6 times/day), as indicated. Demonstrate procedure, then observe return demonstration by the client.

Frequent blood glucose measurements allow client to recognize the impact of her diet and exercise on serum glucose levels and promotes tight control of glucose levels.

Review reasons why oral hypoglycemic medications should be avoided, even though they may have been used by the Class A client, to control diabetes before pregnancy.

Although insulin does not cross the placenta, oral hypoglycemic agents do and are potentially harmful to the fetus, necessitating a change in diabetic management.

Provide information about action and adverse effects of insulin. Assist client to learn administration by injection, insulin pump, or nasal spray (experimental technique) as indicated.

Prenatal metabolic changes cause insulin requirements to change. In the first trimester, insulin requirements are lower, but they double and then quadruple during second and third trimesters.

Explain normal weight gain to client. Encourage her to monitor her own gains at home between visits. Total gain in the first trimester should be 2.5–4.5 lb, then 0.8–0.9 lb/wk thereafter.

Caloric restriction with resulting ketonemia may cause fetal damage and inhibit optimal protein utilization. (Refer to ND: Injury, high risk for, fetal.)

Provide information about need for mild exercise program (regularly, 20 min after meals). Warn against exercising if glucose exceeds 300 mg/dl.

Client should exercise after meals to help prevent hypoglycemia and to stabilize glucose excursion, unless excessive elevation of glucose is present, in which case exercise promotes ketoacidosis.

Provide information regarding the impact of pregnancy on the diabetic condition and future expectations.

Increased knowledge may decrease fear of the unknown, increase likelihood of cooperation, and may help reduce fetal/maternal complications. About 70% of clients diagnosed with GDM will develop NIDDM within 15 years.

Discuss how client can recognize signs of infection.

Important to seek medical help early to avoid complications.

Recommend client maintain a diary of home assessment of serum glucose levels, insulin dosage, diet, exercise, reactions, general feelings of wellbeing, and any other pertinent thoughts.

When reviewed by healthcare practitioner(s), client's diary can assist with evaluation and alteration of therapy.

Provide contact numbers for health team members.

Client needs to be assured that questions will be answered and problems dealt with immediately on a 24 hour a day basis.

Review Hb/Hct levels. Provide dietary information about sources of iron and the need for iron supplements.

Anemias are of greater concern in clients with preexisting diabetes, because elevated glucose levels replace oxygen on the Hb molecule, resulting in reduced oxygen-carrying capacity.

Assist client/family to learn glucagon administration. Instruct client to follow with 8 oz of milk, then recheck glucose level in 15 minutes.

Presence of symptoms of hypoglycemia (diaphoresis, tingling sensation, palpitations) with a blood glucose level under 70 mg/dl requires prompt intervention. Use of glucagon in combination with milk can increase the serum glucose level without the risk of rebound hyperglycemia. Glucagon is also useful during periods of morning sickness/ vomiting when food intake is curtailed and serum glucose levels fall.

Prenatal Hemorrhage

Hemorrhage may occur early or late in pregnancy, owing to certain physiologic problems, each with its own signs and symptoms, which help in establishing differential diagnosis and in creating the plan of care. This general guide for care is meant to treat hemorrhage in the antepartal client, where appropriate, interventions specific to each physiologic problem are identified.

CLIENT ASSESSMENT DATA BASE: GENERAL FINDINGS

CIRCULATION

Hypertension or hypotension may be present.

Pallor.

Dizziness.

EGO INTEGRITY

Anxious, fearful, apprehensive.

FOOD/FLUID

Nausea/vomiting.

SAFETY

Pelvic inflammatory disease.

Repeated episodes of gonorrhea.

SEXUALITY

Multiparity and advanced maternal age.

Previous cesarean sections.

Repeated second- or third-trimester abortions.

Cervical scarring from lacerations, cervical conization, elective abortions, or dilatation and curettage (D and C).

Specific conditions with appropriate signs and symptoms have been listed in the prenatal time sequence in which they might appear.
Ectopic Pregnancy: Timing of rupture depends on location of fetus; i.e., isthmus of fallopian tube may rupture after 4–5 wk; an interstitial implantation may not rupture until the beginning of the second trimester.

CIRCULATION

Hypotension.

Tachycardia.

Delayed capillary refill.

Cold, clammy skin.

Faintness, syncope.

FOOD/FLUID

Abdomen may be tender.

PAIN/DISCOMFORT

Colicky abdominal pain.

Referred shoulder pain may be noted as abdomen fills with blood.

Severe one-sided pain may occur in presence of tubal rupture.

SAFETY

Normal or subnormal temperature.

SEXUALITY

Abdominal tenderness.

Uterine enlargement may be noted.

Adnexal mass is palpable on pelvic examination.

Abortion: Can occur at any time prior to 20 weeks' gestation. (Refer to CP: Spontaneous Termination.) *Hydatidiform Mole:* May occur as early as the 4th week or as late as the second trimester.

CIRCULATION

Hypertensive symptoms and/or edema may have developed prior to 20 weeks' gestation.

FOOD/FLUID

Severe nausea/vomiting (hyperemesis).

Urine may be positive for protein.

SEXUALITY

Uterus enlarged out of proportion to gestation or may be smaller than anticipated.

No fetal heart tones (FHT) or fetal outline palpable; no fetal activity noted.

Clear, grapelike vesicles passed vaginally.

Decrease in breast tissue.

Placenta Previa: May occur after 20 weeks' gestation, usually third trimester; commonly the 8th month.

CIRCULATION

Painless vaginal bleeding (amount dependent on whether previa is marginal, partial, or total); profuse bleeding may occur during labor.

SEXUALITY

Fundal height 28 cm or greater.

FHT within normal limits (WNL).

Fetus may be in transverse lie or unengaged.

Uterus soft.

Abruptio Placentae: This premature separation of placenta occurs during third trimester, usually during labor.

CIRCULATION

Hypertension (predisposing factor).

Bleeding, if present, may be dark or bright; may be concealed.

FOOD/FLUID

Abdomen hard, boardlike; uterus tense with symmetric or asymmetric enlargement.

PAIN/DISCOMFORT

May have pain with retroplacental hemorrhage; marked tenderness to severe general or localized pain; low back pain.

SEXUALITY

Rising uterine fundus.

Progressive decrease of relaxation between contractions.

Hyperactive fetus.

FHT may be WNL or may demonstrate bradycardia or tachycardia.

DIAGNOSTIC STUDIES

Culdocentesis: Positive for free blood.

Complete blood count (CBC): May reveal elevated white blood cell (WBC) count, lowered hemoglobin (Hb) and hematocrit (Hct).

Human chorionic gonadotropin (HCG) titers: Lowered with ectopic pregnancy, elevated with hydatidiform mole.

Activated partial thromboplastin time (APTT), partial thromboplastin time (PTT), prothrombin time (PT), and platelet count: May reveal prolonged coagulation.

Fibrinogen levels: Decreased.

Fibrin split products (FSP) and fibrin degradation products (FDP): Present if disseminated intravascular co-agulation (DIC) develops.

Estrogen and progesterone levels: Decline in spontaneous abortion.

Ultrasonography: Verifies the presence of a fetus, localizes the placenta, and reveals degree of separation; determines fetal age (based on measurement of biparietal diameter, length of femur, crown to rump).

Amniocentesis: Determines lecithin to sphingomyelin (L/S) ratio in cases of placenta previa.

Betke-Kleihauer test on maternal serum, vaginal fluids, amniotic fluid, gastric lavage, or APT test of amniotic fluid: Determines maternal versus fetal blood in amniotic fluid; estimates fetal blood loss.

NURSING PRIORITIES

1. Evaluate client/fetal status.
2. Maintain circulating fluid volume.
3. Assist with efforts to sustain the pregnancy, if possible.
4. Prevent complications.
5. Provide emotional support to the client/couple.
6. Provide client/couple with information about possible short- and long-term implications of the hemorrhage.

DISCHARGE GOALS

1. Homeostasis achieved.
2. Pregnancy maintained.
3. Free of complications.
4. Client/couple dealing constructively with situation.
5. Condition, prognosis, and treatment needs understood.

NURSING DIAGNOSIS:	FLUID VOLUME DEFICIT [ACTIVE LOSS]
May be related to:	Excessive vascular loss.
Possibly evidenced by:	Hypotension, increased pulse rate, decreased pulse pressure, decreased/concentrated urine, decreased venous filling, change in mentation.
DESIRED OUTCOMES— CLIENT WILL:	Demonstrate stabilization/improvement in fluid balance as evidenced by stable vital signs, prompt capillary refill, appropriate sensorium, and individually adequate urine output and specific gravity.

ACTIONS/INTERVENTIONS	RATIONALE

Independent

ACTIONS/INTERVENTIONS	RATIONALE
Evaluate, report, and record amount and nature of blood loss. Initiate pad count; weigh pads/underpad.	Estimation of blood loss helps in differential diagnosis. Each gram of increased pad weight is equal to approximately 1 ml of blood loss.
Institute bedrest. Instruct client to avoid Valsalva's maneuver and intercourse.	Bleeding may stop with a reduction in activity. Increased abdominal pressure or orgasm (which increases uterine activity) may stimulate bleeding.
Position client appropriately, either supine with hips elevated or in semi-Fowler's position for placenta previa. Avoid Trendelenburg position.	Ensures adequate blood available to the brain; elevating hips avoids compression of the vena cava. Semi-Fowler's position allows the fetus to act as a tampon, controlling bleeding in placenta previa. Trendelenburg position may compromise maternal respiratory status.
Note vital signs, capillary refill of nailbeds, color of mucous membranes/skin, and temperature. Measure central venous pressure, if available.	Helps determine severity of blood loss, although cyanosis and changes in blood pressure (BP) and pulse are late signs of circulatory loss and/or developing shock. Also monitors adequacy of fluid replacement.
Monitor uterine activity, fetal status, and any abdominal tenderness.	Helps determine nature of the hemorrhage and possible outcome of hemorrhagic episode. Tenderness is usually present in ruptured ectopic pregnancy or abruptio placentae. Note religious preference; may prohibit use of blood products and establish need for alternative therapy. Client may desire baptism of products of conception in event of inevitable abortion.
Avoid rectal or vaginal examination.	May increase hemorrhage, especially if marginal or total placenta previa is present.
Monitor intake/output. Obtain hourly urine samples; measure specific gravity.	Determines extent of fluid losses and reflects renal perfusion.
Auscultate breath sounds.	Adventitious breath sounds suggest excessive/inappropriate replacement. (Refer to ND: Fluid Volume excess, high risk for.)
Save expelled tissue or products of conception.	Physician needs to evaluate for possible tissue/membrane retention; histologic examination may be necessary.

ACTIONS/INTERVENTIONS

Collaborative

Obtain/review stat blood work: CBC, type and crossmatch, Rh titer, fibrinogen levels, platelet count, APTT, PT, and HCG levels.

Insert indwelling catheter.

Administer intravenous solutions, plasma expanders, whole blood, or packed cells, as indicated.

Prepare for laparotomy in the case of ruptured ectopic pregnancy.

Prepare for D and C in the case of hydatidiform mole or incomplete abortion. (Refer to CP: Spontaneous Termination.)

Prepare for cesarean delivery if any of the following are diagnosed: severe abruptio placentae when the fetus is alive and labor does not ensue; DIC; or placenta previa when fetus is mature, vaginal delivery is not feasible, and bleeding is excessive or unresolved by bedrest.

RATIONALE

Determines amount of blood loss and may provide information regarding cause. Hct should be maintained above 30% to support oxygen and nutrient transport.

Output of less than 30 ml/hr indicates decreased renal perfusion and possible development of tubular necrosis. Appropriate output is determined by individual degree of deficit and rate of replacement.

Increases circulating blood volume and reverses shock symptoms.

Removal of the ruptured fallopian tube, and possibly the ovary, stops the hemorrhage. (Note: If tube is not ruptured, treatment with medication to lyse the products of conception may preserve the tube.)

Removes any chorionic vessels or products of conception that may adhere to endometrium.

Hemorrhage stops once the placenta is removed and venous sinuses are closed.

NURSING DIAGNOSIS:	**TISSUE PERFUSION, ALTERED, uteroplacental**
May be related to:	Hypovolemia.
Possibly evidenced by:	Changes in fetal heart rate (FHR) and/or activity.
DESIRED OUTCOMES— CLIENT WILL:	Demonstrate adequate perfusion, as evidenced by FHR and activity WNL and reactive nonstress test (NST).

ACTIONS/INTERVENTIONS

Independent

Note maternal physiologic status, circulatory status, and blood volume.

Auscultate and report FHR; note bradycardia or tachycardia. Note change in fetal activity (hypoactivity or hyperactivity).

RATIONALE

An episode of bleeding is potentially damaging to the outcome of the pregnancy, possibly causing uteroplacental hypovolemia or hypoxia.

Assesses extent of fetal hypoxia. Initially, the fetus responds to decreased oxygen levels with tachycardia and increased movements. If deficit persists, bradycardia and decreased activity occurs.

ACTIONS/INTERVENTIONS	RATIONALE

Independent

Record maternal blood loss and any uterine contractions.	If uterine contractions are accompanied by cervical dilatation, bedrest and medications may not be effective in maintaining the pregnancy. Excess maternal blood loss reduces placental perfusion.
Note expected date of delivery (EDD) and fundal height.	EDD provides an estimate for determining fetal viability.
Encourage bedrest in left lateral position.	Relieves pressure on the inferior vena cava and promotes placental/fetal circulation and oxygen exchange.

Collaborative

Administer supplemental oxygen to client.	Increases oxygen available for fetal uptake. The fetus has some inherent capacity to cope with hypoxia in that (1) fetal Hb dissociates (releases oxygen at the cellular level) more rapidly than adult Hb, and (2) the fetal red blood cell count is greater than that of the adult, so fetal oxygen-carrying capacity is increased.
Carry out/repeat NST as indicated.	Electronically evaluating the FHR response to fetal movement is useful in determining fetal well-being (reactive test) versus hypoxia (nonreactive).
Replace maternal fluid/blood losses.	Maintains adequate circulating volume for oxygen transport. Maternal hemorrhage negatively affects uteroplacental oxygen transfer, leading to possible loss of pregnancy or worsening fetal status. If oxygen deprivation persists, the fetus may exhaust coping mechanisms, and CNS damage/fetal demise is possible.
Assist with ultrasonography and amniocentesis. Explain procedures.	Determines fetal maturity and gestational age. Aids in determining viability and realistically predicting outcome.
Obtain vaginal specimen for Apt test, or use Kleihauer-Betke test to evaluate maternal serum, vaginal blood, or products of gastric lavage.	Differentiates maternal from fetal blood in amniotic fluid when vaginal bleeding is present; provides rough quantitative estimate of fetal blood loss and indicates implications for fetal oxygen-carrying capacity, and maternal need for Rh immune globulin (RhIgG) injections once delivery occurs. The Betke-Kleihauer test is more sensitive and quantitatively accurate than the APT test.
Prepare client for appropriate surgical intervention	Surgery is necessary if placental separation is severe; or if bleeding is excessive, fetal oxygen deprivation is involved, and vaginal delivery is impossible, as in cases of total placenta previa (a low-lying placenta), where surgery may be indicated to save the life of the fetus.

NURSING DIAGNOSIS:	FEAR
May be related to:	Threat of death (perceived or actual) to self, fetus.
Possibly evidenced by:	Verbalization of specific concerns, increased tension, sympathetic stimulation.
DESIRED OUTCOMES— CLIENT WILL:	Discuss fears regarding self, fetus, and future pregnancies, recognizing healthy versus unhealthy fears.
	Verbalize accurate knowledge of the situation.
	Demonstrate problem-solving and use resources effectively.
	Report/display lessened fear and/or fear behaviors.

ACTIONS/INTERVENTIONS	RATIONALE

Independent

Discuss situation and understanding of situation with client and partner.	Provides information about individual reaction to what is happening.
Monitor client's/couple's verbal and nonverbal responses.	Indicate the degree of fear the client/couple is experiencing.
Listen to and Active-listen of client concerns.	Promotes sense of control over situation and provides opportunity for client to develop own solutions.
Provide information in verbal and written form, and make opportunity for client to ask questions. Answer questions honestly.	Knowledge will help client to cope more effectively with what is happening. Written information allows for review later because client may not be able to assimilate information due to level of anxiety. Honest answers promote better understanding and can reduce fear.
Involve client in planning and participating in care as much as possible.	Being able to do something to help control the situation can reduce the fear.
Explain procedures and what symptoms mean.	Knowledge can help to reduce fear and promote sense of control over situation.

NURSING DIAGNOSIS:	INJURY, HIGH RISK FOR, maternal
Risk factors may include:	Tissue/organ hypoxia, abnormal blood profile, impaired immune system.
Possibly evidenced by:	[Not applicable; presence of signs/symptoms establishes an **actual** diagnosis.]
DESIRED OUTCOMES— CLIENT WILL:	Remain afebrile.
	Display normal blood profile with WBC count, Hb, and coagulation studies WNL.
	Maintain urine output appropriate for individual situation.

ACTIONS/INTERVENTIONS	RATIONALE

Independent

Assess amount of blood loss. Monitor for signs/symptoms of shock. (Refer to ND: Fluid Volume deficit [active loss].)

Persistent, excessive hemorrhage may be life-threatening to the client or may result in postpartal infection, postpartal anemia, DIC, renal failure, or pituitary necrosis attributable to tissue hypoxia and malnutrition.

Note temperature, WBC count, and odor and color of vaginal discharge, obtain culture if appropriate.

Excess blood loss with decreased Hb increases the client's risk of developing an infection.

Record intake/output. Note urine specific gravity.

Reduced kidney perfusion results in reduced output. The anterior pituitary lobe, which enlarges during pregnancy, is at risk for Sheehan's syndrome when hemorrhage occurs. (Refer to Chapter 6, CP: Postpartal Hemorrhage, ND: Tissue Perfusion, altered.)

Monitor for adverse response to administration of blood products, such as allergic or hemolytic reaction; treat per protocol.

Early recognition and intervention may prevent life-threatening situation.

Inspect client for petechiae or for bleeding from gums or I.V. site.

Indicate deficiencies or alterations in coagulation.

Provide information about risks of receiving blood products.

Complications such as hepatitis and human immunodeficiency virus (HIV)/AIDS may not be manifested during hospitalization, but may require treatment at a later date.

Collaborative

Obtain blood type and crossmatch.

Assures correct product will be available if blood replacement required.

Administer fluid replacement.

Maintains circulatory volume to counteract fluid losses or shock.

Monitor coagulation studies (e.g., APTT, platelet count, fibrinogen levels, FSP/FDP).

DIC with an associated drop in fibrinogen levels and a buildup of FSP may occur in response to the release of thromboplastin from placental tissue and/or dead fetus. In order for clot formation to occur, fibrinogen level must be at least 100 mg/dl.

Administer cryoprecipitate and fresh frozen plasma as indicated. Avoid administration of platelets if consumption is still occurring (i.e., if platelet level is dropping).

Cryoprecipitate replaces most clotting factors in clients with DIC. Administration of platelets during period of continued consumption is controversial, because it may perpetuate the clotting cycle, resulting in further reduction of clotting factors and increasing venous congestion and stasis.

Administer heparin, if indicated.

Heparin may be used in DIC in cases of fetal death, or of death of one fetus in a multiple pregnancy, or to block the clotting cycle by preserving clotting factors and reducing hemorrhage until surgical correction occurs.

Administer antibiotic parenterally.

May be indicated to prevent or minimize infection.

Treat underlying problem (e.g., surgery for abruptio placentae or ectopic pregnancy, bedrest at home for placenta previa).

Stops hemorrhage; reduces likelihood of maternal injury.

NURSING DIAGNOSIS:	PAIN [ACUTE]
May be related to:	Muscle contractions/cervical dilatation, tissue trauma (fallopian tube rupture).
Possibly evidenced by:	Reports of pain, distraction behaviors, autonomic responses (changes in pulse/BP).
DESIRED OUTCOMES—CLIENT WILL:	Report pain/discomfort relieved or controlled.
	Demonstrate use of relaxation skills/diversional activities.

ACTIONS/INTERVENTIONS	RATIONALE

Independent

Determine nature, location, and duration of pain. Assess for uterine contractions, retroplacental hemorrhage, or abdominal tenderness.	Aids in diagnosis and choice of treatment. Discomfort associated with spontaneous abortion and hydatidiform mole is due to uterine contractions, which may be augmented by oxytocin infusion. Rupture in ectopic pregnancy results in extreme pain, owing to concealed hemorrhage as the fallopian tube ruptures into the abdominal cavity. Abruptio placentae is accompanied by severe pain, especially when concealed retroplacental hemorrhage occurs.
Assess client's/couple's psychologic stress and emotional response to event.	Anxiety in response to the emergency situation may intensify the degree of discomfort owing to the fear-tension-pain syndrome.
Provide quiet environment and diversional activities. Instruct client in relaxation methods (e.g., deep breathing, visualization, distraction). Explain procedures.	May assist in lowering the level of anxiety and thereby contribute to the reduction of discomfort.

Collaborative

Administer narcotics or sedatives; administer preoperative medications if surgical procedure is indicated.	Promotes comfort; reduces risk of surgical complications.
Prepare for surgical procedure, if indicated.	Treatment of underlying disorder should alleviate pain.

NURSING DIAGNOSIS:	FLUID VOLUME EXCESS, HIGH RISK FOR
Risk factors may include:	Excessive/rapid replacement of fluid losses.
Possibly evidenced by:	[Not applicable; presence of signs/symptoms establishes an **actual** diagnosis.]
DESIRED OUTCOMES—CLIENT WILL:	Display BP, pulse, urine specific gravity, and neurologic signs WNL, without respiratory difficulties.

177

ACTIONS/INTERVENTIONS	RATIONALE

Independent

Monitor for increasing BP and pulse; note respiratory signs such as dyspnea, crackles, or rhonchi.

If fluid replacement is excessive, symptoms of circulatory overload and respiratory difficulties may occur. In addition, the client with abruptio placentae who may already have hypertension is at risk for manifesting negative response to fluid replacement, as is the client with compromised cardiac function.

Carefully monitor infusion rate manually or electronically. Record intake/output. Measure urine specific gravity.

Intake and output should be approximately equal as circulating fluid volume is stabilizing. Urine output increases and specific gravity decreases as kidney perfusion and circulatory volume return to normal.

Assess neurologic status, noting behavior changes or increasing irritability.

Behavior changes may be an early sign of cerebral edema owing to water retention.

Collaborative

Assess Hct level.

Hct level may indicate amount of blood loss and can be used to determine needs and adequacy of replacement.

NURSING DIAGNOSIS:	**KNOWLEDGE DEFICIT [LEARNING NEED], regarding reason for hemorrhage, prognosis, and treatment needs**
May be related to:	Lack of exposure to, and unfamiliarity with, information resources.
Possibly evidenced by:	Request for information, statement of misconceptions, inappropriate or exaggerated behaviors.
DESIRED OUTCOMES— CLIENT/COUPLE WILL:	Participate in learning process.
	Verbalize, in simple terms, the pathophysiology and implications of the clinical situation.

ACTIONS/INTERVENTIONS	RATIONALE

Independent

Explain prescribed treatment and rationale for hemorrhagic condition. Reinforce information provided by other healthcare providers.

Provides information, clarifies misconceptions, and may aid in reducing associated stress.

Allow client opportunity to ask questions and verbalize misconceptions.

Provides for clarification of misconceptions, identification of problems, and opportunity to begin to develop coping skills.

Discuss possible short-term maternal/fetal implications of bleeding episode.

Provides information about possible complications and promotes realistic expectations and cooperation with treatment regimen.

ACTIONS/INTERVENTIONS	RATIONALE

Independent

Review long-term implications for situations requiring follow-up and additional treatment; e.g., hydatidiform mole, dysfunctional cervix, or ectopic pregnancy. (Refer to CP: Premature Dilation of the Cervix.)

HCG levels must be monitored for 1 year after expulsion of a hydatidiform mole. If levels remain high, chemotherapy is indicated, owing to risk of choriocarcinoma. A client with repeated second-trimester spontaneous abortion may have a Shirodkar-Barter procedure performed. A client with an ectopic pregnancy may have difficulty conceiving after removal of the affected tube/ovary.

CLIENT ASSESSMENT DATA BASE

ACTIVITY/REST

Malaise, fatigue.

CIRCULATION

May be jaundiced.

ELIMINATION

Dysuria, urinary frequency, decreased urine output, hematuria.

FOOD/FLUID

Nausea, vomiting, anorexia, weight loss.

Tongue may have visible lesion or sore (hairy leukoplakia seen in AIDS).

PAIN/DISCOMFORT

Backache, flank pain, colicky pain noted with acute pyelonephritis.

Chest pain may occur with tuberculosis.

Severe itching, burning pain with lesions.

May complain of pruritus with active (infectious) hepatitis A or B.

RESPIRATION

Cough may be productive of thick, purulent sputum.

Crackles (rales), wheezes, bronchial breath sounds.

SAFETY

Temperature elevation dependent on type of infection; e.g., low-grade in cystitis, high fever in pyelonephritis.

Chills, night sweats.

History of urinary tract infection (UTI).

Positive cultures, elevated titers, positive screening for infectious disease.

May have visible perineal or genital warts, lesions, or chancres.

Exposure to body fluids or blood products through professional practice or through receiving a transfusion parenterally as a patient; carrier of group B beta-hemolytic streptococci (GBS) or of hepatitis B virus (Hb_sAg, anti-HB_cAg).

SEXUALITY

May have history of early trimester pregnancy loss(es).

May currently have, or may have had exposure to, numerous heterosexual/bisexual partners, which increases risk of exposure to HIV and sexually transmitted diseases (STDs). Husband or sexual partner may be hemophiliac, necessitating blood transfusions and placing him at risk of acquisition of HIV.

Vaginal discharge may be frothy, gray-green (trichomonal infection); whitish (candidal infection); thin, watery, yellow-gray, foul-smelling, "fishy" (*Gardnerella vaginalis* infection).

Strawberry patches on vaginal walls/cervix (trichomonal infection).

Membranes may rupture prematurely.

Fundal height may not be appropriate for gestational age, possibly indicating intrauterine growth retardation (IUGR) associated with rubella or toxoplasmosis, or may correspond with gestational age of less than 37 weeks, indicating increased risk for GBS.

SOCIAL INTERACTION

Immigrants from Africa or Haiti may have increased risk of AIDS; immigrants from Southeast Asia, Central America, or the Caribbean islands may have increased risk of infectious or carrier state of hepatitis B virus (HBV); Native Americans, inner city, lower socioeconomic population, and immigrants from underdeveloped countries also have increased risk of tuberculosis.

TEACHING/LEARNING

Risks factors include diabetes; malnutrition; drug/alcohol addiction; anemia; belonging to lower socioeconomic class, which increases susceptibility/exposure to infectious agents.

DIAGNOSTIC STUDIES

Urinalysis/serum, culture and sensitivity: Detects UTI, asymptomatic bacteremia, or GBS.
RPR (formerly VDRL): Tests for syphilis.
Vaginal, rectal, and cervical smears: Determines presence of gonorrhea, chlamydial infection, bacteria, GBS, or genital herpes.
Viral titers: Identify presence of rubella and cytomegalovirus (CMV).
Purified protein derivative (PPD): Tine test; positive reaction indicates tuberculosis.
Hepatitis/HIV screening: Done in presence of high-risk behaviors.
Complete blood count: Reveals anemia and indicators of infection (elevated WBC, differential shifted to the left).
Chest x-ray: Reveals nodular lesions, patchy infiltrates, cavitation, scar tissue, calcium deposits.
Serial ultrasonography: Detects IUGR.
Specimen of vaginal pool: Determines premature rupture of membranes (PROM).

NURSING PRIORITIES

1. Identify/screen for prenatal infection.
2. Provide information about protocol of care.
3. Promote client/fetal well-being.

DISCHARGE GOALS

1. Individual risks/conditions understood.
2. Condition, prognosis, treatment needs understood.
3. Participates in therapeutic regimen.
4. Pregnancy maintained as appropriate/desired.

NURSING DIAGNOSIS:	INFECTION, HIGH RISK FOR, maternal/fetal
May be related to:	Inadequate primary defenses (e.g., broken skin, stasis of body fluids), inadequate secondary defenses (e.g., decreased hemoglobin, immunosuppression), inadequate acquired immunity, environmental exposure, malnutrition, rupture of amniotic membranes.
Possibly evidenced by:	[Not applicable; presence of signs/symptoms establishes an **actual** diagnosis.]
DESIRED OUTCOMES— CLIENT WILL:	Verbalize understanding of individual causative/risk factors.
	Review techniques and lifestyle changes to reduce risk of infection.
	Achieve timely healing, free of complications.

ACTIONS/INTERVENTIONS	RATIONALE
Independent	
Review lifestyle and profession for presence of associated risk factors.	Drug abusers and healthcare professionals are at risk for exposure to HIV/AIDS and HBV through contact with contaminated needles, body fluids, and blood products.
Obtain information about client's past/present sexual partners and exposure to STDs.	Multiple sexual partners or intercourse with bisexual men increases risk of exposure to STDs and HIV/AIDS.
Assess client's cultural background for risk factors.	Recent arrivals from Asia, South America, and the Caribbean islands have increased risk of exposure to HBV. In Africa, male-to-female ratio of HIV is 1:1 owing to cultural sexual practices.
Assess for signs and symptoms; notify physician if present:	Identifiable signs of infection assist in determining mode of treatment. Some organisms have a predilection for the fetoplacental unit and the neonate, although the client may be asymptomatic; i.e., *Mycoplasma* and *Ureaplasma* organisms affect a significant number of pregnant women and have been cultured in aborted fetuses even though the mothers have been free of symptoms.
Visible lesions/warts.	May indicate herpes simplex virus type II (HSV-II), which can be transmitted to newborn at time of delivery if lesion is present at term or if viral shedding is occurring.
Urinary frequency; dysuria; cloudy, foul-smelling urine.	May be associated with *Escherichia coli* or GBS, or client may have asymptomatic bacteriuria.
Change in color, consistency, and amount of vaginal discharge.	Gray-green discharge may indicate trichomoniasis; thick white discharge may indicate *Candida albicans* infection; thin, watery, yellow-gray foul-smelling ("fishy") discharge suggests *Gardnerella*.

ACTIONS/INTERVENTIONS	RATIONALE

Independent

Determine if viral infection is primary or recurrent.

Both herpesviruses (CMV and HSV-II) recur in times of stress. Yet only primary CMV is problematic to the fetus, and only 50% of fetuses exposed are affected. Although recurrent HSV-II is associated with reduced viral shedding time, the newborn, if exposed to the virus at delivery, can be affected with either visible lesions or a disseminated type of the disease.

Assess status of maternal membranes. If they are ruptured, monitor for signs of maternal/fetal infection (e.g., increased temperature, white blood cell count), and fetal heart rate; or vaginal discharge having an odor.

Infectious organisms transmitted via the ascending route include chlamydiae, mycoplasmas, *Ureaplasma urealyticum*, GBS, and *Haemophilus influenzae*. Fetuses infected via this route are likely to develop bacteremia and pneumonia.

Collaborative

Evaluate fetal growth by monitoring progressive growth of fundal height based on serial ultrasonography.

Infections such as rubella and toxoplasmosis can result in IUGR.

Obtain appropriate specimens and laboratory studies as indicated:
  Urine for routine urinalysis, culture, and sensitivity.

Asymptomatic bacteriuria (colony count greater than 100,000/ml) occurs in as many as 12% of prenatal clients and has been associated with acute and chronic pyelonephritis, preterm delivery, chorioamnionitis, postpartal maternal sepsis, and congenital defects. From 1%–5% UTIs are linked to GBS, which is the leading cause of neonatal meningitis.

  Vaginal/rectal culture for gonococci/chylamydiae.

Approximately 40%–60% of patients with culture positive gonococcus have concomitant chlamydial infection, the most common STD associated with conjunctivitis and pneumonia of the newborn. Gonorrheal infection of the newborn other than ophthalmia neonatorum is infrequent, but does increase rate of neonatal mortality associated with overwhelming infection.

  Vaginal/cervical culture for *Listeria monocytogenes* and GBS.

Fever of nonspecific origin and history of abortions, neonatal meningitis, sepsis, congenital listeriosis, or postpartal maternal sepsis may indicate recurrent listerial infections requiring treatment. From 5%–30% of women have positive cultures for GBS, yet may be asymptomatic. Treatment with antibiotics is indicated at 38 weeks' gestation or later.

  Rubella titer.

From 5%–15% of women of childbearing age are still susceptible to rubella, which has identifiable teratogenic effects on the fetus. If rubella is contracted in the first trimester, the fetus has no chance of escaping teratogenic effects. If rubella is contracted in the second trimester, the fetus has a 50% chance of being affected.

183

ACTIONS/INTERVENTIONS	RATIONALE

Collaborative

Serum for hepatitis B screen for clients in high-risk group (e.g., Asians, Central Americans, natives of Caribbean islands).

Hepatitis in the first and second trimesters rarely affects the fetus. Women who contract hepatitis in the third trimester have a 60% chance of transmitting it to offspring coming in contact with blood products at the time of delivery. Carrier status can be passed on to infants if they are not treated at birth. This can possibly result in cirrhosis and hepatocellular carcinoma.

Serum for HIV screen if high-risk behaviors are present (intravenous drug users, healthcare professionals, laboratory technicians, dialysis workers, those having exposure to bisexual partners, recipients of blood or blood product transfusions).

AIDS destroys the immune system, causing a variety of problems, including HSV-II, CMV, toxoplasmosis, candidiasis, Kaposi's sarcoma, and pneumonia.

Assist as necessary with sputum collection and chest x-rays for client with respiratory symptoms.

Helps in identifying causative organism in bacterial pneumonia and active tuberculosis. (Note: Tuberculosis is not exacerbated by pregnancy.)

Administer antibiotics/medications as indicated:
Penicillin, erythromycin, or spectinomycin.

UTI, listeriosis, gonorrhea, syphilis, bacterial pneumonia, and GBS (in 38th week of gestation or later) all respond to antimicrobial treatment. Prior to 38 weeks' gestation, treatment of client who is carrier of GBS is not effective, because recolonization occurs before birth, with infant still at risk for neonatal sepsis for meningitis.

Acyclovir (Zovirax) capsules or ointments.

Reduces viral shedding for client with HSV-II.

HPA-23 and Zidovudine (AZT).

Although controversial, these drugs are approved by the Food and Drug Administration for prolongation of life in HIV-positive clients.

Pyrimethamine (Daraprim) and sulfadiazine.

Control disease progression in toxoplasmosis, but have known teratogenic effects on fetus.

Folic acid.

Counteracts side effects of pyrimethamine.

Nystatin (Mycostatin) suppositories/vaginal tablets.

Indicated for treatment of *Candida albicans*. (Note: Diabetic client is prone to monilial infection, which may be extremely resistant to prenatal treatment.)

Metronidazole (Flagyl).

Indicated for treatment of trichomonal infections after 20 weeks' gestation. Treatment in the first 20 weeks' is symptomatic; the trichomonal infection may be receptive to clotrimazole vaginal suppositories. (Note: Both partners must be treated to prevent reinfection.)

Isoniazid (INH) in combination with ethambutol hydrochloride or rifampin.

Treatment of choice for tuberculosis, with no known teratogenic effects. Streptomycin is avoided, owing to its association with vestibular and auditory defects; pyrazinamide is also contraindicated.

ACTIONS/INTERVENTIONS

Hepatitis B immune globulin (HBIG).

Gamma globulin.

Prepare for/assist in transfer to tertiary care center as indicated. (Refer to CP: The High-Risk Pregnancy.)

Prepare for termination of pregnancy or labor induction as indicated. (Refer to Chapter 5, CP: Labor: Induced/Augmented.)

RATIONALE

Recommended for exposure to hepatitis B.

Recommended for exposure to hepatitis A.

Availability of staff and equipment ensures optimal care of high-risk client and fetus/newborn.

Pregnancy may be terminated for such conditions as toxoplasmosis occurring prior to 20 weeks' gestation or rubella in the first trimester.

NURSING DIAGNOSIS:	KNOWLEDGE DEFICIT [LEARNING NEED], regarding treatment/prevention, prognosis of condition
May be related to:	Lack of exposure to information and/or unfamiliarity with resources, misinterpretation.
Possibly evidenced by:	Verbalization of problem, inaccurate follow-through of instructions, development of preventable complications/continuation of infectious process.
DESIRED OUTCOMES— CLIENT WILL:	Identify appropriate preventive practices.
	Adopt behaviors/lifestyle changes as indicated.
	Follow-through with individual treatment regimen.
	List signs and symptoms that necessitate evaluation/intervention.
	Verbalize understanding of importance of providing necessary information for data collection.

ACTIONS/INTERVENTIONS

Independent

Identify signs/symptoms of infection. Discuss importance of prompt reporting to healthcare provider.

Discuss mode of transmission of specific infections, as appropriate.

Provide information concerning identified risks associated with client's employment or profession. Stress use of gloves and need for washing hands when client must handle blood products, saliva, or urine.

Identify risk factors associated with client's lifestyle.

RATIONALE

Maternal infection may not be serious, but can have serious implications for the fetus. Timely intervention may prevent complications and enhance likelihood of a positive outcome.

Provides information to assist the client in making decisions relative to lifestyle/behavioral changes; reinforces need for partner to be treated.

Dialysis workers and healthcare professionals who handle body or blood products are at risk for exposure to HSV-II, HIV, and HBV, and need to use universal precautions.

Intravenous drug users are susceptible to percutaneous transmission of HSV-II, HBV, HIV/AIDS, and other STDs. Involvement with multiple sex partners increases risk of being infected.

ACTIONS/INTERVENTIONS	RATIONALE

Independent

Discuss importance of avoiding contact with persons known to have infections, such as upper respiratory infections, tuberculosis, rubella (if not immune), and hepatitis. Stress the need for immunization for rubella after delivery as indicated.

Preventing exposure helps reduce the risk of acquiring infection. From 5%–15% of women of childbearing age are still susceptible to rubella, which is spread by droplets. Immunization after delivery results in immunity during subsequent pregnancies.

Review hygiene measures, including wiping vulva from front to back after urinating and washing hands frequently (including after animal contact).

Helps prevent rectal *E. coli* contaminants from reaching the vagina and reduces contamination with other viruses/bacteria that may be transmitted by poor hygiene practices. Listerial infection is thought to be transmitted via animal contact.

Encourage client to drink 6 to 8 glasses of fluid per day and to void regularly. Discuss results of urine test.

May help prevent UTI associated with stasis. Client with asymptomatic bacteriuria (colony count greater than 100,000/ml) may be at risk for premature delivery, congenital defects in offspring, or anemia.

Suggest client void following intercourse.

May prevent/reduce risk of UTI and transmission of STD, especially CMV, and nongonoccocal urethritis.

Recommend wearing gloves while gardening, avoiding contact with cat litter boxes while pregnant, and cooking meats to appropriate internal temperatures.

Helps prevent toxoplasmosis, most commonly acquired in the United States through contact with cat feces. Some French and Japanese meat dishes are eaten raw or undercooked, thereby increasing the risk of acquiring toxoplasmosis.

Suggest alternative means of sexual gratification for client with active HSV-II, HIV/AIDS, or HBV.

Fondling or masturbation for sexual gratification helps prevent spread of infection to sexual partner.

Provide information about possible effects of infection on client/fetus.

Infection affects approximately 15% of all pregnancies. For some infections, such as rubella, the outcome may be fairly predictable, if the gestational age at which the fetus was exposed is known. For other maternal infections, such as those caused by *Ureaplasma*, *Mycoplasma*, or *Listeria* organisms, it is more difficult to predict the fetal/neonatal outcome, especially because the client may be asymptomatic. Most infections do not pose serious problems to the mother, but can have varying effects on the fetus. Two thirds of these exposed infants are infected in utero, with resultant effects on the liver and brain. Ascending tract infections have a greater chance of resulting in neonatal bacteremia and pneumonia.

Discuss necessary treatments that may have serious fetal implications, such as sulfadiazine and pyrimethamine (used to treat toxoplasmosis), or oral sulfonamides (to treat UTI during the latter weeks of gestation).

These medications have known teratogenic effects on newborn. When toxoplasmosis is present, the fetus is damaged by either the disease or the treatment. Neonatal hyperbilirubinemia and kernicterus may occur with the use of oral sulfonamides.

ACTIONS/INTERVENTIONS	RATIONALE

Independent

Review available options in cases of known teratogenic effects.	Fetus is more susceptible to effects of rubella early in gestation. HBV poses more risks for the fetus in the third trimester. Teratogenic effects of toxoplasmosis include growth retardation, CNS calcification, microcephaly, hydrocephaly, and chorioretinitis. Client/couple may elect to terminate the pregnancy in cases of rubella infection or toxoplasmosis depending on stage of gestation in which exposure occurs.
Discuss possible effects of infection on type and timing of delivery.	Operative delivery may be indicated in the case of certain infections, such as HSV-II if client has active herpes with intact membranes or if membranes are ruptured for more than 4–6 hr. If client or fetus has developed an ascending tract infection following PROM, fetus may need to be delivered prior to term to prevent maternal/fetal sepsis.
Discuss implications of PROM for client and fetus/neonate.	PROM may result in an ascending tract infection with resultant chorioamnionitis and maternal/neonatal sepsis. Common causative organisms in ascending tract infections include GBS, chlamydiae, and *Haemophilus influenzae*.

Discuss implications of specific disease process/treatment as appropriate:

Urinary tract infections.	Client may have asymptomatic bacteriuria with large colony counts (greater than 100,000/ml), and culture may be positive for GBS, *Ureaplasma* organisms, or *Mycoplasma* organisms, placing client at risk for sepsis during and following delivery, and placing the newborn at risk for early- or late-onset infection.
Listeriosis and treatment with penicillin.	It is uncertain how the fetus/infant contracts listeriosis; however, the infection can result in abortion if it is contracted between 17 and 28 weeks' gestation, or cause newborn problems such as meningitis, mental retardation, or hydrocephaly if it is contracted after 28 weeks' gestation.
GBS and antibiotic treatment for the chronic carrier.	GBS, occurring in 5%–30% of pregnant women, is the leading cause of neonatal meningitis and is associated with neonatal sepsis, and with chorioamnionitis if it occurs at less than 37 weeks' gestation and is accompanied by PROM. Treating client with antibiotic (penicillin) prior to 38 weeks' gestation is ineffective, because the bacteria will probably recolonize before delivery. Antibiotics given after 38 weeks' gestation effectively treat the client, but not the fetus.
Chlamydial infection and prenatal treatment with antibiotics.	*Chlamydia* transmitted to the fetus through the ascending route can cause conjunctivitis or pneumonia in the first 3 to 4 months after birth.

ACTIONS/INTERVENTIONS	RATIONALE
Independent	
Neisseria gonorrheae.	Transmission by sexual contact requires that both partners be treated, that condoms be used, and that orogenital sex is avoided until post-treatment cultures are negative at 2 consecutive follow-up visits.
Hepatitis A or B, including designation of hepatitis B carrier state (involving HBV, HB$_s$Ag, anti-Hb$_c$Ag).	Exposure to hepatitis A or B may result in fetal anomalies, preterm birth, intrauterine fetal death, or fetal/neonatal hepatitis. Chronic HBV carrier states can result in cirrhosis and hepatocellular cancer.
HSV-II.	Spread occurs through sexual contact during viral shedding, which lasts 21 days in active primary infections and 12 days in recurrent infections. A stressor such as pregnancy may cause viral shedding.
Positive HIV status.	Incubation periods for HIV range from 6 months to 5 or more years. Because of its immunosuppressive properties, HIV/AIDS results in opportunistic infections, which include pneumonia, meningitis, and encephalitis, caused by CMV, herpesviruses, *Toxoplasma*, *Histoplasma*, *Candida* or *Pneumocystis carinii*.
Primary, secondary, and tertiary stages of syphilis and treatment with penicillin.	Administration of penicillin effectively treats the fetus/newborn. The spirochete does not cross the placenta until 16 to 18 weeks' gestation. Primary and secondary stages of untreated syphilis may lead to stillbirth; tertiary stage results in congenital syphilis of the newborn.
Primary CMV infection during pregnancy.	Although CMV can recur in times of stress, only primary CMV can potentially cause cytomegalic inclusion disease in 50% of the offspring of affected mothers.
Supplemental pyridoxine (vitamin B$_6$).	Helps prevent peripheral neuropathy when isoniazid is used to treat active tuberculosis.
Discuss newborn care and the need for follow-up in infants born to mothers in active or carrier state of HBV.	Bathing the newborn immediately after delivery and administering HBIG and hepatitis B vaccine will prevent the newborn from contracting the virus. Follow-up immunization of the newborn with hepatitis B vaccine at 1 and 6 months are then necessary.
Provide information, specific to infection, regarding possible long-term effects and incubation period.	For example, longitudinal studies of children at age 3.5 to 7 years, show that effects of CMV are ongoing, resulting in learning disabilities, motor deficits, deafness, and lower than normal IQs.
Identify self-help groups and sources of community supports.	May help client in gathering information and resolving issues.

NURSING DIAGNOSIS: **DISCOMFORT***

May be related to: Body response to infective agent, properties of infection (e.g., skin/tissue irritation, development of lesions).

Possibly evidenced by: Verbal reports, restlessness, withdrawal from social contact.

DESIRED OUTCOMES— CLIENT WILL: Identify/use individually appropriate comfort measures.

Report discomfort is relieved/controlled.

Demonstrate use of relaxation skills and diversional activities.

*Authors' note: Currently there is no NANDA diagnostic label that addresses issues of comfort below the level of Pain [acute] or chronic. Although the label of **Discomfort** is not approved, we believe it speaks more directly to the identified problem.

ACTIONS/INTERVENTIONS	RATIONALE
Independent	
Identify source, location, and extent of discomfort; note signs and symptoms of infectious process.	Determines course of treatment and individual interventions.
Suggest increasing fluid intake and voiding in warm sitz bath for client with UTI.	Helps prevent stasis; warmth relaxes perineum and urinary meatus to facilitate voiding.
Provide information about hygienic measures such as frequent bathing, use of cotton underwear, and application of cornstarch for client with vaginal discharge associated with STDs (chlamydial infection or gonorrhea).	Helps promote dryness and prevent skin breakdown.
Provide information regarding use of warm sitz baths, use of hair-dryer on genital area, urinating through an empty toilet paper tube, and the wearing of loose-fitting jeans/pants and cotton underwear for client with HSV-II.	Helps keep genital area, dry/clean; prevents discomfort associated with urine coming in contact with lesions.
Encourage rest for client who has tuberculosis or flulike symptoms associated with listeriosis, rubella, or toxoplasmosis.	Reduces metabolic rate; facilitates response of individual immune system to infection.
Suggest use of humidified air, increased fluid intake, and use of semi-Fowler's position during sleep for clients with respiratory infections, such as tuberculosis.	Helps liquefy secretions and facilitates respiratory functioning. Upright position allows diaphragm to descend, thereby facilitating lung expansion.
Collaborative	
Administer medications as indicated:	
Analgesics (e.g., acetaminophen, codeine).	Relieves discomfort associated with backache, neuralgia, cervical lymphadenopathy, and perineal lesions. (Note: Acetaminophen in toxic levels can cause liver damage. Acetylsalicyclic acid [ASA] can result in alteration of fetal clotting.)

ACTIONS/INTERVENTIONS	RATIONALE
Collaborative	
Antipyretics.	Reduce fever and chills. (Note: In client with PROM, avoid administration of analgesic that may have antipyretic properties [ASA and acetaminophen] because it may mask temperature rise that would signal infection.)
Antibiotics specific to organisms cultured.	Eradicate organisms associated with UTI, bacterial pneumonia, STDs (gonorrhea, syphilis, chylamydial infection), and listeriosis. Relieves flu-like symptoms associated with listeriosis.
Acyclovir (Zovirax) capsules or ointments.	Helps reduce viral shedding time and length of disease associated with HSV-II.
HPA-23.	An experimental anti-AIDS drug that may help reduce discomforts associated with HSV-II, candidiasis, pneumonia, and Kaposi's sarcoma.
Lidocaine hydrochloride (Xylocaine) ointment.	Helps provide local anesthesia to herpetic lesions.

Premature Dilation of the Cervix (Incompetent/Dysfunctional Cervix)

Premature dilation of the cervix often occurs in the fourth or fifth month and is associated with repeated second-trimester spontaneous abortions.

CLIENT ASSESSMENT DATA BASE

EGO INTEGRITY

Feelings of failure at a life event, expressions of shame/guilt.

Expressions/manifestations of anxiety and/or fear.

PAIN/DISCOMFORT

Absence of pain.

SAFETY

May present with premature rupture of membranes during second trimester.

SEXUALITY

History of repeated, relatively painless, bloodless, second-trimester fetal loss (habitual aborter).

Premature shortening, effacement, and dilatation of cervix during current pregnancy.

Cervical trauma associated with previous deliveries with dilatation and curettage, conization, cauterization, or cervical lacerations.

Sterile vaginal examination reveals dilating, effacing cervix.

Membranes may be felt or seen protruding though cervical os.

SOCIAL INTERACTION

Concern about response of others.

TEACHING/LEARNING

Reported previous occurrence of spontaneous abortion.

DIAGNOSTIC STUDIES

Diagnosis is usually made on basis of history of repeated second-trimester abortions.

Serial ultrasonography: Beginning at 6 to 8 weeks' gestation can detect cervical shortening and premature dilatation and aid in diagnosis, especially in women without clear-cut history of cervical dysfunction.
Nitrazine and/or fern test: Detects presence of amniotic fluid, indicating ruptured membranes.

NURSING PRIORITIES

1. Evaluate client/fetal status.
2. Assist with efforts to maintain the pregnancy, if possible.
3. Provide emotional support.
4. Provide appropriate instruction/information.

DISCHARGE GOALS

1. Client/fetal condition stable following procedure.
2. Uterine contractions absent.
3. Therapeutic needs and concerns understood.

NURSING DIAGNOSIS:	ANXIETY [SPECIFY LEVEL]
May be related to:	Situational crisis, threat of death/fetal loss.
Possibly evidenced by:	Increased tension, apprehension, feelings of inadequacy, sympathetic stimulation, and repetitive questioning.
DESIRED OUTCOMES— CLIENT/COUPLE WILL:	Verbalize fears and concerns.
	Report anxiety is reduced to a manageable level.
	Use individually appropriate coping mechanisms to deal with the short- and long-term outcomes of the situation.

ACTIONS/INTERVENTIONS	RATIONALE
Independent	
Provide primary nurse, if possible.	Facilitates continuity of care and increases client's/couple's confidence in care providers.
Review obstetric history.	The degree of anxiety depends on the nature of the situation, the history of fetal loss, the client's understanding of the events and proposed interventions, and the client's coping behaviors, both past and present.
Identify client's perception of the threat represented by this occurrence.	The ambiguity of the outcome can aggravate anxiety.
Determine availability of support systems and psychologic response to event.	Establishes data base and plan of care.
Assess physiologic indicators of anxiety: blood pressure (BP), pulse, respiratory rate, and diaphoresis.	Physiologic changes in vital signs may have psychologic origin.
Remain with couple. Explain what is happening and what can be expected. Provide factual information about causes, implications, and proposed treatment.	May reduce anxiety by increasing awareness of the circumstance.
Provide information on an ongoing basis.	Can allay anxiety.
Collaborative	
Refer to other sources for counseling or support if anxiety is excessive or support systems are inadequate.	May aid in long-term adjustment to situation.

NURSING DIAGNOSIS:	INJURY, HIGH RISK FOR, maternal
Risk factors may include:	Surgical intervention, use of tocolytic drugs.
Possibly evidenced by:	[Not applicable; presence of signs/symptoms establishes an **actual** diagnosis.]
DESIRED OUTCOMES— CLIENT WILL:	Carry pregnancy to stage of fetal viability. Be free of complications.

ACTIONS/INTERVENTIONS	RATIONALE

Independent

ACTIONS/INTERVENTIONS	RATIONALE
Assess for presence of contraindications for cerclage procedure.	The procedure is not done if vaginal bleeding or cramping is present, if membranes are ruptured, if cervical dilatation greater than 3 cm occurs, or if the diagnosis of cervical dysfunction is in question because situation has progressed and spontaneous abortion is inevitable.
Review implication of cerclage procedure on outcome of delivery at term.	A cesarean birth may be planned if the suture is left intact, or the suture may be removed, allowing a vaginal delivery. (Note: Scar tissue may interfere with normal intrapartal cervical dilatation and effacement.)
Note presence of vaginal bleeding, leaking amniotic fluid, or uterine contractions after surgery.	Vaginal bleeding other than slight spotting may be sign of cervical dilatation. Leaking membranes may herald impending delivery and place client at greater risk for infection. Client may experience mild cramping after surgery, but strong uterine contractions may be indication of labor.
Monitor vital signs closely.	Changes in vital signs (e.g., elevated temperature or pulse, decreasing BP) may indicate infection or shock.
Notify physician of abnormal findings or signs of labor.	Prompt intervention lessens likelihood of complications.
Monitor for side effects of drugs used to prevent labor. Provide information to client.	A common side effect is maternal/fetal tachycardia; rare side effects include flushing, pulmonary edema, and congestive heart failure.

Collaborative

ACTIONS/INTERVENTIONS	RATIONALE
Prepare for cerclage procedure (Shirodkar-Barter or McDonald's modification), if indicated. Review information.	Between 14 and 18 weeks' gestation, insertion of a purse-string suture into the cervix may save the pregnancy.
Ensure continued bedrest in supine or Trendelenburg position for 24–48 hr after surgery.	Reduces pressure of presenting part on cervix.
Administer tocolytics as indicated. (Refer to CP: Preterm Labor/Prevention of Delivery.)	Reduces uterine irritability by relaxing smooth muscle.
Avoid contraction stress tests (CST or OCT) for duration of the pregnancy.	CST is contraindicated because it may result in trauma to the uterus and cervical sutures.

ACTIONS/INTERVENTIONS	RATIONALE
Independent	
Auscultate and report fetal heart tones, noting strength, regularity, and rate. Note any changes in fetal movement. Note estimated date of delivery (EDD) and fundal height.	Indicates fetal well-being. EDD provides rough estimate of fetal age to help determine chance of viability.
Assess maternal condition and presence of uterine contractions or other signs of impending delivery. (Refer to CP: Spontaneous Termination.)	If advanced cervical dilatation (4 cm or more) or regular uterine contractions occur, likelihood of preserving pregnancy is small.
Collaborative	
Prepare mother for surgical procedure, as indicated. (Refer to ND: Injury, high risk for, maternal.)	Placement of cervical suture may preserve pregnancy until fetus reaches stage of viability.
Assist with ultrasonography, if indicated.	Provides more accurate picture of fetal maturity and gestational age.

ACTIONS/INTERVENTIONS	RATIONALE
Independent	
Assess client's/couple's emotional response to situation.	The client who has been diagnosed as having premature dilation of cervix may have previously experienced fetal loss. Should delivery occur at this time, fetal survival is extremely doubtful. Previous loss may have left the couple griefstricken, with feelings of guilt.
Note presence of support systems.	Support from family, friends, and others can assist with adjustment to situation.

ACTIONS/INTERVENTIONS

Independent

Encourage client/couple to verbalize feelings surrounding previous/current event.

Discuss normalcy of individual feelings/grief reaction.

Review information about event, and discuss possibility for future pregnancies.

Provide information about community support groups.

RATIONALE

Opens lines of communication and facilitates progress toward successful resolution of feelings.

Client may suffer loss of self-esteem related to her difficulty in carrying a pregnancy to term. Feelings of inadequacy and role failure are frequently present and can have a negative impact on client's future and couple's relationship.

May lessen feelings of guilt and promote future adaptation to situation.

Participation in group activities with others who have been through similar experiences may help client/couple successfully work through grief process.

NURSING DIAGNOSIS:	**KNOWLEDGE DEFICIT [LEARNING NEED], regarding nature of condition, self-care needs**
May be related to:	Lack of exposure/recall or misinterpretation of information.
Possibly evidenced by:	Request for information, statement of misconception, inappropriate or exaggerated behaviors.
DESIRED OUTCOMES— CLIENT WILL:	Verbalize understanding of her own circumstances and treatment.
	Demonstrate self-care behavior to maintain the pregnancy.

ACTIONS/INTERVENTIONS

Independent

Determine level of client's knowledge.

Assess degree of anxiety.

Involve significant other(s) in discussions.

Provide information about future expectations.

Identify signs/symptoms to be reported to the healthcare provider. (Refer to CP: The High-Risk Pregnancy.)

Refer to other resources, such as counseling, group therapy, and childbirth education.

RATIONALE

Provides opportunity to clarify what has been learned previously, to identify cultural myths, and to correct misconceptions.

Anxiety can interfere with learning process.

Helps to reinforce understanding of all individuals involved.

Client may experience concern about whether difficulties may be encountered.

Prompt evaluation/intervention may prevent or limit complications.

May need additional help to deal with individual concerns.

Spontaneous Termination _____

This plan of care applies to the client whose pregnancy is being or has been involuntarily terminated. (To be used in conjunction with Chapter 6, CP: Perinatal Loss.)

CLIENT ASSESSMENT DATA BASE

(Refer to "Client Assessment Data Base" section in CP: Prenatal Hemorrhage.)

CIRCULATION

History of essential hypertension, vascular disease, ABO incompatibility.

ELIMINATION

Chronic nephritis.

EGO INTEGRITY

Pregnancy may/may not have been planned.

May be very anxious/fearful.

FOOD/FLUID

Poor maternal nutritional status.

PAIN/DISCOMFORT

Pelvic cramping, backache.

SAFETY

Exposure to toxic/teratogenic agents.

History of pelvic inflammatory disease, sexually transmitted diseases, or exposure to contagious diseases such as rubella, cytomegalovirus, or active herpes.

SEXUALITY

Vaginal bleeding, ranging from dark spotting to frank bleeding.

Examination may reveal premature dilation of cervix, bicornate or septate uterus, uterine fibroid tumors (leiomyoma), or other abnormalities of the maternal reproductive organs.

Note estimated date of delivery (80% of spontaneous abortions occur in first trimester).

TEACHING/LEARNING

Family history of genetic conditions.

DIAGNOSTIC STUDIES

(Refer to CP: Prenatal Hemorrhage.)

NURSING PRIORITIES

1. Evaluate client status.
2. Prevent complications.

3. Support the grief process.
4. Provide appropriate instruction/information.

DISCHARGE GOALS

1. Free of complications following procedure.
2. Support resources identified/contacted.
3. Specific therapeutic needs and concerns understood.

NURSING DIAGNOSIS:	INJURY, HIGH RISK FOR, maternal
Risk factors may include:	Abnormal blood profile (decreased hemoglobin, altered clotting factors).
Possibly evidenced by:	[Not applicable; presence of signs/symptoms establishes an **actual** diagnosis.]
DESIRED OUTCOMES— CLIENT WILL:	Report any bleeding.
	Be free of negative side effects from termination.

ACTIONS/INTERVENTIONS	RATIONALE

Independent

Assess vital signs and urine output. Note skin color/temperature. Estimate blood loss; conduct pad count/weight.

Early recognition of developing problems is important for prompt treatment.

Assess for and review signs/symptoms of disseminated intravascular coagulation (DIC): abnormal clotting factors, elevated fibrin degradation products levels.

Fetal autolysis of the products of conception, which release thromboplastin, can cause DIC.

Collaborative

Prepare client for hospitalization.

For client with missed abortion, hospitalization is necessary if products of conception are not expelled spontaneously within 1–6 wk after fetal death.

Provide i.v./oral fluids as appropriate. Administer volume expanders/blood products as indicated.

Prevents complications associated with blood loss. (Note: Religious beliefs may limit therapeutic options).

Assist with necessary therapeutic procedures, (e.g., dilatation and curettage [D and C], labor induction with oxytocin or prostaglandin).

The client with incomplete or missed abortion may need D and C to stop bleeding and to remove products of conception. If labor does not spontaneously follow fetal death, induction may be required in the second trimester.

NURSING DIAGNOSIS:	SPIRITUAL DISTRESS (DISTRESS OF THE HUMAN SPIRIT), HIGH RISK FOR
Risk factors may include:	Need to adhere to personal religious beliefs/practices; blame for loss directed at self or God.

ACTIONS/INTERVENTIONS	RATIONALE
Independent	
Determine client's/couple's religious preferences.	Establishes base for creating plan of care.
Ascertain specific client's needs; i.e., baptizing products of conception and/or formal burial.	If the client's/couple's preference for religious rites is not carried out or if desired support is not offered, the client/couple may suffer spiritual distress. (Note: Individual state laws may affect disposition of the fetus.)
Provide information in nonjudgmental manner.	Because of emotional state or lack of knowledge, client may not realize that baptism may be performed.
Be aware of own biases and beliefs about events that are occurring.	Nurses must be aware of their own beliefs and prejudices about religious practices and not impose them on the client.
Provide opportunity for expressions of anger or concern.	Allows detection of self-blame or of alienation from God and/or previously held religious beliefs and values.
Note expressions of hopelessness and/or helplessness.	These feelings may be normal initially. However, they may indicate a need for further evaluation and possible intervention to prevent or treat depression.
Encourage client's participation in development of treatment plan.	Can provide client with sense of control over difficult situation.
Offer clerical support and notify clergy, as desired.	Client may not recognize/verbalize own need for spiritual support.

NURSING DIAGNOSIS:	**KNOWLEDGE DEFICIT [LEARNING NEED], regarding cause of abortion, self-care, contraception/future pregnancy**
May be related to:	Lack of exposure to, or misinterpretation of, information.
Possibly evidenced by:	Request for information, statement of misconception, development of preventable complication.
DESIRED OUTCOMES— CLIENT WILL:	Verbalize the implications of the loss for future pregnancies.
	Explain proper use of desired contraceptive methods.

DESIRED OUTCOMES— CLIENT WILL:	Demonstrate appropriate follow-through with treatment and aftercare.
	Receive Rh$_o$(D) immune globulin within 72 hr of termination when appropriate.

ACTIONS/INTERVENTIONS	RATIONALE

Independent

Provide/review information about the cause of the spontaneous abortion when known; e.g., genetic anomalies, infection, Rh incompatibility.	May enhance understanding and promote positive self-care. Helps client prepare for future pregnancies.
Discuss alternative methods of contraception. Provide written information.	Client needs information to be able to choose a method that will meet her needs. Ovulation may occur before menses resume, so contraception needs to be considered at this time. Because of the anxiety and stress associated with the termination, verbal information may not be retained.
Identify signs/symptoms to be reported to health-care providers.	Prompt evaluation/intervention may prevent or limit complications.
Review need for RhIgG dependent on client's Rh status.	For the Rh$_o$ (D)-negative client, RhIgG prevents formation of anti-Rh-positive antibody so that adverse effects on future pregnancies are avoided.
Identify local support group or couple who have experienced a similar occurrence.	Provides opportunity to share experience with peers; may promote acceptance of loss/hope for the future.
Refer for genetic counseling as appropriate.	May be necessary if the possibility of genetic involvement exists.

NURSING DIAGNOSIS:	SEXUALITY PATTERNS, ALTERED, HIGH RISK FOR
Risk factors may include:	Increasing fear of pregnancy and/or repeat loss, impaired relationship with significant others, self-doubt regarding own femininity.
Possibly evidenced by:	[Not applicable; presence of signs/symptoms establishes an **actual** diagnosis.]
DESIRED OUTCOMES— CLIENT/COUPLE WILL:	Resume sexual activity successfully.
	Use contraception if needed/desired.

ACTIONS/INTERVENTIONS	RATIONALE

Independent

Provide open discussion about sexual activities and future pregnancies.	Client may be reluctant to initiate discussion.

ACTIONS/INTERVENTIONS	RATIONALE
Independent	
Discuss resuming sexual activity, including alternative means of gratification, as indicated.	Safety of resuming sexual activity may depend on the medical regimen. Although the client/couple may find it difficult to talk about this topic, they usually appreciate this information.
Determine past methods of contraception.	Previously used methods of contraception may need to be replaced; client may need new information about contraception in the current situation.
Provide information about contraceptive alternatives, if needed.	May need additional information to make informed decision. Some physicians advise pregnancy be avoided for 2 to 3 months following an abortion.
Provide specific information about contraceptive method chosen.	Client needs to know how to use the method and the possible side effects.
Let client/couple know it is all right to feel what they are feeling and be where they are.	There may be a time during which physiologic healing and grieving need to take place.
Discuss concerns/expectations about future plans, including pregnancies, and feelings about self in this situation.	Because of the client's inability to maintain the pregnancy, one or both partners may have doubts regarding the client's femininity and may fear trying to maintain a pregnancy again.

Elective Termination _____

Therapeutic abortion may be done to safeguard the woman's health, or a voluntary abortion may be a woman's reproductive decision.

CLIENT ASSESSMENT DATA BASE

CIRCULATION

Preexisting maternal health problems placing client at risk.

EGO INTEGRITY

Pregnancy often unplanned; may be result of incest/rape.

May express concern about decision and future expectations.

Possible feelings of abandonment; i.e., loss of contact with male partner.

Stress factors may included inadequate finances, cultural/religious conflicts, and individual plans for the future.

May have strong feelings/beliefs regarding abortion that may be in conflict with present situation (e.g., conception is result of incest or rape); lack of support, or family/other pressures to have abortion.

FOOD/FLUID

Severe nausea and vomiting.

SAFETY

History of pelvic inflammatory disease, sexually transmitted diseases (STDs), or exposure to contagious diseases, such as rubella.

Exposure to toxic/teratogenic agents.

SEXUALITY

Lack of/or inadequate use of birth control measures.

Menstrual history may include problems such as endometriosis, heavy flow, or irregular periods.

Uterus may be in extreme flexion or version.

Absence of adnexal masses (rules out ectopic pregnancy).

Vaginal bleeding may be present.

SOCIAL INTERACTION

Possible lack of support systems or conflict within the family/couple.

TEACHING/LEARNING

Family history of genetic conditions.

Note client's perception of reasons for pregnancy termination, influencing factors, and anticipated effects; note whether alternatives have been considered/discussed.

DIAGNOSTIC STUDIES

Complete blood count, blood type, and Rh determination: Identifies individual needs.
Urine or radioimmunoassay of serum for human chorionic gonadotropin: Verify pregnancy.

Papanicolau smear: Rules out dysplasias.
Gonorrheal culture, rapid plasma reagin (RPR): Determine presence of STD.
Ultrasonography: May be done to confirm the pregnancy, to date the pregnancy, or to localize the placenta, if there is some discrepancy between uterine size and estimated date of delivery.

NURSING PRIORITIES

1. Evaluate biopsychosocial status.
2. Promote/augment coping strategies.
3. Provide emotional support.
4. Prevent postprocedural complications.
5. Provide appropriate instruction/information.

DISCHARGE GOALS

1. Free of complications following procedure.
2. Coping effectively with situation.
3. Specific therapeutic needs and concerns understood.

NURSING DIAGNOSIS:	DECISIONAL CONFLICT, HIGH RISK FOR
Risk factors may include:	Unclear personal values/beliefs, lack of experience or interference with decision making, lack of relevant sources of information or information from multiple or divergent sources, support system deficit.
Possibly evidenced by:	[Not applicable; presence of signs/symptoms establishes an **actual** diagnosis.]
DESIRED OUTCOMES— CLIENT WILL:	Acknowledge feelings of anxiety/distress related to making difficult decision.
	Verbalize confidence in the decision to terminate the pregnancy.
	Meet psychologic needs as evidenced by appropriate expression of feelings, identification of options, and use of resources.
	Display relaxed manner and/or calm demeanor, free of physical signs of distress.

ACTIONS/INTERVENTIONS	RATIONALE
Independent	
Ascertain circumstances of conception and response of family/significant other. Encourage client to talk about the issues and process used to problem-solve and make decision regarding termination.	Allows the nurse to determine whether the client/couple has explored alternatives. The decision to terminate a pregnancy may have been based on an inability to problem-solve or a lack of support and resources.
Note expressions of indecision and dependence on others.	May indicate ambivalence about decision and need for further information and discussion.

ACTIONS/INTERVENTIONS	RATIONALE

Independent

Assist client to look at alternatives and use problem-solving process to validate decision. Involve significant others as appropriate.

Helps client to reinforce reasons for decision and to be comfortable that this is the course she wants to pursue.

Provide explanations about the procedure desired by the client, pre-procedural and post-procedural tests, examinations, and follow-up.

Lack of knowledge about the procedures, reproduction, or self-care may contribute to the client's/family's inability to cope positively with this event, which may be behaviorally manifested by the client canceling appointments or verbalizing ambivalence. Ongoing verbalization can foster positive decision-making by eliminating fear of the unknown and reinforcing reasons for and appropriateness of decision.

Evaluate the influence of family and significant other(s) on the client.

Conflict can arise within the client herself as well as within the family. Allows the nurse to encourage positive forces or provide support where it is lacking.

Remain with the client during examinations and the procedure. Provide both physical and emotional support.

Physical presence of nurse can help client feel accepted and reduce stress.

Act as a liaison and lend support to significant other(s).

Helps reduce stress and encourages significant other(s) to be supportive of the client.

Collaborative

Review safe options available based on gestation.

Assists client in making informed decision.

Obtain/review informed consent.

Depends on agency guidelines. No procedure should be performed unless the client freely consents to it.

Refer for additional counseling or resources, if needed.

Some clients may be more affected by the decision and may require additional support and/or education or genetic counseling.

NURSING DIAGNOSIS:	KNOWLEDGE DEFICIT [LEARNING NEED], regarding reproduction, contraception, self-care, Rh factor
May be related to:	Lack of exposure/recall or misinterpretation of information.
Possibly evidenced by:	Request for information, statement of misconception, inaccurate follow-through of instructions, development of preventable events/complications.
DESIRED OUTCOMES— CLIENT WILL:	Verbalize accurate information about the reproductive system.
	Explain proper use of desired contraceptive methods.
	Demonstrate appropriate follow-through with treatment and aftercare.

ACTIONS/INTERVENTIONS	RATIONALE

Independent

ACTIONS/INTERVENTIONS	RATIONALE
Assess level of client knowledge, and provide information about reproduction. Use charts and diagrams.	Knowledge is essential to prevention of future unplanned pregnancies. Written and visual materials are more concrete and easily understood.
Discuss alternative methods of contraception.	Client needs information to be able to choose a method that is right for her. Ovulation may occur before menses resume, so contraception needs to be considered at this time.
Give specific instructions, preferably written, about the contraceptive chosen.	Client may have a method of contraception prescribed prior to discharge. Because of the anxiety and stress associated with the termination, oral information may not be retained.
Reinforce post-abortion instructions concerning the use of tampons and resumption of sexual activity, exercise, and prescribed antibiotics, if applicable. Provide written instructions.	The stress/anxiety caused by the procedure can diminish the client's ability to retain information. Written instructions can be reviewed when necessary. (Note: Specific time frames vary according to practitioner.)
Provide information about the implications of Rh$_o$(D)-negative blood and the need for RhIgG administration.	The client may not be aware of her blood type or the implications for future pregnancies if she is Rh$_o$(D)-negative. Understanding may promote positive self-care, enhance cooperation, and help prepare client for future pregnancies.
Identify signs/symptoms to be reported to healthcare provider.	Prompt evaluation/intervention may prevent or limit complications.
Verify Rh-negative status and administer RhIgG. Give 50 μg for early abortion; otherwise, dosage is the same as for delivery or fetal hemorrhage in the nonsensitized client.	For the Rh$_o$(D)-negative client, RhIgG prevents anti-Rh-positive antibody formation, so that negative effects on future pregnancies are avoided. Microdoses are given for early abortions and this dose is sufficient up to 12 weeks' gestation. Fetal red blood cells may be noted as early as 38 days after conception.

ACTIONS/INTERVENTIONS

Independent

Note comments indicating feelings of guilt, negative self-concept/self-esteem, and ethical or religious value conflicts.

Discuss alternatives to abortion with the client and significant other(s), if present. Maintain nonjudgmental attitude.

Assist with problem-solving within the client's ethical and religious framework.

Support the client's decision.

Explain the grief response that may occur.

Stress the importance of follow-up visits.

Collaborative

Refer for further counseling. (Refer to CP: The High-Risk Pregnancy, ND: Coping, Individual/Family, ineffective.)

RATIONALE

There may be conflict with family/significant other(s) regarding the morality of the client's decision, which can create confusion for the client.

A decision based on a rational choice is less likely to result in conflict.

The ability to project the consequences of a decision or to explore alternatives may be hampered by anxiety and emotion.

Client may have few, if any, support systems available at this time and may need a nonjudgmental resource.

Client may not expect to feel loss.

There may be delayed psychologic reactions, which can be assessed at the follow-up visit along with the physical status.

Some clients may need additional counseling before and after abortion to help them resolve feelings of conflict or guilt.

NURSING DIAGNOSIS:	ANXIETY [SPECIFY LEVEL]
May be related to:	Situational/maturational crises, unmet needs, unconscious conflict about essential values/beliefs.
Possibly evidenced by:	Increased tension, apprehension, fear of unspecific consequences, sympathetic stimulation, focus on self.
DESIRED OUTCOMES—CLIENT WILL:	Recognize the presence of anxiety.
	Identify the cause of anxiety.
	Begin to use positive coping strategies to adjust to the situation.
	Report anxiety reduced to a manageable level.

ACTIONS/INTERVENTIONS

Independent

Acknowledge the client's anxiety. Encourage ventilation of feelings.

Be empathic and nonjudgmental.

Provide instruction in breathing and relaxation techniques.

RATIONALE

Client may need assistance in recognizing reactions.

Conveys a caring attitude.

Holding the breath and tightening the muscles may influence physiologic responses (blood pressure, pulse, and respiration). Tense muscles may interfere with the procedure.

205

ACTIONS/INTERVENTIONS	RATIONALE

Independent

Explain procedures before they are performed, and stay with the client to provide concurrent feedback.

A physical presence is reassuring and can increase cooperation and promote a sense of security.

Have a support person remain with the client, particularly if she is undergoing a second-trimester procedure requiring induction of labor.

The presence of a familiar person can help reduce anxiety and promote relaxation and coping.

NURSING DIAGNOSIS:	PAIN/DISCOMFORT*
May be related to:	After effects of procedure/drug effect.
Possibly evidenced by:	Report of discomfort, distraction behaviors, changes in muscle tone, autonomic responses/change in vital signs.
DESIRED OUTCOMES— CLIENT WILL:	Identify/use methods that provide relief.
	Report discomfort is minimized and/or controlled.

*Authors' note: Currently there is no NANDA diagnostic label that addresses issues of comfort below the level of Pain [acute] or chronic. Although the label of **Discomfort** is not approved, we believe it speaks more directly to the identified problem.

ACTIONS/INTERVENTIONS	RATIONALE

Independent

Explain to client the nature of discomfort expected.

Knowledge helps the client to cope with reality. Cramping pain during and for 1 week after a first-trimester termination is expected. Clients treated with prostaglandins may experience nausea, vomiting, and diarrhea.

Determine the extent and location of discomfort.

Although some discomfort is expected, severe cramping and abdominal tenderness may indicate complications.

Provide instruction in relaxation and breathing techniques.

May help break the cycle of fear, tension, and pain; provide distraction; and enhance coping.

Collaborative

Administer narcotic/nonnarcotic analgesics, sedatives, and antiemetics, as indicated.

These drugs promote relaxation, decrease pain awareness, and control side effects of treatment (drug therapy).

Provide information about the use of prescription or nonprescription analgesics.

Specific instructions about the use of any drugs increases awareness of safe use and side effects.

NURSING DIAGNOSIS:	INJURY, HIGH RISK FOR, maternal
Risk factors may include:	Surgical procedure/anesthesia.

Possibly evidenced by:	[Not applicable; presence of signs/symptoms establishes an **actual** diagnosis.]
DESIRED OUTCOMES— CLIENT WILL:	Recognize and report signs/symptoms of complications.
	Institute appropriate corrective measures.

ACTIONS/INTERVENTIONS	RATIONALE

Independent

Monitor and assess blood loss. Count and weigh or estimate peripads.	Bleeding is normally like a heavy menstrual period. Excessive loss (more than 1 large pad per hour for 4 hr) may indicate retained tissue or uterine perforation.
Monitor vital signs, noting increased pulse rate, severe headache, or flushed face.	Changes in vital signs are often a late sign of hypovolemic shock from blood loss. If hypertonic saline solution is used in second-trimester procedure and is inadvertently injected into the circulatory system, convulsions and death can occur.
Note dyspnea, wheezing, or agitation.	Prostaglandins may cause vasoconstriction or bronchial constriction.
Evaluate level of discomfort.	Abdominal pain, tenderness, and severe cramping may indicate retained tissue or uterine perforation.
Instruct client to report symptoms indicating complications (e.g., temperature 100.4° F or greater, chills, malaise, abdominal pain or tenderness, severe bleeding, heavy flow with clots, foul-smelling and/or greenish vaginal discharge).	Clients are in the healthcare facility for a short time. Complications, including bleeding and infection, may be manifested days or weeks after the procedure.
Provide information about person to contact in case of emergency.	A specific phone number encourages contact; can save time and anxiety.
Stress importance of returning for a follow-up examination.	Follow-up is necessary to assess healing. A repeat pregnancy test is sometimes done after early first-trimester procedures to assure procedure was complete.

Collaborative

Assess cervical status before procedure. Assist as needed with insertion of *Laminaria* tent or prostaglandin (lamicel) gel.	Aids in softening cervix; may be inserted from 24 to 48 hr before procedure.
Assist with ultrasonography before procedure as indicated.	Helps in confirming gestational age and the size of products of conception.
Assist with any additional treatment or procedures necessary to control complications.	Intravenous therapy may need to be instituted with or without oxytoxics. Additional surgery (dilatation and curettage or hysterectomy) may be needed to control bleeding.

(Refer to Chapter 5, CP: Labor: Induced/Augmented.)

Preterm Labor/Prevention of Delivery _____

Delivery within 2 weeks of the expected date of delivery is desired by both pregnant women and health professionals. *Preterm labor* refers to labor that occurs *after* the fetus has reached the period of viability (at least 20 weeks' gestation but *before* the completion of the 37th week). Carrying the pregnancy to term may be contraindicated if associated client or fetal risks outweigh the risks of delivering a preterm infant.

CLIENT ASSESSMENT DATA BASE

Note: Etiology is unknown in 70%–80% of cases; premature rupture of membranes (PROM) occurs in the remaining 20%–30%.

CIRCULATION

Hypertension, pathologic edema (signs of pregnancy-induced hypertension [PIH]).

Preexisting cardiovascular disease.

EGO INTEGRITY

Moderate anxiety apparent.

FOOD/FLUID

Inadequate or excessive weight gain.

PAIN/DISCOMFORT

Intermittent to regular contractions less than 10 min apart and lasting at least 30 sec for 30–60 min.

RESPIRATORY

May be heavy smoker (7–10 cigarettes/day).

SAFETY

Infection may be present (i.e., urinary tract infection [UTI] and/or vaginal infection).

SEXUALITY

Cervical os dilated/effacing.

Bloody show may be noted.

Membranes may be ruptured (PROM).

Third-trimester bleeding.

Previous abortions, preterm labor/delivery, history of cone biopsy.

Uterus may be overdistended, owing to hydramnios, macrosomia, or multiple gestation.

SOCIAL INTERACTION

May be low socioeconomic class.

TEACHING/LEARNING

Inadequate or no prenatal care.

May be under age 18 or over age 40.

Alcohol/other drug use, diethylstilbesterol (DES) exposure.

DIAGNOSTIC STUDIES

Ultrasonography: Assesses gestation (with fetal weight of 500 to 2499 g).
Nitrazine test: Determines PROM.
White blood cell count: Elevation indicates presence of infection.
Urinalysis and culture: Rule out UTI.
Vaginal culture, rapid plasma reagin (RPR): Identify infection.
Amniocentesis: Lecithin to sphingomyelin (L/S) ratio detects phosphatidylglycerol (pg) for fetal lung maturity; or amniotic infection.
Electronic monitoring: Validates uterine activity/fetal status.

NURSING PRIORITIES

1. Ascertain maternal condition/presence of labor and fetal well-being .
2. Assist with efforts to maintain pregnancy, if possible.
3. Prevent complications.
4. Provide emotional support.
5. Provide necessary information.

DISCHARGE GOALS

1. Cessation of uterine contractions.
2. Free of complications and/or untoward effects.
3. Dealing with situation in a positive manner.
4. Signs of preterm labor/complications and therapy needs understood.

NURSING DIAGNOSIS:	ACTIVITY INTOLERANCE
May be related to:	Muscle/cellular hypersensitivity.
Possibly evidenced by:	Continued uterine contractions/irritability.
DESIRED OUTCOMES— CLIENT WILL:	Reduce activity level.
	Identify/engage in activities appropriate to situation.
	Demonstrate reduction/cessation of uterine contractions.

ACTIONS/INTERVENTIONS	RATIONALE
Independent	
Explain the reasons for requiring bedrest, use of left lateral recumbent/side-lying position, and decreasing activity.	These measures are intended to keep the fetus off the cervix and to enhance uterine perfusion; bed rest may decrease uterine irritability.
Provide comfort measures such as back rubs, changes of position, or decreased stimuli in room (e.g., low lighting).	Decreases muscle tension and fatigue and promotes sense of well-being.
Group activities together as much as possible, such as medication administration, vital signs, and assessments.	Promotes longer opportunities for client to rest between interruptions.

ACTIONS/INTERVENTIONS

Independent

Provide uninterrupted periods for rest/sleep.

Offer diversional activities, such as reading, radio, and television, or visits with selected friends or family.

RATIONALE

Promotes rest, prevents fatigue, and may enhance relaxation.

Assists client in coping with decreased activity.

NURSING DIAGNOSIS:	POISONING, HIGH RISK FOR
Risk factors may include:	Dose-related toxic/side effects of tocolytics.
Possibly evidenced by:	[Not applicable; presence of signs/symptoms establishes an **actual** diagnosis.]
DESIRED OUTCOMES— CLIENT WILL:	Display no evidence of untoward effects of tocolytic therapy.
	Prevent or minimize maternal injury.
	Demonstrate cessation of uterine contractions, dependent on fetal well-being.

ACTIONS/INTERVENTIONS

Independent

Place client in left lateral position. Elevate head during infusion of I.V. drug.

Monitor vital signs. Auscultate lung sounds; note cardiac irregularities and reports of dyspnea/chest tightness.

Measure intake and output. Encourage fluid intake between 2000 and 3000 ml/day, unless restricted (e.g., during administration of magnesium sulfate [$MgSO_4$]).

Weigh client daily.

Monitor for drowsiness, hot flashes, respiratory depression, and depressed deep tendon reflexes, as appropriate.

Have antidote available (calcium gluconate for $MgSO_4$; propranolol for ritodrine or terbutaline sulfate).

RATIONALE

Decreases uterine irritability, increases placental perfusion, and prevents supine hypotension.

Complications, such as pulmonary edema, cardiac dysrhythmias/tachycardia, agitation, dyspnea, chest pain, and increase in plasma volume may occur with administration of beta-receptor agonists (ritodrine, isoxsuprine) and terbutaline sulfate, which stimulates $beta_2$ receptors (especially with concomitant use of steroids).

Promotes adequate hydration and prevents fluid excess, especially when $MgSO_4$ is administered; $MgSO_4$ is excreted through the kidneys, and so urine output must be maintained.

Detects potential alteration in urinary functioning/retention of fluid.

Signs of neuromuscular depression, indicating increasing serum levels of $MgSO_4$.

Administration of antidote may be necessary to reverse or counteract effects of tocolytic agent.

ACTIONS/INTERVENTIONS	RATIONALE
Collaborative	
Assist as needed with sterile vaginal examination.	To assess cervical status. Vaginal examinations are kept to a minimum, because they may contribute to uterine irritability. Safety of tocolytics when cervix is more than 4 cm dilated or 80% effaced is not documented and is generally contraindicated.
Administer I.V. solution or fluid bolus as indicated.	Hydration may decrease uterine activity. Before beginning drug therapy, hydration promotes renal clearance and minimizes hypotension.
Administer I.V. solutions containing tocolytic agents (MgSO4, ritodrine, isoxsuprine, terbutaline sulfate) by infusion pump or microdrip equipment, or by subcutaneous route. (Note: Experimental studies are evaluating the use of prostaglandin synthesis inhibitors such as indomethacin (Indocin), and other beta sympathomimetics such as hexaprenaline.)	$MgSO_4$ acts directly on myometrial tissue to promote relaxation; therefore, there are fewer side effects than other drug choices. For example, unlike I.V. ritodrine, (it produces no change in blood pressure, maternal heart rate or cardiac output. Ritodrine and terbutaline sulfate relax uterine muscle as well as bronchioles and blood vessel walls. Only ritodrine (Yutopar) is currently approved by the Food and Drug Administration (FDA) as a tocolytic agent; however, in some instances, terbutaline sulfate (Brethine) may be preferred.
Administer nifedipine (Procardia) to be chewed and swallowed with food or drink. Nifedipine may be alternated with terbutaline sulfate.	Nifedipine, a calcium channel blocker, is used experimentally when other drugs fail to suppress uterine activity.
Monitor nifedipine levels. Note development of tachycardia, hypotension, peripheral edema, or proteinuria.	The therapeutic dosage of Nifedipine for preterm labor has not been established. Periodic monitoring may prevent development of adverse/toxic effects, such as congestive heart failure.
Apply antiembolic hose, and provide passive range of motion exercises to legs every 1–2 hr.	Prevents pooling of blood in lower extremities, which can occur due to smooth muscle relaxation.
Monitor serum magnesium levels every 6 hr during administration of $MgSO_4$. (Refer to CP: Pregnancy-Induced Hypertension.)	Therapeutic level is 4 to 7 mEq/L or 6 to 8 mg/dl. Toxic signs and symptoms develop above 10 mg/dl.
Insert indwelling catheter, as indicated.	Urine output must be monitored and maintained when administering $MgSO_4$. Output should be at least 30 ml/hr or 100 ml in a 4-hr period.
Monitor serum glucose and potassium levels.	Ritodrine and terbutaline sulfate cause movement of potassium ions into cells, decreasing plasma levels; elevated blood glucose and plasma insulin levels, and release of glycogen from muscle and liver may result in hyperglycemia.
Assess uterine contractions and fetal heart rate (FHR) electronically while I.V. tocolytic agents are administered, or at least twice a day when oral route is used.	Tactile and electronic monitoring of uterine contractions and FHR provides a continuous fetal/uterine assessment and basis for altering or maintaining rate of drug administration. (Note: External monitors may increase contractions with some patients.)

211

ACTIONS/INTERVENTIONS

Collaborative

Decrease i.v. dose of tocolytics and gradually wean client to subcutaneous or oral dose, as indicated.

Arrange for transfer of client to high-risk facility or tertiary care center, if uterine activity persists following administration of tocolytics.

RATIONALE

i.v. therapy should continue for at least 12 hr after contractions cease. Oral/subcutaneous therapy should begin 30 min before stopping i.v. infusion.

Helps ensure availability of appropriate intensive care, which may be needed by newborn following preterm delivery.

NURSING DIAGNOSIS:	INJURY, HIGH RISK FOR, fetal
Risk factors may include:	Delivery of preterm/immature infant.
Possibly evidenced by:	[Not applicable; presence of signs/symptoms establishes an **actual** diagnosis.]
DESIRED OUTCOMES— CLIENT WILL:	Maintain the pregnancy at least to the point of infant maturity.

ACTIONS/INTERVENTIONS

Independent

Assess for maternal conditions that would contraindicate steroid therapy to facilitate fetal lung maturity.

Assess FHR; note presence of uterine activity or cervical changes. Prepare for possible preterm delivery.

Provide information about the actions and side effects of the drug therapy.

Review pros and cons of steroid therapy with client/couple.

Stress necessity of follow-up care.

RATIONALE

In PIH and chorioamnionitis, steroid therapy may aggravate hypertension and mask signs of infection. Steroids may increase blood glucose levels in the patient with diabetes. Drug will not be effective if unable to delay birth for at least 48 hr.

Tocolytics can increase FHR. Delivery may be extremely rapid with small infant if persistent uterine contractions are unresponsive to tocolytics, or if cervical changes continue.

Important for the client/couple to know the purpose of the drug(s) being administered. Ritodrine therapy may cause fetal tachycardia, hyperglycemia, acidosis, and hypoxia. Steroid therapy is most effective when the fetus is between 30 and 32 weeks' gestation (but may be used between 26 and 34 weeks' gestation).

Short-term effects may include hypoglycemia, increased risk of sepsis, and possible suppression of aldosterone for up to 2 wk following delivery. Long-term effects on the development of the child will not be known until longitudinal studies have been completed.

If fetus is not delivered within 7 days of administration of steroids, dose should be repeated weekly.

ACTIONS/INTERVENTIONS

Collaborative

Assist as needed with analysis of amniotic fluid from amniocentesis or vaginal pool specimen; test for ferning.

Administer betamethasone (Celestone) deep I.M.

Initiate tocolytic therapy as ordered.

RATIONALE

L/S ratio, presence of pg, and shake test results indicate fetal lung status. Ferning indicates rupture of membranes with increased risk of infection.

This synthetic cortisol can accelerate fetal lung maturity by stimulating surfactant production and thereby preventing or decreasing the severity of respiratory distress syndrome. (Note: Administration into the deltoid muscle may result in local atrophy.)

Helps reduce myometrial activity to prevent/delay early delivery.

NURSING DIAGNOSIS:	**ANXIETY [SPECIFY LEVEL]; FEAR**
May be related to:	Situational crisis, perceived or actual threats to self and fetus.
Possibly evidenced by:	Increased tension, apprehension, sympathetic stimulation, and extraneous movements.
DESIRED OUTCOMES— CLIENT WILL:	Verbalize understanding of individual situation and possible outcomes.
	Report anxiety is reduced/manageable.
	Appear relaxed; maternal vital signs within normal limits.

ACTIONS/INTERVENTIONS

Independent

Explain procedures, nursing interventions, and treatments. Keep communication open; discuss with client the possible side effects and outcomes, maintaining an optimistic attitude.

Orient client and partner to labor suite environment.

Answer questions honestly, including information regarding contraction pattern and fetal status.

Encourage use of relaxation techniques.

Encourage verbalization of fears or concerns.

Monitor maternal/fetal vital signs.

RATIONALE

Knowledge of the reasons for these activities can decrease fear of the unknown.

Helps client and significant other(s) feel at ease and more comfortable in their surroundings.

Providing clear information can help the client/couple understand what is happening and may reduce anxiety.

Enables the client to obtain maximum benefit from rest periods; prevents muscle fatigue and improves uterine blood flow.

Can help reduce anxiety and stimulate identification of coping behaviors.

Vital signs of client and fetus may be altered by anxiety. Stabilization may reflect reduction of anxiety level.

ACTIONS/INTERVENTIONS

Independent

Assess support systems available to the client/couple.

Collaborative

Administer sedative if other measures are not successful.

RATIONALE

The assistance and caring of significant others, including caregivers, are extremely important during this time of stress and uncertainty.

Provides soothing and tranquilizing effect.

NURSING DIAGNOSIS:	KNOWLEDGE DEFICIT [LEARNING NEED], regarding preterm labor, treatment needs, and prognosis
May be related to:	Misinterpretation or lack of information.
Possibly evidenced by:	Verbalization of questions/concerns, statements of misconceptions.
DESIRED OUTCOMES— CLIENT WILL:	Verbalize awareness of implications and possible outcomes of preterm labor.
	Demonstrate understanding of home therapy and/or self-care needs.
	Identify signs/symptoms requiring evaluation/intervention.

ACTIONS/INTERVENTIONS

Independent

Ascertain client's knowledge about preterm labor and possible outcomes.

Assess client readiness to learn.

Include significant other(s) in teaching-learning process.

Provide information about follow-up care when client is discharged.

Identify signs/symptoms that should be reported immediately to healthcare provider; i.e., sustained uterine contractions, clear drainage from vagina.

Review signs/symptoms of "early" labor. (Refer to CP: The High-Risk Pregnancy, ND: Knowledge Deficit [Learning Need].)

Demonstrate how client is to evaluate contraction activity after discharge, lying down, tilted to one side with a pillow to the back; placing fingertips on the fundus for approximately 1 hr to note hardening/tightening of the uterus.

RATIONALE

Establishes data base and identifies needs.

Factors such as anxiety or lack of awareness of need for information can interfere with readiness to learn. Retention of information is enhanced when client is motivated and ready to learn.

Support from significant others can help allay anxiety as well as reinforce principles of teaching and learning.

Client may need to return on a regular basis for monitoring and/or treatments.

Prompt evaluation and interventions can improve the outcome of the pregnancy.

Assists client to recognize preterm labor so that therapy to suppress this labor can be instituted or reinstituted promptly.

Although uterine contractions commonly occur periodically, contractions occurring 10 min or less apart for an hour can result in cervical dilation and labor without prompt intervention.

ACTIONS/INTERVENTIONS	RATIONALE

Independent

Arrange for client to visit neonatal intensive care unit.	Helps alleviate fears and facilitates adjustment to situation.
Discuss need to restrict lifestyle by stopping smoking and possibly by restricting sexual activity and nipple stimulation.	Nicotine has adverse effect on fetoplacental growth and on uterine circulation. Orgasm release of oxytocin may stimulate uterine activity.
Encourage regular rest periods 2 to 3 times daily in left side-lying position after discharge. If bedrest is to be continued, suggest client spend part of day on couch/recliner.	Enhances relaxation and reduces fatigue. If client is up and about, resting in the bedroom may maximize rest; however, the client on full bedrest may feel isolated and bored without a "change of scenery."
Review daily routine, employment, and activity schedule to identify alternatives and ways to compensate for limitations.	Pacing activities, avoidance of heavy chores/lifting, and modification in work duties or cessation of employment may help prevent recurrence of preterm labor.
Recommend client empty bladder every 2 hr while awake.	Prevents pressure of a full bladder on the irritable uterus.
Review daily fluid needs; i.e., 2 to 3 quarts of liquid and avoidance of caffeine.	Dehydration and caffeine both lead to increased uterine muscle irritability.
Obtain permit, if necessary, for administration of terbutaline.	Currently only ritodrine is FDA-approved as a tocolytic agent; terbutaline sulfate is still considered an experimental drug.
Stress avoidance of over-the-counter (OTC) drugs while tocolytic agents are administered unless approved by physician.	Concurrent use of OTC drugs may cause deleterious effects, especially if OTC drug has similar side effects to tocolytic agent (e.g., antihistamines or inhalers with bronchodilating effects such as epinephrine [Primatene Mist]).
Recommend adhering to a predetermined schedule for oral drug therapy.	Maintains blood level of drug for optimum effect. (Note: Recent studies are evaluating the effectiveness and safety of low-dose continuous subcutaneous infusion and intermittent high-dose bolus administration of terbutaline in place of oral therapy.
Provide information about taking oral tocolytics with food.	Food improves tolerance to drug and reduces side effects.
Identify drug side effects requiring medical evaluation.	Pulse rate greater than 120 bpm; presence of tremors, palpitations, chest pain, or dyspnea; or feelings of nervousness and agitation may require alteration/discontinuation of drug.

Collaborative

Refer client to other resources, as indicated (e.g., community health nurse, childbirth classes, groups such as Parents of Twins, or other couple who have had a successful outcome).	May need additional help in coping with situation, especially if client returns home to await delivery.

NURSING DIAGNOSIS:	**PAIN [ACUTE]/DISCOMFORT***
May be related to:	Muscle contractions, effects of medications.

Possibly evidenced by:	Reports of pain/discomfort, muscle tension, narrowed focus.
DESIRED OUTCOMES—CLIENT WILL:	Report discomfort is minimized, controlled.
	Use relaxation techniques.
	*Authors' note: Currently there is no NANDA diagnostic label that addresses issues of comfort below the level of Pain [acute] or chronic. Although the label of **Discomfort** is not approved, we believe it speaks more directly to the identified problem.

ACTIONS/INTERVENTIONS	RATIONALE
Independent	
Expedite the admissions process and institute bed rest for client, using left lateral position.	Left lateral position improves uterine blood flow and may decrease uterine irritability.
Review relaxation techniques.	Helps reduce client's perception of discomfort and promotes sense of control. (Refer to ND: Anxiety [specify level]; Fear.)
Use nursing comfort measures such as changes of linen and position, back rug, and Therapeutic Touch.	Relieve muscle tension and fatigue.
Assess mucous membranes for ulceration or reaction to chewing of nifedipine.	Nifedipine may be irritating to oral cavity, in which case it should be swallowed whole.
Monitor maternal and fetal vital signs.	Reflects effectiveness of interventions.
Collaborative	
Administer analgesics, as indicated.	Mild analgesics decrease muscle tension and discomfort.

(Refer to CP: The High-Risk Pregnancy, and other CPs as appropriate; e.g., Chapter 5, Cesarean Birth; Chapter 7, Preterm Infant.)

CHAPTER 5

INTRAPARTAL CONCEPTS

INTRAPARTAL ASSESSMENT TOOL

The client should undergo a basic assessment at the time of admission because not all clients will arrive with a prenatal history/physical or will have been seen prenatally. Furthermore, with the increase in early release, discharge planning must be implemented as soon as feasible.

Date: _____ Name: _____ DOB: _____ Age: _____
Reason for Admission: _____
Health Care Provider: Maternal: _____ Infant: _____
Father of Child: _____ Age: _____ Race: _____
Source of information: _____ Reliability: _____ (1–4 with "4" very reliable)

ACTIVITY/REST

Subjective
Sleep/rest last 24 hr: _____
Occupation: _____
Usual activities/hobbies: _____

Objective
Neuromuscular assessment: Quality of
   extremities: _____
  Posture: _____ Tremors: _____
  ROM: _____ Strength: _____
  Deformity: _____ Other: _____

CIRCULATION

Subjective
History of: Elevated BP: _____ Heart trouble: _____
  Rheumatic fever: _____ Ankle/leg edema: _____
  Phlebitis: _____ Slow healing: _____
Extremities: Numbness: _____ Tingling: _____
Cough/character of sputum: _____

Objective
BP: R: Sitting: _____ Lying: _____ Standing: _____
  L: Sitting: _____ Lying: _____ Standing: _____
Pulse (palpation): Carotid: _____ Temporal: _____
  Jugular: _____ Peripheral: _____
Heart sounds: _____ Rate: _____
  Rhythm: _____ Quality: _____
Extremities: Temperature: _____ Color: _____
  Capillary refill: _____
  Homans' sign: _____ Varicosities: _____
Color/cyanosis: Mucous membranes: _____
  Nail beds: _____
  Conjunctiva: _____ Sclera: _____

ACTIVITY/REST
EGO INTEGRITY

Subjective
Pregnancy planned (Y/N): _____
Previous childbirth experience: _____
Attitude toward this pregnancy: Client: _____
   Father: _____
Client's perceptions of her mother's childbirth experience: _____
   Support person(s) (identify): _____
Expectations during labor/delivery of: Self: _____
   Support person(s): _____
   Primary nurse: _____ Physician/midwife: _____
Relationship with father of the baby: _____
Fathers: Education: _____ Occupation: _____
Financial concerns: _____
Religion: Maternal: _____ Paternal: _____
Cultural factors: _____
Presence of risk factors: _____
Preparation for childbirth: _____

Objective
Response to labor (check those that apply):
   Calm: _____ Anxious: _____ Excited: _____
   Depressed: _____ Fearful: _____ Irritable: _____
   Restive: _____ Intense: _____ Tired: _____
Observed interaction with support person(s): _____
   Physical contact: _____ Verbal: _____
Management of labor: _____
   Frequency of coaching required: _____
   Use of support person(s): _____
   Breathing/relaxation techniques: _____
   Copes with contraction effectively: _____

ELIMINATION

Subjective:
Usual bowel pattern: _____ Laxative use: _____
   Character of stool: _____ Bleeding: _____
   Hemorrhoids: _____
Character of urine: _____
Pain/burning/difficulty voiding: _____
History of kidney/bladder disease: _____

Objective
Bowel sounds: _____
Hemorrhoids (per pelvic exam): Internal: _____
   External: _____
Bladder palpable: _____ Overflow voiding: _____
Urinalysis report: _____ Albuminuria: _____

FOOD/FLUID

Subjective
Oral intake last 4 hr: _____
Nausea/vomiting: _____
Dentures: _____
Headache: _____ Visual disturbance: _____
Epigastric pain: _____
Use of diuretics: _____
Diabetes/onset: _____
Thyroid disorder: _____

Objective
Current weight: _____ Total prenatal gain: _____
   Height: _____
Skin turgor: _____
Edema (degree): Legs: _____ Sacrum: _____
   Hands: _____ Face: _____
Deep tendon reflexes: _____
Jugular distention: _____
Appearance of tongue: _____
   Mucous membranes: _____
   Teeth/gums: _____
Breath sounds: _____
Hb/Hct (anemia): _____
Diabetic screening: GTT: _____
Urine sugar/acetone: _____
Thyroid studies: _____

HYGIENE

Subjective
Activities of daily living: Independent: _____
   Dependent (specify): _____

Objective
General appearance: _____
Body odor: _____ Condition of scalp: _____
Presence of vermin: _____

NEUROSENSORY

Subjective

Fainting spells/dizziness: _____
Tingling/numbness (location): _____
Seizures: _____ How controlled: _____
Eyes: Vision loss: R: _____ L: _____
Ears: Hearing loss: R: _____ L: _____

Objective

Mental status (e.g., alert/oriented): _____
Pupils: R: _____ L: _____ Glasses: _____
   Contacts: _____
Hearing aid: _____
Unusual speech pattern/impairment: _____

PAIN/DISCOMFORT

Subjective

Uterine contractions began: _____
   Became regular: _____
Location of contractile pain:
   Front: _____ Sacral area: _____
Degree of discomfort: Mild: _____ Moderate: _____
   Severe: _____
How relieved: Breathing/relaxation techniques: _____
   Positioning: _____ Sacral rubs: _____
   Effleurage: _____

Objective

Facial expression: _____ Narrowed focus: _____
Body movement: _____

RESPIRATORY

Subjective

Dyspnea/cough: _____
History: Bronchitis: _____ Asthma: _____
   Tuberculosis: _____ Other: _____
Smoker: _____ Pk/day: _____ No. of yr: _____

Objective

Respiratory status: Rate: _____ Depth: _____
   Quality: _____
Breath sounds: _____
Sputum characteristics: _____
Chest x-ray results: _____

SAFETY

Subjective

Allergies/sensitivity: _____ Reaction (specify): _____
History of STD (date/type): _____
Health status of living children: _____
Month of first prenatal visit: _____
Previous/current obstetric problems and treatment:
   PIH: _____ Kidney: _____
   Hemorrhage: _____ Cardiac: _____
   Diabetes: _____ Infection (specify)/UTI: _____
   ABO/Rh sensitivity: _____ Uterine surgery: _____
   Anemia: _____
Length of time since last pregnancy: _____
Type of previous delivery: _____
Blood transfusion: _____ When: _____
   Reaction (describe): _____
Maternal stature/build: _____
Fractures/dislocations: _____
Pelvis: _____
Arthritis/unstable joints: _____
Spinal problems/deformity:
   Kyphosis: _____ Scoliosis: _____
   Trauma: _____ Surgery: _____
Prosthesis: _____
Ambulatory Devices: _____

Objective

Temperature: _____
Skin integrity: _____ Rashes: _____ Sores: _____
   Bruises: _____ Scars: _____
Paresthesia/paralysis: _____
Fetal status: Heart rate: _____ Location: _____
   Method of auscultation: _____
   Fundal height: _____ Estimated gestation: _____
   Activity/movement: _____
   Fetal assessment testing (Y/N): _____
      Date: _____
      Test: _____ Results: _____
Labor status: Cervical dilation: _____
   Effacement: _____
   Fetal descent: _____ Engagement: _____
   Presentation: _____ Lie: _____
   Position: _____
Membranes: Intact: _____ Ruptured (time): _____
   Nitrazine test: _____ Amount of drainage: _____
   Character: _____
Blood type/Rh: Maternal: _____ Paternal: _____
Screens: Sickle cell: _____ Rubella: _____
   Hepatitis: _____ HIV: _____
Serology: Syphilis: Pos _____ Neg _____
Cervical/rectal culture: Pos _____ Neg _____
Vaginal warts/lesions: _____
Perineal varicosities: _____

SEXUALITY

Subjective

Last menstrual period: _____
 EDD: _____
Practices breast self-exam (Y/N): _____
Obstetric history: Gravida: _____ Para: _____
 Abortions: _____ Living children: _____
 Full term: _____ Premature: _____
 Multiple births: _____
Delivery history: Year: _____ Place: _____
 Length gestation: _____ Length labor: _____
 Type delivery: _____ Born A/D: _____ Wt: _____
 Complications Maternal/Fetal: _____

Objective

Pelvis: Adequate: _____ Borderline: _____
 Contracted: _____
 Inlet: _____ Mid: _____ Outlet: _____
 Pelvimetry: _____
Prognosis for delivery: _____
Breast exam: _____ Nipples: _____
Serology test: _____

SOCIAL INTERACTION

Subjective

Marital status: _____ No. of years in relationship:
 _____
 Members of family: _____
Living with: _____ Extended family: _____
 Other support person(s): _____
Report of problems: _____

Objective

Verbal/nonverbal communication with family/SOs:
 _____
Family interaction (behavior) pattern: _____

TEACHING/LEARNING

Subjective

Education level: Maternal: _____ Paternal: _____
 Occupations: _____
Dominant language (specify): _____
Literate: _____ Cognitive limitations: _____
Familial risk factors (maternal/paternal; indicate relationship):
 Tuberculosis: _____ Diabetes: _____
 High BP: _____ Epilepsy: _____
 Heart disease: _____ Stroke: _____
 Kidney disease: _____ Cancer: _____
 Multiple births: _____
 Genetic problems (specify): _____
 Other (specify): _____
Prescribed medications (note last dose):
 Drug: _____ Dose: _____ Schedule: _____
 Take regularly (Y/N): _____
Nonprescription drugs: OTC: _____
 Street drugs: _____
 Use of alcohol (amount/frequency): _____
Relevant illnesses and/or hospitalizations/surgeries: _____
Plans/expectations for: Labor site (choice): _____
 Support person(s) for labor: _____
 For delivery: _____
Medications: During labor: _____ During
 delivery: _____
Position: During labor: _____ During
 delivery: _____

Discharge Plan Considerations

Date information obtained: _____
Anticipated date of discharge: _____
Availability of maternity leave: _____
Resources available: Persons: _____
Financial: _____
Anticipated needs/assistance required: _____

Procedures: I.V. fluids: _____   Fetal monitor: _____
   Enema: _____   Episiotomy: _____
   Type of delivery: _____
   Type of infant feeding: _____
Preparation for:
   Prenatal/intrapartal period and infant care/feeding:
   Classes: _____   Books: _____
   Other (specify): _____
Support person(s) preparation: _____

Labor: Stage I—Latent Phase

The latent phase, or the first phase of stage I labor, begins with the onset of true labor and ends with the cervix dilated 4 cm. The phase averages approximately 8–10 hr, up to 20 hr for nulliparas, and 3–6 hr, up to 14 hr for multiparas.

CLIENT ASSESSMENT DATA BASE

EGO INTEGRITY

May be excited or anxious.

PAIN/DISCOMFORT

Regular contractions, increasing in frequency, duration, and severity.

Contractions are mild, 5–30 min apart, lasting 10–30 sec.

SAFETY

Fetal heart tones best heard at level of umbilicus (dependent on fetal position).

SEXUALITY

Membranes may or may not have ruptured.

Cervix is dilated from 0–4 cm.

Fetus may be at station 0 (primigravida) or from 0–+2 cm (multigravida).

Scant vaginal discharge, may be pink mucus ("show"), brownish, or may consist of mucus plug.

NURSING PRIORITIES

1. Enhance client's/couple's emotional and physical preparedness for labor.
2. Promote and facilitate normal labor progress.
3. Support client's/couple's coping abilities.
4. Prevent maternal/fetal complications.

NURSING DIAGNOSIS:	ANXIETY, HIGH RISK FOR
Risk factors may include:	Situational crisis, interpersonal transmission, unmet needs.
Possibly evidenced by:	[Not applicable; presence of signs/symptoms establishes an **actual** diagnosis.]
DESIRED OUTCOMES— CLIENT WILL:	Report anxiety is at a manageable level.
	Use breathing and relaxation techniques proficiently.
	Appear relaxed appropriate to the labor situation.
	Remain normotensive.

ACTIONS/INTERVENTIONS	RATIONALE
Independent	
Provide primary nurse or continuous intrapartum professional support as indicated.	Continuity of care and assessment may decrease stress. Research studies suggest that these clients require less pain medication, which may result in shorter labor.
Orient client to environment, staff, and procedures. Provide information about psychologic and physiologic changes in labor as needed.	Education may reduce stress and anxiety and promote labor progress.
Assess level and causes of anxiety, preparedness for childbirth, cultural background, and role of significant other/coach.	Provides baseline information. Anxiety magnifies pain perception, interferes with use of coping techniques, and stimulates the release of aldosterone, which may increase sodium and water resorption.
Monitor blood pressure (BP) and pulse as indicated. (If BP is elevated on admission, repeat procedure in 30 min to obtain true reading once client is relaxed.)	Stress activates the hypothalamic-pituitary-adrenocortical system, which increases retention and resorption of sodium and water and increases excretion of potassium. Sodium and water resorption may contribute to development of intrapartal toxemia/hypertension. Loss of potassium may contribute to reduction of myometrial activity.
Monitor uterine contractile pattern; report dysfunctional labor. (Refer to CP: Dysfunctional Labor/Dystocia.)	A hypertonic or hypotonic contractile pattern may develop if stress persists and causes prolonged catecholamine release.
Encourage client to verbalize feelings, concerns, and fears.	Stress, fear, and anxiety have a profound effect on the labor process, often prolonging the first phase owing to utilization of glucose reserves; causing excess epinephrine release from adrenal stimulation, which inhibits myometrial activity; and increasing norepinephrine levels, which tends to increase uterine activity. Such an imbalance of epinephrine and norepinephrine can create a dysfunctional labor pattern.
Demonstrate breathing and relaxation methods. Provide comfort measures. (Refer to CP: Labor: Stage I—Active Phase, ND: Pain [acute].)	Reduces stressors that might contribute to anxiety; provides coping strategies.
Promote privacy and respect for modesty; reduce unnecessary exposure. Use draping during vaginal examination.	Modesty is a concern in most cultures. Support person may or may not desire to be present while client is examined or treated.
Be aware of client's need or preference for female caregivers.	Cultural practices may prohibit presence of men during labor and/or delivery.
Provide opportunity for conversation to include choice of infant names, expectations of labor, and perceptions/fears during pregnancy.	Presents opportunity for client to verbalize excitement about herself, the pregnancy, and her baby. Serves as a diversion to help pass time during what is commonly the longest phase of labor.
Determine diversional needs; encourage variety of activities (e.g., television, books, cards, walking).	Helps divert attention away from labor, making time pass more quickly. If condition permits, walking usually promotes cervical dilatation, shortens labor, and lowers the incidence of fetal heart rate (FHR) abnormalities.

ACTIONS/INTERVENTIONS

Independent

Prepare for and/or assist with discharge from hospital setting, as indicated.

RATIONALE

During very early latent phase with no apparent progress of labor, the comfort and familiarity of the home environment may decrease anxiety, thereby hastening the labor process, and allow opportunity for a variety of acceptable diversional activities.

NURSING DIAGNOSIS:	KNOWLEDGE DEFICIT [LEARNING NEED], regarding progression of labor, available options
May be related to:	Lack of exposure/recall, information misinterpretation.
Possibly evidenced by:	Questions, statements of misconception, inaccurate follow-through of instruction.
DESIRED OUTCOMES— CLIENT WILL:	Verbalize understanding of psychologic and physiologic changes.
	Participate in decision-making process.
	Demonstrate correct breathing and relaxation techniques.

ACTIONS/INTERVENTIONS

Independent

Assess client's preparation, knowledge level, and expectations.

Provide information about procedures (especially fetal monitor and telemetry) and normal progression of labor.

Discuss options for care during the labor/delivery process. Provide information about birthing alternatives if available and appropriate.

Review roles of staff members.

Demonstrate breathing/relaxation techniques appropriate to each phase of labor; teach and review pushing positions for stage II.

Review appropriate activity levels and safety precautions, whether client remains in hospital/clinic or returns home.

Obtain informed consent for procedures. Explain usual procedures and the possible risks associated with labor and delivery.

Refer to ND: Coping, Individual, ineffective, high risk for.

RATIONALE

Helps establish information/learning needs.

Antepartal education can facilitate the labor and delivery process, assist the client in maintaining control during labor, help promote a positive attitude and/or sense of control, and may decrease reliance on medication.

Necessary for the client/couple to participate actively in the decision-making process.

Identifies resources for specific needs/situations.

Unprepared couples need to learn coping mechanisms on admission to reduce stress and anxiety. Couples with prior preparation can benefit from review and reinforcement.

Provides guidelines for client to make appropriate self-care choices; allows client to engage in safe diversional activities to refocus attention/pass time.

When procedures involve client's body, it is necessary for client to have appropriate information to make informed choices.

NURSING DIAGNOSIS:	FLUID VOLUME DEFICIT, HIGH RISK FOR
Risk factors may include:	Decreased intake, increased losses (e.g., mouth breathing, hormonal shifts).
Possibly evidenced by:	[Not applicable; presence of signs/symptoms establishes an **actual** diagnosis.]
DESIRED OUTCOMES— CLIENT WILL:	Maintain fluid intake as able.
	Demonstrate adequate hydration (e.g., moist mucous membranes, yellow/amber urine of appropriate amount, absence of thirst, lack of fever, stable vital signs/FHR).

ACTIONS/INTERVENTIONS	RATIONALE

Independent

Monitor intake/output. Note urine specific gravity. Encourage client to empty bladder at least once every $1^1/_2$–2 hr.	Intake and output should be approximately equal, dependent on degree of hydration. Concentration of urine increases as urine output decreases and may warn of dehydration. Fetal descent may be impaired if bladder is distended.
Monitor temperature every 4 hr, more frequently if elevated. Monitor vital signs/FHR as indicated.	Dehydration may cause increases in temperature, BP, pulse, respirations, and FHR.
Assess production of mucus, amount of tearing within eyes, and skin turgor.	Additional signs of adequacy of hydration or development of dehydration.
Provide clear fluids and ice chips, as permitted.	Helps promote hydration and may provide some calories.
Assess cultural practices regarding intake.	Some cultures (e.g., some African tribes, residents of the southern region of the United States) drink special teas, believing they stimulate continued progression of labor.
Provide mouth care and hard candy, as permitted.	Reduces discomfort of a dry mouth.

Collaborative

Administer bolus of parenteral fluids, as indicated.	May be needed if oral intake is inadequate or restricted. Acts as a safeguard in the event of dehydration or hemorrhage; counteracts some negative effects of anesthesia or analgesia.
Monitor hematocrit (Hct) level.	Hct increases as the plasma component decreases in the presence of severe dehydration.

NURSING DIAGNOSIS:	COPING, INDIVIDUAL, INEFFECTIVE, HIGH RISK FOR
Risk factors may include:	Situational crisis, personal vulnerability, inadequate support systems and/or coping methods.
Possibly evidenced by:	[Not applicable; presence of signs/symptoms establishes an **actual** diagnosis.]

ACTIONS/INTERVENTIONS	RATIONALE
Independent	
Determine client's cultural background, coping abilities, and verbal and nonverbal responses to pain. Determine past experiences and antepartal preparation.	Each client responds in a unique manner to the stresses of labor and associated discomfort based on these factors. The appearance of appropriate or inappropriate coping may actually be a manifestation of one's culture; e.g., Asian or African-American women may be stoic because of fear of shaming self or family, whereas Hispanic and Middle Eastern cultures typically encourage verbal expression of suffering. For this reason, it is important to compare both verbal and nonverbal responses when assessing coping ability.
Note age of client and presence of partner/support person(s).	Negative coping may result in increased anxiety, in which case the client may request medication too early in the labor process. Younger clients and those unattended may exhibit more vulnerability to stress/discomfort and have difficulty maintaining composure/control.
Stay with/provide companion for client who is alone.	Unmet needs and fear of being abandoned at a time of increased dependence may interfere with ability to focus on the task at hand.
Support client/couple during contractions by reinforcing breathing and relaxation techniques.	Reduces anxiety and provides distraction, which may block perception of pain impulses within the cerebral cortex.
Establish rapport and accept behavior without judgment. Make verbal contract about expected behaviors of client and nurse.	Facilitates cooperation; provides an opportunity for the client to leave the experience with positive feelings and enhanced self-esteem. Nurse may need to set limits if inappropriate behavior occurs or may need to assist the client in maintaining/regaining control of breathing and relaxation.
Assess uterine contraction/relaxation pattern, fetal status, vaginal bleeding, and cervical dilatation.	Rule out possible complications that could be causing or contributing to the discomfort/reduced coping ability.
Collaborative	
Discuss types of regional or systemic analgesics or anesthetics when available in birth setting.	Helps client make informed choice about methods to relieve pain/promote comfort and maintain control.
Discuss administration of sedatives such as secobarbital.	Occasionally, a barbiturate may be administered during early labor to promote rest/sleep, so that the client enters the active phase more relaxed and rested and better able to cope.

NURSING DIAGNOSIS:	INFECTION, HIGH RISK FOR, maternal
Risk factors may include:	Invasive procedures, repeat vaginal examinations, fecal contamination, rupture of amniotic membranes.
Possibly evidenced by:	[Not applicable; presence of signs/symptoms establishes an **actual** diagnosis.]
DESIRED OUTCOMES— CLIENT WILL:	Identify/use techniques to minimize risk of infection.
	Be free of signs of infection (e.g., afebrile; amniotic fluid clear, nearly colorless and odorless).

ACTIONS/INTERVENTIONS

Independent

Perform initial vaginal examination; repeat when contractile pattern or client's behavior indicates significant progress of labor.

Emphasize importance of good handwashing as appropriate.

Use aseptic technique during vaginal examination.

Provide/encourage perineal care after elimination; every 4 hr and as indicated, change underpad/ linen when wet.

Assess vaginal secretions using phenaphthazine (nitrazine paper). Perform microscopic examination for positive ferning.

Monitor and describe character of amniotic fluid.

Monitor temperature, pulse, respirations, and white blood cell count (WBC), as indicated.

Collaborative

Provide oral and parenteral fluids as indicated.

Carry out perineal preparation when indicated.

Administer cleansing enema, if indicated.

RATIONALE

Repeated vaginal examinations contribute to the incidence of ascending tract infections.

Reduces risk of acquiring/spreading infective agents.

Helps prevent growth of bacteria; limits contaminants from reaching the vagina.

Reduces risk of ascending tract infection.

Spontaneous rupture of membranes 1 hr or more before onset of labor increases risk of chorioamnionitis during the intrapartal period. Color changes of nitrazine paper from yellow to dark blue indicate presence of alkaline amniotic fluid; ferning indicates rupture of membranes. (Note: Excess bloody show, which is more alkaline than vaginal secretions, may cause similar changes on nitrazine paper.)

With infection, amniotic fluid becomes thicker and yellow-tinged and has a strong, detectable odor.

Within 4 hr after rupture of membranes, the incidence of chorioamnionitis increases progressively with the passage of time, reflected by elevations of vital signs and WBC count.

Maintains hydration and general sense of wellbeing.

May facilitate perineal repair at delivery and cleaning of perineum in the postpartal period, thereby reducing risk of infection.

Although not often done, bowel evacuation may promote progression of labor and prevent or reduce risk of infection due to contamination of the sterile field during delivery.

227

ACTIONS/INTERVENTIONS	RATIONALE
Collaborative	
Administer prophylactic antibiotic i.v. if indicated.	Although antibiotic administration in the intrapartal period is somewhat controversial because of antibiotic load for the fetus, it may help protect against development of chorioamnionitis in the client at risk.
Administer oxytocin infusion, as ordered. (Refer to CP: Labor: Induced/Augmented.)	If client is at 36 weeks' gestation, and labor does not ensue within 24 hr after rupture of membranes, infection may occur. Onset of labor reduces risk of negative effects on client/fetus.
Obtain blood cultures if symptoms of sepsis are present.	Detects and identifies causative organism(s).

NURSING DIAGNOSIS:	INJURY, HIGH RISK FOR, fetal
Risk factors may include:	Tissue hypoxia/hypercapnia or infection.
Possibly evidenced by:	[Not applicable; presence of signs/symptoms establishes an **actual** diagnosis.]
DESIRED OUTCOMES— CLIENT WILL:	Display FHR and beat-to-beat variability within normal limits, with no ominous periodic changes in response to uterine contractions.

ACTIONS/INTERVENTIONS	RATIONALE
Independent	
Perform Leopold's maneuvers to determine fetal position, lie, and presentation.	A transverse lie or breech presentation may necessitate cesarean birth. Other abnormalities, such as face, chin, and posterior presentations, may also require special interventions to prevent prolongation of labor.
Obtain baseline FHR manually and/or electronically. Monitor frequently. Note FHR variability and periodic changes in response to uterine contractions.	FHR should range from 120 to 160 bpm with average variability, accelerating in response to maternal activity, fetal movement, and uterine contractions.
Note progress of labor.	Prolonged/dysfunctional labor with an extended latent phase can contribute to problems of maternal exhaustion, severe stress, infection, and hemorrhage due to uterine atony/rupture, placing the fetus at greater risk for hypoxia and injury.
Inspect maternal perineum for vaginal warts, herpetic lesions, or chlamydial discharges.	Sexually transmitted diseases (STDs) can be acquired by the fetus during the delivery process; therefore, cesarean birth may be indicated, especially for clients with herpes simplex virus type II. (Refer to Chapter 4, CP: Prenatal Infection.)
Administer perineal care to mother according to protocol; change underpad when wet.	Helps prevent growth of bacteria; eliminates contaminants that might contribute to maternal chorioamnionitis or fetal sepsis.

ACTIONS/INTERVENTIONS	RATIONALE

Independent

Note FHR when membranes rupture, then every 15 min × 3. Monitor periodic changes in FHR after rupture.

Changes in amniotic fluid pressure with rupture, and/or variable decelerations of FHR after rupture, may reflect compression of the umbilical cord, which reduces oxygen transfer to the fetus.

Assess for visible cord prolapse at vaginal introitus. If present:

Calm the couple, explain the prolapse and its implications.

Helps couple understand the significance of prolapse, and promotes cooperation with emergency measures.

Elevate client's hips (elevated Sims' position), or help client to assume knee-chest position.

Relieves pressure of presenting part on cord.

Check cord for pulsations; wrap cord in sterile gauze soaked in saline solution.

Keeps cord moist and helps decrease chance of uterine infection.

Monitor FHR and periodic changes if a problem is detected with fetoscopy or external monitor. Note presence of sinusoidal pattern.

Any decrease in baseline FHR variability—severe and untreatable variable decelerations, recurrent late decelerations, or persistent bradycardia—indicates fetal decompensation, hypoxia, or acidosis resulting from anaerobic metabolism. Sinusoidal pattern is often associated with fetal anemia or severe fetal hypoxia just prior to death.

Position client in left lateral position.

Increases placental perfusion; prevents supine hypotensive syndrome.

Collaborative

Prepare for transfer to hospital setting as indicated, if client is at home, or in alternative birth center.

Compromised fetal status or identification of maternal conditions such as STD requires closer observation and may indicate need for therapeutic interventions such as cesarean birth.

Rule out maternal problems or medications that could effect an increase in FHR (e.g., fever, anxiety, anemia, beta-sympathomimetic drugs).

These factors can increase maternal and fetal heart rate.

Turn off oxytocin if infusing, and increase plain intravenous solution.

Promotes greater periods of uterine relaxation and increases uteroplacental blood flow; increases circulating blood volume available for oxygen transfer within maternal circulation of the placenta.

Administer oxygen via face mask.

Increases maternal oxygen available for fetal uptake.

Assist as needed with obtaining fetal scalp blood sample when indicated.

Scalp samples between 7.20 and 7.25 pH require constant monitoring and may possibly require immediate surgical intervention.

Prepare for surgical intervention, as indicated. (Refer to CP: Cesarean Birth.)

CNS damage occurs if fetal hypoxia/acidosis persists for more than 30 min. Cesarean birth is treatment of choice for prolapsed cord prior to full cervical dilatation, in order to avoid fetal compromise/demise.

Labor: Stage I—Active Phase

As contractions increase to moderate intensity in the active phase, and as the cervix dilates from 4 to 8 cm, the client becomes more involved and focused on the labor process. The active phase lasts approximately 1–2 hr in the multipara and 3–4 hr in the nullipara. The fetus descends in the birth canal at approximately 2 cm/hr in the multipara and 1 cm/hr in the nullipara.

CLIENT ASSESSMENT DATA BASE

ACTIVITY/REST

May show evidence of fatigue.

EGO INTEGRITY

May appear more serious and absorbed with labor process.

Apprehensive about ability to control breathing and/or perform relaxation techniques.

PAIN/DISCOMFORT

Contractions are moderate, occurring every 2.5–5 min and lasting 30–45 sec.

SAFETY

Fetal heart tone detected slightly below umbilicus in vertex position.

Fetal heart rate (FHR) variability and periodic changes commonly noted in response to contractions, abdominal palpation, and fetal movement.

SEXUALITY

Cervix dilates from approximately 4 to 8 cm (1.5 cm/hr multipara, 1.2 cm/hr nullipara).

Moderate amount of bloody show present.

Fetus descends to +1–+2 cm below ischial spines.

NURSING PRIORITIES

1. Promote and facilitate normal progression of labor.
2. Support client's/couple's coping abilities.
3. Promote maternal and fetal well-being.

NURSING DIAGNOSIS:	PAIN [ACUTE]
May be related to:	Tissue dilation/hypoxia, pressure on adjacent structures, stimulation of both parasympathetic and sympathetic nerve endings.
Possibly evidenced by:	Verbalizations, distraction behaviors (restlessness), muscle tension.

DESIRED OUTCOMES—CLIENT WILL:	Identify/use techniques to control pain/discomfort.
	Report discomfort is minimized.
	Appear relaxed/resting between contractions.
	Be free of side effects if analgesia/anesthetic agents are administered.

ACTIONS/INTERVENTIONS	RATIONALE
Independent	
Assess degree of discomfort through verbal and nonverbal cues; note cultural influences on pain response.	Attitudes and reactions to pain are individual and based on past experiences, understanding of physiologic changes, and cultural background.
Assist in use of appropriate breathing/relaxation techniques and in abdominal effleurage.	May block pain impulses within the cerebral cortex through conditioned responses and cutaneous stimulation. Facilitates progression of normal labor.
Assist with comfort measures (e.g., back/leg rubs, sacral pressure, back rest, mouth care, repositioning, perineal care, and linen changes).	Promotes relaxation and hygiene; enhances feeling of well-being. (Note: Left lateral position reduces uterine pressure on the vena cava, but periodic repositioning prevents tissue ischemia and/or muscle stiffness and promotes comfort.)
Encourage client to void every 1–2 hr. Palpate above symphysis pubis to determine distention, especially after nerve block.	Keeps bladder free of distention, which can increase discomfort, result in possible trauma, interfere with fetal descent, and prolong labor. Epidural or paracervical analgesia may interfere with sensations of fullness.
Provide information about available analgesics, usual responses/side effects (client and fetal), and duration of analgesic effect in light of current situation.	Allows client to make informed choice about means of pain control. (Note: If conservative measures are not effective and increasing muscle tension impedes progress of labor, minimal use of medication may enhance relaxation, shorten labor, limit fatigue, and prevent complications.)
Support client's decision about the use or nonuse of medication in a nonjudgmental manner. Continue encouragement for efforts and use of relaxation techniques.	Helps reduce feelings of failure in the client/couple who may have anticipated an unmedicated birth and did not follow through with that plan. Enhances sense of control and may prevent/decrease need for medication.
Instruct client in use of patient-controlled analgesia; monitor her use.	Enables the client to manage own pain control, usually with less medication.
Time and record the frequency, intensity, and duration of uterine contractile pattern every 30 min.	Monitors labor progress and provides information for client. (Note: Anesthetic agents may alter uterine contractile pattern.) (Refer to CP: Dysfunctional Labor/Dystocia.)
Assess nature and amount of vaginal show, cervical dilation, effacement, fetal station, and fetal descent.	Cervical dilatation should be 1.2 cm/hr in the nullipara and 1.5 cm/hr in the multipara; vaginal show increases with fetal descent. Choice and timing of medication is affected by degree of dilatation and contractile pattern.

231

ACTIONS/INTERVENTIONS	RATIONALE

Independent

Provide safety measures; e.g., encourage client to move slowly, keep side rails up after drug administration, and support legs during transfer.

Regional block anesthesia produces vasomotor paralysis, so that sudden movement may precipitate hypotension. Analgesics alter perception, and client may fall trying to get out of bed.

Assess blood pressure (BP) and pulse every 1–2 min after regional injection for first 15 min, then every 10–15 min for remainder of labor. Position in left lateral position with head flat and feet elevated, or elevate knees and manually displace uterus to the left as indicated.

Maternal hypotension, the most common side effect of regional block anesthesia, may interfere with fetal oxygenation. Supine hypotension may occur owing to lithotomy position during administration of paracervical anesthetic. Left lateral positioning increases venous return and enhances placental circulation. Assesses FHR variability. Agents such as bupivacaine (Marcaine) and chloroprocaine hydrochloride (Nesacaine) have little effect on FHR variability; alterations should be investigated thoroughly. (Note: Risks associated with caudal anesthesia include perforation of fetal scalp, as well as maternal rectum.)

Engage client in conversation to assess sensorium; monitor breathing patterns and pulse.

Systemic toxic responses with altered sensorium occur if medication is absorbed into the vascular system. Altered sensorium may also be an early indicator of developing hypoxia. Interference with respiratory functioning occurs if analgesia is too high, paralyzing the diaphragm.

Assess for warmth, redness of large toe or ball of foot, and equal distribution of spinal medication.

Ensures proper placement of catheter for continuous block and adequate levels of anesthetic agent.

Collaborative

Administer analgesic such as alphaprodine hydrochloride (Nisentil) or meperidine hydrochloride (Demerol) with potentiating tranquilizers, by I.V. or deep I.M. between contractions, if indicated.

I.V. route is preferred because it ensures more rapid and equal absorption of analgesic. Medication administered by I.M. route may require up to 45 min to reach adequate plasma levels, and maternal uptake may be variable, especially if drug is injected into subcutaneous fat instead of muscle.

Initiate or assist with paracervical block when cervix is 4–5 cm dilated. (Anesthetic may be administered in a single dose or on a continuous basis using an indwelling catheter.)

Anesthetizes the inferior hypogastric plexus and ganglia, providing relief during cervical dilatation. (Note: Paracervical block may cause severe fetal bradycardia.)

Administer oxygen, and increase plain fluid intake if systolic pressure falls below 100 mm Hg or falls more than 30% below baseline pressure.

Increases circulating fluid volume, placental perfusion, and oxygen available for fetal uptake.

Monitor FHR electronically, and note decreased variability or bradycardia. Obtain fetal scalp sample if bradycardia persists for 30 min or more.

Fetal bradycardia and decreased variability is a common side effect of paracervical block. These side effects can begin 2–10 min after administration of anesthetic, and may last for 5–10 min.

Administer I.V. bolus of 500 to 1,000 ml of lactated Ringer's solution just before administration of peridural block.

Increased circulating fluid level helps prevent side effects of hypotension associated with block.

ACTIONS/INTERVENTIONS

Collaborative

Administer peridural, epidural, or caudal block anesthesia using an indwelling catheter.

Administer succinylcholine chloride and assist with intubation if convulsion occurs.

RATIONALE

Provides relief once active labor is established; reinforcement through catheter provides sustained comfort during delivery. Such analgesia does not interfere with uterine activity and/or Ferguson reflex. It relaxes the cervix and facilitates the labor process, but may alter internal fetal rotation and diminish client's ability to bear down when needed.

Systemic toxic reaction to epidural anesthetic may alter sensorium or cause convulsions if medication is absorbed into the vascular system.

NURSING DIAGNOSIS:	**URINARY ELIMINATION, ALTERED**
May be related to:	Altered intake, fluid shifts, hormonal changes, mechanical compression of bladder, effects of regional anesthesia.
Possibly evidenced by:	Changes in amount/frequency of voiding, urinary urgency, urine retention, slowed progression of labor.
DESIRED OUTCOMES— CLIENT WILL:	Empty bladder appropriately. Be free of bladder injury.

ACTIONS/INTERVENTIONS

Independent

Palpate above symphysis pubis.

Record and compare intake and output. Note amount, color, concentration, and specific gravity of urine.

Encourage frequent attempts to void, at least every 1–2 hr.

Position client upright, run water from the faucet, pour warm water over the perineum, or have client blow bubbles through a straw.

Take temperature and pulse, noting increases. Assess dryness of skin and mucous membranes.

RATIONALE

Detects presence of urine in bladder and degree of fullness. Incomplete emptying of the bladder may occur due to decreased sensation and tone.

Output should approximate intake. Increased output may reflect excessive fluid retention prior to the onset of labor and/or effects of bedrest; i.e., increased glomerular filtration rate and decreased adrenal stimulation. Specific gravity reflects kidney's ability to concentrate urine and the client's hydration status. Decreased output may occur with dehydration, hemorrhage, and pregnancy-induced hypertension (PIH). (Refer to CP: Intrapartal Hypertension.)

Pressure of the presenting part on the bladder often reduces sensation and interferes with complete emptying. Regional anesthesia also may contribute to voiding difficulties.

Facilitates voiding/enhances emptying of bladder.

Monitors degree of hydration.

ACTIONS/INTERVENTIONS	RATIONALE

Collaborative

Catheterize as indicated.	An overdistended bladder can cause atony, impede fetal descent, or become traumatized by presenting part of the fetus.

NURSING DIAGNOSIS:	ANXIETY, HIGH RISK FOR
Risk factors may include:	Situational crisis, interpersonal transmission of other(s), unmet needs.
Possibly evidenced by:	[Not applicable; presence of signs/symptoms establishes an **actual** diagnosis.]
DESIRED OUTCOMES—CLIENT WILL:	Report anxiety minimized/manageable.
	Appear relaxed and/or in control.
	Self-initiate breathing/relaxation techniques.
	Follow instructions of coach/nurse.

ACTIONS/INTERVENTIONS	RATIONALE

Independent

Assess client's anxiety level through verbal and nonverbal cues.	Identifies level of intervention necessary. Excess anxiety increases pain perception and can have negative impact on the outcome of labor.
Provide continuous intrapartal professional support. Inform client that she will not be left alone.	Fear of abandonment can intensify as labor progresses. The client may experience increased anxiety and/or loss of control when left unattended.
Encourage use of breathing and relaxation techniques. Breathe with client/couple as necessary.	Assists in reduction of anxiety and of perception of pain within the cerebral cortex, enhancing sense of control.
Monitor FHR and its variability; monitor maternal BP.	Prolonged anxiety can result in endocrine imbalances, with excess release of epinephrine and norepinephrine, elevating BP and pulse. (Note: Medications relaxing smooth muscle may reduce FHR variability and maternal BP.)
Evaluate contractile pattern/progression of labor.	Increasing force/intensity of uterine contractions can heighten client's concerns about personal capabilities and outcome of labor. In addition, increased levels of epinephrine may also inhibit myometrial activity. Excess anxiety and stress levels can deplete glucose reserves, thereby decreasing the amount available for adenosine triphosphate synthesis, which is necessary for uterine contractions.
Refer to CP: Labor: Stage 1—Latent Phase, ND: Anxiety, high risk for.	If client is admitted during the active phase, interventions usually accomplished during the latent phase need to be addressed at this time.

ACTIONS/INTERVENTIONS

Collaborative

Administer combination of narcotic and tranquilizer (e.g., meperidine hydrochloride and hydroxyzine pamoate [Vistaril]) I.M.

RATIONALE

Tranquilizers potentiate the action of the narcotic, reduce anxiety, and assist client in focusing on breathing/relaxation techniques.

NURSING DIAGNOSIS:	COPING, INDIVIDUAL/COUPLE, INEFFECTIVE, HIGH RISK FOR
Risk factors may include:	Situational crises, personal vulnerability, inadequate support systems.
Possibly evidenced by:	[Not applicable; presence of signs/symptoms establishes an **actual** diagnosis.]
DESIRED OUTCOMES— CLIENT/COUPLE WILL:	Identify effective coping behaviors.
	Engage in activities to maintain/enhance control.

ACTIONS/INTERVENTIONS

Independent

Ascertain client's understanding and expectations of the labor process.

Encourage verbalization of feelings.

Reinforce positive coping mechanisms and aids to relaxation.

Note withdrawn behavior.

Assess effectiveness of significant other/coach. Provide role modeling as indicated.

Demonstrate behaviors coach can use to assist with pain control and relaxation. Provide information and correct misconceptions.

Limit verbalization/instruction during contractions to a single coach.

RATIONALE

The client's/couple's coping skills are most challenged during the active and transition phases as contractions become increasingly intense. Lack of knowledge, misconceptions, or unrealistic expectations can have a negative impact on coping abilities.

Helps nurse gain insight into individual needs, and assists client/couple to deal with concerns.

Assists client in maintaining or gaining control. Enhances feelings of competence, and fosters self-esteem. The stressors that accompany labor can be threatening to a woman's self-esteem, especially if she has not coped positively with past experiences and/or successfully accomplished the tasks of pregnancy.

Adolescents, in particular, may become withdrawn and not express needs to be nurtured.

The client is influenced by those around her and may respond positively when others remain calm and in control.

Enhances coping and self-esteem of coach/couple.

Allows client to focus attention and may enhance ability to follow directions. Multiple coaches may actually result in decreased concentration, confusion, and loss of control.

ACTIONS/INTERVENTIONS	RATIONALE

Independent

Provide positive reinforcement for efforts. Use touch and soothing words of encouragement.	Encourages repetition of appropriate behaviors. Enhances individual's confidence in own ability to cope with or handle labor, while also meeting her needs for dependency.

NURSING DIAGNOSIS:	**INJURY, HIGH RISK FOR, maternal**
Risk factors may include:	Effects of medication, delayed gastric motility, physiologic urges.
Possibly evidenced by:	[Not applicable; presence of signs/symptoms establishes an **actual** diagnosis.]
DESIRED OUTCOMES— CLIENT WILL:	Verbalize understanding of individual risks and reasons for specific interventions.
	Follow directions to protect self/fetus from injury.
	Be free of preventable injury/complications.

ACTIONS/INTERVENTIONS	RATIONALE

Independent

Monitor uterine activity manually or electronically, noting frequency, duration, and intensity of contraction. (Refer to CP: Dysfunctional Labor/Dystocia.)	The uterus is susceptible to possible rupture if a hypertonic contractile pattern develops spontaneously or in response to oxytocin administration. Placental separation and hemorrhage can also occur if contraction persists.
Institute bedrest as labor intensifies or following administration of medication. Avoid leaving client unattended.	Promotes safety should dizziness or precipitous delivery occur following administration of medication.
Place client in left lateral or semi-upright position.	Increases placental perfusion and prevents supine hypotensive syndrome. (Note: Some women may prefer an upright position during the phase of maximum slope of labor [4–9 cm dilation]). Studies suggest this position may shorten this phase of labor without increasing discomfort or producing adverse effects on fetal well-being.)
Administer perineal care every 4 hr and p.r.n.	Reduces risk of ascending infection, which can occur, especially with prolonged rupture of membranes.
Monitor temperature and pulse.	Elevation of temperature and pulse are indicators of developing infection.
Offer client ice chips or clear liquids, as appropriate; avoid solid foods.	Delayed gastric motility inhibits digestion during labor, placing the client at risk for aspiration.
Monitor urine for ketones.	Urinary ketones indicate metabolic acidosis resulting from a deficiency in glucose metabolism, which may reduce uterine activity and cause myometrial fatigue that prolongs labor.

ACTIONS/INTERVENTIONS	RATIONALE

Independent

Have client pant or blow out when she feels the urge to bear down.

Panting during the active phase or the transition phase prevents bearing down too early, and can thereby prevent lacerations or edema of the cervix/birth canal.

Collaborative

Discontinue or decrease flow rate of oxytocin if contraction lasts longer than 60 sec, or if the uterus fails to relax between contractions.

Helps to prevent hypertonic contractile pattern with resultant decreased placental blood flow and risk of uterine rupture. (Refer to CP: Dysfunctional Labor/Dystocia.)

Administer i.v. antibiotics, if indicated.

Administration of antibiotics during labor is somewhat controversial, but may protect against infection in cases of prolonged rupture of membranes.

NURSING DIAGNOSIS:	**GAS EXCHANGE, IMPAIRED, HIGH RISK FOR, fetal**
Risk factors may include:	Altered oxygen supply/blood flow.
Possibly evidenced by:	[Not applicable; presence of signs/symptoms establishes an **actual** diagnosis.]
DESIRED OUTCOMES— FETUS WILL:	Display FHR and beat-to-beat variability within normal limits (WNL).
	Be free of adverse effects from hypoxia during labor.

ACTIONS/INTERVENTIONS	RATIONALE

Independent

Assess for presence of maternal factors or conditions that compromise uteroplacental circulation (e.g., diabetes, PIH, kidney or cardiac disorders). Note prenatal testing of placental functioning by nonstress test or contraction stress test.

High-risk situations that negatively affect circulation are likely to be manifested in late decelerations and fetal hypoxia.

Monitor FHR every 15–30 min if WNL. Monitor FHR electronically if it is less than 120 bpm, or greater than 160 bpm.

Fetal tachycardia or bradycardia is indicative of possible compromise, which may necessitate intervention.

Check FHR immediately if membranes rupture, and then again 5 min later. Observe maternal perineum for visible cord prolapse.

Detects fetal distress due to visible or occult cord prolapse.

Instruct client to remain on bedrest if presenting part does not fill the pelvis (station +4).

Reduces risk of cord prolapse.

Note and record color and amount of amniotic fluid and time of membrane rupture.

In a vertex presentation, prolonged hypoxia results in meconium-stained amniotic fluid owing to vagal stimulation, which relaxes the fetal anal sphincter. Hydramnios may be associated with fetal anomalies and poorly controlled maternal diabetes.

ACTIONS/INTERVENTIONS	RATIONALE

Independent

Monitor fetal descent in birth canal through vaginal examination. Plot progress on Friedman graph. In cases of breech presentation, assess FHR more frequently.

Prolonged head compression stimulates vagal responses and results in fetal bradycardia if the rate of descent is not at least 1 cm/hr for primipara or 1.5 cm/hr for multiparas. Fundal pressure in breech presentation may cause vagal stimulation and head compression.

Assess FHR changes during a contraction, noting decelerations and accelerations.

Detects severity of hypoxia and possible cause. The fetus is vulnerable to potential injury during labor, owing to situations that reduce oxygen levels, such as cord prolapse, prolonged head compression, or uteroplacental insufficiency

Monitor uterine activity manually or electronically.

Development of hypertonicity can compromise uteroplacental circulation and fetal oxygenation.

Talk to client/couple as care is being given, and provide information about situation, as appropriate.

Provides psychologic support and assurance to reduce anxiety related to increased monitoring.

Collaborative

If late or variable decelerations occur:

Transfer to acute care setting if client is in an alternative birth setting.

May require specialized monitoring or interventions available only in acute care setting.

Discontinue oxytocin if it is being administered.

Strong contractions caused by oxytocin may inhibit or reduce uterine relaxation and lower fetal oxygen levels.

Place client in left lateral position.

Increases placental perfusion, which may correct problem if due to uteroplacental insufficiency.

Turn client from side to side as indicated.

Helps take pressure from the presenting part off the umbilical cord if cord is being compressed.

Increase I.V. infusion rate.

Increases circulating fluid volume and placental perfusion.

Administer oxygen to client.

Increases available oxygen for placental transfer.

Prepare for and assist with fetal scalp sampling, repeating as indicated.

Prolonged, decreased variability may indicate acidosis, diagnosed using the pH value obtained by scalp sampling.

Prepare for delivery by the most expeditious means or by surgical intervention if no improvement occurs.

Repetitive late decelerations over a 30-min period accompanied by decreased variability may warrant a cesarean birth to prevent fetal injury and/or death from hypoxia.

(Refer to CP: Labor Stage I—Latent Phase, NDs: Knowledge Deficit [Learning Need]; Infection, high risk for, maternal; Injury, high risk for, fetal; and Fluid Volume deficit, high risk for.)

Labor: Stage I—Transition Phase (Deceleration) _____

The transition phase is the most intense of the three phases of stage I labor. It is also the shortest phase, lasting approximately 2–3 hr in nulliparas and 1 hr in multiparas. The cervix dilates from 8 to 10 cm as the fetus descends approximately 1 cm/hr in nulliparas and 2 cm/hr in multiparas.

CLIENT ASSESSMENT DATA BASE

CIRCULATION

Blood pressure (BP) elevated 5–10 mm Hg above client's normal.

Pulse elevated.

EGO INTEGRITY

Irritable behavior.

May have difficulty maintaining control, requiring reminders about breathing.

May be amnesic.

May state, "I can't stand it anymore," or may desire to "leave the hospital and come back later."

ELIMINATION

Urge to void or defecate throughout phase (fetus in posterior position).

FOOD/FLUID

Nausea or vomiting may occur.

PAIN/DISCOMFORT

Strong uterine contractions occurring every 2–3 min and lasting 45–60 sec.

Intense level of discomfort in abdominal/sacral area.

May become very restless, thrash with pain, or be fearful.

May report being "too hot"; tingling sensation of fingertips, toes, and face.

Leg tremors may occur.

SAFETY

Diaphoretic.

Fetal heart tones heard just above symphysis pubis.

Fetal heart rate (FHR) may display late decelerations (uterine circulation is compromised) or early decelerations (head compression).

SEXUALITY

Cervix dilates from 8–10 cm.

Fetus descends from +2–+4 cm.

Copious amounts of bloody show.

239

NURSING PRIORITIES

1. Promote fetal and maternal well-being.
2. Provide physical and emotional support.

NURSING DIAGNOSIS:	PAIN [ACUTE]
May be related to:	Mechanical pressure of presenting part; tissue dilation/stretching and hypoxia; stimulation of parasympathetic and sympathetic nerves; emotional tension.
Possibly evidenced by:	Verbalizations, distraction behavior (e.g., restlessness), facial mask of pain, narrowed focus, autonomic responses.
DESIRED OUTCOMES— CLIENT WILL:	Verbalize reduction of pain.
	Use appropriate techniques to maintain control.
	Rest between contractions.

ACTIONS/INTERVENTIONS	RATIONALE
Independent	
Assess degree of discomfort through verbal and nonverbal cues. Assess personal and cultural implications of pain.	Attitudes toward pain and reactions to pain are individual and based on past experiences, cultural background, and self-concept.
Assess client's need for physical touch during contractions.	Touch may serve as a distraction, provide supportive reassurance, and encouragement, and may aid in maintaining control/reducing pain. (Note: Desire for touch may change from one contraction to the next.)
Monitor frequency, duration, and intensity of uterine contractions.	Detects progress and screens for abnormal uterine response.
Inform client of onset of contractions.	Client may "sleep" and/or encounter partial amnesia between contractions. This can impair her ability to recognize contractions as they begin and can have a negative impact on her control.
Assist client and coach with changing to more rapid breathing; (i.e., pant-blow, Lamaze level 3).	Redirects and focuses attention; helps reduce perception of pain within the cerebral cortex.
Provide for a quiet environment that is adequately ventilated, dimly lit, and free of unnecessary personnel. Carry out nursing procedures between contractions.	Nondistracting environment provides optimal opportunity for rest and relaxation between contractions.
Assist client with comfort measures, including sacral/back rubs, positioning, mouth care, perineal care, change of pads/linens, sponge baths to face and neck, or bath/whirlpool.	Such measures promote hygiene, relaxation, and physical comfort. (Note: Individual needs/preference can change quickly during transition; i.e., client may request sacral rub, then the next moment demand everyone move away from her.)
Monitor cervical dilation. Note perineal bulging or vaginal show.	Discomfort levels increase as cervix dilates, fetus descends, and small blood vessels rupture.

ACTIONS/INTERVENTIONS

Independent

Encourage client to void.

Offer encouragement, provide information about labor progress, and provide positive reinforcement for client's/couple's efforts.

Provide break for coach as appropriate.

Observe client for tingling of lips, face, hands, or feet. If present, have client breathe into cupped hands or paper bag.

Monitor maternal vital signs and FHR variability after drug administration. Note drug's effectiveness and the physiologic response.

Collaborative

Administer analgesic, if ordered. Assist anesthesiologist if epidural or caudal anesthetic is to be used.

RATIONALE

May enhance labor progress and reduce risk of trauma to bladder.

Provides emotional support, which can reduce fear, lower anxiety levels, and minimize pain.

Coach may be reluctant to leave, but does need a break for renewal of energy and relaxation, which can enhance ability to help partner.

Discomfort caused by respiratory alkalosis can be relieved by increasing carbon dioxide levels through the rebreathing process.

Narcotics have a depressant effect on the fetus. Therefore, they should not be administered within 1 hour of anticipated delivery.

Judicious use of a pharmacologic agent assists the client in coping with contractions and may facilitate labor.

NURSING DIAGNOSIS:	CARDIAC OUTPUT, DECREASED, HIGH RISK FOR
Risk factors may include:	Decreased venous return, hypovolemia, changes in systemic vascular resistance.
Possibly evidenced by:	[Not applicable; presence of signs/symptoms establishes an **actual** diagnosis.]
DESIRED OUTCOMES— CLIENT WILL:	Maintain vital signs appropriate for stage of labor, free of pathologic edema and excessive albuminuria.
	Display FHR within normal limits (WNL).

ACTIONS/INTERVENTIONS

Independent

Assess BP and pulse between contractions, as indicated. Note abnormal readings.

Note presence and extent of edema. Monitor FHR during and between contractions.

RATIONALE

During contractions, blood pressure usually increases 5–10 mm Hg, except during transition phase, when the blood pressure remains elevated. Increased resistance to cardiac output can occur if intrapartal hypertension develops, further elevating blood pressure. Finally, cardiac output/blood pressure may be negatively affected by uterine pressure on the inferior vena cava, reducing venous return, or by a decrease in circulating blood volume caused by dehydration or occasionally hemorrhage.

Excess fluid retention places the client at risk for circulatory changes, with possible uteroplacental insufficiency manifested as late decelerations.

ACTIONS/INTERVENTIONS

Independent

Accurately record parenteral and oral intake and output. Measure specific gravity if kidney function is decreased.

Test urine for albumin. Report levels above +2.

Monitor BP and pulse every 15 min, or continually if hypotension is severe after administration of analgesia.

Note any hypertensive responses to oxytocin administration. (Refer to CPs: Labor: Induced/Augmented; Intrapartal Hypertension.)

RATIONALE

Bedrest promotes increases in cardiac and urine output with a corresponding decrease in urine specific gravity. An elevation of specific gravity and/or reduction in urine output suggests dehydration or possibly developing hypertension.

Indicates glomerular spasms, which reduce the reabsorption of albumin. Levels greater than +2 indicate kidney involvement; levels +1 or lower may be due to muscle catabolism occurring with exercise or to increased metabolism in the intrapartal period.

Analgesics relax smooth muscles within the blood vessels, reducing resistance to cardiac output and lowering BP and pulse.

Oxytocin increases cardiac circulating volume (sodium/water absorption) and cardiac output, and may also increase BP and pulse.

NURSING DIAGNOSIS:	FLUID VOLUME DEFICIT, HIGH RISK FOR [fluctuation]
Risk factors may include:	Excess fluid loss/hemorrhage, reduced intake, excess fluid retention, rapid parenteral fluid administration.
Possibly evidenced by:	[Not applicable; presence of signs/symptoms establishes an **actual** diagnosis.]
DESIRED OUTCOMES— CLIENT WILL:	Maintain vital signs and urine output/concentration WNL. Be free of thirst.

ACTIONS/INTERVENTIONS

Independent

Monitor BP and pulse every 15 min and more frequently during oxytocin infusion.

Assess client's anxiety level.

Take temperature every 4 hr as indicated (every 2 hr after membranes rupture). Assess skin and mouth for dryness.

Record intake and output. Note concentration of urine. Measure urine specific gravity, as indicated.

RATIONALE

Increased BP and pulse may indicate fluid retention; decreased BP and increased pulse may be late signs of fluid volume loss or dehydration.

Anxiety may alter BP and pulse, affecting assessment findings.

Dehydration can result in elevated body temperature, dry skin, and reduced production of saliva.

Bedrest results in decreased adrenal cortex activity, increased glomerular filtration rate, and increased urine output. When fluid volume is decreased, aldosterone acts to reabsorb water and sodium from the kidney tubules, reducing urine output.

ACTIONS/INTERVENTIONS	RATIONALE
Independent	
Measure amount and character of emesis.	Nausea and vomiting contribute to fluid losses. With reduced gastric motility, food may remain in the stomach for up to 12 hr after ingestion and pose a risk for aspiration.
Remove excess clothing, keep environment cool, and wipe client's face/body with cool washcloth.	Limits diaphoreses; provides comfort.
Assess amount and location of edema; hematocrit (Hct) level, changes in behavior, and reflex irritability. (Refer to CP: Intrapartal Hypertension.)	Intrapartal hypertension can develop, causing fluid shifts from the intravascular spaces and increasing Hct levels. Cerebral edema/vasospasms/hypoxia can cause increased reflex irritability and/or behavior changes.
Assess amount of vaginal bloody show; observe for excess blood loss.	Bloody show increases as the presenting part moves down in the birth canal; excess bleeding may indicate placental separation.
Position client on left side as appropriate.	Increases venous return by taking pressure of the gravid uterus off the inferior vena cava and descending aorta.
Collaborative	
Administer and monitor i.v. fluid infusion.	Maintains hydration by replacing fluid losses. Rate may be adjusted to meet individual needs, but too-rapid administration can lead to fluid overload, especially in a compromised client.

NURSING DIAGNOSIS:	**FATIGUE**
May be related to:	Discomfort/pain, overwhelming psychologic/emotional demands, increased energy requirements, changes in energy production.
Possibly evidenced by:	Verbalizations, impaired ability to concentrate, emotional lability or irritability, lethargy, altered coping ability.
DESIRED OUTCOMES— CLIENT/COUPLE WILL:	Use techniques to conserve energy between contractions.
	Report sense of control.
	Appear moderately relaxed.

ACTIONS/INTERVENTIONS	RATIONALE
Independent	
Assess degree of fatigue.	Fatigue may interfere with the client's physical and psychologic abilities to maximally participate in labor process and to master and carry out self-care and infant care after delivery.
Provide dimly lit, nondistracting environment.	Reducing stressors helps promote rest.
Keep client informed of progress of labor. Provide encouragement for efforts client makes.	Provides reinforcement for desired behaviors. Realizing that labor is progressing toward goal may help client maintain maximal effort.

243

ACTIONS/INTERVENTIONS	RATIONALE

Independent

Provide comfort measures (Refer to ND: Pain [acute].)	Promotes relaxation, enhances sense of control, and may strengthen coping.
Plan care to limit interruptions.	Maximizes opportunities for rest.
Encourage client to close eyes, extend legs, and relax between contractions.	A comfortable position facilitates muscle relaxation.
Monitor urine for ketones.	Urinary ketones indicate metabolic acidosis resulting from a deficiency in glucose metabolism, which may reduce uterine activity and cause myometrial fatigue that can prolong labor.
Monitor energy level of partner. Assume coaching responsibilities as needed.	Allows coach to have a brief break and refresh self, enhancing ability to maintain focus and support client.
Administer an analgesic if ordered and if delivery is not anticipated within 1 hour.	May help the client cope with contractions and facilitate relaxation between contractions. Use with caution, because analgesics may cause fetal depression.

NURSING DIAGNOSIS:	**COPING, INDIVIDUAL/COUPLE, INEFFECTIVE, HIGH RISK FOR**
Risk factors may include:	Sense of "work overload," personal vulnerability, inadequate support system.
Possibly evidenced by:	[Not applicable; presence of signs/symptoms establishes an **actual** diagnosis.]
DESIRED OUTCOMES— CLIENT/COUPLE WILL:	Identify effective coping behaviors.
	Engage in activities to maintain/enhance control.

ACTIONS/INTERVENTIONS	RATIONALE

Independent

Reinforce information that labor is progressing; encourage client to cope with one contraction at a time.	Provides reassurance that baby will soon be born. A natural response in the transition phase is for the client to feel that she has had enough and wants to "quit and go home."
Inform client/coach of initiation of each contraction.	Allows client to rest/relax and still maintain control of breathing pattern as contraction begins.
Ensure that client, under direction of coach, initiates breathing patterns. Breathe with client if necessary.	A more complex breathing pattern initiated at the beginning of a contraction is necessary as a distraction and helps reduce pain perception within the cerebral cortex. Client may have difficulty understanding directions because of inward focus.

ACTIONS/INTERVENTIONS	RATIONALE

Independent

Acknowledge reality of irritable feelings of both client and coach.	The increase in intensity and frequency of contractions and the premature urge to push may add to sense of loss of control. The client's hostility may be manifested as anger at the nurse or coach. In addition, general fatigue of both client and coach further impair their ability to cope.
Encourage client and coach to verbalize doubts about ability to continue and fear of being left alone.	When these thoughts are expressed, they can be acknowledged and the client/coach can realize that they are coping and can continue.
Provide support to coach.	May feel helpless and require more support as the coach becomes less able to relieve partner's pain.

(Refer to CP: Labor Stage 1—Active Phase: NDs: Coping, individual/couple, ineffective, high risk for; Infection, high risk for, maternal; Gas Exchange, impaired, high risk for, fetal.)

Labor: Stage II (Expulsion) _____

Stage II of labor, the stage of expulsion, begins with full cervical dilatation (10 cm) and ends with the birth of the newborn. Maternal efforts to bear down occur involuntarily during contractions that are 1.5–2 min apart, lasting 60–90 sec. Average rate of fetal descent is 1 cm/hr for nulliparas, 2 cm or more an hour for multiparas.

CLIENT ASSESSMENT DATA BASE

ACTIVITY/REST

Reports of fatigue.

May report inability to self-initiate pushing/relaxation techniques.

Lethargic.

Dark circles under eyes.

CIRCULATION

Blood pressure may rise 5–10 mm Hg in between contractions.

EGO INTEGRITY

Emotional responses may range from feelings of fear/irritation/relief/joy.

May feel a loss of control or the reverse as she is now actively involved in bearing down.

ELIMINATION

Involuntary urge to defecate/push with contractions, combining intraabdominal pressure with uterine pressure.

May have fecal discharge while bearing down.

Bladder distention may be present, with urine expressed during pushing efforts.

PAIN/DISCOMFORT

May moan/groan during contractions.

Amnesia between contractions may be noted.

Reports of burning/stretching sensation of the perineum.

Legs may tremble during pushing efforts.

Uterine contractions strong, occurring 1.5–2 min apart and lasting 60–90 sec.

May fight contractions, especially if she did not participate in childbirth classes.

RESPIRATORY

Respiratory rate increases.

SAFETY

Diaphoresis is often present.

Fetal bradycardia (appearing as early decelerations on electric monitor) may occur during contractions (head compression).

SEXUALITY

Cervix fully dilated (10 cm) and 100% effaced.

Increased vaginal bloody show.

Rectal/perineal bulging with fetal descent.

Membranes may rupture at this point if still intact.

Increased expulsion of amniotic fluid during contractions.

Crowning occurs, caput is visible just before birth in vertex presentation.

NURSING PRIORITIES

1. Facilitate normal progression of labor and fetal descent.
2. Promote maternal and fetal well-being.
3. Support client's/couple's wishes regarding delivery experience, maintaining safety as a priority.

NURSING DIAGNOSIS:	**PAIN [ACUTE]**
May be related to:	Mechanical pressure of presenting part, tissue dilation/stretching, nerve compression, intensified contractile pattern.
Possibly evidenced by:	Verbalizations, distraction behavior (e.g., restlessness), facial mask of pain, narrowed focus, autonomic responses.
DESIRED OUTCOMES— CLIENT WILL:	Verbalize reduction of pain.
	Use appropriate technique to maintain control.
	Rest between contractions.

ACTIONS/INTERVENTIONS	RATIONALE
Independent	
Identify degree of discomfort and its sources.	Clarifies needs; allows for appropriate intervention.
Provide comfort measures, such as mouth care; perineal care/massage; clean, dry linen and underpads; cool environment (68° to 72° F) cool moist cloths to face and neck; or hot compresses to perineum, abdomen, or back as desired.	Promotes psychologic and physical comfort, allowing client to focus on labor, and may reduce the need for analgesia or anesthesia.
Provide information to client/couple about type of anesthesia available at this stage specific to the delivery setting (e.g., local, subarachnoid, or pudendal block anesthetics; epidural or caudal reinforcement) or transcutaneous electrical nerve stimulation (TENS). Review advantages/disadvantages as appropriate.	Although client is under the stress of labor and discomfort levels may interfere with normal decision-making skills, she still needs to be in control and make her own informed decisions regarding anesthesia. (Note: The option of a nerve root block should be restricted to a hospital setting where emergency equipment is available.)

ACTIONS/INTERVENTIONS	RATIONALE

Independent

Monitor and record uterine activity with each contraction.	Provides information/legal documentation about continued progress; helps identify abnormal contractile pattern, allowing prompt assessment and intervention. (Refer to CP: Dysfunctional Labor/Dystocia.)
Provide information and support related to progress of labor.	Keeps couple informed of proximity of delivery; reinforces that efforts are worthwhile and the "end is in sight."
Encourage client/couple to manage efforts to bear down with spontaneous, rather than sustained, pushing during contractions. Stress importance of using abdominal muscles and relaxing pelvic floor.	Anesthetics may interfere with client's ability to feel sensations associated with contractions, resulting in ineffective bearing down. Spontaneous, rather than sustained, efforts to bear down avoid negative effects of Valsalva's maneuver associated with reduced maternal and fetal oxygen levels. Relaxation of the pelvic floor reduces resistance to pushing efforts, maximizing effort to expel the fetus.
Monitor perineal and rectal bulging, opening of vaginal introitus, and fetal station.	Anal eversion and perineal bulging occur as the fetal vertex descends, indicating need to prepare for delivery.
Assist client in assuming optimal position for bearing down; (e.g., squatting or lateral recumbent, semi-Fowler's position (elevated 30–60 degrees), or use of a birthing chair. Assess effectiveness of efforts to bear down; help client to relax all muscles and rest between contractions. (Refer to ND: Skin/Tissue Integrity, impaired, high risk for.)	Proper positioning with relaxation of perineal tissue optimizes bearing-down efforts, facilitates labor progress, reduces discomfort, and reduces need for forceps application. Complete relaxation between contractions promotes rest and helps limit muscle strain/fatigue.
Monitor maternal blood pressure (BP) and pulse, and fetal heart rate (FHR). Watch for unusual adverse reactions to medication, such as antigen–antibody reactions, respiratory paralysis, or spinal blockage. Note adverse reactions such as nausea, vomiting, urine retention, delayed respiratory depression, and pruritus of face, eyes, or mouth. (Refer to ND: Gas Exchange, impaired, high risk for, fetal.)	Maternal hypotension caused by decreased peripheral resistance as vascular tree dilates is the main adverse reaction to subarachnoid or peridural block. Fetal hypoxia or bradycardia is possible, owing to decreased circulation within the maternal portion of the placenta. Other adverse reactions may occur after administration of spinal or peridural anesthetic, especially when morphine is used.

Collaborative

Assess bladder fullness. Catheterize between contractions if distention is noted and client is unable to void.	Promotes comfort, facilitates fetal descent, and reduces risk of bladder trauma caused by presenting part of fetus.
Support and position for saddle block, spinal, local, or pudendal anesthesia, as indicated:	Proper positioning ensures proper placement of medication and helps prevent complications.

Local Anesthesia:

Assist as needed with administration of local anesthetic before episiotomy.	Anesthetizes local perineal tissue for repair purposes.

248

ACTIONS/INTERVENTIONS	RATIONALE

Collaborative

Regional Anesthesia:

Assist with reinforcement of medication via indwelling peridural block catheter when caput is visible. Monitor vital signs and adverse responses. (Refer to CP: Labor: Stage I—Active Phase, ND: Pain [acute].)

Reduces discomfort associated with episiotomy, forceps application, and fetal expulsion. Adverse reactions include maternal hypotension, muscle twitching/convulsions, loss of consciousness, reduced FHR, and beat-to-beat variability.

Position client in dorsal lithotomy position and assist as necessary with administration of pudendal anesthetic.

Anesthetizes lower two thirds of vagina and perineum during delivery and for episiotomy repair. May interfere with efforts to bear down but has no effect on maternal BP, FHR, or FHR variability.

Spinal Anesthesia:

Administer I.V. fluid bolus of 1,000 ml, as indicated, before administration of intrathecal anesthetic for subarachnoid block (spinal, low spinal, or saddle block).

Increases maternal circulating fluid as a means of preventing adverse reactions of anesthetic such as maternal hypotension, fetal hypoxia, and fetal bradycardia.

Assist with administration of intrathecal subarachnoid anesthetic with client in sitting or lateral recumbent position with head sharply flexed on chest and back arched. Identify beginning and ending of contractions. Administer anesthetic between contractions when fetal head is on the perineum.

Anesthetizes nerve endings at lumbar spaces L3-4 and L4-5. Administration of medication during a contraction may cause the level of the anesthetic to rise too high, anesthetizing the diaphragm.

Administer oxygen and increase plain I.V. fluid. Displace uterus to the left and elevate legs if hypotension occurs.

Enhances venous return and circulating blood volume, and increases placental perfusion and oxygenation.

Assist with administration of opiates (e.g., morphine) into epidural space via indwelling catheter. Have naloxone 0.4 mg available as an antidote.

Intraspinal narcotic, acting on opiate receptors within the spinal column, blocks pain for as long as 11 hr. Literature reveals mixed results regarding use of morphine via indwelling catheter in stage II labor (may be more effective in the active phase of stage I labor).

Administer promethazine hydrochloride or metoclopramide hydrochloride when indicated.

May relieve pruritus, a side effect of morphine administration.

Transcutaneous Electrical Nerve Stimulation (TENS)

Apply two pairs of electrodes on either side of thoracic and sacral vertebrae.

Electrical stimulation of pain receptors within the skin may block pain sensations by causing release of endorphins. Has no adverse effect on client or fetus and may reduce need for analgesia/anesthesia.

Encourage and assist client/couple with operation of control knobs on battery-operated transcutaneous electrical stimulation device.

Ability to turn on mild electrical currents during a contraction promotes a feeling of control for the client.

General Anesthesia:

Assist with general anesthesia (inhalation or I.V. administration), as indicated.

Because of maternal and fetal side effects, general anesthesia should only be used in obstetric emergencies, such as hemorrhage, internal version with a second twin, or delivery of the aftercoming head in a breech presentation.

249

ACTIONS/INTERVENTIONS	RATIONALE

Collaborative

Assist with monitoring BP, pulse, respirations, FHR, and variability. Watch for vomiting reaction.

General anesthesia has a depressant effect on the client and fetus, and poses a risk of maternal aspiration.

NURSING DIAGNOSIS:	CARDIAC OUTPUT, ALTERED [fluctuation]
May be related to:	Fluctuation in venous return, changes in systemic vascular resistance.
Possibly evidenced by:	Variations in blood pressure, changes in pulse rate, decreased urine output, fetal bradycardia.
DESIRED OUTCOMES— CLIENT WILL:	Maintain vital signs appropriate for stage of labor.
	Use techniques to sustain/enhance vascular return.
	Display FHR and variability within normal limits (WNL).

ACTIONS/INTERVENTIONS	RATIONALE

Independent

Monitor BP and pulse frequently (every 5–15 min). Note amount and concentration of urine output; test for albuminuria.

Increases in cardiac output of 30%–50% occur in the expulsion stage, peaking at the acme of uterine contractions and slowly returning to a precontractile state as the contraction diminished or ceases. Intrapartal toxemia due to stress, excess sodium and fluid retention, or oxytocin administration may be manifested by increased BP, decreased urine output, and increased concentration of urine.

Encourage client to inhale/exhale during bearing-down efforts, using an open glottis technique and holding breath no longer than 5 sec at a time. Instruct client to push only when she feels the urge to do so. (Pushing should not be forced.)

Repeated, prolonged Valsalva's maneuvers, occurring when the client holds her breath while pushing against a closed glottis, eventually interrupt venous return, and reduce cardiac output, BP, and pulse pressure. Avoiding Valsalva's maneuver minimizes fall of maternal Po_2 and rise in Pco_2 levels, which would have a negative impact on fetus.

Monitor FHR after every contraction or bearing-down effort.

Detects fetal bradycardia and hypoxia associated with reduction in maternal circulation and reduced placental perfusion caused by anesthesia, Valsalva's maneuver, or incorrect positioning. (Refer to ND: Gas Exchange, impaired, high risk for, fetal.)

Encourage client/couple to select laboring position that optimizes circulation, such as the lateral recumbent position, Fowler's position, or squatting.

Upright and lateral recumbent positions prevent occlusion of the inferior vena cava and obstruction of the aorta, sustaining venous return and preventing hypotension.

ACTIONS/INTERVENTIONS

Independent

Monitor BP and pulse immediately after administration of anesthesia, and repeat until client is stable. (Refer to ND: Pain [acute] for information about anesthesia and side effects.)

Collaborative

Regulate I.V. infusion as indicated; monitor oxytocin administration, and decrease rate if necessary.

RATIONALE

Hypotension is the most common adverse reaction to lumbar epidural or subarachnoid block as vascular dilation slows venous return and reduces cardiac output.

I.V. line should be available in case the need to correct hypotension or administer emergency drugs arises. Excess fluid retention (a possible adverse reaction of oxytocin) may contribute to development of intrapartal toxemia.

NURSING DIAGNOSIS:	**GAS EXCHANGE, IMPAIRED, HIGH RISK FOR, fetal**
Risk factors may include:	Mechanical compression of head/cord, reduced placental perfusion, prolonged labor, maternal hyperventilation.
Possibly evidenced by:	[Not applicable; presence of signs/symptoms establishes an **actual** diagnosis.]
DESIRED OUTCOMES— FETUS WILL:	Be free of variable or late decelerations with FHR WNL.
CLIENT WILL:	Maintain control of respiratory pattern.
	Use positions promoting venous return/placental circulation.

ACTIONS/INTERVENTIONS

Independent

Assess fetal station, presentation, and position. If fetus is in occiput posterior position, place client on her side.

Position client in lateral recumbent or upright position, or turn side to side as indicated.

Avoid placing client in dorsal recumbent position.

RATIONALE

During stage II labor, the fetus is most vulnerable to bradycardia and hypoxia, which are associated with vagal stimulation during head compression. Malpresentations such as face, mentum (chin), or brow may prolong labor and increase risk of hypoxia and the likelihood of the need for a cesarean birth. Posterior position increases duration of stage II labor. Lateral recumbent position facilitates rotation from occiput posterior (OP) position to occiput anterior (OA) position.

Increases placental perfusion, prevents supine hypotensive syndrome, and takes pressure from presenting part off cord, enhancing fetal oxygenation and improving FHR patterns.

Contributes to fetal hypoxia and acidosis; reduces baseline variability and placental circulation.

251

ACTIONS/INTERVENTIONS	RATIONALE

Independent

Assess client's breathing pattern. Note reports of tingling sensation of face or hands, dizziness, or carpopedal spasms.

Identifies ineffective (inappropriate) respiratory pattern. Initially, hyperventilation results in respiratory alkalosis and an increase in serum pH; toward the end of labor, the pH falls and acidosis develops owing to lactic acid buildup from myometrial activity.

Have client breathe into cupped hands or small paper bag, as indicated.

Increases carbon dioxide levels and corrects respiratory alkalosis caused by hyperventilation.

Assist coach in helping with verbal control of respirations. Remind client to focus on an object.

Provides opportunity for client and partner to work together to maintain/regain control of situation and maintain state of relaxation during contractions.

Monitor client for fruity breath odor.

Indicates acidosis associated with hyperventilation. As shifts in acid-base levels occur, fetal status can be compromised, with resultant acidosis and hypoxia.

Encourage client/couple to inhale and exhale every 10–20 sec during bearing-down efforts. Monitor response to pushing efforts.

Helps maintain adequate oxygen levels. Exhaling while pushing minimizes physiologic effects of Valsalva's maneuver, which can decrease maternal heart rate and Po_2, and increases Pco_2, potentially resulting in placental and fetal hypoxia and acidosis.

Assess FHR, with fetoscope or fetal monitor, during and after each contraction or pushing effort.

Early decelerations due to vagal stimulation from head compression should return to baseline patterns between contractions.

Monitor periodic changes in FHR for severe, moderate, or prolonged decelerations. Note presence of variable or late decelerations.

Variable decelerations indicate hypoxia due to possible cord entrapment or to nuchal or short cord. Late decelerations indicate uteroplacental insufficiency, which should not be allowed to persist for more than 30 min. Late decelerations are more likely to occur in clients with pregnancy-induced hypertension, diabetes, kidney problems, or placental aging or following maternal anesthesia.

Note short- and long-term FHR variability.

Average beat-to-beat changes should range from 6 to 10 bpm, indicating integrity of fetal CNS.

Collaborative

Perform sterile vaginal examination, feeling for prolapse. If prolapse is present, lift vertex off cord.

Elevation of vertex helps free umbilical cord, which may be compressed between presenting part and birth canal.

Transfer to acute care setting, if client is in alternative birth center.

In cases of bradycardia or reduced FHR variability, more invasive monitoring, acute care equipment, or a cesarean birth may be needed.

Monitor FHR electronically with internal lead. If severe bradycardia, late decelerations, or prolonged variable decelerations appear:

Electronic monitoring allows continued, accurate assessment. Direct scalp electrodes accurately detect abnormal fetal responses and reduction in beat-to-beat variability.

ACTIONS/INTERVENTIONS	RATIONALE
Collaborative	
Position client in left lateral position; increase plain i.v. fluid.	Increases maternal circulating blood volume and placental perfusion.
Administer oxygen to client.	Increases circulating oxygen available for fetal uptake. During this stage of labor, enhanced metabolic processes increase oxygen consumption by twice the normal level.
Assist as needed with intermittent fetal scalp sampling.	Determines trends in fetal acid-base status, and diagnoses fetal acidosis. The pH of fetal blood falls rapidly during stage II labor, and prolonged hypoxia may result in anaerobic metabolism with buildup of lactic acid.
Prepare for surgical intervention if spontaneous vaginal or low forceps delivery is not immediately possible after approximately 30 min, and fetal pH is 7.20 or less.	The fastest means of delivery must be implemented when the fetus has severe or irreversible hypoxia or acidosis.

NURSING DIAGNOSIS:	SKIN/TISSUE INTEGRITY, IMPAIRED, HIGH RISK FOR
Risk factors may include:	Precipitous labor, hypertonic contractile pattern, adolescence, large fetus, forceps application.
Possibly evidenced by:	[Not applicable; presence of signs/symptoms establishes an **actual** diagnosis.]
DESIRED OUTCOMES— CLIENT WILL:	Relax perineal musculature during bearing-down efforts.
	Be free of preventable lacerations.

ACTIONS/INTERVENTIONS	RATIONALE
Independent	
Assist client/couple with proper positioning, breathing, and efforts to relax. Ensure that client relaxes the perineal floor while using abdominal muscles in pushing.	Helps promote gradual stretching of perineal and vaginal tissue. If maternal tissue within the birth canal or perineum resists gradual stretching as the presenting part of the fetus descends, trauma or lacerations of the cervix, vagina, perineum, urethra, and clitoris are possible.
Offer use of birthing chair, if available. Encourage squatting, Fowler's position, or standing while pushing, if these positions are not contraindicated.	Upright positions reduce duration of labor, enhance forces of gravity, reduce need for episiotomy, and maximize uterine contractility.
Place client in left lateral Sims' position for delivery, if comfortable.	Reduces perineal tension, promotes gradual stretching, and reduces need for episiotomy.
Help client as needed in transfer to delivery table between contractions. Monitor safety, and support legs, especially if epidural (caudal) catheter is in place.	Reduces risk of injury, especially if client is unable to assist with transfer.

253

ACTIONS/INTERVENTIONS	RATIONALE

Independent

Lift legs simultaneously, if stirrups are used, and place feet and legs properly in low position. Avoid pressure on popliteal space; support feet.

Reduces muscle strain; prevents pressure on calf and popliteal space that could contribute to development of postpartal thrombophlebitis.

Collaborative

Assess for bladder fullness; catheterize prior to delivery as appropriate. (Refer to CP: Labor: Stage I—Active Phase, ND: Urinary Elimination, altered, high risk for.)

Reduces bladder trauma from presenting part.

Assist as needed with hand maneuvers; apply pressure to fetal chin through maternal perineum while exerting pressure on the occiput with the other hand (modified Ritgen maneuver).

Allows slow delivery once the fetal head has distended the perineum 5 cm; reduces trauma to maternal tissues.

Assist with midline or mediolateral episiotomy, if necessary.

Although controversial, episiotomy may prevent tearing of perineum in cases of a large infant, rapid labor, and insufficient perineal relaxation. It may shorten stage I of labor, especially when forceps are used.

Assist with forceps application to fetal head, if necessary. Record type of forceps used.

Maternal tissue trauma is increased with forceps application, which may result in possible lacerations or extension of episiotomy.

Maintain accurate delivery records of location of episiotomy and/or lacerations.

Ensures proper documentation of events occurring during delivery process; identifies specific problems affecting postpartal recovery.

NURSING DIAGNOSIS:	FLUID VOLUME DEFICIT, HIGH RISK FOR
Risk factors may include:	Active loss, reduced intake, fluid shifts.
Possibly evidenced by:	[Not applicable; presence of signs/symptoms establishes an **actual** diagnosis.]
DESIRED OUTCOMES— CLIENT WILL:	Maintain vital signs WNL, adequate urine output, moist mucous membrane.
	Be free of thirst.

ACTIONS/INTERVENTIONS	RATIONALE

Independent

Measure intake/output and urine specific gravity. Assess skin turgor and production of mucus. Note albuminuria.

In presence of dehydration, urine output decreases, specific gravity increases, and skin turgor and mucus production decrease. Proteinuria may be due to dehydration or exhaustion, or may indicate preeclampsia.

Monitor temperature as indicated.

Elevated temperature and pulse may indicate dehydration or, on occasion, infection.

ACTIONS/INTERVENTIONS

Independent

Assess FHR and baseline; note periodic changes and variability (if internal scalp electrode is used).

Reduce excess clothing, cool body with wet cloths, and maintain cool environment. Protect from chilling.

Place client in upright or lateral recumbent position.

Collaborative

Administer fluids orally (sips of clear fluids or ice chips), as allowed, or parenterally.

RATIONALE

Initially, FHR may increase with maternal dehydration and fluid losses. Prolonged maternal acidosis may result in fetal acidosis and hypoxia. (Refer to ND: Gas Exchange, impaired, high risk for, fetal.)

Cools the body through evaporation; may reduce diaphoretic losses. Muscle tremors associated with chilling increase body temperature and general discomfort. (Note: Diaphoresis, blood loss at delivery, hyperventilation, reduced oral intake, and vomiting all contribute to possible alterations in maternal fluid-electrolyte balances.)

Optimizes placental perfusion.

Replaces fluid losses. Solutions such as lactated Ringer's solution administered intravenously help correct or prevent electrolyte imbalances.

NURSING DIAGNOSIS:	INFECTION, HIGH RISK FOR, maternal
Risk factors may include:	Repeated invasive procedures, traumatized tissues, exposure to pathogens, prolonged labor or rupture of membranes.
Possibly evidenced by:	[Not applicable; presence of signs/symptoms establishes an **actual** diagnosis.]
DESIRED OUTCOMES— CLIENT WILL:	Be free of infection.

ACTIONS/INTERVENTIONS

Independent

Perform perineal care every 4 hr (more often if membranes have been ruptured for a prolonged time), using medical asepsis. Remove fecal contaminants expelled during pushing; change linens/underpad as needed.

Note date and time of rupture of membranes. (Refer to Chapter 4, CP: Prenatal Infection.)

Perform vaginal examination only when absolutely necessary, using aseptic technique.

Monitor temperature, pulse, and white blood cell (WBC) count, as indicated.

RATIONALE

Helps promote cleanliness; prevents development of an ascending uterine infection and possible sepsis.

Within 4 hr after rupture of membranes, the client and fetus become vulnerable to ascending tract infections and possible sepsis.

Repeated vaginal examination increases the risk of endometrial infections.

Increased temperature or pulse greater than 100 bpm may indicate infection. Normal protective leukocytosis with WBC count as high as 25,000/mm^3 must be differentiated from elevated WBC count due to infection.

ACTIONS/INTERVENTIONS

Independent

Use surgical asepsis in preparing equipment. Clean perineum with sterile water and soap or surgical disinfectant at delivery.

Assist coach with dressing in scrub apparel (if indicated), washing hands, and so forth, as required by setting. Reduce number of persons present at delivery, giving consideration to wishes of client and family members.

Collaborative

Administer antibiotics, as indicated.

Provide aseptic conditions for delivery.

RATIONALE

Reduces risk of contamination.

Reduces risk of infection resulting from cross-contamination.

Used only occasionally, prophylactic antibiotics are somewhat controversial and must be used with caution because they may stimulate overgrowth of resistant organisms.

Helps prevent postpartal infection and endometritis.

NURSING DIAGNOSIS:	INJURY, HIGH RISK FOR, fetal
Risk factors may include:	Malpresentations/positions, precipitous delivery, or cephalopelvic disproportion (CPD).
Possibly evidenced by:	[Not applicable; presence of signs/symptoms establishes an **actual** diagnosis.]
DESIRED OUTCOMES— FETUS WILL:	Be free of preventable trauma or other complications.

ACTIONS/INTERVENTIONS

Independent

Assess fetal position, station, and presentation.

Monitor labor progress and rate of fetal descent.

Assess amount of amniotic fluid expelled at the time membranes rupture and then during contractions.

RATIONALE

Malpresentations such as face, mentum (chin), or brow may prolong labor and increase the likelihood that cesarean delivery will be necessary, because lack of neck flexion increases the diameter of the fetal head as it passes through the pelvic outlet. Breech presentation usually necessitates surgical intervention, owing to the high risk of spinal cord injuries resulting from hyperextension of the fetal head during vaginal delivery.

Precipitous labor increases the risk of fetal head trauma because skull bones do not have adequate time to adjust to dimensions of the birth canal.

Hydramnios is associated with fetal disorders such as anencephaly, disorders of the gastrointestinal tract, kidney dysfunction, and maternal diabetes. Oligohydramnios is associated with postmaturity and intrauterine growth retardation secondary to placental insufficiency.

ACTIONS/INTERVENTIONS	RATIONALE

Independent

Note color of amniotic fluid.

Meconium-stained amniotic fluid, greenish in color, may indicate fetal distress due to hypoxia in a vertex presentation or to compression of fetal intestinal tract in breech presentation.

Transfer to delivery room, as appropriate, when vertex is visible at introitus in nullipara, or when multipara is 8 cm dilated.

If delivery is to occur in area separate from the labor setting, transfer at this time ensures that infant is born where emergency medications and equipment are available if needed.

Remain with client and monitor pushing efforts as head emerges. Instruct client to pant during process.

Ensures that trained personnel are present and reduces possibility of trauma to fetal vertex; allows gradual accommodation of skull bones to birth canal and overriding of sutures.

Obtain emergency delivery kit if delivery not usually done in labor room. (Refer to CP: Precipitous Labor/Delivery or Unplanned Out-of-Hospital Delivery.) Ensure proper functioning of equipment and availability of supplies needed in case of either uncomplicated or complicated delivery.

Assures the availability of needed equipment and supplies in the event that labor progresses too rapidly for a planned delivery. When precipitous delivery is imminent, transfer to the delivery table is postponed until the neonate is delivered and the cord is clamped and cut.

Maintain record of events.

Accurate documentation provides information about neonate/client status and postpartal needs.

Collaborative

Assist with vaginal delivery when fetus is in posterior position.

Posterior position increases possibility of fetal trauma due to neck injuries.

Assist with vertex rotation from OP to OA (Scanzoni maneuver).

Manual rotation from OP to OA is possible (if no CPD exists). Double application of forceps to vertex may increase risk of fetal injury, yet OA position is preferred position for delivery.

Prepare for surgical intervention if indicated. (Refer to CP: Cesarean Birth.)

Cesarean birth may be necessary in cases of CPD, persistent OP position, or deep transverse arrest of the head with prolonged stage II labor or fetal distress, or with breech or shoulder presentation. Fetus with anencephaly may not dilate maternal tissues effectively and may therefore require surgical intervention.

NURSING DIAGNOSIS:	FATIGUE, HIGH RISK FOR
Risk factors may include:	Decreased metabolic energy production, increased energy requirements, overwhelming psychologic/emotional demands, presence of pain.
Possibly evidenced by:	[Not applicable; presence of signs/symptoms establishes an **actual** diagnosis.]
DESIRED OUTCOMES— CLIENT WILL:	Effectively participate in bearing-down activities.
	Relax/rest between efforts.

257

ACTIONS/INTERVENTIONS	RATIONALE

Independent

Assess fatigue level, and note activities/rest immediately before onset of labor.

The amount of fatigue is cumulative, so that the client who has experienced a longer-than-average stage I of labor, or one who was not rested at the onset of labor, may experience greater feelings of exhaustion.

Encourage rest/relaxation between contractions. Provide environment conducive to rest. (Refer to ND: Pain [acute].)

Conserves energy needed for pushing efforts and delivery. Stage II can be extremely exhausting because of the muscular effort involved in bearing down, the intensity of the emotional response to the birth experience, inadequate rest, and/or length of labor.

Keep client/couple informed of progress.

Helps provide needed psychologic energy. Spontaneous efforts to bear down tend to lengthen stage II of labor, but do not negatively affect the fetus.

Encourage use of relaxation techniques. Review them with client/coach, as necessary.

Tense muscles increase feelings of exhaustion and resistance to fetal descent and may prolong labor.

Monitor fetal descent, presentation, and position. (Refer to ND: Injury, high risk for, fetal.)

Malposition and malpresentation may prolong labor and cause/increase fatigue.

Collaborative

Supply fluids with glucose orally if desired/allowed or parenterally if client is in acute care setting. Test urine for ketones, as indicated.

Replenishes reserves that may have been depleted in labor, and that may have resulted in hypoglycemia or ketonuria.

Assist with anesthesia or use of forceps if client's efforts do not rotate fetal vertex and promote fetal descent.

Low forceps delivery may be necessary in the event of extreme maternal feelings and/or when maternal efforts to deliver are unsuccessful. Midforceps delivery with rotation (Scanzoni maneuver) helps rotate fetus from OP to OA position. (Refer to ND: Injury, high risk for, fetal.)

Prepare for cesarean birth if vaginal delivery is not possible.

Maternal fatigue and lack of progress may result from CPD or fetal malposition.

NURSING DIAGNOSIS:	**COPING, INDIVIDUAL, INEFFECTIVE, HIGH RISK FOR**
Risk factors may include:	Situational crisis, personal vulnerability, inadequate support system, unrealistic perceptions/expectations.
Possibly evidenced by:	[Not applicable; presence of signs/symptoms establishes an **actual** diagnosis.]
DESIRED OUTCOMES— CLIENT WILL:	Verbalize feelings congruent with behavior.
	Demonstrate effective coping skills by the use of self-directed techniques for bearing-down efforts.

ACTIONS/INTERVENTIONS	RATIONALE
Independent	
Determine client's/couple's perception of behavioral response to labor. Encourage verbalization of feelings. Note cultural influences.	Helps nurse gain insight into couple's feelings and identifies needs. Depending on ethnic background and childbirth preparation, involvement in the birth process can be ego-enhancing for the father or support person who desires active participation. Conversely, negative feelings or disappointment about performance arise if active involvement is not allowed or encouraged.
Discuss normal emotional and physical changes as well as variation in emotional responses.	Understanding helps client cope with situation and cooperate with pushing efforts. Emotional responses in this stage of labor vary from excitement at being able to participate more actively/control the forces of labor through pushing efforts, to embarrassment, irritability, or fear resulting from loss of control. This may be manifested by a lack of cooperation or ineffective pushing during contractions.
Monitor response to contraction. Provide gentle but firm instructions for efforts to bear down when the urge to push arises.	Active involvement provides positive means of coping and assists in descent of the fetus. Negative coping can result in prolonged labor and increases the likelihood that anesthesia and/or forceps may be needed for the delivery.
Discuss options for pain control/reduction. (Refer to ND: Pain [acute].)	Client may require anesthesia or analgesia to promote relaxation and facilitate coping.
Support client/couple in their decision to use analgesia or anesthesia.	The client's perception of her performance may be influenced by her own goals for coping with pain. If she has planned an unmedicated birth, she may feel a sense of failure if she resorts to anesthesia as fatigue and pain become intense. The client may be concerned about the support person's sense of failure as a coach if she resorts to medication. The nurse can reduce these feelings of "failure" by accepting the decision in a nonjudgmental manner.
Point out tense or furrowed brow, clenched fists, and so forth, and suggest that coach touch tense areas.	Helps client focus on tension reduction, and allows client and coach to work together to regain control of situation.
Provide comfort measures (e.g., applying cool cloths to face, neck, and extremities; eliminating excess clothing; positioning properly; providing perineal care; and providing a quiet, nonstimulating environment).	Reduction of discomforts and distractions allows couple to focus on labor efforts.
Encourage client to rest between contractions with eyes closed.	Conserves strength needed for pushing, thereby facilitating the coping process.
Facilitate coach's participation in meeting client's needs regarding comfort, pushing, and emotional support.	Active participation fosters positive sense of self and may actually strengthen and enhance couple's future relationship and their relationship to the child.

ACTIONS/INTERVENTIONS	RATIONALE
Independent	
Provide positive reinforcement; inform couple of labor progress, appearance of fetal vertex, and that their efforts are helpful. Provide mirror for visualization of emerging infant.	Helps couple to feel positive about their participation and rewarded for their cooperation. Encourages continuation of efforts.

Labor: Stage III (Placental Expulsion)

Stage III of labor begins with the birth of the baby and is completed with placental separation and expulsion. Lasting anywhere from 1 to 30 minutes, with an average length of 3–4 minutes in the nullipara, and 4–5 minutes in the multipara, this stage is the shortest. Careful management and monitoring are necessary, however, to prevent short- and long-term negative outcomes.

CLIENT ASSESSMENT DATA BASE

ACTIVITY/REST

Behaviors may range from excitement to fatigue.

CIRCULATION

Blood pressure (BP) increases as cardiac output increases, then returns to normal levels shortly thereafter.

Hypotension may occur in response to analgesics and anesthetics.

Pulse rate slows in response to change in cardiac output.

FOOD/FLUID

Normal blood loss is approximately 250–300 ml.

PAIN/DISCOMFORT

May complain of leg tremors/chills.

SAFETY

Manual inspection of uterus and birth canal determines presence of tears or lacerations.

Extension of the episiotomy or birth canal lacerations may be present.

SEXUALITY

Dark vaginal bleeding occurs as the placenta separates from the endometrium, usually within 1–5 min after delivery of the infant.

Umbilical cord lengthens at vaginal introitus.

Uterus changes from discoid to globular shape and rises in abdomen.

NURSING PRIORITIES

1. Promote uterine contractility.
2. Maintain circulating fluid volume.
3. Promote maternal and newborn safety.
4. Support parental-infant interaction.

NURSING DIAGNOSIS:	FLUID VOLUME DEFICIT, HIGH RISK FOR
Risk factors may include:	Lack/restriction of oral intake, vomiting, diaphoresis, increased insensible water loss, uterine atony, lacerations of the birth canal, retained placental fragments.

ACTIONS/INTERVENTIONS	RATIONALE

Independent

Instruct the client to push with contractions; help direct her attention toward bearing down.	Client attention is naturally on the newborn; in addition, fatigue may affect individual efforts, and she may need help in directing her efforts toward assisting with placental separation. Bearing down helps promote separation and expulsion, reduces blood loss, and enhances uterine contraction.
Assess vital signs before and after administering oxytocin.	Hypertension is a frequent side effect of oxytocin.
Palpate uterus; note "ballooning."	Suggests uterine relaxation with bleeding into uterine cavity.
Monitor for signs and symptoms of excess fluid loss or shock (i.e., check BP, pulse, sensorium, skin color, and temperature). (Refer to Chapter 6 CP: Postpartal Hemorrhage.)	Hemorrhage associated with fluid loss greater than 500 ml may be manifested by increased pulse, decreased BP, cyanosis, disorientation, irritability, and loss of consciousness.
Place infant at client's breast if she plans to breastfeed.	Suckling stimulates release of oxytocin from the posterior pituitary, promoting myometrial contraction and reducing blood loss.
Massage uterus gently after placental expulsion.	Myometrium contracts in response to gentle tactile stimulation, thereby reducing lochial flow and expressing blood clots.
Record time and mechanism of placental separation; i.e., Duncan's mechanism versus Schulze's mechanism.	Separation should occur within 5 min after birth. Failure to separate may require manual removal. The more time it takes for the placenta to separate, and the more time in which the myometrium remains relaxed, the greater the blood loss.
Inspect maternal and fetal surfaces of placenta. Note size, cord insertion, intactness, vascular changes associated with aging, and calcification (which possibly contributes to abruption).	Helps detect abnormalities that may have an impact on maternal or newborn status.
Obtain and record information related to inspection of uterus and placenta for retained placental fragments.	Retained placental tissue can contribute to postpartal infection and to immediate or delayed hemorrhage. If detected, the fragments should be removed manually or with appropriate instruments.

Collaborative

Avoid excessive traction on umbilical cord.	Force may contribute to breakage of the cord and retention of placental fragments, increasing blood loss.

ACTIONS/INTERVENTIONS

Collaborative

Administer fluids through parenteral route.

Administer oxytocin through I.M. route, or dilute I.V. drip in electrolyte solution, as indicated. I.M. ergot preparation may be given at the same time.

Obtain and record information related to inspection of birth canal for lacerations. Assist with repair of cervix, vagina, and episiotomy extension.

Assist as needed with manual removal of placenta under general anesthesia and sterile conditions.

Elevate fundus by dipping fingers down behind and moving uterine body up away from symphysis pubis.

RATIONALE

If fluid loss is excessive, parenteral replacement helps restore circulating volume and oxygenation of vital organs.

Promotes vasoconstrictive effect within the uterus to control postpartal bleeding after placental expulsion. i.v. bolus may result in maternal hypertension. Water intoxication may occur if electrolyte-free solution is used.

Lacerations contribute to blood loss; can cause hemorrhage.

Manual intervention may be necessary to facilitate expulsion of placenta and stop hemorrhage.

May be requested by practitioner to facilitate internal examination.

NURSING DIAGNOSIS:	INJURY, HIGH RISK FOR, maternal
Risk factors may include:	Positioning during delivery/transfers, difficulty with placental separation, abnormal blood profile.
Possibly evidenced by:	[Not applicable; presence of signs/symptoms establishes an **actual** diagnosis.]
DESIRED OUTCOMES— CLIENT WILL:	Observe safety measures. Be free of maternal injury.

ACTIONS/INTERVENTIONS

Independent

Palpate fundus, and massage gently.

Gently massage fundus after placental expulsion. (Refer to ND: Fluid Volume deficit, high risk for.)

Assess respiratory rhythm and excursion.

Clean vulva and perineum with sterile water and antiseptic solution; apply sterile perineal pad.

Lower client's legs simultaneously from stirrups.

Assist in transfer from delivery table to bed or stretcher, as appropriate.

RATIONALE

Facilitates placental separation.

Avoids overstimulation/trauma to fundus.

With placental separation, danger exists that an amniotic fluid emboli may enter maternal circulation, causing pulmonary emboli, or that fluid changes may result in emboli mobilization.

Removes possible contaminants that might result in an ascending tract infection during postpartal period.

Helps avoid muscle strain.

Client may be unable to move lower limbs due to continued effects from anesthesia. Post spinal or saddle block care may dictate keeping client flat for several hours after delivery, although such precautions are controversial.

ACTIONS/INTERVENTIONS	RATIONALE

Independent

Assess client's behavior, noting CNS changes.

Increased intracranial pressure during pushing and a rapid increase in cardiac output place the client with preexisting cerebral aneurysm at risk for rupture.

Obtain sample of cord blood; send to laboratory for blood typing of newborn. Record information regarding the sample being sent.

If infant is Rh-positive and client is Rh-negative, the client will require immunization with Rh immune globulin (Rh-Ig) in the postpartal period. (Refer to Chapter 6, CP: The Client at 4 Hours to 3 Days Post Partum.)

Collaborative

Use ventilatory assistance if needed.

Respiratory failure may occur following amniotic or pulmonary emboli.

If uterine inversion occurs:

Administer volume replacement, insert indwelling urinary catheter; obtain blood type and cross match; monitor vital signs, and maintain careful intake/output records.

Rapid maternal hemorrhage and shock follows inversion, and immediate lifesaving interventions may be necessary. Kidney function is a useful indicator of fluid volume levels/tissue perfusion.

Administer oxytocin i.v., replace uterus under anesthesia, and give ergonovine maleate (ergotrate) i.m. after replacement. Assist with packing of uterus as indicated.

Promotes contractility of uterine myometrium.

Administer prophylactic antibiotics.

Limits potential for endometrial infection.

NURSING DIAGNOSIS:	FAMILY PROCESSES, ALTERED, HIGH RISK FOR
Risk factors may include:	Developmental transition (gain of a family member), situational crisis (change in roles/responsibilities).
Possibly evidenced by:	[Not applicable; presence of signs/symptoms establishes an **actual** diagnosis.]
DESIRED OUTCOMES— CLIENT WILL:	Demonstrate behaviors indicative of readiness to actively participate in the acquaintance process when both mother and infant are physically stable.

ACTIONS/INTERVENTIONS	RATIONALE

Independent

Facilitate interaction between the client/couple and the newborn as soon as possible after delivery.

Fosters the beginning of lifelong emotional ties between family members. Both mother and infant have a critically sensitive period during which interactional capabilities are enhanced.

Provide client and the father the opportunity to hold baby immediately after birth if infant's condition is stable.

Early physical contact helps foster attachment. Fathers are also more likely to participate in infant caretaking activities and feel stronger emotional ties if they are actively involved with the infant soon after birth.

ACTIONS/INTERVENTIONS

Independent

Delay installation of eye prophylaxis ointments (containing erythromycin or tetracycline) until client/couple and infant have interacted.

(Refer to Chapter 7, CP: The First Hour of Life.)

RATIONALE

Allows infant to establish eye contact with parent(s) and actively participate in the interaction, free from the blurred vision caused by medication.

NURSING DIAGNOSIS:	KNOWLEDGE DEFICIT [LEARNING NEED], regarding labor process
May be related to:	Lack of information and/or misinterpretation of information.
Possibly evidenced by:	Verbalizations of questions/concerns, lack of cooperation.
DESIRED OUTCOMES— CLIENT WILL:	Verbalize understanding of physiologic responses.
	Actively engage in efforts to push to promote placental expulsion.

ACTIONS/INTERVENTIONS

Independent

Discuss/review normal processes of stage III labor.

Explain reason for such behavioral responses as chills and leg tremors.

Discuss routine for recovery period during the first 4 hr following delivery. Orient client to new staff and unit if transfer occurs at the end of this stage.

RATIONALE

Provides opportunity to answer questions/clarify misconceptions, enhancing cooperation with regimen.

Understanding helps client accept such changes without anxiety or undue concern.

Provides continuity of care and reassurance; enhances cooperation.

NURSING DIAGNOSIS:	PAIN [ACUTE]
May be related to:	Tissue trauma, physiologic response following delivery.
Possibly evidenced by:	Verbalizations, changes in muscle tone, restlessness.
DESIRED OUTCOMES— CLIENT WILL:	Verbalize management/reduction of pain.

ACTIONS/INTERVENTIONS

Independent

Assist with use of breathing techniques during surgical repair, as appropriate.

Apply ice bags to perineum after delivery.

Change wet clothing and bedding.

RATIONALE

Breathing helps direct attention away from the discomfort, promotes relaxation.

Constricts blood vessels, reduces edema, and provides local comfort and anesthesia.

Promotes warmth, comfort, and cleanliness.

ACTIONS/INTERVENTIONS	RATIONALE
Independent	
Provide a heated blanket.	Postdelivery tremors/chills may be due to sudden release of pressure on pelvic nerves or may possibly be related to a fetus-to-mother transfusion occurring with placental separation. Warmth promotes muscle relaxation and enhances tissue perfusion, reducing fatigue and enhancing sense of well-being.
Collaborative	
Assist with episiotomy repair, as necessary.	Approximation of edges facilitates healing.
Administer testosterone cypionate/estradiol valecate (Deladumone or Ditate) immediately after placental delivery, if client chooses not to breastfeed. Provide information about adverse effects, and ensure that client understands effects of estrogen and testosterone.	Although still used by some physicians to suppress lactation, estrogen preparations have been associated with serious adverse effects, such as liver tumors and increased clotting. Client needs to be aware of such risks. (Note: Current drug of choice is bromocriptine (Parlodel), and administration is usually begun 4 hr after delivery.)

Dysfunctional Labor/Dystocia

CLIENT ASSESSMENT DATA BASE

ACTIVITY/REST

Report of fatigue, lack of energy.

Lethargy, decreased performance.

CIRCULATORY

Blood pressure may be elevated.

May have received magnesium sulfate for pregnancy-induced hypertension.

ELIMINATION

Bowel or bladder distention may be evident.

EGO INTEGRITY

May be extremely anxious, fearful.

PAIN/DISCOMFORT

May have received narcotic or peridural anesthesia early in labor process.

May have noted false labor at home.

Infrequent contractions, mild to moderate in intensity (less than three contractions in a 10-min period).

May occur prior to the onset of labor (primary latent-phase dysfunction) or after labor is well established (secondary active phase dysfunction).

Latent phase of labor may be prolonged: 20 hours or longer in nullipara (average is 8$\frac{1}{2}$ hours.), or 14 hours in multipara (average is 5$\frac{1}{2}$ hours).

Myometrial resting tone may be 8 mm Hg or less, and contractions may measure less than 30 mm Hg or may occur more than 5 minutes apart. Alternatively, resting tone may be greater than 15 mm Hg, with contractions rising to 50 to 85 mm Hg with increased frequency and decreasing intensity.

SAFETY

May have had external version after 34 weeks' gestation in attempt to convert breech to cephalic presentation.

Fetal descent may be less than 1 cm/hr in nullipara or less than 2 cm/hr in multipara (protracted descent). No progress may occur within 1 or more hr for nullipara or within 30 min in multipara (arrest of descent).

Vaginal examination may reveal fetus to be in malposition (i.e., chin, face, or brow position).

Cervix may be rigid/"not ripe."

Dilation may be less than 1.2 cm/hr in primipara or less than 1.5 cm/hr for multipara, in active phase (protracted active phase).

SEXUALITY

May be primigravida or grand multipara.

Uterus may be overdistended owing to hydramnios, multiple gestation, a large fetus, or grand multiparity.

May have identifiable uterine tumors.

DIAGNOSTIC STUDIES

Prenatal testing: May have confirmed polyhydramnios, large fetus, or multiple gestation.
Nonstress test/contraction stress test: Assess fetal well-being.
X-ray pelvimetry or ultrasound: Evaluates pelvic architecture, fetal presentation, position, and formation.
Fetal scalp sampling: Detects or rule out acidosis.

NURSING PRIORITIES

1. Identify and treat abnormal uterine pattern.
2. Monitor maternal/fetal physical response to contractile pattern and length of labor.
3. Provide emotional support for the client/couple.
4. Prevent complications.

NURSING DIAGNOSIS:	**INJURY, HIGH RISK FOR, maternal**
Risk factors may include:	Alteration of muscle tone/contractile pattern, mechanical obstruction to fetal descent, maternal fatigue.
Possibly evidenced by:	[Not applicable; presence of signs/symptoms establishes an **actual** diagnosis.]
DESIRED OUTCOMES— CLIENT WILL:	Accomplish cervix dilation at least 1.2 cm/hr for primipara, 1.5 cm/hr for multipara in active phase, with fetal descent at least 1 cm/hr for primipara, 2 cm/hr for multipara.

ACTIONS/INTERVENTIONS	RATIONALE
Independent	
Review history of labor, onset, and duration.	Helpful in identifying possible causes, needed diagnostic studies, and appropriate interventions. Uterine dysfunction may be caused by an atonic or a hypertonic state. Uterine atony is classified as primary when it occurs before the onset of labor (latent phase) or secondary when it occurs after well-established labor (active phase).
Note timing/type of medication(s). Avoid administration of narcotics or of epidural block anesthetics until cervix is 4 cm dilated.	A hypertonic contractile pattern may occur in response to oxytocin stimulation; sedation given too early (or in excess of needs) can inhibit or arrest labor.
Evaluate current level of fatigue, as well as activity and rest, prior to onset of labor.	Excess maternal exhaustion contributes to secondary dysfunction, or may be the result of prolonged labor/false labor.
Assess uterine contractile pattern manually or electronically.	Dysfunctional contractions prolong labor, increasing the risk of maternal/fetal complications. A *hypotonic* pattern is reflected by frequent, mild contractions measuring less than 30 mm Hg. A *hypertonic* pattern is reflected by increased frequency and decreased intensity of contractions, with an elevated resting tone greater than 15 mm Hg.

ACTIONS/INTERVENTIONS	RATIONALE

Independent

Note condition of cervix. Monitor for signs of amnionitis. Note elevated temperature or white blood cell count; note odor and color of vaginal discharge.

A rigid or unripe cervix will not dilate, impeding fetal descent/labor progress. Development of amnionitis is directly related to length of labor, so that delivery should occur within 24 hr after rupture of membranes.

Note effacement, fetal station, and fetal presentation.

These indicators of labor progress may identify a contributing cause of prolonged labor. For example, breech presentation is not as effective a wedge for cervical dilatation as is vertex presentation.

Palpate abdomen of thin client for presence of pathologic retraction ring between uterine segments. (These rings are not palpable through the vagina, or through the abdomen in the obese client).

In obstructed labor, a depressed pathologic ring (Bandl's ring) may develop at the juncture of lower and upper uterine segments, indicating impending uterine rupture.

Place client in lateral recumbent position and encourage bedrest or ambulation, as tolerated.

Relaxation and increased uterine perfusion may correct a hypertonic pattern. Ambulation may assist gravitational forces in stimulating normal labor pattern and cervical dilatation.

Encourage client to void every 1–2 hr. Assess for bladder fullness over symphysis pubis.

A full bladder may inhibit uterine activity and interfere with fetal descent.

Assess degree of hydration. Note amount and type of intake. (Refer to ND: Fluid Volume deficit, high risk for.)

Prolonged labor can result in a fluid-electrolyte imbalance as well as depletion of glucose reserves, resulting in exhaustion and prolonged labor with increased risk of uterine infection, postpartal hemorrhage, or precipitous delivery in the presence of hypertonic labor.

Review bowel habits and regularity of evacuation.

Bowel fullness may inhibit uterine activity and interfere with fetal descent.

Remain with client; provide quiet environment as indicated.

Reduction of outside stimuli may be necessary to allow sleep after administration of medication to client in the hypertonic state. Also helpful in reducing level of anxiety, which can contribute to both primary and secondary uterine dysfunction.

Have emergency delivery kit available.

May be needed in the event of a precipitous labor and delivery, which are associated with uterine hypertonicity.

Collaborative

Prepare client for amniotomy, and assist with the procedure, when cervix is 3–4 cm dilated.

Rupture of membranes relieves uterine overdistention (a cause of both primary and secondary dysfunction) and allows presenting part to engage and labor to progress in the absence of cephalopelvic disproportion (CPD).

ACTIONS/INTERVENTIONS

Collaborative

Use nipple stimulation to produce endogenous oxytocin, or initiate infusion of exogenous oxytocin or prostaglandins. (Refer to CP: Labor: Induced/Augmented.)

Administer narcotic or sedative, such as morphine, phenobarbital, or secobarbital, for sleep, as indicated.

Assist with preparation for cesarean section, as indicated, for malposition, CPD, or Bandl's ring. (Refer to CP: Cesarean Birth.)

Prepare for forceps delivery, as necessary.

RATIONALE

Oxytocin may be necessary to augment or institute myometrial activity for hypotonic uterine pattern. It is usually contraindicated in hypertonic labor pattern because it can accentuate the hypertonicity, but may be tried with amniotomy if latent phase is prolonged and if CPD and malpositions are ruled out.

May help distinguish between true and false labor. With false labor, contractions cease; with true labor, more effective pattern may ensue following rest. Morphine helps promote heavy sedation and eliminate hypertonic contractile pattern. A period of rest conserves energy and reduces utilization of glucose to relieve fatigue.

Immediate cesarean delivery is indicated for Bandl's ring for fetal distress due to CPD.

Excessive maternal fatigue, resulting in ineffective bearing-down efforts in Stage II labor, necessitates use of forceps.

NURSING DIAGNOSIS:	**INJURY, HIGH RISK FOR, fetal**
Risk factors may include:	Prolonged labor, fetal malpresentations, tissue hypoxia/acidosis, abnormalities of the maternal pelvis, CPD.
Possibly evidenced by:	[Not applicable; presence of signs/symptoms establishes an **actual** diagnosis.]
DESIRED OUTCOMES— FETUS WILL:	Display fetal heart rate (FHR) within normal limits, with good variability, no late decelerations noted.
CLIENT WILL:	Participate in interventions to improve labor pattern and/or reduce identified risk factors.

ACTIONS/INTERVENTIONS

Independent

Assess FHR manually or electronically. Note variability, periodic changes, and baseline rate. If in alternative birth center (ABC), check fetal heart tones between contractions using Doptone. Count for 10 min, break for 5 min, and count again for 10 min. Continue this pattern throughout the contraction to midway between it and the following contraction.

Note uterine pressures during resting and contractile phases via intrauterine pressure catheter if available.

RATIONALE

Detects abnormal responses, such as exaggerated variability, bradycardia, and tachycardia, which may be caused by stress, hypoxia, acidosis, or sepsis.

Resting pressure greater than 30 mm Hg or contractile pressure greater than 50 mm Hg reduce or compromise oxygenation within intervillous spaces.

ACTIONS/INTERVENTIONS	RATIONALE
Independent	
Identify maternal factors such as dehydration, acidosis, anxiety, or vena caval syndrome.	Sometimes, simple procedures (such as turning client to lateral recumbent position) increase circulating blood and oxygen to uterus and placenta and may prevent or correct fetal hypoxia.
Note frequency of uterine contractions. Notify physician if frequency is 2 min or less.	Contractions occurring every 2 min or less do not allow for adequate oxygenation of intervillous spaces.
Assess for malpositioning using Leopold's maneuvers and findings on internal examination (location of fontanels and cranial sutures). Review results of ultrasonography.	Determining fetal lie, position, and presentation may identify factor(s) contributing to dysfunctional labor.
Monitor fetal descent in birth canal in relation to ischial spines.	Descent that is less than 1 cm/hr for a primipara, or less than 2 cm/hr for a multipara, may indicate CPD or malposition.
Arrange transfer to acute care setting if malposition is detected in client in ABC.	Risk of fetal/neonatal injury or demise increases with vaginal delivery if presentation is other than vertex.
Prepare for the most expedient method of delivery, if fetus is in brow, face, or chin presentation.	Such presentations increase the risk of CPD, owing to a larger diameter of the fetal skull entering the pelvis (11 cm in brow or face presentation, 13 cm in chin presentation), often necessitating cesarean delivery because of failure to progress and ineffective labor pattern. (Fetal skull diameter for vertex presentation is 9.5 cm).
Assess for deep transverse arrest of the fetal head.	Failure of the vertex to rotate fully from an occiput posterior (OP) to an occiput anterior (OA) position may result in a transverse position, arrested labor, and the need for cesarean delivery.
Have client assume hands-and-knees position, or lateral Sims' position on side opposite that to which fetal occiput is directed, if fetus is in OP position.	These positions encourage anterior rotation by allowing fetal spine to fall toward the client's anterior abdominal wall (70% of fetuses in OP position rotate spontaneously).
Note color and amount of amniotic fluid when membranes rupture.	Excess amniotic fluid causing uterine overdistention is associated with fetal anomalies. Meconium-stained amniotic fluid in a vertex presentation results from hypoxia, which causes vagal stimulation and relaxation of the anal sphincter. Noting characteristics of amniotic fluid alerts staff to potential needs of newborn.
Observe for visible or occult cord prolapse when membranes rupture, and for variable decelerations on monitor strip, especially if fetus is in breech presentation.	Cord prolapse is more likely to occur in breech presentation, because the presenting part is not firmly engaged, nor is it totally blocking the os, as in vertex presentation.
Note odor and change in color of amniotic fluid with prolonged rupture of membranes. Obtain culture if findings are abnormal.	Ascending infection and sepsis with accompanying tachycardia may occur with prolonged rupture of membranes.

271

ACTIONS/INTERVENTIONS

Collaborative

Administer antibiotic to client, as indicated.

Prepare for delivery in posterior position, if fetus fails to rotate from OP to OA position (face to pubis). Alternatively, double application of forceps (Scanzoni maneuver) may be used to rotate and deliver fetus.

Prepare for cesarean delivery if breech presentation is present, if fetus fails to descend, labor progress ceases, or CPD is identified.

RATIONALE

Prevents/treats ascending infection and will protect fetus as well.

Delivering the fetus in a posterior position results in a higher incidence of maternal lacerations. Delivery using double application of forceps (midforceps delivery) may be necessary.

Vaginal delivery of a breech is associated with injury to the fetal spinal column, brachial plexus, clavicle, and brain structures, increasing neonatal mortality and morbidity. Risk of hypoxia due to prolonged vagal stimulation with head compression, and trauma such as intracranial hemorrhage, can be alleviated or prevented if CPD is identified and surgical intervention follows immediately.

NURSING DIAGNOSIS:	FLUID VOLUME DEFICIT, HIGH RISK FOR
Risk factors may include:	Hypermetabolic state, vomiting, profuse diaphoresis, restricted oral intake, mild diuresis associated with oxytocin administration.
Possibly evidenced by:	[Not applicable; presence of signs/symptoms establishes an **actual** diagnosis.]
DESIRED OUTCOMES— CLIENT WILL:	Maintain fluid balance, as evidenced by moist mucous membranes, appropriate urine output, and palpable pulses. Be free of complications.

ACTIONS/INTERVENTIONS

Independent

Keep accurate intake/output, test urine for ketones, and assess breath for fruity odor.

Monitor vital signs. Note reports of dizziness with change of position.

Assess lips and oral mucous membranes and degree of salivation.

Note abnormal FHR response. (Refer to ND: Injury, high risk for, fetal.)

RATIONALE

Decreased urine output and increased urine specific gravity reflect dehydration. Inadequate glucose intake results in a breakdown of fats and presence of ketones.

Increased pulse rate and temperature, and orthostatic blood pressure changes may indicate decrease in circulating volume.

Dry oral mucous membranes/lips and decreased salivation are further indicators of dehydration.

May reflect effects of maternal dehydration and decreased perfusion.

ACTIONS/INTERVENTIONS	RATIONALE

Collaborative

Review laboratory data: hemoglobin/hematocrit (Hb/Hct), serum electrolytes, and serum glucose.

Increased Hct suggests dehydration. Serum electrolyte levels detect developing electrolyte imbalances; serum glucose levels detect hypoglycemia.

Administer fluids intravenously.

Parenteral solutions containing electrolytes and glucose can correct or prevent maternal and fetal imbalances and may reduce maternal exhaustion.

NURSING DIAGNOSIS:	COPING, INDIVIDUAL, INEFFECTIVE
May be related to:	Situational crisis, personal vulnerability, unrealistic expectations/perceptions, inadequate support systems.
Possibly evidenced by:	Verbalizations and behavior indicative of inability to cope (loss of control, inability to problem-solve and/or meet role expectations), irritability, reports of tension/fatigue.
DESIRED OUTCOMES— CLIENT WILL:	Verbalize understanding of what is happening. Identify/use effective coping techniques.

ACTIONS/INTERVENTIONS	RATIONALE

Independent

Determine progress of labor. Assess degree of pain in relation to dilation/effacement.

Prolonged labor with resultant fatigue can reduce the client's ability to cope/manage contractions. Increasing pain when the cervix is not dilating/effacing can indicate developing dysfunction. Extreme pain may indicate developing anoxia of the uterine cells.

Acknowledge reality of client's reports of pain/discomfort.

Discomfort and pain may be misunderstood in the presence of lack of progression that is not recognized as a dysfunctional problem. Feeling listened to and supported can reduce discomfort and help client to relax and cope with situation.

Determine anxiety level of client and coach. Note evidence of frustration.

Excess anxiety increases adrenal activity/release of catecholamines, causing endocrine imbalance. Excess epinephrine inhibits myometrial activity. Stress also depletes glycogen stores, reducing glucose available for adenosine triphosphate (ATP) synthesis, which is needed for uterine contraction.

Discuss possibility of discharge of client to home until active labor starts.

Client may be able to relax better in familiar surroundings. Provides opportunity to divert/refocus attention and to attend to tasks that may be contributing to level of anxiety/frustration.

Provide comfort measures and reposition client. Encourage use of relaxation techniques and learned breathing.

Reduces anxiety, promotes comfort, and assists client to cope positively with the situation.

ACTIONS/INTERVENTIONS	RATIONALE
Independent	
Provide encouragement for client/couple efforts to date.	May be useful in correcting misconception that client is overreacting to labor or is somehow to blame for alteration of anticipated birth plan.
Give factual information about what is happening.	Can assist with reduction of anxiety and promote coping.
(Refer to CPs: Labor: Stage I—Latent Phase; Labor: Stage I—Active Phase.)	

Labor: Induced/Augmented _____

This plan of care concerns the induction of labor for maternal health problems, fetal compromise, or post-maturity, and the augmentation of labor in uterine dysfunction (medically indicated inductions). For optimal use of this plan of care, combine it with the previous plans of care in this chapter, concerning the normal stages of labor and dysfunctional labor, as appropriate.

CLIENT ASSESSMENT DATA BASE

CIRCULATION

Blood pressure (BP) elevation, which may indicate anxiety or pregnancy-induced hypertension (PIH); a BP decrease may indicate supine hypotension or dehydration.

FOOD/FLUID

Maternal weight loss of 2.5–3 lb may be associated with postmaturity or fetal weight loss.

NEUROSENSORY

Deep tendon reflexes may be brisk 3+ with PIH; presence of clonus indicates severe excitability.

PAIN/DISCOMFORT

Uterine palpation may reveal contractile pattern.

SAFETY

May experience spontaneous rupture of membranes without contractions (at or near term).

Elevated temperature (infection in presence of prolonged rupture of membranes).

Fetal heart rate (FHR) may be greater than 160 bpm if preterm, hypoxic, or septic.

Fetal size may indicate weight loss; fetal demise.

Greenish amniotic fluid indicates fetal distress in vertex presentation.

Fundus may be lower than anticipated for term, with intrauterine growth retardation associated with maternal vascular involvement.

History/presence of Rh isoimmunization, chorioamnionitis, diabetes, PIH not controlled by medical therapy, chronic hypertension, postmaturity, cyanotic maternal cardiac disease, or renal disease.

SEXUALITY

Precipitous (or rapid) labor with previous pregnancy; client lives a distance from the hospital.

Cervix may be ripe (approximately 50% effacement and 2–3 cm dilated).

Uterine inertia may occur.

Bloody show may be present with dilation.

Increased vaginal bleeding may indicate placenta previa or abruptio placentae.

May be more than 42 weeks' gestation.

DIAGNOSTIC STUDIES

Complete blood count with differential: Determines presence of anemia and infection, as well as level of hydration.
Blood type and Rh factor if not previously done.

Urinalysis: Reveals urinary tract infection, protein, or glucose.
Lecithin to sphingomyelin (L/S ratio): Determine fetal maturity.
Nitrazine paper and/or fern test: Confirms rupture of membranes.
Scalp pH: Indicates degree of fetal hypoxia.
Ultrasonography: Determines gestational age, fetal size, presence of fetal heart motion, and location of the placenta.
Pelvimetry: Identifies cephalopelvic disproportion (CPD) or fetal position.
Nonstress test or contraction stress test: Evaluates fetal/placental functioning.

NURSING PRIORITIES

1. Promote maternal and fetal well-being.
2. Provide client/couple with information about induction and augmentation of labor.
3. Provide emotional support.
4. Promote comfort.

NURSING DIAGNOSIS:	KNOWLEDGE DEFICIT [LEARNING NEED], regarding procedure, possible outcomes
May be related to:	Lack of exposure/unfamiliarity with information resources, misinterpretation of information.
Possibly evidenced by:	Verbalization of questions/concerns, exaggerated behaviors.
DESIRED OUTCOMES— CLIENT WILL:	Verbalize understanding of procedures/situation. Participate in decision-making process.

ACTIONS/INTERVENTIONS	RATIONALE

Independent

Review the need for induction or argumentation of labor.	Informed consent and cooperation depend on the client's understanding of the situation and choices.
Explain the expected procedures to client/couple: Contractions and FHR will be monitored continuously. BP will be checked every 15 min. Administration of oxytocin may result in increased discomfort as contractions become more intense. Onset of labor will be more rapid. Analgesics may need to be administered after 5 cm dilatation or when good labor pattern is established.	Anxiety is allayed when client/couple know what is happening and what to expect. Cooperation and involvement are also enhanced.
Review amniotomy procedure; explain that it is no more uncomfortable than sterile vaginal examination.	Amnihook is guided into the vagina by the examiner's fingers during the sterile vaginal examination. Membranes, which do not contain nerves, are hooked or nicked to rupture, stimulating labor. Amniotomy can be a successful means of inducing labor when used alone or in conjunction with oxytocin. However, amniotomy commits the client to delivering within 24 hr.
Demonstrate and explain use of equipment (i.e., external or internal fetal monitor and i.v. infusion pump). Point out safety features and alarms.	Knowledge can alleviate anxiety, enhance coping with false alarms, and give a sense of control over the situation.

ACTIONS/INTERVENTIONS	RATIONALE

Independent

Instruct client/coach in basic interpretation of fetal monitor, differentiating changes in pattern that occur on movement.	Encourages involvement, gives a sense of control, and lessens anxiety regarding normal variations of tracing.
Explain oxytocin infusion.	Oxytocin may be used prior to amniotomy or may be implemented after a trial of amniotomy that fails to induce labor.
Prepare for possibility of failed induction and/or operative intervention if fetal distress occurs.	Depending on the degree of cervical ripening and the client's response to procedures, induction may not be successful. If membranes are ruptured, and induction fails, a cesarean birth is indicated. Cesarean delivery may also be performed, and induction discontinued, if severe fetal distress is apparent. Providing this information to the client/couple in advance can prepare them psychologically and may diminish disappointment.

NURSING DIAGNOSIS:	FEAR; ANXIETY [SPECIFY LEVEL]
May be related to:	Situational "crisis," perceived threat to client/fetus, unanticipated deviation from expectations.
Possibly evidenced by:	Identification of specific concerns, increased tension, apprehension, feelings of inadequacy, decreased self-awareness, sympathetic stimulation
DESIRED OUTCOMES— CLIENT WILL:	Use support systems effectively.
	Report anxiety diminished and/or managed.
	Appear relaxed.
	Accomplish successful labor.

ACTIONS/INTERVENTIONS	RATIONALE

Independent

Assess psychologic and emotional status.	Any interruption of the normal progression of labor can contribute to feelings of anxiety and failure. These feelings can interfere with client cooperation and hamper the induction process.
Encourage verbalization of feelings.	Client may be frightened or may not clearly understand the need for inducing labor. A sense of failure of being unable to "labor naturally" may occur. (Note: In cases of fetal demise, going through labor is especially disturbing and requires extensive support; Refer to Chapter 6, CP: Perinatal Loss.)
Use positive terminology; avoid use of terms that indicate abnormality of procedures or processes.	Helps client/couple accept the situation without self-recrimination.

ACTIONS/INTERVENTIONS

Independent

Listen to client's comments that may indicate loss of self-esteem.

Provide opportunities for client input into decision-making process.

Encourage use/continuation of breathing techniques and relaxation exercises.

RATIONALE

Client may believe that any intervention to aid the labor process is a negative reflection on her own abilities.

Enhances client's sense of control even though much of what is happening may be beyond her control.

Helps to reduce anxiety and enable client to participate actively.

NURSING DIAGNOSIS:	INJURY, HIGH RISK FOR, maternal
Risk factors may include:	Adverse effects/response to therapeutic interventions.
Possibly evidenced by:	[Not applicable; presence of signs/symptoms establishes an **actual** diagnosis.]
DESIRED OUTCOMES— CLIENT WILL:	Develop/maintain a good labor pattern; i.e., contractions 2–3 min apart, lasting 40–50 sec, with uterine relaxation to normal tone between contractions.
	Accomplish delivery without complications.

ACTIONS/INTERVENTIONS

Independent

Review prenatal record for history of previous pregnancies and outcomes, prenatal laboratory studies, pelvic measurements, allergies, weight gain, vital signs, last menstrual period, and estimated date of delivery (EDD).

Obtain history regarding insertion of laminaria tent or prostaglandin vaginal suppository.

Perform sterile vaginal examination to determine readiness or ripeness of cervix and fetal station. Repeat as indicated by client's reaction and contraction pattern.

RATIONALE

Provides information needed in formulating plan of care. Alerts nurse to the possibility of existing or developing problem(s).

Insertion of laminaria tent the evening before the induction softens the cervix and facilitates labor induction. (Note: Development of adverse reactions such as hypertonicity/activity of the uterus or nausea/vomiting require discontinuation/removal of the prostaglandin gel.)

A soft, partially effaced (more than 50%) and/or dilated (at least 3 cm) "ripe" cervix is a good indication that induction will be successful. A firm, thick "unripe" cervix with little or no dilatation may require 2 or 3 trials before induction is successful. Time of amniotomy depends on fetal station. Repeat examinations determine labor progress, but to avoid infection, they should be limited as much as possible after membranes are ruptured.

ACTIONS/INTERVENTIONS	RATIONALE

Independent

Check BP and pulse every 15 min after induction begins and before increasing oxytocin.

Assesses maternal well-being and detects development of hypotension/hypertension. Oxytocin is given slowly in increasing amounts. Fifteen to 20 minutes of infusion are necessary to reach therapeutic blood levels of oxytocin. It is rapidly metabolized and excreted by the kidneys, so constant infusion should be maintained. Regular, consistent contractions of good quality are needed to dilate the cervix effectively.

Evaluate monitor tracing constantly. Note rate and reactivity of FHR.

Careful monitoring is essential to determine client/fetal response to procedure, to identify adverse reactions, and to produce an effective labor pattern.

Palpate fundus to evaluate frequency and duration of contractions. Observe for overstimulation of uterus (tetanic contraction). Note intensity and resting tone between contractions when intrauterine catheter is used.

External uterine monitoring indicates the frequency, not intensity, of contractions. Rapid labor/delivery may occur, increasing risk of cervical and soft tissue trauma. Overstimulation causes fetal hypoxia, uterine rupture, and premature separation of placenta. If contraction lasts more than 60 sec or occurs more than 2–3 min apart, oxytocin should be discontinued.

Document vital signs, medications, oxytocin onset and dosage increases, change of position, oxygen administration, and times of sterile vaginal examinations on monitor tracing.

Monitor tracing is a legal document, showing progress of induction, fetal/maternal response, and actions taken by healthcare staff.

Monitor intake and output. Measure urine specific gravity. Palpate bladder.

Decreased output with increased specific gravity reflects fluid deficit. Urine retention may impede labor and fetal descent.

Note reports of abdominal cramping, dizziness, and nausea/vomiting; presence of lethargy, hypotension, tachycardia, and cardiac dysrhythmia.

Water intoxication may develop dependent on rate/type of fluid administration.

Provide perineal care as indicated. Monitor temperature every 2 hr. Note color and odor of vaginal drainage.

Reduces risk of infection and/or provides early detection of developing infection. Presence of meconium staining indicates fetal distress.

Collaborative

Review prenatal laboratory work. Perform nitrazine paper or fern test, if indicated.

Evaluates maternal and fetal status, and determines whether membranes have ruptured.

Assist with application of prostaglandin gel.

Facilitates cervical ripening; may stimulate labor and/or enhance effectiveness of oxytocin infusion.

Assist with amniotomy. Place client in low semi-Fowler's position with knees bent as for vaginal examination.

Rupture of membranes may stimulate labor without need of drug infusion (successful in approximately 80% of clients at term), or it may be done in conjunction with oxytocin administration. Amniotomy is contraindicated if presenting part is high.

ACTIONS/INTERVENTIONS	RATIONALE

Collaborative

Start primary I.V. line with large-gauge indwelling catheter.	Large-gauge catheter is preferred in case of the need for surgical intervention, blood transfusion, or emergency fluid/drug administration.
Assist as necessary with insertion of intrauterine catheter.	Internal monitoring accurately quantitates intensity and frequency of contractions and helps identify overstimulation and possible uterine rupture due to overadministration of oxytocin.
Dilute and administer oxytocin in electrolyte solution with a two-bottle I.V. system, piggybacking oxytocin close to I.V. site, according to unit policy and procedures.	The synthetic hormone oxytocin stimulates the uterine smooth muscle, increasing the excitability of the muscle cells, which increases the strength of contractions. Oxytocin can be discontinued if necessary, and the primary site can be quickly cleared and available for other infusions when solution is infused close to I.V. site. Additionally, water intoxication can result from excessive or rapid fluid administration, especially when D_5W is used instead of electrolyte solutions.
Observe safety precautions related to the use of infusion and to proper labeling of oxytocin solution.	Errors or fluctuations in rate of administration may cause undermedication or overmedication, resulting in inadequate contractions or uterine rupture. Drug delivery is verified by closely monitoring the pump and the decreasing level of fluid. Confusing solutions in two-bottle system could result in drug overdose.
Discontinue oxytocin, as indicated, and increase infusion of plain I.V. solution. Notify physician.	Hyperstimulation of the uterus (intrauterine pressure greater than 75 mm Hg) leads to abruptio placentae, uterine tetany, and possible rupture.
Administer 1 to 2 g magnesium sulfate ($MgSO_4$) slowly, as necessary.	Although the circulatory half-life of oxytocin is 3–4 min, uterine activity from effects of oxytocin administration may last 20–30 min after infusion is stopped. $MgSO_4$ may be indicated to relieve oxytocin-induced uterine tetany.

NURSING DIAGNOSIS:	**GAS EXCHANGE, IMPAIRED, HIGH RISK FOR, fetal**
Risk factors may include:	Altered blood flow to placenta or through umbilical cord (prolapse).
Possibly evidenced by:	[Not applicable; presence of signs/symptoms establishes an **actual** diagnosis.]
DESIRED OUTCOMES— FETUS WILL:	Display FHR within normal limits, free of late decelerations. Engage in behaviors that enhance fetal safety.

ACTIONS/INTERVENTIONS	RATIONALE
Independent	
Note fetal maturity based on client's history, EDD, and uterine measurements.	Gestational age of fetus should be 36 weeks or more for induction or augmentation of labor to be performed unless maternal condition warrants intervention before this time.
Perform Leopold's maneuvers and sterile vaginal examination. Note presentation and station of fetus.	Determines whether fetus is in vertex presentation and rules out CPD. If presenting part is too high (−2 cm), amniotomy may need to be postponed, owing to risk of prolapsed cord.
Position client on back with head of bed elevated and a pillow or wedge placed under one hip, preferably the right, so that client tilts to side.	Aids in obtaining an adequate external fetal monitor strip to evaluate contraction pattern and fetal heart tones. Wedge relieves pressure of fetus on vena cava and enhances placental circulation.
Apply EFM 15–20 min before induction procedure.	Determines fetal well-being, and provides baseline assessment of FHR and uterine activity.
Monitor FHR, as indicated, in conjunction with amniotomy.	Determining FHR prior to and following procedure provides information to ensure fetal well-being. Acceleration for a short period after amniotomy is normal; however, signs of distress may indicate fetal hypoxia from compression of cord or late decelerations.
Apply fundal pressure, as indicated.	May be required for firm positioning of presenting part on cervix to prevent cord prolapse during amniotomy.
Note time of rupture of membranes and character and consistency of fluid.	A mature fetus should be delivered within 24 hr of rupture of membranes to reduce risk of ascending infection. (Note: If fetus is not mature, measures may be taken to avoid delivery as long as possible unless signs of infection/distress are noted.)
Assess reaction of FHR to contractions, noting bradycardia and late or variable decelerations.	Proper assessment is needed to avoid hypoxia. Normal range for FHR is 120–160 bpm. To ensure fetal well-being, oxytocin may need to be discontinued and different measures taken, depending on interpretation of EFM tracing.
Collaborative	
Review results of ultrasonography and amniocentesis, pelvimetry, and L/S ratio.	Determines fetal age and presentation; helps identify CPD and other needs of fetus/neonate during and following delivery.
Assist as needed in application of internal fetal electrode.	Internal fetal electrode should be used for more accurate observation, especially if signs of fetal distress or meconium are present.
Have client void before administration of oxytocin and before application of fetal electrode.	A full bladder can interfere with fetal position and placement of monitor.

NURSING DIAGNOSIS:	PAIN [ACUTE]
May be related to:	Altered characteristics of chemically stimulated contractions, psychologic concerns.
Possibly evidenced by:	Verbalizations, increased muscle tone, distraction behaviors (restlessness, moaning, crying), facial mask of pain.
DESIRED OUTCOMES— CLIENT WILL:	Participate in behaviors to diminish pain sensations and enhance comfort.
	Appear relaxed between contractions.
	Report pain is reduced/manageable.

ACTIONS/INTERVENTIONS	RATIONALE
Independent	
Establish a rapport that enables client/coach to feel comfortable asking questions.	Answers to questions can alleviate fear and promote understanding.
Discuss anticipated changes/difference in labor pattern and contractions.	Helps prepare client because induction procedures and use of oxytocin result in rapid onset of strong, frequent contractions, which often interfere negatively with the client's ability to use learned coping techniques, which a slower buildup in the contractile pattern would allow.
Review/provide instruction in simple breathing techniques.	Encourages relaxation and gives client a means of coping with and controlling the level of discomfort.
Encourage client to use relaxation techniques. Provide instruction as necessary.	Relaxation can aid in reducing tension and fear, which magnify pain and hamper labor progress.
Provide comfort measures (e.g., effleurage, back rub, propping with pillows, applying cool washcloths, offering ice chips/lip balm).	Promotes relaxation, reduces tension and anxiety, and enhances client's coping and control.
Encourage and assist client with change of position, and adjust EFM.	Prevents/limits muscle fatigue; enhances circulation.
Review analgesics that are available and appropriate for client, and explain their time factors and restrictions.	Enhances client's control of situation and provides information necessary for making an informed choice. If client is medicated before she is 5 cm dilated, labor progress may be slowed; if delivery is imminent (within 2–4 hr), medication may depress the newborn.
Give encouragement; keep client informed on progress.	Reassures client/coach. Provides positive reinforcement for efforts and promotes focus on the future.
Collaborative	
Administer analgesic medications once dilation and contractions are established.	Relieves pain; promotes relaxation and coping with contractions, allowing client to remain focused on work of labor.

Cesarean Birth _____

Cesarean birth is an alternative to vaginal birth when the safety of the mother and/or fetus is compromised.

CLIENT ASSESSMENT DATA BASE

CIRCULATION

Hypertension.

Vaginal bleeding may be present.

EGO INTEGRITY

May view anticipated procedure as a sign of failure and/or as a negative reflection on abilities as a female.

FOOD/FLUID

Epigastric pain, visual disturbance, edema (signs of pregnancy-induced hypertension [PIH]).

PAIN/DISCOMFORT

Dystocia.

Prolonged/dysfunctional labor, failed induction.

Uterine tenderness may be present.

SAFETY

Active sexually transmitted disease (e.g., herpes).

Severe Rh incompatibility.

Presence of maternal complication such as PIH, diabetes, renal or cardiac disease, or ascending infection; prenatal abdominal trauma.

Prolapsed cord, fetal distress.

Impending delivery of premature fetus.

Unsuccessful external cephalic version to rotate breech presentation.

Membranes may have been ruptured for 24 hr or longer.

SEXUALITY

Cephalopelvic disproportion (CPD).

Multiple pregnancies or gestations (overdistended uterus).

Previous cesarean delivery, previous uterine or cervical surgery.

Tumor/neoplasm obstructing the pelvis/birth canal.

TEACHING/LEARNING

Cesarean birth may or may not be planned, affecting client's preparation and understanding of procedure.

DIAGNOSTIC STUDIES

Complete blood count, blood typing (ABO) and cross match, Coombs' test.
Urinalysis: Determines albumin/glucose levels.
Cultures: Identify presence of herpes simplex virus type II.

Pelvimetry: Determines CPD.
Amniocentesis: Assesses fetal lung maturity.
Ultrasonography: Locates placenta; determines fetal growth, lie, and presentation.
Nonstress test or contraction stress test: Assesses fetal response to movement/stress of uterine contractions/abnormal pattern.
Continuous electronic monitoring: Validates fetal status/uterine activity.

NURSING PRIORITIES

1. Promote maternal/fetal well-being.
2. Provide client/couple with necessary information.
3. Support client's/couple's desires to participate actively in birth experience.
4. Prepare client for surgical procedure.
5. Prevent complications.

NURSING DIAGNOSIS:	KNOWLEDGE DEFICIT [LEARNING NEED], regarding surgical procedure, expectations, postoperative regimen
May be related to:	Lack of exposure/unfamiliarity with information, misinterpretation.
Possibly evidenced by:	Request for information, statement of misconception, exaggerated behaviors.
DESIRED OUTCOMES— CLIENT WILL:	Verbalize understanding of indications for cesarean birth. Recognize this as an alternative childbirth method.

ACTIONS/INTERVENTIONS	RATIONALE
Independent	
Assess learning needs.	This alternative birth method is discussed in prepared childbirth classes, but many clients fail to retain the information because it has no personal significance at the time. Clients having a repeat cesarean delivery may not clearly remember or understand the details of their previous delivery.
Note stress level and whether procedure was planned or unplanned.	Identifies client's/couple's readiness to incorporate information.
Provide accurate information in simple terms. Encourage couple to ask questions and verbalize their understanding.	Provides information and clarifies misconceptions. Provides an opportunity to evaluate client's/couple's understanding of situation.
Review indications for alternative birth option.	Approximately one in 5 or 6 deliveries is a cesarean birth; should be viewed as an alternative, not an abnormal situation, to enhance maternal/fetal safety and well-being.
Describe preoperative procedures in advance, and provide rationale as appropriate.	Information allows client to anticipate events and understand reasons for interventions/actions.

ACTIONS/INTERVENTIONS

Independent

Provide postoperative teaching; include instructions in leg exercise, coughing, and deep breathing; splinting techniques; and abdominal tightening exercises.

Discuss anticipated sensations during delivery and recovery period.

RATIONALE

Provides techniques to prevent complications related to venous stasis and hypostatic pneumonia, and to decrease stress on operative site. Abdominal tightening decreases discomfort associated with gas formation and abdominal distention.

Knowing what to expect and what is "normal" helps prevent unnecessary concern.

NURSING DIAGNOSIS:	ANXIETY [SPECIFY LEVEL]
May be related to:	Situational crisis, threat to self-concept, perceived/actual threat of maternal and fetal well-being, interpersonal transmission.
Possibly evidenced by:	Increased tension, distress, apprehension, feelings of inadequacy, sympathetic stimulation, restlessness.
DESIRED OUTCOMES— CLIENT/COUPLE WILL:	Verbalize fears for the safety of client and infant.
	Discuss feelings about cesarean birth.
	Appear appropriately relaxed.
	Use resources/support system effectively.

ACTIONS/INTERVENTIONS

Independent

Assess psychologic response to event and availability of support system(s).

Ascertain whether procedure is planned or unplanned.

Stay with client, and remain calm. Speak slowly. Convey empathy.

Reinforce positive aspects of maternal and fetal condition.

Encourage client/couple to verbalize and/or express feelings (cry).

RATIONALE

The greater the client perceives the threat, the greater the level of her anxiety.

With unplanned cesarean birth, the client/couple usually has no time for physiologic or psychologic preparation. Even when planned, cesarean birth can create apprehension in the client/couple owing to an actual or perceived physical threat to the mother and infant related to the condition necessitating the procedure and to the surgery itself.

Helps to limit interpersonal transmission of anxiety, and demonstrates caring for the client/couple.

Focuses on possibility of successful outcome and helps to bring perceived/actual threat into perspective.

Helps to identify negative feelings/concerns and provides opportunity to cope with ambivalent or unresolved feelings/grief. The client may also feel an emotional threat to her self-esteem, owing to her feelings that she has failed, that she is weak as a woman, and that her expectations have not been met. Coach may question own abilities in assisting client and providing needed support.

ACTIONS/INTERVENTIONS	RATIONALE
Independent	
Support/redirect expressed coping mechanisms.	Supports basic and automatic coping mechanisms, increases self-confidence and acceptance, and reduces anxiety. (Note: Some client actions may be viewed as ineffective [e.g., screaming and throwing things] and need to be redirected to enhance client sense of control.)
Discuss past childbirth experience/expectations, as appropriate.	Client may have distorted memories of past delivery or unrealistic perceptions of abnormality of cesarean birth that will increase anxiety.
Provide period of privacy. Reduce environmental stimuli, such as the number of people present, as indicated by client's desires.	Allows client/couple opportunity to internalize information, marshal resources, and cope effectively.

NURSING DIAGNOSIS:	**SELF ESTEEM, SITUATIONAL LOW, HIGH RISK FOR**
Risk factors may include:	Perceived "failure" at a life event.
Possibly evidenced by:	[Not applicable; presence of signs/symptoms establishes an **actual** diagnosis.]
DESIRED OUTCOMES— CLIENT WILL:	Identify and discuss negative feelings.
	Verbalize confidence in herself and in her abilities.

ACTIONS/INTERVENTIONS	RATIONALE
Independent	
Determine client's usual feelings about self and pregnancy.	Diagnosis of a change in self-concept is based on knowledge of past self-perceptions and experiences. Cesarean birth, whether planned or unplanned, has the potential to alter the way the client feels about herself. The client sees that the birth plan has been altered, and that surgical intervention is needed to deliver the infant, while most women are able to deliver without any such intervention.
Encourage verbalization of feelings.	Identifies areas to be addressed. Clients' reactions vary and may be difficult to diagnose in the preoperative period. Feelings of negative self-image related to disappointment in the birth experience may interfere with postpartal activities related to successful breastfeeding and infant care.
Encourage questions and provide information/reinforce previous learning.	Enhances understanding and clarifies misconceptions.
Refer to cesarean birth as an alternative method of childbirth.	Terms such as "C-section" and "normal delivery" imply that the cesarean birth is different and unnatural, and that the client is therefore not normal.

ACTIONS/INTERVENTIONS

Independent

Provide verbal communication of assessment and interventions. Written information can be provided at a later time.

Identify other couples/resources to refer to after delivery.

Collaborative

Encourage partner's presence at the delivery as appropriate.

Encourage the client/couple to participate in delivery room bonding activities (e.g., breastfeeding and holding the infant).

RATIONALE

When a problem of self-esteem arises for the client, it may become more severe in the postpartal period. During the preoperative period, client is focusing on the here and now and may not be ready to read or deal with additional information.

At this crucial time, the nature of the situation usually does not allow opportunity to talk with others who have shared the same experience. However, these activities may be beneficial in the future to help with resolution of feelings/perceptions.

Provides support for the mother, promotes parental bonding, and provides additional input to the client's recall of the birth experience, because memory lapses are more common during periods of crisis.

Provides reinforcement of the birth experience and deemphasizes the surgical nature of the delivery.

NURSING DIAGNOSIS:	POWERLESSNESS
May be related to:	Interpersonal interaction, perception of illness-related regimen, lifestyle of helplessness.
Possibly evidenced by:	Verbalization of lack of control, lack of participation in care or decision making, passivity.
DESIRED OUTCOMES—CLIENT/COUPLE WILL:	Verbalize fears and feelings of vulnerability.
	Express individual needs/desires.
	Participate in decision-making process whenever possible.

ACTIONS/INTERVENTIONS

Independent

Assess factors contributing to sense of powerlessness.

Present options in care when possible (e.g., choice of anesthesia, I.V. placement, and use of mirror).

RATIONALE

Unplanned (and sometimes planned) cesarean birth may be characterized by the client's/couple's sense of loss of control over the birth experience. The client becomes subjected to the procedures and equipment used in illness. For those clients experiencing their first hospitalization, which involves fear of the unknown, powerlessness becomes a major stress factor.

Allows the client/couple to have some sense of input/control over the situation.

ACTIONS/INTERVENTIONS	RATIONALE
Independent	
Identify client's/couple's expectations and desires regarding the delivery experience.	Provides opportunity to accommodate needs and promote positive experience.
Provide personal space and time alone for the couple prior to surgery. (Note: Remain with client if partner is absent.)	Creates sense of control and lets couple have time to talk about their situation. Leaving client alone may result in feelings of abandonment and increased level of anxiety.
Provide information, and discuss client's/couple's perceptions.	Reduces stress caused by misconceptions/unfounded fears as well as fear of the unknown.

NURSING DIAGNOSIS:	PAIN [ACUTE], HIGH RISK FOR
Risk factors may include:	Increased/prolonged muscle contractions, psychologic reactions.
Possibly evidenced by:	[Not applicable; presence of signs/symptoms establishes an **actual** diagnosis.]
DESIRED OUTCOMES— CLIENT WILL:	Verbalize reduced discomfort/pain.

ACTIONS/INTERVENTIONS	RATIONALE
Independent	
Assess location, nature, and duration of pain, especially as it relates to the indication for cesarean birth.	Indicates the appropriate choice of treatment. The client awaiting imminent cesarean birth may experience varying degrees of discomfort, depending on the indication for the procedure.
Eliminate anxiety-producing factors (e.g., loss of control), provide accurate information, and encourage presence of partner.	Levels of pain tolerance are individual and are affected by various factors. Excessive anxiety in response to the emergency situation may enhance discomfort because fear, tension, and pain are interrelated and alter client's ability to cope.
Instruct in relaxation techniques; position for comfort as possible. Use Therapeutic Touch.	May assist in reduction of anxiety and tension and promote comfort.
Collaborative	
Administer sedative, narcotics, or preoperative medication.	Promotes comfort by blocking pain impulses. Potentiates the action of anesthetic agents.

NURSING DIAGNOSIS:	INFECTION, HIGH RISK FOR
Risk factors may include:	Invasive procedures, rupture of amniotic membranes, break in the skin, decreased hemoglobin (Hb), exposure to pathogens.

Possibly evidenced by:	[Not applicable; presence of signs/symptoms establishes an **actual** diagnosis.]
DESIRED OUTCOMES— CLIENT WILL:	Be free of infection.
	Achieve timely wound healing without complications.

ACTIONS/INTERVENTIONS	RATIONALE

Independent

Review history for preexisting conditions/risk factors. Note time of rupture of membranes.	Underlying maternal conditions, such as diabetes or hemorrhage, potentiate the risk of infection or poor wound healing. Risk of chorioamnionitis increases with the passage of time, placing mother and fetus at risk. Presence of infectious process may increase fetal risk of contamination.
Assess for signs/symptoms of infection (e.g., elevated temperature, pulse, white blood cell count, or odor/color of vaginal discharge).	Rupture of membranes occurring 24 hr prior to surgery may result in chorioamnionitis prior to surgical intervention and may alter wound healing.
Provide perineal care at least every 4 hr if membranes have ruptured.	Reduces risk of ascending infection.

Collaborative

Carry out preoperative skin preparation; scrub according to protocol.	Reduces risk of skin contaminants entering the incision, reducing risk of postoperative infection.
Obtain blood, vaginal, and placental cultures, as indicated.	Identifies infecting organism and degree of involvement.
Note hemoglobin (Hb) and hematocrit (Hct); note estimated blood loss during surgical procedure.	Risk of postdelivery infection and poor healing is increased if Hb levels are low and blood loss is excessive. (Note: Greater blood loss is associated with classic incision than with lower uterine segment incision.)
Administer parenteral broad-spectrum antibiotic preoperatively.	Prophylactic antibiotic may be ordered to prevent development of an infectious process, or as treatment for an identified infection, especially if the client has had prolonged rupture of membranes. (Note: Research suggests administration of antibiotic up to 2 hours before start of procedure provides the most protection from infection.)

(Refer to CP: Labor: Stage 1—Latent Phase, ND: Infection, high risk for, maternal.)

NURSING DIAGNOSIS:	GAS EXCHANGE, IMPAIRED, HIGH RISK FOR, fetal
Risk factors may include:	Altered blood flow to placenta and/or through umbilical cord.
Possibly evidenced by:	[Not applicable; presence of signs/symptoms establishes an **actual** diagnosis.]

ACTIONS/INTERVENTIONS

Independent

Note presence of maternal factors that negatively affect placental circulation and fetal oxygenation.

Continue monitoring FHR, noting beat-to-beat changes or decelerations during and following contractions.

Note presence of variable decelerations; change client's position from side to side.

Note color and amount of amniotic fluid when membranes rupture.

Auscultate the fetal heart when membranes rupture.

Monitor fetal heart response to preoperative medications or regional anesthesia.

Collaborative

Apply internal lead, and monitor fetus electronically as indicated.

Assist physician with elevation of vertex, if required.

Arrange for presence of pediatrician and neonatal intensive care nurse in delivery room for both scheduled and emergency cesarean births.

RATIONALE

Reduced circulating volume or vasospasms within the placenta reduce oxygen available for fetal uptake.

Fetal distress may occur, owing to hypoxia; may be manifested by reduced variability, late decelerations, and tachycardia followed by bradycardia. (Note: Infection from prolonged rupture of membranes increases FHR.)

Compression of cord between birth canal and presenting part may be relieved by position changes.

Fetal distress in vertex presentation is manifested by meconium staining, which is the result of a vagal response to hypoxia.

Occult or visible prolapse of the umbilical cord in the absence of full cervical dilatation may necessitate cesarean birth.

Narcotics usually reduce FHR variability and may require administration of naloxone (Narcan) following delivery to reverse narcotic respiratory depression. Maternal hypotension in response to anesthesia commonly causes transient fetal bradycardia, reduced variability, and sleep.

Provides more accurate measurement of fetal response and condition.

Position changes may relieve pressure on cord.

Infant may be preterm or may experience altered responses, owing to underlying maternal condition(s) and/or alternative birth process, necessitating immediate care/resuscitation.

Possibly evidenced by:	[Not applicable; presence of signs/symptoms establishes an **actual** diagnosis.]
DESIRED OUTCOMES— CLIENT WILL:	Be free of injury.

ACTIONS/INTERVENTIONS	RATIONALE

Independent

Remove prosthetic devices (e.g., contact lenses, dentures/bridges) and jewelry.	Reduces risk of accidental injury.
Determine time and content of last meal. Report information to anesthesiologist. Ensure availability and functioning of resuscitation equipment.	If client has eaten just before surgical procedure, risks of vomiting and aspiration increase, and general anesthesia may be contraindicated.
Restrict oral intake once decision for cesarean birth is made.	Reduces possibility of aspiration from vomiting.
Review labor record, noting voiding frequency, output, appearance, and time of last voiding.	May indicate urine retention or reflect fluid imbalance or dehydration in client who has been in labor.
Monitor urine output and color following insertion of indwelling catheter. Note any blood-tinged urine.	Reflects hydration level, circulatory status, and possible bladder trauma associated with surgical procedure.
Assist with positioning for anesthesia; support legs in postoperative transfer to stretcher. Note client's response during and after anesthesia. (Refer to Chapter 6, CP: Care Following Cesarean Birth [4 Hours to 5 Days].)	Essential for placement of anesthesia. Client with saddle block or spinal anesthesia will be unable to move or detect temperature extremes in lower extremities. Idiosyncratic responses to anesthesia can occur, such as anaphylaxis or respiratory paralysis if anesthetic block rises too high.
Keep accurate instrument and sponge counts at critical times during closure according to hospital protocol.	Ensures that all equipment and sponges are accounted for and not accidentally left in client's body.

Collaborative

Obtain urine specimen for routine analysis, protein, and specific gravity. Ensure that laboratory results are available before surgery is started.	Client is at increased risk if infectious process or hypertensive state is present.
Insert indwelling catheter to continuous gravity drainage system either just before surgical procedure or in the operating room.	Reduces risk of bladder injury during surgical procedure.
Administer preprocedural medication (e.g., atropine).	Reduces oral secretions, limiting risk of aspiration.

NURSING DIAGNOSIS:	CARDIAC OUTPUT, DECREASED, HIGH RISK FOR
Risk factors may include:	Decreased venous return, alteration in systemic vascular resistance.

ACTIONS/INTERVENTIONS	RATIONALE
Independent	
Note length of labor, if applicable. Assess for dehydration or excess intrapartal fluid losses.	Decreased intake and/or increased fluid losses lead to reduced circulating volume and cardiac output.
Remove nail polish on fingernails/toenails.	Allows clear visualization of nailbeds for assessing circulatory status.
Monitor respirations, blood pressure (BP), and pulse before, during, and after administration of anesthesia.	Hypotension is an anticipated side effect of regional anesthesia (e.g., saddle block or spinal anesthesia) because such anesthesia relaxes smooth muscles within vascular walls, affecting circulating volume and reducing placental perfusion.
Place towel or wedge under client's right hip.	Shifts uterus off inferior vena cava and increases venous return. Compression caused by obstruction of the inferior vena cava and aorta by the gravid uterus in a supine position may cause as much as a 50% decrease in cardiac output.
Note change in behavior or mental status, or cyanosis of mucous membranes.	Oxygen deficits are manifested first by changes in mental status, later by cyanosis.
Collaborative	
Administer supplemental oxygen through nasal cannula, as indicated.	Increases oxygen available for maternal and fetal uptake.
Initiate i.v. infusion of electrolyte solution. Administer bolus, as indicated.	Expands circulatory volume; provides route for emergency medication in the event of a complication.
Note alteration in vital signs; assist anesthetist as needed. Estimate and record blood losses.	Excess fluid losses and hemorrhage during labor and the intraoperative period may reduce cardiac output and promote vasoconstriction with shunting of blood to major organs. Diminished cardiac output and shock are manifested by decreased BP, increased or thready pulse, and cool/clammy skin.
Assist with isotonic fluid replacement using whole blood, plasma expanders, cryoprecipitate, platelets, or packed cells. (Refer to Chapter 6, CP: Postpartal Hemorrhage, ND: Fluid Volume deficit [active loss].)	Replaces lost fluids, increases circulating blood volume, and increases oxygen-carrying capacity.
Prepare and administer oxytocin infusion.	Aids myometrium contraction and reduces blood loss from exposed endometrial blood vessels once delivery of infant and placenta is completed.

NURSING DIAGNOSIS:	SENSORY-PERCEPTUAL ALTERATIONS, overload
May be related to:	Multiple environmental stimuli, increased number of personnel, excessive noise level, psychologic stress.
Possibly evidenced by:	Exaggerated emotional response, irritability, muscle tension.
DESIRED OUTCOMES— CLIENT WILL:	Verbalize understanding of need for increased level of activity.
	Appear appropriately relaxed.
	Maintain focus, tuning out extraneous distractions.

ACTIONS/INTERVENTIONS	RATIONALE

Independent

Assess environment for factors causing sensory overload.	Identifies factors, which may or may not be controllable. Cesarean delivery necessitates many medical and nursing activities necessary to assuring the health of mother and infant. Client tends to focus on the procedures being performed and the conversations going on in the room. The birth experience may be compromised by invasive technologic methods, shifting the focus from the birth of the infant to the surgical procedure.
Provide information about the surgical routine, including sounds, lights, dress, and instruments.	Knowledge about procedures, instruments, and alarms can help decrease anxiety.
Decrease noise levels, limit conversations, and use equipment/alarms judiciously.	Client may be keenly aware of sounds. Conversation, noise from equipment, and alarms may cause unnecessary anxiety.
Include client/couple in operating room conversation or silence, using concerned communication.	Ignoring the client can increase fear, which detracts from a positive birth experience.
Maintain eye contact, especially when wearing mask.	Conveys feeling of caring and includes the client/couple in activities/conversation.

Collaborative

Eliminate unnecessary personnel from the environment.	Avoids intrusions into personal space, which could increase anxiety. Individuals who are not involved in care of the client may detract from the intimacy of the birth experience.

Precipitous Labor/Delivery or Unplanned/Out-of-Hospital Delivery

Rapid progression of labor, lasting less than 3 hr from onset to delivery, and out-of-hospital delivery are emergency situations that place the client/fetus at increased risk for complications and/or untoward outcomes. The attending nurse may have primary responsibility for the safety of the mother and fetus.

CLIENT ASSESSMENT DATA BASE

EGO INTEGRITY

Irritability.

FOOD/FLUID

Nausea/vomiting.

PAIN/DISCOMFORT

May have an unusually high pain threshold or not be aware of abdominal contractions.

Possible absence of palpable contractions, as occurs with maternal obesity.

Low back discomfort (may not be recognized as a sign of progressing labor).

Intense/prolonged uterine contractions, inadequate uterine relaxation between contractions.

Involuntary urge to bear down.

SAFETY

Accelerated cervical dilation and fetal descent.

Preterm or small-for-gestational age infant (increases potential for rapid labor/delivery).

Rectal/perineal bulging.

Increased vaginal show.

SEXUALITY

History of short or rapid labor.

Young maternal age; large pelvis.

Multiparity or previous vaginal surgery (decreases soft-tissue resistance).

NURSING PRIORITIES

1. Promote maternal and fetal/newborn well-being.
2. Provide a physiologically and psychologically safe experience for client and newborn.
3. Prevent complications.

NURSING DIAGNOSIS:	ANXIETY [SPECIFY LEVEL]
May be related to:	Situational crisis, threat to self/fetus, interpersonal transmission.

Possibly evidenced by:	Increased tension; scared, fearful, restless/jittery; sympathetic stimulation.
DESIRED OUTCOMES— CLIENT WILL:	Use breathing and relaxation techniques effectively.
	Cooperate with necessary preparations for a rapid delivery.
	Follow directions and/or actively participate in delivery process.

ACTIONS/INTERVENTIONS	RATIONALE

Independent

Maintain calm, deliberate manner. Offer clear, concise instructions and explanations.	An emergency or extremely rapid delivery occurring out of the hospital or in a hospital setting without the presence of a clinician (physician or nurse midwife) can be extremely anxiety-provoking for the client/couple, who had anticipated an orderly progression through labor and delivery. Reactions may include hostility, fear, and disappointment when the actual birth event is not in keeping with their expectations. Composure of nurse reassures client and prevents transmission of undue concern and anxiety.
Provide a quiet environment; position client for optimal comfort.	Reduces distractions/discomfort, allowing client to focus attention.
Encourage coach/significant other to remain with client, provide support, and assist as needed.	Allowing full participation by a support person enhances self-esteem, furthers cohesion of family unit, reduces anxiety, and provides assistance for the professional.
Remain with client. Provide ongoing information regarding labor progress and anticipated delivery.	Reduces anxiety, fosters positive coping and cooperation, and reduces fear associated with the unknown.
Support appropriate coping/relaxation techniques.	Enhances sense of control; optimizes participation in the birth process.
Arrange for services of medical/nursing staff as soon as possible. Inform client that help has been requested.	The arrival of assistance helps the client/couple to feel less anxious and more secure.
Conduct delivery in a calm manner; provide ongoing explanations.	Helps client/couple remain calm and cooperate with instructions.
Place newborn on maternal abdomen once newborn respirations are established. Allow coach to hold infant.	Helps promote bonding and establishes a positive feeling about the experience.

Collaborative

Administer sedation as appropriate.	May help slow labor progress and allow client to regain control.

NURSING DIAGNOSIS:	SKIN/TISSUE INTEGRITY, IMPAIRED, HIGH RISK FOR, maternal
Risk factors may include:	Rapid progress of labor, lack of necessary equipment.
Possibly evidenced by:	[Not applicable; presence of signs/symptoms establishes an **actual** diagnosis.]
DESIRED OUTCOMES— CLIENT WILL:	Be free of lacerations/tears.

ACTIONS/INTERVENTIONS	RATIONALE
Independent	
Assess level of preparedness and knowledge. Provide information as necessary regarding the labor process and breathing/relaxation techniques.	Information helps nurse to manage the situation effectively, promotes client cooperation with necessary emergency measures, and reduces risk of injury.
Perform Leopold's maneuvers to determine fetal position. If abnormal presentation or position is detected, arrange for immediate transfer as appropriate.	If presentation and position are other than vertex/occiput anterior, complications could arise, so that transportation to hospital or delivery setting is imperative.
Perform vaginal examination, as appropriate and situation permits.	Determines cervical effacement, dilatation, fetal station, and imminence of delivery.
Stay with client continuously. Send for help in hospital setting, or enlist the aid of the most competent bystander or significant other in out-of-hospital setting.	Constant monitoring ensures nurse will be present should delivery occur.
Discontinue oxytocin if being administered.	Reduces uterine stimulation; may enhance uterine relaxation between contractions.
Observe client for rectal distention, fecal discharge, or increased vaginal flow.	These signs indicate labor progress as descending presenting part compresses sigmoid and rectum.
Encourage client to pant, rather than push, when crowning occurs.	Decreases urge to push and helps reduce likelihood/degree of lacerations and perineal trauma.
Gently massage perineum ("ironing") with index finger on inside of vagina and thumb on outer portion.	Aids in stretching perineal tissue, reducing risk of tearing.
Apply gentle pressure against fetal head; support perineum with other hand. Facilitate delivery of the shoulders with gentle upward traction.	Helps prevent fetal head from delivering too rapidly, which can contribute to lacerations of the birth canal.

NURSING DIAGNOSIS:	FLUID VOLUME DEFICIT, HIGH RISK FOR
Risk factors may include:	Presence of nausea/vomiting, lack of intake, excessive vascular loss.

Possibly evidenced by:	[Not applicable; presence of signs/symptoms establishes an **actual** diagnosis.]
DESIRED OUTCOMES—CLIENT WILL:	Maintain adequate level of hydration as evidenced by palpable pulses, prompt capillary refill, moist mucous membranes.

ACTIONS/INTERVENTIONS

Independent

Note characteristics of labor pattern and uterine tone. Monitor uterine activity manually or electronically. Assess for any abnormal vaginal bleeding or uterine rigidity.

Place newborn on client's abdomen following delivery once respiratory pattern is well established.

Monitor for signs of placental separation; avoid exerting force on umbilical cord. Save placenta for inspection by physician or nurse midwife. If out-of-hospital setting, wrap up placenta to be sent with client on transfer to hospital.

Monitor degree of uterine contractility and the color and amount of vaginal flow. Massage fundus gently; place infant to breast.

Inspect perineum for lacerations. If they are present, press clean perineal pad against perineum. Instruct client to keep thighs together.

Arrange for transportation to acute care setting in out-of-hospital birth.

Record time/method of placental expulsion and client's condition.

RATIONALE

Abruptio placentae can be a complication of emergency childbirth.

Weight of newborn stimulates uterine contractions and aids in placental separation.

A complete inspection of the placenta can be carried out later to ensure that no tissue remains in utero.

Stimulates uterine contractility, reducing vaginal flow, and helps to prevent hemorrhage due to uterine atony. Potential for abruptio placentae exists in the presence of rapid, severe uterine contractions without a sufficient period of relaxation between them.

Pressure limits bleeding until help is available to make needed repairs.

Examination of client by physician or nurse midwife is necessary to rule out retained placental tissue, and possibly to repair perineal or vaginal lacerations.

Accurate record aids in identification of potential for complications.

NURSING DIAGNOSIS:	INFECTION, HIGH RISK FOR
Risk factors may include:	Broken skin/traumatized tissue, increased environmental exposure, rupture of amniotic membranes.
Possibly evidenced by:	[Not applicable; presence of signs/symptoms establishes an **actual** diagnosis.]
DESIRED OUTCOMES—CLIENT WILL:	Be free of infection.

ACTIONS/INTERVENTIONS	RATIONALE

Independent

Provide as much privacy as possible in cases of unplanned out-of-hospital delivery. Prepare clean delivery surface using clean towels, clothes turned inside out, or unread newspapers placed under the client's buttocks.	Reduces possibility of contamination.
Scrub hands, don sterile gloves, place sterile towels under buttocks, and spray perineum with povidone-iodine (Betadine) solution if time permits in hospital setting.	Reduces likelihood of postdelivery infection.
Remove undergarments/newspapers when soiled.	Removes media that would support growth of pathogens.
Record time of rupture of membranes. Note amount and color of drainage.	Rupture of membranes increases risk of ascending infection. Characteristics of drainage may indicate presence of infection.

NURSING DIAGNOSIS:	PAIN [ACUTE]
May be related to:	Occurrence of rapid, strong muscle contractions; psychologic issues.
Possibly evidenced by:	Verbalizations of inability to use learned pain-management techniques, sympathetic stimulation, distraction behaviors (moaning, restlessness).
DESIRED OUTCOMES— CLIENT WILL:	Relax between contractions.
	Report discomfort/pain is reduced.

ACTIONS/INTERVENTIONS	RATIONALE

Independent

Note character and location of pain. Evaluate strength and intensity of contractions and duration of relaxation period.	Contractions may be of unexpected severity. Excess myometrial hypoxia may result from a tumultuous labor, intensifying discomfort.
Initiate breathing and relaxation techniques. Have coach/significant other provide effleurage and sacral back rub. Encourage client to assume position of comfort, preferably left lateral or semi-upright.	Helps reduce discomfort through gate control theory, cutaneous stimulation, and counterpressure. Increases circulation to myometrium.
Remove excess or constrictive clothing. Provide cool/comfortable environment, if possible. Change underpad/linens, as needed.	Promotes relaxation and comfort; enhances sense of well-being. Reduces discomfort.
Use physical restraint cautiously, using verbal commands, or have significant other(s) hold gently if necessary.	Provides safety in an "uncontrolled" setting.
Monitor bladder distention; encourage voiding.	Urine retention and consequent bladder distention may increase discomfort, impede labor, and result in bladder trauma.

NURSING DIAGNOSIS:	INJURY, HIGH RISK FOR, fetal
Risk factors may include:	Rapid descent/pressure changes, compromised circulation, environmental exposure.
Possibly evidenced by:	[Not applicable; presence of signs/symptoms establishes an **actual** diagnosis.]
DESIRED OUTCOMES— NEWBORN WILL:	Display Apgar score of 7 or better at 1 min and at 5 min.
	Be free of injury.

ACTIONS/INTERVENTIONS	RATIONALE
Independent	
Assess fundal height and uterine size. If possible, obtain information from client interview or chart regarding prior testing to determine or confirm gestational age. Ascertain expected date of delivery.	Helps predict size and needs of infant at birth.
Monitor fetal heart rate electronically or with fetoscope in hospital setting. In any setting, assess fetal activity level.	Provides data regarding condition of fetus.
Remain with client. In hospital setting, send for emergency delivery kit. Have staff person notify attending physician or nurse midwife of imminent delivery.	Kit contains equipment necessary for management of newborn in precipitate labor and delivery.
Place client in left lateral position.	Helps promote adequate placental perfusion; prevents supine hypotensive syndrome.
Have client pant rather than push as crowning occurs.	Helps prevent dural or subdural tears during rapid descent and delivery.
Assess for nuchal cord. If present, loop cord over newborn's head before delivery of body. (Note: In hospital setting, place two clamps on cord and cut cord before delivery of body if cord is too tight. In out-of-hospital setting, clean shoelaces or cloth strips can be used.)	Nuchal/short cord may cause hypoxia/anoxia to newborn during delivery process.
Rupture membranes if they are intact following delivery of head, suction (if available) nasal passages, and clear mouth.	Prevents aspiration of amniotic fluid. Removes secretions and facilitates initial respiration efforts.
Support newborn during delivery of body.	Vernix and amniotic fluid covering the body may make newborn difficult to grasp.
Hold newborn at the level of or slightly lower than the uterus.	While controversial, it is believed to facilitate blood flow through the umbilical cord, thereby providing an additional amount of blood to the newborn. (Note: Holding the newborn above the uterus causes blood to flow from the cord by force of gravity.)
Suction or clear oropharynx again. Place infant on client's abdomen, with infant's head slightly lower than body.	Helps clear airway; facilitates drainage of mucus.

ACTIONS/INTERVENTIONS	RATIONALE
Independent	
Dry newborn immediately (especially head); wrap infant in blanket, coat, or unused plastic food wrap; and give to client to hold next to her own body or place at client's breast. Without unwrapping infant, reassess temperature by feeling infant's stomach with back of fingers.	Reduces likelihood of cold stress. Mother's body warmth helps warm the newborn. Early feedings help prevent hypoglycemia.
Determine infant's condition at birth, noting Apgar score at 1 min and at 5 min. Keep accurate record of time of delivery, sex and condition of newborn, and resuscitative measures used.	Provides information that is needed by medical personnel for later evaluation of the newborn.
Prepare for transfer to hospital setting. Placenta can be left attached to newborn during the transfer (wrapped in newspaper or towel).	Client and newborn need to be evaluated by medical personnel.
(Refer to Chapter 7, CP: The First Hour of Life.)	

Intrapartal Hypertension

Pregnancy-induced hypertension (PIH) may have been diagnosed during the prenatal period, necessitating induction of labor/cesarean birth, or onset of symptoms may occur during labor (or early post partum). Early recognition and prompt intervention promotes optimal outcomes for client and fetus.

This plan of care is to be used in conjunction with the first five care plans in this chapter, which concern the three stages of labor, or with CP: Cesarean Birth, as indicated.

CLIENT ASSESSMENT DATA BASE

(Refer to Chapter 4, CP: Pregnancy-Induced Hypertension; and to the intrapartal assessment tool at the beginning of this chapter.)

CIRCULATION

May have been monitored/treated for prenatal hypertension either at home or in hospital setting.

May have been normotensive throughout the pregnancy.

Blood pressure may or may not be elevated at the onset of labor.

Progressive fluid retention may be present.

SAFETY

May be receiving an oxytocin infusion for induction or to offset tocolytic effects of magnesium sulfate ($MgSO_4$).

SEXUALITY

May be scheduled for induction (if cervix is favorable) or cesarean birth (preferably after 36 weeks' gestation) because of deteriorating maternal and placental status.

Pregnancy may or may not be full term (with uterus at xiphoid process).

DIAGNOSTIC STUDIES

Kidney, liver, and coagulation studies may show altered function (Refer to CP: Pregnancy-Induced Hypertension.)

NURSING PRIORITIES

1. Reduce/alleviate maternal hypertension.
2. Monitor client and fetal status.
3. Maintain/increase placental circulation.
4. Prevent eclamptic state.

NURSING DIAGNOSIS:	FLUID VOLUME EXCESS
May be related to:	Compromised regulatory mechanism (pathologic state with fluid shifts), excessive fluid intake, effects of drug therapy (oxytocin infusion).
Possibly evidenced by:	Blood pressure changes, edema, weight gain, changes in mentation.
DESIRED OUTCOMES— CLIENT WILL:	Display usual mentation; blood pressure (BP), pulse, urine output, and specific gravity within normal limits (WNL); deep tendon reflexes (DTRs) 2+ (normal); free of headache and visual disturbances.

ACTIONS/INTERVENTIONS	RATIONALE

Independent

Assess location and extent of edema. Note hemoglobin and hematocrit levels.

Helps determine degree of fluid retention and possible shifts to extracellular tissues. If the pathologic state is excessive, involving vasospasms and hypertension, fluid that has shifted from the intravascular space to extracellular tissue may begin to reenter the circulatory system, contributing to fluid overload and significant increase in BP.

Assess BP and pulse as indicated, especially if client is receiving oxytocin.

Preexisting elevated BP may rise even higher in the intrapartal period, or a normotensive client may become hypertensive during labor in response to increased basal metabolic rate, anxiety, and/or sodium and water retention from oxytocin infusion.

Assess ankle clonus, DTRs, lung sounds, visual acuity, presence of right upper quadrant (RUQ) pain. (Refer to Chapter 4, CP: Pregnancy-Induced Hypertension, ND: Fluid Volume deficit [regulatory failure].)

Progressive edema may be manifested by hyperreflexia or by cerebral, liver, or lung involvement.

Monitor urine output. Measure specific gravity; check albumin by dipstick test.

Kidney function is directly correlated to circulatory fluid volume, so that if fluid is trapped in third spaces, output decreases and specific gravity increases.

Position client on left side during stage I and II labor, or place wedge underneath right buttock.

Prevents compression of aorta and inferior vena cava; increases venous return, placental circulation, and kidney perfusion.

Collaborative

Administer antihypertensives (e.g., hydralazine [Apresoline], sodium nitroprusside [Nipride]) intravenously by infusion pump, if diastolic readings are greater than 110 mm Hg.

Vasodilator drugs relax smooth muscle of blood vessels, thereby reducing BP immediately. Sodium nitroprusside acts within 30 sec in emergency situations, providing a rapid decline in blood pressure.

Insert indwelling urinary catheter.

Provides accurate hourly totals of urine output, and monitors client for developing renal problems or oliguria. (Refer to Chapter 4, CP: Pregnancy-Induced Hypertension, ND: Tissue Perfusion, altered, renal.)

Administer furosemide (Lasix) if indicated.

On occasion, circulatory overload/failure may cause pulmonary edema requiring aggressive therapy. Otherwise, it is contraindicated as it may cause dehydration.

NURSING DIAGNOSIS:	GAS EXCHANGE, IMPAIRED, HIGH RISK FOR, fetal
Risk factors may include:	Altered blood flow, vasospasms and/or prolonged uterine contractions.

Possibly evidenced by:	[Not applicable; presence of signs/symptoms establishes an **actual** diagnosis].
DESIRED OUTCOMES— FETUS WILL:	Be free of late deceleration.
	Manifest good variability.
	Demonstrate a baseline heart rate of 120–150 bpm.

ACTIONS/INTERVENTIONS	RATIONALE

Independent

Assess fetal heart rate; note periodic changes (accelerations and decelerations) and patterns of short- or long-term variability. Report reduced variability and late decelerations, if present.	Recurrent or late decelerations combined with reduced variability or tachycardia then bradycardia may indicate uteroplacental insufficiency or potential fetal compromise/demise.
Position client on left side; use wedge under right buttock if client is supine, or raise client to semi-sitting position.	Prevents supine hypotensive syndrome; increases placental perfusion, which is especially critical in the hypertensive client who has low fetal reserve manifested as late decelerations.

Collaborative

Note findings of prenatal testing, especially amniocentesis, nonstress test, contraction stress test, gestational age of fetus, and fetal lung maturity.	Helps in predicting fetal response to labor and in evaluating newborn's ability to establish respiratory function in the early neonatal period.
Apply internal electrode to presenting part.	Accurately monitors fetal response and variability.
Note administration of $MgSO_4$ or diazepam (Valium) to client.	May reduce beat-to-beat variability and depress newborn.
In the event of late decelerations:	Continuation of pattern for more than 30 min markedly increases risk of negative effects of fetal hypoxia, acidosis, and asphyxia.
Increase plain i.v. fluid and discontinue oxytocin infusion. Notify physician immediately, especially if sinusoidal pattern is present.	Stopping oxytocin and increasing plain i.v. fluid may increase placental circulating volume/oxygenation. (Oxytocin infusion may reduce periods of maternal uterine relaxation between contractions, thereby reducing oxygen levels.) (Note: A sinusoidal pattern with minimal to absent short-term variability may occur just prior to death in a severely hypoxic fetus.)
Elevate client's legs; administer oxygen through nasal cannula at 10–12 L/min.	Increases venous return, circulating blood volume, and oxygen available for fetal uptake.
Assist as necessary with obtaining fetal scalp sample.	Fetal scalp pH should range between 7.30 and 7.35. A preacidotic value of 7.20 to 7.24 should be repeated in 15 min, with expeditious delivery carried out if values are less than 7.20.
Arrange for presence of pediatrician or neonatal/pediatric intensive care unit nurse at delivery.	May be needed to provide resuscitation or immediate care of the newborn.
Prepare for vaginal delivery or cesarean birth depending on fetal status and cervical dilatation.	Intervention may be necessary to prevent fetal/neonatal compromise due to asphyxia.

303

NURSING DIAGNOSIS:	URINARY ELIMINATION, ALTERED
May be related to:	Fluid shifts, hormonal changes, effects of medication.
Possibly evidenced by:	Decreased amount/frequency of voiding; bladder distention, changes in urine specific gravity, presence of albumin.
DESIRED OUTCOMES—CLIENT WILL:	Display individually adequate urine output with specific gravity WNL and urinary albumin not greater than 1+.

ACTIONS/INTERVENTIONS	RATIONALE
Independent	
Monitor intake and output.	Increased diuresis may occur, resulting in loss of 4 lb or more of retained fluid in a 24-hr period owing to bedrest, which reduces adrenal functioning.
Note color, amount, specific gravity, and albumin levels in each voiding.	Increasing urine output is reflected in less concentrated urine with decreasing specific gravity. Albumin greater than 2+ indicates glomerular spasms.
Assess bladder fullness; assist as necessary in emptying. (Refer to CP: Labor: Stage 1—Active Phase, ND: Urinary Elimination, altered.)	A full bladder may impede fetal descent and increases risk of maternal injury.
Collaborative	
Insert indwelling urinary catheter for continuous drainage.	In severe PIH, there may be extensive kidney involvement requiring close and accurate monitoring of renal function. In many cases, the client with severe PIH requires a cesarean delivery because of deteriorating maternal, fetal, and placental status and usually has an indwelling catheter inserted prior to surgery to prevent bladder trauma.

(Refer to Chapter 4, CP: Pregnancy-Induced Hypertension, ND: Tissue Perfusion, altered, renal.)

NURSING DIAGNOSIS:	INJURY, HIGH RISK FOR, maternal
Risk factors may include:	Tonic-clonic convulsions, altered clotting factors (release of thromboplastin from the placenta).
Possibly evidenced by:	[Not applicable; presence of signs/symptoms establishes an **actual** diagnosis].
DESIRED OUTCOMES—CLIENT WILL:	Restrict activities as indicated.
	Be free of seizure activity and related complications.

ACTIONS/INTERVENTIONS	RATIONALE

Independent

Assess for CNS involvement (i.e., headache, irritability, visual disturbances) and presence of RUQ pain.

Suggestive of cerebral edema and vasoconstriction, indicating progression of condition. Multiorgan involvement (e.g., liver distention creating epigastric pain) reflects HELLP syndrome, increasing mortality and morbidity.

Provide quiet environment, limit visitors, reduce room lighting, and maintain bedrest.

Helps reduce stimuli that might precipitate a seizure.

Measure urine output prior to and during administration of $MgSO_4$.

Output of at least 30 ml/hr is required for administration of $MgSO_4$.

Elicit deep tendon reflexes (DTRs) (brachial, wrist, knee); note ankle clonus. Note signs of hyperactivity, convulsion, or coma. Discontinue $MgSO_4$ in absence of patellar reflex.

Labor may precipitate eclamptic state, with hyperreflexia and progressive edema occurring just prior to the convulsion. Reduced DTRs suggest toxic levels of $MgSO_4$, which is administered to depress CNS.

Monitor respiratory rate/depth during $MgSO_4$ administration. Stop administration if respirations are less than 12/min.

$MgSO_4$ may depress respirations if drug levels reach toxic level.

Evaluate uterine activity and response to $MgSO_4$.

$MgSO_4$ has tocolytic properties that may reduce myometrial contractility, possibly necessitating oxytocin augmentation. (Refer to CP: Labor: Induced/Augmented.)

Give client nothing by mouth if seizure activity is suspected.

Reduces risk of aspiration.

Obtain emergency equipment (suction, oxygen, medications, emergency delivery pack).

May be needed in the event of a seizure or precipitous delivery.

Implement seizure precautions per protocol.

Reduces risk of injury if convulsions occur. An eclamptic episode may initiate the onset of labor, or labor may need to be artificially induced following an eclamptic seizure.

Palpate for uterine tenderness/rigidity; check for vaginal bleeding. Note history of concurrent medical conditions.

Client is at increased risk for abruptio placentae, especially if there is a preexisting medical problem such as diabetes mellitus or renal or cardiac conditions causing vascular involvement.

Monitor for signs of disseminated intravascular coagulation (DIC): easy/spontaneous bruising, prolonged bleeding.

Abruptio placentae with release of thromboplastin predisposes client to DIC.

Collaborative

Administer $MgSO_4$ by infusion pump or intramuscularly. Have calcium gluconate (10%) available. (Refer to Chapter 4, CP: Pregnancy-Induced Hypertension, ND: Injury, high risk for, maternal.)

Acts on myoneural junction to depress CNS activity; helps prevent seizure intrapartally. Calcium gluconate is an antidote to $MgSO_4$.

Initiate oxytocin infusion using piggyback setup with isotonic solution as indicated.

May be necessary for labor induction or augmentation to overcome tocolytic effects of $MgSO_4$. (Note: May cause additional elevation of BP owing to sodium/water retention, thereby increasing risk of seizure activity.)

ACTIONS/INTERVENTIONS	RATIONALE

Collaborative

Review laboratory studies.

Liver enzymes (AST, ALT).	Determines progression of condition, development of HELLP syndrome.
Platelet count, clotting factors. (Refer to Chapter 4, CP: Prenatal Hemorrhage.)	Release of thromboplastin from abruptio placentae may initiate DIC.
Administer diazepam (Valium) intravenously as indicated.	Depresses thalamus and hypothalamus and effectively manages eclamptic convulsion.

NURSING DIAGNOSIS:	**KNOWLEDGE DEFICIT [LEARNING NEED], regarding conditions, prognosis, treatment needs**
May be related to:	Lack of exposure/unfamiliarity with information resources, misinterpretation.
Possibly evidenced by:	Request for information, statement of misconception, inappropriate behaviors, development of preventable complications.
DESIRED OUTCOMES—CLIENT WILL:	Verbalize understanding of situation and treatment plan.

ACTIONS/INTERVENTIONS	RATIONALE

Independent

Assess client's level of knowledge and degree of anxiety.	Determines specific information needs and readiness to learn.
Explain the impact of procedures, nursing activities, and medications on client and fetus. Clarify misconceptions and elicit questions.	Reduces fear associated with the unknown; even those who have had problems previously may benefit from review of information throughout the labor and delivery process.
Provide simple explanations about actual and potential physiologic changes associated with prenatal and intrapartal hypertension.	Increases client awareness of the seriousness of her condition, and allows her to make informed decisions about her care.
Discuss impact of labor progress on hypertensive state.	Allows client to recognize that her hypertensive state may escalate during labor, requiring more intense interventions and possibly a rapid delivery (either vaginal or cesarean).

(Refer to CPs: Labor: Stage I—Latent Phase; Labor: Stage II (Expulsion), Labor: Stage III (Placental Expulsion), ND: Knowledge Deficit [Learning Need].)

NURSING DIAGNOSIS:	**ANXIETY [SPECIFY LEVEL]**
May be related to:	Situational crisis, interpersonal transmission/contagion, threat of death.

Possibly evidenced by:	Increased tension, apprehension, uncertainty, restlessness, sympathetic stimulation.
DESIRED OUTCOMES— CLIENT WILL:	Verbalize awareness of feelings of anxiety.
	Report reduction in level of anxiety.
	Appear relaxed between contractions.

ACTIONS/INTERVENTIONS	RATIONALE
Independent	
Assess client's/couple's source and level of anxiety.	All clients approach labor and delivery with a certain degree of anxiety, which becomes even greater in a high-risk situation. Such anxiety is directly related to fear of the unknown and lack of predictable outcomes for the client and her fetus.
Encourage verbalization of feelings; provide appropriate emotional support.	Aids client/couple in identifying specific concerns and helps relieve anxiety.
Inform client that pediatrician will be present at delivery; if possible, introduce client to pediatrician prior to delivery.	Assures client/couple that at delivery, the infant will be in competent hands and receive appropriate care.

(Refer to CPs: Labor: Stage I—Latent Phase, Labor: Stage I—Active Phase; ND: Anxiety, high risk for.)

NURSING DIAGNOSIS:	**PAIN [ACUTE]**
May be related to:	Intensification of uterine activity, discomfort associated with hypertension or oxytocin infusion; myometrial hypoxia (abruptio placentae) and anxiety.
Possibly evidenced by:	Verbalizations, altered muscle tone, distraction behaviors (restlessness, moaning, crying), facial mask of pain, autonomic responses.
DESIRED OUTCOMES— CLIENT WILL:	Use appropriate breathing and relaxation techniques.
	Report reduction of pain/discomfort.

ACTIONS/INTERVENTIONS	RATIONALE
Independent	
Assess source and nature of pain/discomfort.	Helps in determining appropriate nursing responses. Discomfort levels associated with uterine activity may be intensified in the client with hypertension, owing to high anxiety levels; myometrial hypoxia, which may be associated with placental separation (abruptio placentae); and/or intense onset of labor associated with oxytocin infusion, which has a negative impact on client's ability to cope with contractions.

307

ACTIONS/INTERVENTIONS	RATIONALE

Independent

Review/encourage use of relaxation techniques and controlled breathing.	Client may not have completed/participated in childbirth classes, or stress of situation may interfere with her ability to recall/perform these activities.
Provide comfort measures; e.g., cool cloth, dry linens, back/sacral rub.	Promotes relaxation and may enhance ability to cope with contractions.
Discuss available anesthesia and analgesia.	Knowledge enables client to make informed choices and maintain a sense of control.
Investigate report of acute abdominal pain. Note increased vaginal bleeding. (Refer to Chapter 4, CP: Prenatal Hemorrhage.)	Client with hypertension is more prone to abruptio placentae because of vasospasm and fibrin deposits.

Collaborative

Assess uterine response to labor using intrauterine catheter, if available, in place of tocotransducer.	Accurately measures intensity and resting tone of contractions and detects hyperstimulation caused by oxytocin induction.
Reduce/discontinue oxytocin infusion in presence of hyperactive uterine response or reduced relaxation between contractions.	Helps to terminate hypersensitive response. Tetanic contraction may cause uterine rupture.
Provide/assist with administration of meperidine hydrochloride (Demerol), fentanyl (Sublimaze), or pudendal block or local anesthetic.	Demerol administered in stage I labor and pudendal or local anesthetic administered in stage II labor are recommended; epidural or saddle block anesthesia may be contraindicated because of its known hypotensive effect, which further reduce placental perfusion.

Intrapartal Diabetes Mellitus _____

Although most diabetic clients go to term with spontaneous labor, close management of the intrapartal period is necessary for optimal outcome.

This plan of care is to be used in conjunction with the first five plans of care in this chapter, concerning the three stages of labor, or with CP: Cesarean Birth, as indicated.

CLIENT ASSESSMENT DATA BASE

(Refer to Chapter 4, CP: Diabetes Mellitus, Prepregnancy/Gestational; and to the intrapartal assessment tool at the beginning of this chapter.)

CIRCULATION

Blood pressure may or may not be elevated.

History of ankle/leg edema.

Rapid pulse, pallor, diaphoresis (hypoglycemia).

EGO INTEGRITY

Reports concerns regarding labor, impending delivery, and possible effects of diabetes on outcome.

Anxious, irritable, increased tension.

FOOD/FLUID

May report episodes of hypoglycemia, glycosuria.

Polydipsia, polyuria, hunger (hyperglycemia).

Dependent edema.

Ketonuria, elevated serum glucose.

SEXUALITY

Large amount of amniotic fluid on rupture of membranes (suggests hydramnios).

TEACHING/LEARNING

May have been hospitalized during the prenatal period for complications such as poor diabetic control, pregnancy-induced hypertension (PIH), and preterm labor due to polyhydramnios.

DIAGNOSTIC STUDIES

Serum glucose: May or may not be elevated.
Glycosylated hemoglobin (HbA$_{1c}$): Reflects diabetic control during the preceding 5 weeks.
Urinalysis: Reveals presence of glucose and ketones (hyperglycemia, ketoacidosis, and nutritional status) and albumin (PIH).
Ultrasonography and pelvimetry: Evaluates fetal size, and risk of macrosomia and shoulder dystocia.
Amniocentesis for lecithin to sphingomyelin (L/S) ratio and saturated phosphatidylcholine (SPG): Determines fetal lung maturity. SPG levels are better predictors of lung maturity than L/S ratio.

NURSING PRIORITIES

1. Monitor client/fetal status and progress of labor.
2. Maintain normoglycemia (euglycemia).
3. Provide emotional support to the client/couple.
4. Promote successful delivery of an appropriate-for-gestational-age (AGA) infant.

NURSING DIAGNOSIS:	TRAUMA, HIGH RISK FOR; GAS EXCHANGE, IMPAIRED, HIGH RISK FOR, fetal
Risk factors may include:	Inadequate maternal diabetic control, presence of macrosomia or intrauterine growth retardation (IUGR).
Possibly evidenced by:	[Not applicable; presence of signs/symptoms establishes an **actual** diagnosis.]
DESIRED OUTCOMES— NEONATE WILL:	Be full term, AGA, free of injury.
	Display normal levels of glucose, free of signs of hypoglycemia.

ACTIONS/INTERVENTIONS	RATIONALE
Independent	
Review prenatal course and maternal diabetic control.	Maternal hyperglycemia in the prenatal period promotes macrosomia, placing the fetus at risk for birth injury due to shoulder dystocia or cephalopelvic disproportion (CPD). If the client has severe vascular involvement associated with diabetes (Class C to F), the fetus often suffers IUGR and is at risk for hypoxia during the stress of labor, owing to uteroplacental ischemia. In addition, a high maternal glucose level at delivery stimulates the fetal pancreas, resulting in hyperinsulinemia, which can result in potentially severe neonatal hypoglycemia when the fetus is delivered and removed from the hyperglycemic environment.
Check maternal urine at each voiding for glucose/ketones, and albumin. Monitor blood pressure (BP). (Refer to Chapter 4, CP: Pregnancy-Induced Hypertension.)	Elevated glucose and ketone levels indicate maternal ketoacidosis, which can result in fetal acidosis and potential CNS injury. Elevated ketone levels alone suggest malnutrition/starvation affecting fetal growth. Elevated protein levels may indicate maternal vascular changes associated with PIH (occurs in 12%–13% of pregnant diabetics), which may reduce oxygen transfer to the fetus.
Monitor temperature as indicated. Note character of vaginal discharge.	Increased risk of ascending infection in diabetic clients; may result in neonatal sepsis.
Encourage lateral recumbent position for client during labor.	Promotes placental perfusion and increases oxygen available for fetal uptake.
Perform or assist with vaginal examination to determine progress of labor.	Prolonged labor may increase risk of fetal distress. Also with prolonged labor, diabetic control may deteriorate, resulting in negative effects on the fetus.
Collaborative	
Review results of prenatal tests such as biophysical profile (BPP), nonstress test (NST), and contraction stress test (CST).	Provides information about placental reserve for fetal oxygenation during intrapartal period.

ACTIONS/INTERVENTIONS	RATIONALE

Collaborative

Obtain or review results from amniocentesis and ultrasonography.	Provides information about fetal lung maturity; helps predict intensity of medical support needed in delivery room. Because fetal hyperinsulinemia interferes with surfactant production, the L/S ratio is not a good predictor of fetal maturity in the diabetic client; the presence of SPG is considered a reliable indicator.
Monitor maternal serum glucose level via fingerstick every hour until stable, then every 2–4 hr as indicated.	Varies during labor, owing to increased energy needs, depletion of glycogen levels, and a medically induced fasting state.
Monitor fetal heart rate with continuous fetal monitoring device, preferably with an internal electrode.	Tachycardia, bradycardia, or late decelerations with reduced variability indicate fetal hypoxia possibly related to diabetic vascular changes, which reduce uteroplacental perfusion.
Initiate i.v. infusion of 5% dextrose solution, as indicated.	It may be possible to maintain euglycemia without administering glucose until active labor starts. Glucose needs vary in the active phase, and some sources recommend dextrose infusion to equal 2.55 mg/kg/min. (Refer to ND: Injury, high risk for, maternal.)
Prepare for induction of labor using oxytocin (Pitocin) or for cesarean birth if medically indicated as a result of complications such as hypertension, IUGR, poor metabolic control, macrosomia, or CPD.	Delivery is indicated when medical evidence supports belief that intrauterine environment is potentially more harmful to the fetus than the extrauterine environment. Cesarean birth may be indicated in presence of macrosomia/CPD or rapidly deteriorating fetal status. (Refer to Chapter 7, CP: The Preterm Infant, for discussion of newborn complications.)
Arrange for pediatrician, neonatologist, or neonatal intensive care unit nurse to be present in delivery room, as indicated.	Helps ensure that the best-qualified professionals are available for assisting with or carrying out any necessary emergency measures.

NURSING DIAGNOSIS:	**INJURY, HIGH RISK FOR, maternal**
Risk factors may include:	Inadequate diabetic control (hypertension, severe edema, ketoacidosis, uterine atony/overdistention and dystocia).
Possibly evidenced by:	[Not applicable; presence of signs/symptoms establishes an **actual** diagnosis.]
DESIRED OUTCOMES— CLIENT WILL:	Maintain serum glucose levels below 100 mg/dl.
	Display stable vital signs.
	Be free of injury/complications.

ACTIONS/INTERVENTIONS	RATIONALE

Independent

Note time/content of last meal; amount/type/time of last dose of insulin. Ascertain recent serum glucose levels and any fluctuations. Observe for signs and symptoms of hypoglycemia

Useful in predicting client's needs. As client progresses into active labor, her metabolism increases, making her more prone to a hypoglycemic episode.

Check urine at each voiding for glucose, ketones, and protein.

Elevated ketone levels alone indicate a state of starvation. Elevated glucose and ketones reflect ketoacidosis. Elevated protein levels accompanied by edema and elevated blood pressure (BP) suggest PIH.

Monitor vital signs every hour during induction. Monitor BP every 15 min.

Clients with diabetes mellitus are at risk for developing PIH. Pitocin increases sodium/water reabsorption from the kidney tubules, possibly elevating BP readings.

Assess quality, duration, and frequency of contractions.

Dystocia may occur as a result of CPD related to macrosomia.

Evaluate skin turgor, pulse and temperature, and condition of mucous membranes.

If serum glucose is initially elevated, dehydration may occur as a result of osmotic diuresis (glycosuria) and restriction of oral intake.

Note presence, quality, and consistency of bloody show. Notify physician if excess bleeding is present.

Clients with diabetes are prone to hemorrhage, owing to abruptio placentae or overdistention of the uterus resulting from polyhydramnios or macrosomia.

Have glucagon available at the bedside.

If serum glucose falls rapidly below 60 mg/dl, administration of glucagon may be necessary to trigger conversion of glycogen to glucose.

Collaborative

Review results of ultrasonography and pelvimetry.

Macrosomic infant may cause prolonged labor and necessitate operative vaginal or cesarean birth.

Monitor serum glucose level every hour until stable, then every 2–4 hr. Use client's own glucose reflectance meter if available.

Levels vary during labor, owing to increased energy needs, depletion of glycogen levels, and medically induced state of fasting. Self-monitoring promotes involvement/sense of control, is more economical and faster than laboratory testing.

Maintain glucose level between 60 and 100 mg/dl:

Intrapartal glucose levels play a crucial role in outcome of pregnancy.

Initiate intravenous infusion of 5% dextrose solutions as indicated.

I.V. infusion prevents dehydration and maintains serum glucose, avoiding depletion of glycogen stores.

Administer subcutaneous or I.V. insulin infusion as appropriate.

Labor increases sensitivity to insulin, and low doses (up to 2.0 units/hr) are usually sufficient to maintain normoglycemia. Additional insulin may not be required during stage II labor and immediately post delivery; I.V. infusion of insulin is discontinued at the end of stage III labor.

Double rate of infusing dextrose for subsequent hour if blood glucose levels fall below 60 mg/dl.

Provides glucose to counteract hypoglycemia.

ACTIONS/INTERVENTIONS	RATIONALE
Collaborative	
Use Biostator Glucose Controller (Miles Laboratories), if available.	This is a closed-loop system that delivers insulin or dextrose, depending on the individual's needs, and eliminates need for repeated serum glucose sampling.
Prepare for induction of labor by administration of Pitocin, or cesarean birth, if indicated. (Refer to CPs: Cesarean Birth; Labor: Induced/Augmented.)	May be necessary to ensure maternal and newborn well-being.
Obtain complete blood count, blood type, and cross match if surgical procedure is planned.	Ensures availability of blood products in the event that replacement is needed as a result of hemorrhage.
Avoid use of solutions that contain glucose to expand the maternal plasma volume prior to regional block anesthesia or if cesarean birth is indicated.	Solutions containing glucose rapidly elevate serum glucose levels beyond normoglycemia.

NURSING DIAGNOSIS:	**ANXIETY [SPECIFY LEVEL]**
May be related to:	Situational "crisis"/threat to health status (maternal or fetal).
Possibly evidenced by:	Increased tension, apprehension, fear of unspecific consequences, sympathetic stimulation.
DESIRED OUTCOMES— CLIENT/COUPLE WILL:	Verbalize awareness of feelings concerning diabetes and labor.
	Use appropriate coping strategies.

ACTIONS/INTERVENTIONS	RATIONALE
Independent	
Arrange for continued presence of primary nurse during labor. Position call light for easy access if couple must be left unattended, and inform them summons will be answered promptly. Notify couple of substitute personnel and introduce them.	Enhances continuity of care. Client/couple needs to know they are not alone and that immediate help is available, especially who will respond in absence of primary nurse.
Ascertain present response to labor and to medical management; assess effectiveness of support systems.	Provides baseline assessment for future comparisons; identifies strengths and potential problems.
Involve couple in activities as much as possible. Encourage use of relaxation and breathing techniques.	Provides a feeling of control over situation.
Explain all procedures; reinforce information from other healthcare providers.	Knowledge of what is occurring helps to decrease fears.
Encourage questions and verbalization of concerns.	An open and encouraging atmosphere decreases intimidation by procedures or equipment, allowing concerns to be expressed and dealt with.

ACTIONS/INTERVENTIONS	RATIONALE
Independent	
Keep couple informed concerning progress of labor. Be positive, providing accurate information.	Information on labor progress, given in a straightforward, open manner, can be helpful in diminishing concerns about the unknown. Provides reinforcement for efforts.
Keep couple informed of fetal status.	Helps to alleviate/minimize concerns and fosters trust.

CHAPTER 6

MATERNAL POSTPARTAL CONCEPTS

POSTPARTAL ASSESSMENT TOOL (Continuation of Intrapartal Assessment Tool)

ACTIVITY/REST

Subjective

Activity/sleep prior to onset of labor: _____
Length of labor: _____
Energy level: _____

Objective

Mental status (e.g., euphoric, withdrawn, lethargic): ____

CIRCULATION

Objective

BP: ____ Pulse: ____
Extremities: Temperature: ____ Color: _____
 Homans' sign: _____
Blood loss during delivery: ____

EGO INTEGRITY

Subjective

Reality of labor/delivery experience compared with
 expectations of self: _____
 Support person: _____
 Primary nurse: _____
 Physician/midwife: _____

Objective

Emotional reaction: ____

ELIMINATION

Subjective

Time of last void: _____
Last bowel movement: _____

Objective

Presence of hemorrhoids: ____
Bladder palpable: ____
Presence of catheter: ____
 Color of urine: ____
Bowel sounds: ____

FOOD/FLUID

Subjective

Recent oral intake: _____
Specific requests: _____
Nausea/vomiting: _____

Objective

Skin turgor: _____
Edema: Legs: _____ Sacrum: _____
   Hands: _____ Face: _____
Appearance of tongue: _____
   Mucous membranes: _____

NEUROSENSORY

Subjective

Sensation of lower extremities: _____

Objective

Movement of lower extremities: _____
Deep tendon reflexes: _____

PAIN/DISCOMFORT

Subjective

Location: _____ Intensity: _____
Frequency: _____ Quality: _____
Duration: _____ Radiation: _____
Precipitating factors: _____

Objective

Facial expression: _____
Body movement: _____

SAFETY

Subjective

Time of ROM: _____
Intrapartal obstetrical problems/treatment:
   PIH: _____ Hemorrhage: _____
Blood transfusion: _____

Objective

Temperature: _____
Condition of perineum: _____
Surgical repair: Episiotomy: _____
   Lacerations: _____

SEXUALITY

Subjective

Expression of feelings: _____

Objective

Fundus: Position: _____ Firm: _____ Boggy: _____
Lochia: Color: _____ Flow: _____
   Presence of clots: _____
Breasts: Soft: _____ Firm: _____
   Presence of colostrum: _____

SOCIAL INTERACTIONS

Subjective

Perceptions regarding neonate: _____

Objective

Family interaction: _____
Presence of attachment behaviors (specify): _____

TEACHING/LEARNING

Subjective

Choice of infant feeding: _____
Response to initial feeding interaction: _____

Discharge Considerations

(As noted in intrapartal history.)

Stage IV (First 4 Hours Following Delivery of the Placenta) ___

CLIENT ASSESSMENT DATA BASE

ACTIVITY/REST

May appear "energized" or fatigued/exhausted, sleepy.

CIRCULATION

Pulse usually slow (50 to 70 bpm), owing to vagal hypersensitivity.

Blood pressure (BP) variable; may be lower in response to analgesia/anesthesia, or elevated in response to oxytocin administration or pregnancy-induced hypertension (PIH).

Edema, if present, may be dependent (e.g., confined to lower extremities); or may include upper extremities and facies, or may be generalized (signs of PIH).

Blood loss during labor and delivery up to 400–500 ml for vaginal delivery or 600–800 ml for cesarean birth.

EGO INTEGRITY

Emotional reactions varied and changeable; e.g., excitation or behaviors showing lack of attachment, disinterest (exhausted), or disappointment.

May express concern or apologize for intrapartal behavior or loss of control; may express fears regarding condition of newborn and immediate neonatal care.

ELIMINATION

Hemorrhoids often present and protruding.

Bladder may be palpable over symphysis pubis, or urinary catheter may be in place.

Diuresis may occur if pressure of presenting part obstructs urinary flow, and/or i.v. fluids are administered during labor and delivery.

FOOD/FLUID

May report thirst, hunger, or nausea.

NEUROSENSORY

Sensation and movement of lower extremities decreased in presence of spinal anesthesia or caudal/epidural analgesia.

Hyperreflexia may be present (suggests developing or persistent hypertension, especially in diabetic, adolescent, or primiparous client).

PAIN/DISCOMFORT

May report discomfort from various sources; e.g., afterpains, tissue trauma/episiotomy repair, bladder fullness, or feeling cold/muscle tremors with "chills."

SAFETY

Slight temperature elevation initially (exertion, dehydration).

Episiotomy repair intact, with tissue edges closely approximated.

SEXUALITY

Fundus firmly contracted, midline and located at the level of the umbilicus.

Moderate amount of vaginal drainage or lochia, dark red, with only a few small clots at most (up to small plum size).

Perineum free of redness, edema, ecchymosis, or discharge.

Striae may be present on abdomen, thighs, and breasts.

Breasts soft, with nipples erect.

TEACHING/LEARNING

Note medications given, including time and amount.

DIAGNOSTIC STUDIES

Hemoglobin/hematocrit (Hb/Hct), complete blood count, urinalysis, other studies: May be done as indicated by physical findings.

NURSING PRIORITIES

1. Promote family unity and bonding.
2. Prevent or control bleeding.
3. Enhance comfort.

NURSING DIAGNOSIS:	FAMILY PROCESSES, ALTERED, bonding
May be related to:	Developmental transition/gain of a family member.
Possibly evidenced by:	Hesitance to hold/interact with infant, verbalization of concerns.
DESIRED OUTCOMES— CLIENT/COUPLE WILL:	Hold infant, as maternal and neonatal conditions permit.
	Demonstrate appropriate attachment and bonding behaviors.

ACTIONS/INTERVENTIONS	RATIONALE

Independent

Encourage client to hold, touch, and examine the infant, preferably touching skin to skin.

The first hours after delivery offer a unique opportunity for family bonding to occur, because both mother and infant are emotionally receptive to cues from each other, which initiates the attachment and acquaintance. Close physical contact soon after birth facilitates the bonding process and capitalizes on infant's receptivity during the first period of reactivity, which coincides with a maternal period of heightened awareness ("ecstasy") in the first hour postpartum. (Note: Even if the client has chosen to relinquish her child, interacting with the newborn may facilitate the grieving process.)

ACTIONS/INTERVENTIONS	RATIONALE
Independent	
Encourage father to touch and hold infant and assist with infant care, as allowed by the situation.	Helps facilitate bonding/attachment between father and infant. Fathers who actively participate in the birth process and early infant interactional activities commonly report feeling a special bond to the infant.
Observe and record family-infant interactions, noting behaviors thought to indicate bonding and attachment within specific culture.	Eye-to-eye contact, use of en face position, talking in a high-pitched voice, and holding infant closely are associated with attachment in American culture. On first contact with the infant, a mother manifests a progressive pattern of behaviors whereby she initially uses fingertips to explore the infant's extremities and progresses to use of the palm before enfolding the infant with whole hand and arms.
Note verbalizations/behaviors suggesting disappointment or lack of interest/attachment.	The arrival of a new family member, even when wanted and anticipated, creates a transient period of disequilibrium, requiring incorporation of the new child into the existing family.
Welcome family and siblings during recovery period if desired by client and if allowed by maternal/neonatal condition and setting.	Promotes family unit, and helps siblings to begin process of positive adaptation to new roles and incorporation of new member into family structure.
Ensure family privacy between examinations during initial interaction with the newborn, as conditions of mother and infant permit.	Client, father, siblings, and infant need time to become acquainted with one another.
Encourage and assist with breastfeeding dependent on client's choice and cultural beliefs/practices.	Early contact has a positive effect on duration of breastfeedings; skin-to-skin contact and initiation of maternal tasks promotes bonding. Some cultures (e.g., Hispanic, Navajo, Filipino, Vietnamese) refrain from breastfeeding until the milk flow is established.
Answer client's questions regarding protocol of care during immediate postdelivery period.	Information relieves anxiety that may interfere with bonding or result in self-absorption rather than in attention to newborn.
Collaborative	
Notify appropriate healthcare team members (e.g., nursery staff or postpartal nurse) of observations, as indicated.	Inadequate bonding behaviors or poor interaction between client/couple and infant necessitates support and further evaluation. (Refer to CP: The Client at 4 Hours to 3 Days Postpartum, NDs: Parenting, altered, high risk for; Family Coping: potential for growth.)

NURSING DIAGNOSIS:	**FLUID VOLUME DEFICIT, HIGH RISK FOR**
Risk factors may include:	Myometrial fatigue/failure of homeostatic mechanisms (e.g., continued uteroplacental circulation, incomplete vasoconstriction, inadequate fluid shifts, effects of PIH).

ACTIONS/INTERVENTIONS	RATIONALE
Independent	
Place client in recumbent position.	Optimizes cerebral blood flow, and facilitates monitoring of fundus and vaginal flow.
Assess contributing intrapartal events, especially induced/augmented labor or prolonged labor.	In many cases, oxytocin-stimulated labor requires increased amounts of oxytocin in the postpartal period to maintain myometrial contractility. Prolonged labor results in myometrial fatigue, increasing risk of uterine atony.
Note type of delivery and anesthesia, blood loss at delivery, and length of stage III labor.	Excess uterine manipulation, operative delivery, anesthesia, or problems with placental separation may contribute to blood loss and myometrial fatigue. The postdelivery client may incur loss of as much as 300–400 ml of blood during a vaginal delivery, and twice that amount in a cesarean delivery, with no negative effects. Blood loss during delivery is quickly replaced by mobilization of extravascular fluid (physiologic edema), so that total blood volume changes are minimal unless losses exceed normal fluid shifts.
Note location and consistency of the fundus every 15 min (advance per protocol/client's condition), and record findings.	Uterine myometrial activity contributes to hemostasis by compressing the endometrial blood vessels. The fundus should be firm and located at the umbilicus. Displacement may indicate a full bladder, retained blood clots, or uterine relaxation.
Gently massage fundus if it is soft (boggy). Hold or support uterus with one hand just above the symphysis pubis while massaging the fundus with the other hand. Use a firm, steady, downward pressure on the fundus. Record results of intervention.	Fundal massage stimulates uterine contractions and controls bleeding. Overstimulation can cause uterine relaxation owing to muscle exhaustion. Downward pressure enhances expulsion of clots that may have interfered with uterine contractility.
Place infant at client's breast if client has chosen to breastfeed.	Infant suckling stimulates posterior pituitary release of oxytocin, which promotes myometrial contractility.
Assess for bladder fullness above symphysis pubis. Notify physician if distention is noted and client is unable to void. (Refer to CP: The Client at 4 Hours to 3 Days Postpartum, ND: Urinary Elimination, altered.)	A full bladder displaces the fundus and interferes with uterine contractility.

ACTIONS/INTERVENTIONS	RATIONALE
Independent	
Assess amount (using a predetermined scale), color, and nature of lochial flow every 15 min (advance per protocol and client's condition).	Helps identify potential lacerations of vagina and cervix, which could result in excessive, bright red flow. (Saturation of a perineal pad in a 15-min period is considered excessive flow and requires prompt evaluation.) Uterine atony increases lochial flow.
Assess BP and pulse every 15 min.	As fluid shifts occur and blood is redistributed into the venous bed, a moderate drop in the systolic and diastolic BP and mild tachycardia may be noted. More marked changes may occur in response to anesthesia, magnesium sulfate, or shock, or may be elevated in response to oxytocin or PIH. Bradycardia may occur normally in response to increased cardiac output and increased stroke volume, and vagal hypersensitivity following delivery. Sustained tachycardia may accompany shock.
Examine perineum every 15 min per protocol, noting condition of episiotomy repair, excess edema, ecchymosis, or intense internal pressure.	Excess edema may cause loss of approximation of episiotomy repair. Ecchymosis, excess perineal edema, signs or symptoms of shock in presence of well-contracted uterus, and no visible vaginal blood loss may indicate hematoma formation.
Notify physician or healthcare provider if blood loss is excessive and/or vital signs are unstable. Prepare for transfer to hospital if client is in an alternative birth center or home setting.	Medical intervention may be needed to identify or treat underlying problems.
Collaborative	
Review initial Hb and Hct levels. Obtain stat levels as indicated. (Refer to CP: Postpartal Hemorrhage, ND: Tissue Perfusion, altered.)	Aids in estimating amount of blood loss. Pregnancy-induced hypervolemia acts as a safeguard against hemorrhage. Client with lower-than-normal Hb (10 mg or less) or Hct (30% or less) is less able to tolerate blood loss. Usually, as much as 10% of total blood volume can be lost with no negative effects.
Start or maintain i.v. infusion of isotonic solution.	Increases blood volume and provides open vein for administration of emergency medication if needed.
Administer oxytocin or ergot preparation. Increase rate of intravenous oxytocin infusion per protocol if uterine bleeding persists.	Stimulates contractility of myometrium, closing off exposed blood vessels at former placental site, and reduces blood loss.
Obtain platelet count, levels of fibrinogen and fibrin split products, prothrombin time, and activated partial thromboplastin time.	Alterations may suggest developing coagulation disorders.
Replace fluid losses with plasma, packed cells, or whole blood as indicated.	Replacement of fluid losses may be needed to increase circulating volume and prevent shock.
Assist in preparation, as necessary, for further treatment such as dilatation and curettage, laparotomy, evacuation of hematoma, repair of birth canal lacerations, or hysterectomy.	If bleeding does not respond to conservative measures/oxytocin administration, surgery may be indicated.

ACTIONS/INTERVENTIONS	RATIONALE
Independent	
Assess nature and degree of discomfort, type of delivery, nature of intrapartal events, length of labor, and anesthesia or analgesia administered.	Helps identify factors that intensify discomfort/pain.
Congratulate the client/couple on birth of newborn. Provide opportunity for talking about childbirth experience.	Promotes a sense of accomplishment, positive self-esteem, and emotional well-being. Allows client/couple opportunity to work through and accept intrapartal events.
Provide appropriate information about routine care during postpartal period.	Information may lessen anxiety associated with fear of the unknown, which could intensify perception of pain.
Inspect episiotomy repair or lacerations. Evaluate approximation of wound repair; note presence of edema or hemorrhoids. Apply ice pack.	Trauma and edema increase degree of discomfort and may cause stress on suture line. Ice provides local anesthesia, promotes vasoconstriction, and reduces edema formation.
Assess for leg or body tremors or uncontrollable shaking. Place warm blankets on client.	Postdelivery tremors (chills) may be due to sudden release of pressure on pelvic nerves or may possibly be related to fetus-to-mother transfusion occurring with placental separation. Warm blankets may promote muscle relaxation and a feeling of well-being.
Institute comfort measures (e.g., mouth care; partial bath; clean, dry linen; periodic perineal care).	Promotes comfort, feeling of cleanliness, and well-being. Higher-level psychologic needs can be met only after basic physical needs are satisfied.
Offer clear fluids as appropriate.	Relieves thirst associated with fluid losses in delivery, side effects of anesthesia, and breathing through mouth.
Assess for bladder fullness by palpating above symphysis pubis. Determine time of last voiding; note prenatal fluid retention.	Intrapartal bed rest, postdelivery mobilization of fluids, and I.V. fluid support may result in diuresis and discomfort associated with a full bladder.
Massage uterus gently as indicated. Note presence of factors that intensify the severity and frequency of afterpains.	Gentle massage promotes contractility but should not cause excessive discomfort. Multiparity, uterine overdistention, oxytocin stimulation, and breastfeeding increase degree of afterpains associated with myometrial contractions.

ACTIONS/INTERVENTIONS

Independent

Encourage use of breathing/relaxation techniques.

Position or reposition client as needed. Assess for combined effects of anesthesia.

Provide quiet environment; encourage rest between assessments.

Collaborative

Administer analgesic as needed.

RATIONALE

Enhances sense of control and may reduce severity of discomfort associated with afterpains (contractions) and fundal massage.

Sensation and movement of lower extremities may still be affected by subarachnoid or peridural block, which interferes with client's ability to assume a comfortable position.

Labor and delivery are exhausting processes. Although client may be "too excited to sleep," quiet and rest may prevent undue fatigue.

Analgesics act on higher brain centers to reduce perception of pain.

CLIENT ASSESSMENT DATA BASE

Progressive continuation of data base for Stage IV.

ACTIVITY/REST

Insomnia may be noted.

CIRCULATION

Diaphoretic episodes more often occur during night.

EGO INTEGRITY

Irritability, tearful/crying ("postpartum blues" often noted about day 3 following delivery).

ELIMINATION

Diuresis between day 2 and 5.

FOOD/FLUID

Loss of appetite may be reported about day 3.

PAIN/DISCOMFORT

Breast tenderness/engorgement may occur between days 3 to 5 postpartum.

SEXUALITY

Uterus 1 cm above umbilicus at 12 hr following delivery, descending approximately 1 fingerbreadth daily thereafter.

Lochia rubra continues for 2–3 days, progressing to lochia serosa with flow dependent on position (e.g., recumbent versus up ambulating) and activity (e.g., breastfeeding).

Breasts: Production of colostrum first 48 hours, progressing to mature milk, usually by day 3; may be earlier, dependent on when breastfeeding is begun.

NURSING PRIORITIES

1. Promote comfort and general well-being.
2. Prevent complications.
3. Support family bonding.
4. Provide information and anticipatory guidance.

DISCHARGE GOALS

1. Physiologic/psychologic needs being met.
2. Complications prevented/resolving.
3. Family bonding initiated.
4. Postpartal needs understood.

NURSING DIAGNOSIS:	PAIN [ACUTE]/DISCOMFORT*
May be related to:	Mechanical trauma, tissue edema/engorgement or distention, hormonal effects.
Possibly evidenced by:	Reports of cramping (afterpains), headache, perineal discomfort, and breast tenderness; guarding/distraction behaviors, facial mask of pain.
DESIRED OUTCOMES—CLIENT WILL:	Identify and use appropriate interventions to manage discomfort.
	Verbalize lessening of discomfort.
	*Authors' note: Currently there is no NANDA diagnostic label that addresses issues of comfort below the level of Pain [acute] or chronic. Although the label of **Discomfort** is not approved, we believe it speaks more directly to the identified problem.

ACTIONS/INTERVENTIONS	RATIONALE
Independent	
Determine presence, location, and nature of discomfort. Review labor and delivery record.	Identifies specific needs and appropriate interventions.
Inspect perineum and episiotomy repair. Note edema, ecchymosis, localized tenderness, purulent exudate, or loss of approximation of suture line. (Refer to ND: Infection, high risk for.)	May reflect excess trauma to perineal tissue and/or developing complications requiring further evaluation/intervention.
Apply ice pack to perineum, especially during the first 24 hours following delivery.	Provides localized anesthesia, promotes vasoconstriction, and reduces edema and vasodilation.
Encourage use of moist heat (e.g., sitz/tub bath) between 100° and 105° F (38.0° to 43.2° C) for 20 min, 3 to 4 times daily, after the first 24 hours.	Increases circulation to perineum, enhances oxygenation and nutrition of tissues, reduces edema, and promotes healing.
Recommend sitting with gluteal muscles contracted over episiotomy repair.	Use of gluteal tightening while sitting reduces stress and direct pressure on perineum.
Inspect perineum for hemorrhoids. Suggest application of ice for 20 min every 4 hr, use of witch hazel compresses, and elevation of pelvis on pillow. (Refer to ND: Constipation, high risk for.)	Aids in regression of hemorrhoids and vulvar varicosities by promoting localized vasoconstriction; reduces discomfort and itching, enhancing return to normal bowel function.
Assess uterine tenderness; determine presence and frequency/intensity of afterpains. Note contributing factors.	During the first 12 hours postpartum, uterine contractions are strong and regular, and they continue for the next 2–3 days, although their frequency and intensity is reduced. Factors intensifying afterpains include multiparity, uterine overdistention, breastfeeding, and administration of ergot and oxytocin preparations.
Suggest client lie prone with pillow under abdomen, and that she engage in visualization techniques or diversional activities.	Promotes comfort, enhances sense of control, and refocuses attention.

ACTIONS/INTERVENTIONS	RATIONALE

Independent

Inspect breast and nipple tissue; assess for presence of engorgement and/or cracked nipples.

At 24 hours postpartum, breasts should be soft and nontender, and nipples should be free of cracks or reddened areas. Breast engorgement, nipple tenderness, or presence of cracks on nipple (if client is lactating) may occur 2 or 3 days postpartum.

Encourage wearing of supportive bra.

Lifts breasts inward and upward, resulting in a more comfortable position.

Provide information regarding increasing the frequency of feedings, applying heat to breasts before feedings, positioning the infant properly, and expressing milk manually.

These measures can help the lactating client stimulate the flow of milk and relieve stasis and engorgement. (Refer to ND: Breastfeeding [specify].)

Suggest client initiate feedings on nontender nipple for several feedings in succession if only one nipple is sore or cracked.

Initial suckling response is strong and may be painful. Starting feeding with unaffected breast and then proceeding to involved breast may be less painful and may enhance healing.

Apply ice to axillary area of breasts if the client is not planning to breastfeed. Provide tight compression with binder for 72 hr or use of well-fitting supportive bra. Avoid excess exposure of breasts to heat or stimulation of breasts by infant, sexual partner, or client until suppression process is completed (approximately 1 wk).

Binding and ice prevent lactation by mechanical means and are the preferred method for suppression of lactation. Discomfort lasts approximately 48–72 hr, but eases or ceases with avoidance of nipple stimulation.

Assess client for bladder fullness; implement measures to facilitate voiding. Instruct client in use of Kegel exercise after anesthesia wears off. (Refer to ND: Urinary Elimination, altered, high risk for.)

Return of normal bladder function may take 4–7 days, and overdistention of bladder may create feelings of urgency and discomfort. Kegel exercise aids in healing and recovery of tone of pubococcygeal muscle and prevents urinary stress incontinence.

Evaluate for headache, especially following subarachnoid anesthesia. Avoid medicating client before nature and cause of headache are determined. Note character of headache (e.g., deep location behind the eyes, with pain radiating to both temples and occipital area; relieved in supine position but increased in sitting or standing position) to distinguish from headache associated with anxiety or pregnancy-induced hypertension (PIH). Encourage bed rest, increase oral fluids, and notify physician or anesthesiologist, as indicated.

Leakage of cerebrospinal fluid (CSF) through the dura into the extradural space reduces volume needed to support brain tissue, causing the brain stem to fall onto the base of the skull when client is in an upright position. Fluids help stimulate production of CSF. PIH may result in cerebral edema, necessitating other interventions. (Refer to ND: Fluid Volume excess, high risk for.)

Collaborative

Administer bromocriptine mesylate (Parlodel) twice daily with meals for 2–3 wk. Assess client for hypotension; remain with client during first ambulation. Provide information about the possibility of rebound breast engorgement or congestion when use of medication is discontinued.

Acts to suppress secretion of prolactin, yet is a potent dopamine agonist receptor and can cause severe hypotension. Therefore, it should be initiated only after vital signs are stable and no sooner than 4 hours following delivery. Up to 40% of women experience problems of rebound congestion and engorgement.

ACTIONS/INTERVENTIONS

Collaborative

Administer analgesic 30–60 min prior to breast-feeding. For nonlactating client, administer analgesics every 3–4 hr for breast engorgement and afterpains.

Provide anesthetic sprays, topical ointments, and witch hazel compresses for perineum as appropriate.

Assist as needed with saline injection or administration of "blood patch" over site of dural puncture. Keep client in horizontal position following the procedure.

RATIONALE

Provides comfort, especially during lactation, when afterpains are most intense owing to the release of oxytocin. When client is free of discomfort, she can focus on care of herself and her infant, and on mastering mothering tasks.

Promotes localized comfort.

Effective for relief of severe spinal headache. The blood patch procedure has a 90%–100% success rate; creates a blood clot that produces pressure and seals the leak.

NURSING DIAGNOSIS:	**BREASTFEEDING (specify) [depending on whether mother-infant dyad exhibits satisfaction or dissatisfaction with breastfeeding experience]**
May be related to:	Level of knowledge, previous experiences, infant gestational age, level of support, physical structure/characteristics of the maternal breasts.
Possibly evidenced by:	Maternal verbalization regarding level of satisfaction, observations of breastfeeding process, infant response/weight gain.
DESIRED OUTCOMES— CLIENT WILL:	Verbalize understanding of breastfeeding process/situation.
	Demonstrate effective techniques for breastfeeding.
	Display mutually satisfactory breastfeeding regimen, with infant content after feedings.

ACTIONS/INTERVENTIONS

Independent

Assess client's knowledge and previous experience with breastfeeding.

Determine support systems available to client, and attitude of partner/family.

Provide information, verbal and written, regarding physiology and benefits of breastfeeding, nipple and breast care, special dietary needs, and factors that facilitate or interfere with successful breastfeeding.

RATIONALE

Helps in identifying current needs and developing plan of care.

Having sufficient support enhances opportunity for a successful breastfeeding experience. Negative attitudes and comments interfere with efforts and may cause client to abandon attempt to breastfeed.

Helps to ensure adequate milk supply, prevents nipple cracking and soreness, facilitates comfort, and establishes role of breastfeeding mother. Pamphlets and books provide resources that client can refer to as needed.

327

ACTIONS/INTERVENTIONS	RATIONALE

Independent

Demonstrate and review breastfeeding techniques. Note positioning of infant during feeding and length of feedings.

Proper positioning usually prevents sore nipples, regardless of the length of feedings.

Assess client's nipples; recommend that client inspect nipples after each feeding.

Early identification and intervention may prevent/limit development of nipple soreness or cracking, which could impair breastfeeding process.

Encourage client to air-dry nipples for 20–30 min after feedings and to apply lanolin preparation after feedings, or to use heat lamp with 40-watt bulb placed 18 inches from breast for 20 min. Instruct client to avoid the use of soaps or the use of plastic liners inside bra pads, and to change nursing pad when wet or moist.

Exposure to air or heat helps toughen nipples, whereas soaps may cause drying. Keeping nipples in a wet medium promotes bacterial growth and skin breakdown. (Note: Studies suggest applying a small amount of breast milk to the nipple area may be useful for treating cracked nipples by keeping the area soft and pliable.)

Instruct client to avoid use of nipple shield unless specifically indicated.

These have been found to contribute to lactation failures. Shields prevent the infant's mouth from coming into contact with the mother's nipple, which is necessary for continued release of prolactin (promoting milk production), and can interfere with or prevent establishment of adequate milk supply. (Note: Temporary use of shield may be beneficial in the presence of severe nipple cracking.)

Provide special nipple breast shields (e.g., Eschmann shields) for lactating client with flat, inverted nipples. Suggest application of ice prior to feedings and exercise of nipple by rolling between thumb and forefinger and using Hoffman technique.

Lacted cups/breast shields, exercises, and ice help make nipple more erect; Hoffman technique breaks adhesions, which cause inversion of nipple.

Collaborative

Refer client to support groups; e.g., La Leche League.

Provides ongoing help to promote a successful outcome.

Identify available community resources as indicated; e.g., Women, Infants, and Children (WIC) program.

WIC and other federal agencies support breastfeeding through client education and nutritional

---

NURSING DIAGNOSIS: **INJURY, HIGH RISK FOR**

Risk factors may include: Biochemical, regulatory function (e.g., orthostatic hypotension, development of PIH or eclampsia); effects of anesthesia; thromboembolism; abnormal blood profile (anemia, rubella sensitivity, Rh incompatibility).

Possibly evidenced by: [Not applicable; presence of signs/symptoms establishes an **actual** diagnosis.]

DESIRED OUTCOMES— CLIENT WILL: Demonstrate behaviors to reduce risk factors/protect self.

Be free of complications.

ACTIONS/INTERVENTIONS	RATIONALE

Independent

Review hemoglobin (Hb) level and blood loss at delivery. Note signs of anemia (e.g., fatigue, dizziness, pallor).

Anemia or excessive blood loss predisposes client to syncope or fainting spells, owing to inadequate delivery of oxygen to the brain.

Encourage early ambulation and exercise except in client who has received subarachnoid anesthesia, who may remain flat for 6–8 hr, without use of pillow or raising head, as indicated by protocol and return of sensation/muscle control. (Refer to ND: Pain [acute]/Discomfort.)

Enhances circulation and venous return of lower extremities, reducing risk of thrombus formation, which is associated with stasis. Although recumbent position after subarachnoid anesthesia is controversial, it may aid in prevention of CSF leakage and resultant headache.

Assist client with initial ambulation. Provide adequate supervision in shower or sitz bath. Leave call bell within client's reach.

Orthostatic hypotension may occur when changing from supine to upright position on initial ambulation, or it may result from vasodilation caused by the heat of the shower or sitz bath.

Have client sit on floor or chair with head between legs, or have her lie down in a flat position, if she feels faint. Use ammonia capsule (smelling salts).

Helps maintain or enhances circulation and delivery of oxygen to brain.

Assess client for hyperreflexia, right upper quadrant (RUQ) pain, headache, or visual disturbances. Maintain seizure precautions, and provide quiet environment as indicated. (Refer to ND: Fluid Volume excess, high risk for; Chapter 4, CP: Pregnancy-Induced Hypertension, ND: Injury, high risk for, maternal.)

Danger of eclampsia due to PIH exists for up to 72 hours postpartum, although literature suggests the convulsive state has occurred as late as the fifth day postpartum.

Note effects of magnesium sulfate (MgSO$_4$), if administered. Assess patellar response, and monitor respiratory rate.

Absence of patellar reflex and respiratory rate below 12/min indicate toxicity and a need to reduce or discontinue drug therapy.

Inspect lower extremities for signs of thrombophlebitis (e.g., redness, warmth, pain/tenderness). Note presence or absence of Homans' sign. (Refer to CP: Postpartal Thrombophlebitis.)

Elevated fibrin split products (possibly released from placental site), reduced mobility, trauma, sepsis, and extensive activation of blood clotting following delivery predispose the client to the development of thromboembolism. Homans' sign may be present with deep venous thrombus, but may be absent with superficial phlebitis.

Apply local heat; promote bedrest with affected limb elevated.

Stimulates circulation and decreases venous pooling in lower extremities, reducing edema and promoting healing.

Evaluate rubella status on prenatal chart (less than 1:10 titer indicates susceptibility). Assess client for allergies to eggs or feathers; if present, withhold vaccine. Provide written and oral information, and obtain informed consent for vaccination after reviewing side effects, risks, and the necessity to prevent conception for 2–3 mo following the vaccination.

Helps prevent teratogenic effects in subsequent pregnancies. Administration of vaccine in the immediate postpartal period may cause side effects of transient arthralgia, rash, and cold symptoms during incubation period of 14–21 days. Allergic anaphylactic or hypersensitivity response may occur, necessitating administration of epinephrine.

Collaborative

Administer MgSO$_4$ by infusion pump, as indicated.

Helps reduce cerebral irritability in presence of PIH or eclampsia. (Refer to ND: Fluid Volume excess, high risk for.)

ACTIONS/INTERVENTIONS

Collaborative

Apply support hose or elastic wrap to legs when risk or symptoms of phlebitis are present.

Administer anticoagulant; evaluate coagulation factors, and note signs of failure to clot. (Refer to CP: Postpartal Thrombophlebitis.)

Administer $Rh_o(D)$ immune globulin (RhIgG) I.M. within 72 hours postpartum, as indicated, for Rh-negative mother who has not been previously sensitized and who delivers an Rh-positive infant whose direct Coombs' test on cord blood is negative. Obtain Betke-Kleihauer smear if significant fetal-maternal transfusion is suspected at delivery.

RATIONALE

Reduces venous stasis, enhancing venous return.

Although usually not required, anticoagulant may help prevent further development of thrombus.

Dose of 300 μg is usually sufficient to promote lysis of fetal Rh-positive red blood cells (RBCs) that may have entered maternal circulation during delivery, and that may potentially cause sensitization and problems of Rh incompatibility in subsequent pregnancies. Presence of 20 ml or more of Rh-positive fetal blood in maternal circulation necessitates higher dose of RhIgG.

NURSING DIAGNOSIS:	INFECTION, HIGH RISK FOR
Risk factors may include:	Tissue trauma and/or broken skin, decreased Hb, invasive procedures and/or increased environmental exposure, prolonged rupture of amniotic membranes, malnutrition.
Possibly evidenced by:	[Not applicable; presence of signs/symptoms establishes an **actual** diagnosis.]
DESIRED OUTCOMES— CLIENT WILL:	Demonstrate techniques to reduce risks/promote healing.
	Display wound free of purulent drainage.
	Be free of infection, be afebrile, and have normal lochial flow and character.

ACTIONS/INTERVENTIONS

Independent

Assess prenatal and intrapartal records, noting frequency of vaginal examinations and complications such as premature rupture of membranes (PROM), prolonged labor, lacerations, hemorrhage, or retained placenta.

Monitor temperature and pulse routinely and as indicated; note signs of chills, anorexia, or malaise.

Assess location and contractility of uterus; note involutional changes or presence of extreme uterine tenderness.

RATIONALE

Helps identify risk factors that may impair healing and/or retard epithelial growth of endometrial tissue and predispose client to infection.

Elevation of temperature to 101° F (38.3°C) within the first 24 hours is highly indicative of infection; an elevation to 100.4° F (38.0°C) on any 2 of the first 10 days postpartum is significant.

The fundus, which is initially 2 cm below the umbilicus, rises to the level of the umbilicus and involutes at the rate of 1–2 cm/day (one fingerbreadth per day). Failure of the myometrium to involute at this rate, or development of extreme tenderness, signals possible retained placental tissue or infection. (Note: Size of the uterus is influenced by the size of the infant just delivered.) (Refer to CP: Puerperal Infection.)

ACTIONS/INTERVENTIONS	RATIONALE

Independent

Note amount and odor of lochial discharge or change in normal progression from rubra to serosa.

Lochia normally has a fleshy odor; however, in endometritis the discharge may be purulent and foul-smelling, and may fail to demonstrate normal progression from rubra to serosa to alba.

Evaluate condition of nipples, noting presence of cracks, redness, or tenderness. Recommend routine examination of breasts. Review proper care and infant feeding techniques. (Refer to ND: Pain [acute]/Discomfort.)

The development of nipple fissures/cracks potentiates risk of mastitis.

Inspect site of episiotomy repair every 8 hr. Note excessive tenderness, redness, purulent exudate, edema, gapping at suture line (loss of approximation), or presence of lacerations.

Early diagnosis of localized infection may prevent spread to uterine tissue. (Note: Presence of third- to fourth-degree lacerations increases risk of infection.)

Note frequency/amount of voidings.

Urinary stasis increases the risk of infection.

Assess for signs of urinary tract infection (UTI) or cystitis (e.g., increased frequency, urgency, or dysuria). Note color and appearance of urine, visible hematuria, and presence of suprapubic pain.

Symptoms of UTI may appear on day 2 to 3 postpartum owing to ascending tract infection from urethra to bladder and possibly to kidney.

Encourage perineal care using perineal bottle or sitz bath 3 to 4 times daily or after voiding/defecation. Recommend that client shower daily and change perineal pads at least every 4 hr, applying them from front to back.

Frequent cleaning from front to back (symphysis pubis to anal area) helps prevent rectal contaminants from entering vagina or urethra. Sitz or tub baths stimulate perineal circulation and promote healing.

Encourage and use careful handwashing technique and appropriate disposal of soiled underpads, perineal pads, and contaminated linen. Discuss with client the importance of continuing these measures after discharge.

Helps prevent or retard spread of infection.

Assess client's nutritional status. Note appearance of hair, fingernails, skin, and so forth. Note prepregnancy weight and prenatal weight gain.

Client who is 20% below normal weight, or who is anemic or malnourished, is more susceptible to postpartal infection and may have special dietary needs for protein, iron, and calories.

Provide information about selecting foods high in protein, vitamin C, and iron. Encourage client to increase fluid intake to 2000 ml/day.

Protein helps promote healing and regeneration of new tissue and overcomes delivery losses. Iron is necessary for hemoglobin synthesis. Vitamin C facilitates iron absorption and is necessary for cell wall synthesis. Increased fluid helps prevent urinary stasis and kidney problems.

Promote sleep and rest.

Reduces metabolic rate and allows nutrition and oxygen to be used for healing process rather than for energy needs.

Collaborative

Assess white blood cell (WBC) count.

An increase in WBC count the first 10 to 12 days postpartum normally occurs as a protective mechanism and is associated with an increase in neutrophils and a shift to the left, which may interfere initially with identification of infection.

ACTIONS/INTERVENTIONS	RATIONALE

Independent

Note Hb and Hct. Administer iron preparations and vitamins, as necessary.

Determines whether anemic state is present. Helps correct deficiencies.

Administer methylergonovine maleate (Methergine) or ergonovine maleate (Ergotrate) every 3 to 4 hr, as appropriate.

Fosters myometrial contraction and uterine involution, reducing risk of infection.

Assist with or obtain cultures from vagina, serum, and site of episiotomy repair as indicated.

To identify causative organism, if present, and determine appropriate antibiotic.

Encourage client to apply antibiotic creams to perineum, as indicated.

Eradicates local infectious organisms.

Obtain clean catch (midstream) urine specimen for routine analysis.

Urine retention, bacteria introduced by catheterization, and/or bladder trauma during delivery combine to create an excellent environment for bacterial growth. Bacterial concentrations of 100,000 microorganisms per 100 ml of fresh urine usually indicate an infection.

Administer antipyretic after cultures are obtained.

When administered before identification of infectious process, antipyretics may mask signs and symptoms necessary for a differential diagnosis.

Administer broad-spectrum antibiotic until culture/sensitivity report is returned, then alter therapy as indicated. (Note: Parenteral route via heparin lock is preferred for treatment of endometritis and sepsis.)

Prevents infection from spreading to surrounding tissues or bloodstream. Choice of antibiotic depends on sensitivity of infecting organism.

Contact appropriate community agencies, such as visiting nurse services, for follow-up on diet, antibiotic course, possible complications, and return medical examination.

Any postpartal infection places the client in a debilitated state that requires more rest, closer monitoring, and assistance with home maintenance and self-care.

NURSING DIAGNOSIS:	URINARY ELIMINATION, ALTERED
May be related to:	Hormonal effects (fluid shifts/increased renal plasma flow), mechanical trauma, tissue edema, effects of anesthesia.
Possibly evidenced by:	Increased bladder filling/distention, changes in amount/frequency of voiding.
DESIRED OUTCOMES— CLIENT WILL:	Void unassisted within 6–8 hr after delivery. Empty bladder with each void.

ACTIONS/INTERVENTIONS	RATIONALE

Independent

Assess current fluid intake and urine output. Note intrapartal fluid intake and urine output and length of labor.

In the early postpartal period, approximately 9 lb of fluid is lost through urine output and insensible losses, including diaphoresis. Prolonged labor and ineffective fluid replacement may result in dehydration and reduced urine output.

ACTIONS/INTERVENTIONS	RATIONALE
Independent	
Palpate bladder. Monitor fundal height and location, and amount of lochial flow.	Renal plasma flow, which increases by 25%–50% during the prenatal period, remains elevated in the first week postpartum, resulting in increased bladder filling. Bladder distention, which can be assessed by degree of uterine displacement, causes increased uterine relaxation and lochial flow.
Note presence of edema or lacerations/episiotomy, and type of anesthesia used.	Trauma to bladder or urethra, or edema, may hinder voiding; anesthesia may interfere with sensation of fullness.
Test urine for albumin and acetone. Distinguish between proteinuria associated with PIH and that associated with normal processes. (Refer to ND: Fluid Volume excess, high risk for.)	Catalytic process associated with uterine involution may result in normal proteinuria (+1) for the first 2 days postpartum. Acetone may indicate dehydration associated with prolonged labor and/or delivery.
Encourage voiding within 6–8 hr postpartum, and every 4 hr thereafter. If condition permits, have client walk to bathroom. Pour warm water over the perineum, run water from the faucet, add spirits of peppermint to bedpan, or have client sit in sitz bath or take a warm shower, as indicated.	A variety of nursing interventions may be necessary to stimulate or facilitate voiding. A full bladder interferes with uterine motility and involution, and increases lochial flow. Prolonged bladder overdistention can damage the bladder wall and result in atony.
Instruct client to use Kegel exercise daily after effects of anesthesia subside.	Performing Kegel exercise 100 times per day increases circulation to perineum, aids in healing and recovery of tone of pubococcygeal muscle, and prevents or reduces stress incontinence.
Encourage drinking 6 to 8 glasses of fluid per day.	Helps prevent stasis and dehydration, and replaces fluid lost at delivery.
Assess for signs of UTI (e.g., burning on urination, increased frequency, cloudy urine).	Stasis, poor hygiene, and introduction of bacteria may predispose client to UTI. (Refer to ND: Infection, high risk for.)
Collaborative	
Catheterize, using straight or indwelling catheter, as indicated.	May be necessary to reduce bladder distention, allow for uterine involution, and prevent bladder atony associated with bladder overdistention.
Obtain urine specimen, using clean catch technique or catheterization, if client has symptoms of UTI.	Presence of bacteria or positive culture and sensitivity are diagnostic for UTI.
Monitor laboratory test results, such as blood urea nitrogen (BUN) and 24-hour urine for total protein, creatinine clearance, and uric acid as indicated.	In the client who has had PIH, kidney or vascular involvement may persist, or it may appear for the first time during the postpartal period. As steroid levels decrease following delivery, renal function, reflected by BUN and creatinine clearance, begins to return to normal within 1 week; anatomic changes (e.g., dilation of ureters and renal pelvis) may take up to 1 month to return to normal.

NURSING DIAGNOSIS:	FLUID VOLUME DEFICIT, HIGH RISK FOR
Risk factors may include:	Reduced intake/inadequate replacement, excessive losses (vomiting, diaphoresis, increased urine output and insensible losses, hemorrhage).
Possibly evidenced by:	[Not applicable; presence of signs/symptoms establishes an **actual** diagnosis.]
DESIRED OUTCOMES— CLIENT WILL:	Remain normotensive with fluid intake and urine output appropriately balanced, and Hb/Hct within normal levels.

ACTIONS/INTERVENTIONS	RATIONALE

(Refer to CP: Stage IV [First 4 Hours Following Delivery of Placenta].)

Independent

Note fluid losses at delivery; review intrapartal history. (Refer to CP: Postpartal Hemorrhage.)	Potential hemorrhage or excess blood loss at delivery that continues into the postpartal period may result from prolonged labor, oxytocin stimulation, retained tissue, uterine overdistention, or general anesthesia.
Evaluate location and contractility of uterine fundus, amount of vaginal lochia, and condition of perineum every 2 hr for the first 8 hr, as appropriate, then every 8 hr for the remainder of hospitalization. Note administration of medication, such as MgSO$_4$, that would cause uterine relaxation.	Differential diagnosis may be needed to determine cause of fluid deficit and protocol of care. A relaxed or boggy uterus with increased lochial flow may result from myometrial fatigue or retained placental tissue. Immediately after delivery the fundus should be firm and located at the umbilicus, and then involute approximately one fingerbreadth per day.
Gently massage fundus if uterus is boggy.	Stimulates uterine contraction; may control bleeding.
Note presence of thirst; provide liquids as tolerated.	Thirst may be a homeostatic means of replacing fluid losses through increased oral intake.
Evaluate status of bladder; promote emptying if bladder is full. (Refer to ND: Urinary Elimination, altered.)	A full bladder interferes with uterine contractility and causes displacement and relaxation of fundus.
Monitor temperature.	Increased temperature may signify dehydration; if it is 100.4°F (38°C) in the first 24 hours following delivery and recurs for 2 days, it may indicate infection. (Refer to CP: Puerperal Infection.)
Monitor pulse.	Tachycardia may occur, maximizing fluid circulation, in the event of dehydration or hemorrhage.
Assess blood pressure (BP), as indicated.	Elevated BP may be due to the effects of oxytocin vasopressor drugs, or to preexisting or newly developed PIH. Falling BP may be a late sign of excess fluid loss, especially if accompanied by other signs or symptoms of shock.

ACTIONS/INTERVENTIONS	RATIONALE

Independent

Evaluate fluid intake and urine output during I.V. infusion, or until normal voiding patterns are reestablished.

Helps in analyzing fluid balance and degree of deficit.

Evaluate Hb/Hct levels on prenatal records; compare with postpartal levels.

Hb/Hct usually return to normal within 3 days. Hb should not drop more than 2 g/100 ml unless blood loss is excessive. Elevation of Hct levels occurs normally by the third to seventh day postpartum, owing to plasma loss in excess of blood cell decreases that occurs during the first 72 hours. However such elevation may also indicate excess shift of intravascular fluids to extracellular spaces.

Monitor filling of breasts and milk supply if lactating.

The dehydrated client is unable to produce sufficient milk supply.

Collaborative

Replace fluid losses with I.V. infusion containing electrolytes.

Helps reestablish circulating blood volume and replace losses from delivery and diaphoresis.

Administer ergot products such as ergonovine maleate (Ergotrate) or methylergonovine maleate (Methergine) parenterally or orally, or administer I.M./I.V. synthetic oxytocin preparations (Syntocinon, Pitocin). Assess BP before administering ergot preparations; withhold medication and notify physician if BP is elevated.

These products act directly on the myometrium to promote uterine contraction. Ergot, a vasoconstrictor, may cause hypertension and should be withheld if BP is 140/90 mm Hg or greater.

Initiate or increase rate of I.V. fluid such as lactated Ringer's solution with 10 to 20 units oxytocin.

Oxytocin (Pitocin) may be needed to stimulate the myometrium if excess bleeding persists and uterus fails to contract. Persistent bleeding in presence of firm fundus may indicate lacerations and the need for further investigation. (Refer to CP: Postpartal Hemorrhage.)

NURSING DIAGNOSIS: **FLUID VOLUME EXCESS, HIGH RISK FOR**

Risk factors may include: Fluid shifts following placental delivery, inappropriate fluid replacement, effects of oxytocin infusion, presence of PIH.

Possibly evidenced by: [Not applicable; presence of signs/symptoms establishes an **actual** diagnosis.]

DESIRED OUTCOMES— CLIENT WILL: Display BP and pulse within normal limits, be free of edema and visual disturbances, with clear breath sounds.

ACTIONS/INTERVENTIONS	RATIONALE

Independent

Review prenatal and intrapartal history for PIH, noting elevated BP, proteinuria, and edema.

Helps determine likelihood of similar complications persisting/developing in postpartal period.

ACTIONS/INTERVENTIONS	RATIONALE

Independent

Monitor BP and pulse. Auscultate breath sounds, noting moist cough, rales, or rhonchi. Note presence of dyspnea or stridor.

Circulatory overload is manifested by increases in BP and pulse, and by fluid accumulation in the lungs. Elevated BP may also be related to PIH and fluid retention associated with oxytocin infusion.

Monitor fluid intake and urine output; measure specific gravity.

Indicates fluid needs/adequacy of therapy.

Note dosage of oxytocin (Pitocin) when it is administered parenterally.

Oxytocin increases sodium/water resorption from the kidney tubules and may result in elevated BP.

Assess presence, location, and extent of edema. Monitor for signs of progressive edema (e.g., visual disturbances, hyperreflexia, clonus, RUQ pain, and headache). (Note: Assess for headache prior to administering any analgesics.)

Danger of eclampsia or convulsive state exists for 72 hours, but can actually occur as late as 5 days after delivery. Medication may mask signs of headache caused by cerebral edema.

Test for presence of proteinuria by dipstick every 4 hr.

Postpartal proteinuria of 1+ is normal, owing to catalytic process of uterine involution. Levels of 2+ or greater may be associated with glomerular spasms of PIH.

Evaluate client's neurologic status. Note hyperreflexia, irritability, or personality changes.

Cerebral intoxication is an early indicator of excess fluid retention.

Have client monitor weight daily, especially if postpartal toxemia is present.

Client should lose up to 12 lb at delivery attributable to infant, products of conception, urine, and insensible losses, and 5 lb more in the postpartal period through fluid and electrolyte shifts.

Collaborative

Note test results for uric acid, 24-hour protein and creatinine clearance, and serum creatinine levels.

Abnormal results, such as increasing uric acid (greater than 7 mg/100 ml) and elevated creatinine levels, indicate deterioration of renal function.

Insert indwelling catheter, as indicated.

May be needed to monitor urine output on hourly basis if warranted by client's condition (e.g., severe PIH or oliguria).

Evaluate for HELLP syndrome (hemolysis of RBCs, elevated liver enzyme levels, and low platelet count).

HELLP syndrome is a potential postpartal consequence of PIH with liver involvement or with hemorrhage of hepatic vessels.

Administer $MgSO_4$ per infusion pump when indicated. (Refer to Chapter 4, CP: Pregnancy-Induced Hypertension, ND: Injury, high risk for, maternal.)

$MgSO_4$ acts at myoneural junction and may have transient effects of lowering BP and increasing urine output.

Administer antihypertensives such as hydralazine (Apresoline) or methyldopa (Aldomet) per protocol (e.g., if diastolic readings are 110 mm Hg or greater).

Hydralazine relaxes peripheral arterioles and promotes vasodilation; methyldopa acts on postganglionic nerve endings and interferes with chemical neurotransmission, reducing peripheral vascular resistance.

Administer furosemide (Lasix) as indicated.

Furosemide acts on loop of Henle to increase urine output and relieve pulmonary edema.

336

ACTIONS/INTERVENTIONS

Collaborative

Administer mannitol in presence of PIH with decreased urine output.

RATIONALE

For client with PIH, impending renal failure, or oliguria, mannitol acts as osmotic diuretic to draw fluids into vascular bed and increase renal plasma flow and urine output.

NURSING DIAGNOSIS:	CONSTIPATION
May be related to:	Decreased muscle tone (diastasis recti), effects of progesterone, dehydration, excess analgesia or anesthesia, prelabor diarrhea, lack of intake, perineal/rectal pain.
Possibly evidenced by:	Reported abdominal/rectal fullness or pressure, nausea, less than usual amount of stool, straining at stool, decreased bowel sounds.
DESIRED OUTCOMES— CLIENT WILL:	Resume usual/optimal bowel habits within 4 days after delivery.

ACTIONS/INTERVENTIONS

Independent

Auscultate for presence of bowel sounds; note normal evacuation habits or diastasis recti.

Assess for presence of hemorrhoids. Provide information about reinserting hemorrhoid into anorectal canal with lubricated finger cot or rubber glove, and applying ice or witch hazel compresses or local anesthetic creams.

Provide appropriate dietary information about importance of roughage, increased fluids, and the attempt to establish normal evacuation pattern.

Encourage increase in activity level and ambulation, as tolerated.

Assess episiotomy; note presence of laceration and degree of tissue involvement.

Collaborative

Administer laxatives, stool softeners, suppositories, or enemas.

RATIONALE

Evaluates bowel function. Presence of severe diastasis recti (separation of the two rectus muscles along the median line of the abdominal wall) reduces abdominal muscle tone needed for efforts to bear down during evacuation.

Reduces size of hemorrhoid, relieves itching and discomfort, and promotes localized vasoconstriction.

Roughage (e.g., fruits and vegetables, especially with seeds and skins) and increased fluids provide bulk and stimulate elimination.

Helps promote gastrointestinal peristalsis.

Excess edema or perineal trauma with third- and fourth-degree lacerations may cause discomfort and prevent client from relaxing perineum during evacuation for fear of further injury.

May be necessary to promote return to normal bowel habits and to prevent straining or perineal stress during evacuation. (Note: Administration of suppositories or enemas in presence of third- or fourth-degree perineal laceration may be contraindicated because further trauma may occur).

NURSING DIAGNOSIS:	PARENTING, ALTERED, HIGH RISK FOR
Risk factors may include:	Lack of support between/from significant other(s), lack of knowledge, ineffective and/or no available role model, unrealistic expectations for self/infant/partner, unmet social/emotional maturation needs of client/partner, presence of stressor (e.g., financial, housing, employment).
Possibly evidenced by:	[Not applicable; presence of signs/symptoms establishes an **actual** diagnosis.]
DESIRED OUTCOMES— CLIENT WILL:	Verbalize concerns and questions about parenting.
	Discuss parenting role realistically.
	Begin to actively engage in newborn care tasks as appropriate.
	Identify available resources.

ACTIONS/INTERVENTIONS	RATIONALE

Independent

ACTIONS/INTERVENTIONS	RATIONALE
Assess strengths, weaknesses, age, marital status, available sources of support, and cultural background.	Identifies potential risk factors and sources of support, which influence the client's/couple's ability to take on the challenging role of parenthood. For example, the adolescent may still be formulating goals and an identity. She may have difficulty accepting the infant as a person and coping with full-time parenting responsibility. The single parent who lacks support systems may have difficulty assuming sole responsibility for parenting. Cultures in which the extended family live together may provide more emotional and physical support, facilitating adoption of the new role.
Note client's/partner's response to birth and to parenting role.	Client's ability to adapt positively to parenting may be strongly influenced by the father's reaction.
Initiate primary nursing care for mother and baby as a unit.	Promotes family-centered care, continuity and individualization of care, and may facilitate development of positive family bonds.
Evaluate nature of emotional and physical parenting that client/couple received during childhood.	Parenting role is learned, and individuals use their own parents as role models. Those who experienced a negative upbringing or poor parenting are at greater risk for failing to meet the challenge than those who received positive parenting.
Assess partners' interpersonal communication skills and their relationship to one another.	A strong relationship characterized by honest communication and good interpersonal and listening skills fosters growth.
Review intrapartal record for length of labor, presence of complications, and role of partner in labor.	Long, difficult labor may temporarily deplete the physical and emotional energy necessary for learning the mothering role and may negatively affect lactation. (Note: It often takes 24 hr following delivery for the mother to leave her own "taking in" phase.)

ACTIONS/INTERVENTIONS	RATIONALE

Independent

Evaluate past and present physical status and occurrence of prenatal, intrapartal, or postpartal complications.

Events such as preterm labor, hemorrhage, infection, or any maternal complication may influence client's psychologic status, reducing her ability to learn new parenting skills and undermining her attachment to the newborn.

Evaluate infant's condition; communicate with nursery staff as indicated. Note any special problems or concerns.

Mothers often undergo grief for the loss of the idealized perfect infant in contrast with their own infant. Emotional problems and the inability to adjust positively to parenting may result from the infant's temporary birth disfigurement, the birth of a high-risk infant, or the mother's inability to reconcile differences between prenatal fantasies and postnatal reality.

Administer the Neonatal Perception Inventory (NPI), Part I, within the first 2 days postpartum. Arrange for the follow-up inventory, Part II, to be administered at 1 month postpartum.

The NPI assesses adaptive potential of mother-infant pair by evaluating the mother's perceptions of average baby versus her own. This tool is particularly helpful in assessing the mothering potential of the adolescent, who often fantasizes about the infant's behaviors and capabilities, and who may not cope positively with stressor of caring for a newborn. This inventory provides a statistically significant relationship between its indications at 1 month and the emotional development of children at age $4\frac{1}{2}$ years and later at age 10 to 11 years.

Monitor and document the client's/couple's interactions with infant. Note presence of bonding (acquaintance) behaviors: making eye contact, using high-pitched voice and en face (face to face) position, calling infant by name, and holding infant closely. Determine family cultural background.

Few mothers or fathers experience significant love at first; instead, they become acquainted with the infant gradually. Infant and parent who do not develop positive attachment are at risk for physical or emotional abuse. Cultural background often determines type of bonding and acquaintance behaviors.

Provide "rooming-in" or physical space and privacy for contact between mother, father, and infant.

Facilitates attachment behaviors; fosters acquaintance process.

Encourage couple/siblings to visit and hold the infant and to participate in infant care activities as permitted. If baby remains in the hospital for observation or procedures, provide telephone number of special care nursery; take pictures of the infant for the couple.

Helps promote bonding and prevent feelings of helplessness. Emphasizes the reality of baby's existence.

Assess client's readiness and motivation to learn.

Many factors influence individual learning (e.g., understanding of need for information, anxiety, postdelivery euphoria).

Provide formal and informal educational opportunities followed by staff demonstration, staff assistance, and educational videotapes on infant care, infant feeding, and parenting.

Helps parents learn the fundamentals of infant care, promotes discussion and mutual problem-solving, and provides group support. Helps parents to become more comfortable and gain skills and comfort in handling and caring for infant prior to discharge.

ACTIONS/INTERVENTIONS

Independent

Have client demonstrate learned behaviors associated with infant feeding and care. Provide written information and telephone number of contact person for client to take home.

Initiate follow-up telephone call or home visit by primary nurse, if possible, at 1 week, and at 4 to 6 weeks postpartum.

Collaborative

Refer to community support groups, such as visiting nurse services, social services, parenting groups, or adolescent clinics.

Refer for counseling if family is at high risk for parenting problems or if positive bonding between client/couple and infant is not occurring.

RATIONALE

Helps reinforce teaching program and prevent anxiety related to unanswered questions, especially if family is part of early discharge program or if delivery took place in an alternative birth center.

Some maternity centers now include such follow-up, especially for the adolescent or for the family at high risk for parenting problems.

Helps promote positive parenting through group support and mutual problem-solving experience. Adolescents, particularly, may benefit from such support.

Negative parenting behaviors and ineffective coping may need to be corrected through counseling, nurturing, or even lengthy psychotherapy, and new behaviors and role models incorporated, to avoid repetition of parenting mistakes and child abuse.

NURSING DIAGNOSIS:	COPING, INDIVIDUAL, INEFFECTIVE, HIGH RISK FOR
Risk factors may include:	Maturational crisis of pregnancy/childbearing and assuming the role of motherhood and parenting (or relinquishing for adoption), personal vulnerability, inadequate support systems, unrealistic perceptions.
Possibly evidenced by:	[Not applicable; presence of signs/symptoms establishes an **actual** diagnosis.]
DESIRED OUTCOMES— CLIENT WILL:	Verbalize anxieties and emotional responses.
	Identify individual strengths and own coping abilities.
	Seek appropriate resources as needed.

ACTIONS/INTERVENTIONS

Independent

Assess client's emotional response during prenatal and intrapartal periods and client's perception of her performance during labor. (Refer to Chapter 4, CP: First Trimester, ND: Role Performance, altered, high risk for.)

Encourage discussion by client/couple of perceptions of birth experience.

RATIONALE

There is a direct correlation between positive acceptance of the feminine role and uniquely feminine functions and positive adaptation to childbirth, mothering, and lactation. Additionally, the client who is relinquishing her child encounters these issues in a different context and needs support for her decisions.

Assists client/couple to work through process and clarify reality from fantasized experience.

ACTIONS/INTERVENTIONS	RATIONALE

Independent

Assess for symptoms of transitory depression (postpartal "blues") at 2 to 3 days postpartum (e.g., anxiety, tearfulness, despondency, poor concentration, and mild or severe depression). Provide information about the normalcy of this condition and associated mood swings and emotional lability.

As many as 80% of mothers experience a transitory depression or a feeling of emotional letdown following delivery, perhaps related to genetics, social or environmental factors, or physiologic endocrine responses. These symptoms usually resolve spontaneously within a week or so following discharge. For some, however, initial feelings of discouragement may be replaced by excessive depression caused by a cycle of anxiety, anorexia, and excessive fatigue beginning soon after discharge.

Evaluate client's past coping abilities, cultural background, support systems, and plans for domestic help on discharge.

Helps in assessing client's ability to handle stress. The ability to cope positively is also influenced by father's reaction. The emotional and physical support offered by extended families or other home assistance may facilitate coping.

Provide emotional support and anticipatory guidance to help client learn new roles and strategies for coping with newborn. Discuss the normal emotional responses that occur after discharge.

Mothering/parenting skills are not instinctive but must be learned. Coping with interrupted sleep and meeting the infant's needs on a 24-hour basis may be difficult, and coping strategies must be developed.

Evaluate and document client-infant interaction. Note presence or absence of bonding (attachment) behaviors. (Refer to ND: Parenting, altered, high risk for.)

Mother and infant are equal participants in the attachment process, and both must receive rewarding responses during the interaction. A lack of maternal attachment or absence of maternal behaviors evident in the postpartal period can lead to serious long-term consequences.

Encourage verbalization of feelings of guilt, personal failure, or doubt about individual parenting abilities, especially if family is at high risk for problems with parenting. (Refer to CP: The Parents of a Child with Special Needs.)

Helps couple to evaluate strengths and problem areas realistically and recognize the need for appropriate professional help.

Provide opportunity for client to review decision to relinquish child.

Following delivery, the normal emotional responses are compounded by the previous decision to have child adopted. The client may experience conflict and requires nonjudgmental support to facilitate coping at this time.

Collaborative

Refer client/couple to parenting support group, social service, community groups, or visiting nurse services.

Approximately 40% of women with mild postpartal depression have symptoms that persist for up to 1 year and that may require further follow-up.

Refer client/couple to psychiatric counselor, if appropriate.

From 1%–2% of clients suffer severe postpartal depression necessitating hospitalization for psychoses such as affective disorders (e.g., depression or depression with manic episode) and schizophrenia.

Administer diazepam (Valium), promethazine hydrochloride (Phenergan), or lithium carbonate, as indicated.

Severe/prolonged difficulties may require additional intervention. Selection of drug therapy depends on whether short- or long-term control is needed.

<table>
<tr><td>NURSING DIAGNOSIS:</td><td>SLEEP PATTERN DISTURBANCE</td></tr>
<tr><td>May be related to:</td><td>Hormonal and psychologic responses (intense exhilaration, anxiety, excitement), pain/discomfort, exhausting process of labor and delivery.</td></tr>
<tr><td>Possibly evidenced by:</td><td>Verbal reports of difficulty falling asleep/not feeling well rested, irritability, dark circles under eyes, frequent yawning.</td></tr>
<tr><td>DESIRED OUTCOMES— CLIENT WILL:</td><td>Identify adjustments to accommodate changes required by demands of new family member.

Report increased sense of well-being and feeling rested.</td></tr>
</table>

ACTIONS/INTERVENTIONS	RATIONALE
Independent	
Assess level of fatigue and need for rest. Note length of labor and type of delivery.	Long, difficult labor or delivery, especially when it occurs during the night, increases the level of fatigue.
Assess factors, if any, interfering with rest. Organize care to allow minimum disturbances and extra resting or sleeping periods. Encourage verbalization about birth experience. Provide quiet environment.	Helps promote rest, sleep, and relaxation and reduces stimuli. If mother does not get needed sleep, "sleep hunger" may result, prolonging the restorative processes of the postpartal period.
Provide information about needs for sleep/rest following discharge.	Creative planning to allow retiring early with the baby and napping during the day helps meet bodily needs and overcome excess fatigue.
Provide information about effects of fatigue and anxiety on milk supply.	Fatigue may negatively affect psychologic adjustment, milk supply, and let-down reflex.
Assess home environment, home assistance, and presence of siblings and other family members.	The multipara with children at home may need more sleep in the hospital to overcome sleep deficits and meet her needs and the needs of her family.
Collaborative	
Administer medications (e.g., analgesics).	May be needed to promote needed relaxation and sleep.

<table>
<tr><td>NURSING DIAGNOSIS:</td><td>KNOWLEDGE DEFICIT [LEARNING NEED], regarding self-care and infant care</td></tr>
<tr><td>May be related to:</td><td>Lack of exposure/recall, misinterpretation, unfamiliarity with resources.</td></tr>
<tr><td>Possibly evidenced by:</td><td>Verbalizations of concerns/misconceptions, hesitancy in or inadequate performance of activities, inappropriate behaviors (e.g., apathy).</td></tr>
<tr><td>DESIRED OUTCOMES— CLIENT WILL:</td><td>Verbalize understanding of physiologic changes, individual needs, expected outcomes.

Perform necessary activities/procedures correctly and explain reasons for the actions.</td></tr>
</table>

ACTIONS/INTERVENTIONS	RATIONALE
Independent	
Ascertain client's perception of labor and delivery, length of labor, and client's fatigue level.	There is a correlation between length of labor and the ability to assume responsibility for self-care/infant care tasks and activities. The longer the labor is, the more negative the client's perception of her performance in labor, and the longer it may take her to assume responsibility for her own care and to synthesize new information and learn new roles.
Assess client's readiness and motivation for learning. Assist client/couple in identifying needs.	The postpartal period can be a positive experience if opportune teaching is provided to foster maternal growth, maturation, and competence. However, the client needs time to move from a "taking in" to a "taking hold" phase, in which her receptiveness and readiness is heightened and she is emotionally and physically ready for learning new information to facilitate mastery of her new role.
Initiate written teaching plan using standardized format or checklist. Document information given and client's response.	Helps standardize the information parents receive from staff members, and reduces client confusion caused by dissemination of conflicting advice or information.
Provide information about role of a progressive postpartal exercise program.	Exercise helps tone musculature, increases circulation, produces a trimmer figure, and enhances feelings of general well-being.
Provide information about self-care, including perineal care and hygiene; physiologic changes, including normal progression of lochial discharge; needs for sleep and rest; role changes; and emotional changes. Have client demonstrate the material learned, when appropriate.	Helps prevent infection, fosters healing and recuperation, and contributes to positive adaptation to physical and emotional changes.
Discuss sexuality needs and plans for contraception. Provide information about available methods, including advantages and disadvantages. (Refer to CP: Maternal Assessment: 1 Week Following Discharge, ND: Knowledge Deficit [Learning Need].)	Couple may need clarification regarding available contraceptive methods and the fact that pregnancy could occur even prior to the 6-week visit.
Reinforce importance of 6-week postpartal examination with healthcare provider.	Follow-up visit is necessary to evaluate recovery of reproductive organs, healing of incision/episiotomy repair, general well-being, and adaptation to life changes.
Identify potential problems necessitating physician's evaluation prior to the scheduled 6-week visit (e.g., a return to bright red vaginal bleeding, foul-smelling lochia, elevated temperature, malaise, prolonged feelings of anxiety/depression).	Further intervention or treatment may be needed before the 6-week visit to prevent or minimize potential complications.
Discuss normal physical and psychologic changes and needs associated with the postpartal period.	Client's emotional state may be somewhat labile at this time and often is influenced by physical well-being. Anticipating such changes may reduce the stress associated with this transition period that necessitates learning new roles and taking on new responsibilities.

ACTIONS/INTERVENTIONS	RATIONALE

Independent

Identify available resources; e.g., visiting nurse services, Public Health Service, WIC program, La Leche League.

Promotes independence and provides support for adaptation to multiple changes.

NURSING DIAGNOSIS:	FAMILY COPING: POTENTIAL FOR GROWTH
May be related to:	Sufficiently meeting individual needs and adaptive tasks, enabling goals of self-actualization to surface.
Possibly evidenced by:	Family member(s) moving in direction of health-promoting and enriching lifestyle.
DESIRED OUTCOMES— CLIENT/FAMILY WILL:	Verbalize desire to undertake tasks leading to incorporation of new family member.
	Express feelings of self-confidence and satisfaction with progress and adaptation being made.

ACTIONS/INTERVENTIONS	RATIONALE

Independent

Assess relationship of family members to one another; establish primary nurse.

The nurse can help to provide a positive hospital experience and prepare the family for growth through the developmental stages that accompany acquisition of a new family member.

Provide for unlimited visiting opportunities for father and siblings. Ascertain whether siblings attended an orientation program.

Facilitates family development and ongoing process of acquaintance and attachment. Helps family members feel comfortable caring for newborn.

Initiate parent support group and individual or group instruction in breastfeeding, infant care, and the physical and emotional changes during the postpartal period.

Verbalization and discussion in group setting fosters sharing of ideas, opportunities for problem solving, and group support. Aids development of positive self-esteem, mastery, comfort, and understanding of new role.

Encourage equal participation of parents in infant care.

Flexibility and sensitization to family needs help foster self-esteem and sense of competence in caring for newborn following discharge.

Provide anticipatory guidance regarding the normal emotional changes associated with postpartal period.

Helps prepare couple for possible changes they may experience; reduces stress associated with the unknown or with unexpected events, and may promote positive coping.

Provide written information regarding suggested books for children (siblings) about the new baby. Encourage siblings to verbalize feelings of replacement or abandonment. Encourage parents to spend extra time with older children.

Helps children to identify and cope with feelings of possible replacement or abandonment. Parents should know that feelings of jealousy are normal.

Suggest that friends include older children in activities outside of the home.

School-age children probably adjust more easily to a new baby, as their horizons are already expanded to include attachment activities outside of the home.

ACTIONS/INTERVENTIONS

Collaborative

Refer client/couple to postpartal parent groups in community.

RATIONALE

Increases parents' knowledge of childrearing and child development, and provides supportive atmosphere while parents incorporate new roles.

Care Following Cesarean Birth (4 Hours to 5 Days Postpartum

CLIENT ASSESSMENT DATA BASE

Review prenatal and intraoperative record, and the indication(s) for cesarean delivery.

CIRCULATION

Blood loss during surgical procedure approximately 600–800 ml.

EGO INTEGRITY

May display emotional lability, from excitation, to apprehension, anger, or withdrawal.

Client/couple may have questions or misgivings about role in birth experience.

May express inability to deal with current situation.

ELIMINATION

Indwelling urinary catheter may be in place; urine clear amber.

Bowel sounds absent, faint, or distinct.

FOOD/FLUID

Abdomen soft with no distention initially.

NEUROSENSORY

Impaired movement and sensation below level of spinal epidural anesthesia.

PAIN/DISCOMFORT

May report discomfort from various sources; e.g., surgical trauma/incision, afterpains, bladder/abdominal distention, effects of anesthesia.

Mouth may be dry.

RESPIRATORY

Lung sounds clear and vesicular.

SAFETY

Abdominal dressing may have scant staining or be dry and intact.

Parenteral line, when used, is patent, and site is free of erythema, swelling, and tenderness.

SEXUALITY

Fundus firmly contracted and located at the umbilicus.

Lochia flow moderate and free of excessive/large clots.

DIAGNOSTIC STUDIES

Complete blood count, hemoglobin/hematocrit (Hb/Hct): Assesses changes from preoperative levels and evaluates effect of blood loss in surgery.
Urinalysis; urine, blood, vaginal, and lochial cultures: Additional studies are based on individual need.

NURSING PRIORITIES

1. Promote family unity and bonding.
2. Enhance comfort and general well-being.
3. Prevent/minimize postoperative complications.
4. Promote a positive emotional response to birth experience and parenting role.
5. Provide information regarding postpartal needs.

DISCHARGE GOALS

1. Family bonding initiated.
2. Pain/discomfort easing.
3. Physical/psychologic needs being met.
4. Complications prevented/resolving.
5. Positive self-appraisal regarding birth and parenting roles expressed.
6. Postpartal needs understood.

NURSING DIAGNOSIS:	FAMILY PROCESSES, ALTERED, bonding
May be related to:	Developmental transition/gain of a family member, situational crisis (e.g., surgical intervention, physical complications interfering with initial acquaintance/interaction, negative self-appraisal).
Possibly evidenced by:	Hesitancy to hold/interact with infant, verbalization of concerns/difficulty coping with situation, does not deal with traumatic experience constructively.
DESIRED OUTCOMES— CLIENT WILL:	Hold infant, as maternal and neonatal conditions permit.
	Demonstrate appropriate attachment and bonding behaviors.
	Begin to actively engage in newborn care tasks as appropriate.

ACTIONS/INTERVENTIONS	RATIONALE

Independent

Encourage client to hold, touch, and examine the infant, depending on condition of client and the newborn. Assist as needed.	The first hours after birth offer a unique opportunity for family bonding to occur because both mother and infant are emotionally receptive to cues from each other, which initiates the attachment and acquaintance process. Assistance in first few interactions or until intravenous line is removed prevents client from feeling discouraged or inadequate. (Note: Even if the client has chosen to relinquish her child, interacting with the newborn may facilitate the grieving process.)
Provide opportunity for father/partner to touch and hold infant and assist with infant care as allowed by situation.	Helps facilitate bonding/attachment between father and infant. Provides a resource for the mother, validating the reality of the situation and the newborn at a time when procedures and her physical needs may limit her ability to interact.

ACTIONS/INTERVENTIONS	RATIONALE
Independent	
Observe and record family-infant interactions, noting behaviors thought to indicate bonding and attachment within specific culture.	Eye-to-eye contact, use of en face position, talking in a high-pitched voice, and holding infant closely are associated with attachment in American culture. On first contact with the infant, a mother manifests a progressive pattern of behaviors whereby she initially uses fingertips to explore the infant's extremities and progresses to use of the palm before enfolding the infant with whole hand and arms.
Discuss need for usual progression and interactive nature of bonding. Note normalcy of variation of response from one time to another and among different children.	Helps client/couple understand significance and importance of the process and provides reassurance that differences are to be expected.
Note verbalizations/behaviors suggesting disappointment or lack of interest/attachment.	The arrival of a new family member, even when wanted and anticipated, creates a transient period of disequilibrium, requiring incorporation of the new child into the existing family.
Allow parents the opportunity to verbalize negative feelings about themselves and the infant.	Unresolved conflicts during the early parent-infant acquaintance process may have long-term negative effects on the future parent-child relationship.
Note circumstances surrounding cesarean birth, parents' self-appraisal and perception of birth experience, their initial reaction to infant, and their participation in birth experience.	Parents need to work through meaning attributed to stressful events surrounding childbirth and orient themselves to reality before they can focus on infant. Effects of anesthesia, anxiety, and pain can alter the client's perceptual abilities during and following operation.
Encourage and assist with breastfeeding dependent on client's choice and cultural beliefs/practices.	Early contact has a positive effect on duration of breastfeedings; skin-to-skin contact and initiation of maternal tasks promotes bonding. Some cultures (e.g., Hispanic, Navajo, Filipino, Vietnamese) refrain from breastfeeding until the milk flow is established.
Welcome family and siblings for brief visit as soon as maternal/newborn condition permits. (Refer to CP: The Client at 4 Hours to 3 Days Postpartum, ND: Family Coping: potential for growth.)	Promotes family unity, and helps siblings begin process of positive adaptation to new roles and incorporation of new member into family structure.
Provide information, as desired, about infant's safety and condition. Support couple as needed.	Helps couple to process and evaluate necessary information, especially if initial acquaintance period has been delayed.
Answer client's questions regarding protocol of care during early postdelivery period.	Information relieves anxiety that may interfere with bonding or result in self-absorption rather than in attention to newborn.
Collaborative	
Notify appropriate healthcare team members (e.g., nursery staff or postpartal nurse) of observation as indicated.	Inadequate bonding behaviors or poor interaction between client/couple and infant necessitates support and further evaluation. (Refer to CP: The Client at 4 Hours to 3 Days Postpartum, ND: Parenting, altered, high risk for.)

ACTIONS/INTERVENTIONS

Collaborative

Prepare for ongoing support/follow-up after discharge; e.g., visiting nurse services, community agencies, and parent support group.

RATIONALE

Many couples have unresolved conflicts regarding initial parent-infant acquaintance process that require resolution after discharge.

NURSING DIAGNOSIS:	PAIN [ACUTE]/DISCOMFORT*
May be related to:	Surgical trauma, effects of anesthesia, hormonal effects, bladder/abdominal distention.
Possibly evidenced by:	Reports of incisional pain, cramping (afterpains), headache, abdominal bloating, breast tenderness; guarding/distraction behaviors, facial mask of pain.
DESIRED OUTCOMES—CLIENT WILL:	Identify and use appropriate interventions to manage pain/discomfort.
	Verbalize lessening of pain.
	Appear relaxed, able to sleep/rest appropriately.
	Appear
	*Authors' note: Currently there is no NANDA diagnostic label that addresses issues of comfort below the level of Pain [acute] or chronic. Although the label of **Discomfort** is not approved, we believe it speaks more directly to the identified problem.

ACTIONS/INTERVENTIONS

Independent

Determine characteristics and location of discomfort. Note verbal and nonverbal cues such as grimacing, rigidity, and guarding or restricted movement.

Provide information and anticipatory guidance regarding causes of discomfort and appropriate interventions.

Evaluate blood pressure (BP) and pulse; note behavior changes (distinguish between restlessness associated with excessive blood loss from that associated with pain).

Note uterine tenderness and presence/characteristics of afterpains; note postoperative infusion of oxytocin.

RATIONALE

Client may not verbally report pain and discomfort directly. Comparing specific characteristics of pain aids in differentiating postoperative pain from developing complications (e.g., ileus, bladder retention or infection, wound dehiscence).

Promotes problem-solving, helps reduce pain associated with anxiety and fear of the unknown, and provides sense of control.

In many clients pain may cause restlessness and an increase in BP and pulse. Analgesia may lower BP.

During the first 12 hours postpartum, uterine contractions are strong and regular, and they continue for the next 2–3 days, although their frequency and intensity are reduced. Factors intensifying afterpains include multiparity, uterine overdistention, breastfeeding, and administration of ergot and oxytocin preparations.

ACTIONS/INTERVENTIONS	RATIONALE

Independent

Reposition client, reduce noxious stimuli, and offer back rubs. Encourage use of breathing and relaxation techniques and distraction (stimulation of cutaneous tissue) as learned in childbirth classes. Encourage presence and participation of partner as appropriate.

Relaxes muscles, and distracts from painful sensations. Promotes comfort, and reduces unpleasant distractions, enhancing sense of well-being.

Initiate deep-breathing exercises, incentive spirometry, and coughing using splinting procedures as appropriate, 30 min after administration of analgesics.

Deep breathing enhances respiratory effort. Splinting reduces strain and stretching of incisional area and lessens pain and discomfort associated with movement of abdominal muscles. Coughing is indicated when secretions or rhonchi are auscultated.

Encourage early ambulation. Recommend avoidance of gas-forming foods or fluids; e.g., beans, cabbage, carbonated beverages, whole milk, very hot or very cold beverages, or use of straws for drinking. (Refer to ND: Constipation.)

Decreases gas formation and promotes peristalsis to relieve discomfort of gas accumulation, which often peaks on third day after cesarean delivery.

Recommend use of left lateral recumbent position.

Allows gas to rise from descending to sigmoid colon, facilitating expulsion.

Inspect perineum for hemorrhoids. Suggest application of ice for 20 min every 4 hr, use of witch hazel compresses, and elevation of pelvis on pillow as appropriate.

Aids in regression of hemorrhoids and vulvar varicosities by promoting localized vasoconstriction, reducing discomfort and itching, and enhancing return to normal bowel function.

Palpate bladder, noting fullness. Facilitate periodic voiding after removal of indwelling catheter.

Return of normal bladder function may take 4–7 days, and overdistention of bladder may create feelings of urgency and discomfort.

Evaluate for headache, especially following subarachnoid anesthesia. Avoid medicating client before nature and cause of headache are determined. Note character of headache (e.g., deep location behind the eyes, with pain radiating to both temples and occipital area; relieved in supine position but increased in sitting or standing position) to distinguish from headache associated with anxiety or pregnancy-induced hypertension (PIH).

Leakage of cerebrospinal fluid (CSF) through the dura mater into the extradural space reduces volume needed to support brain tissue, causing the brain stem to fall onto the base of the skull when client is in an upright position. PIH may result in cerebral edema, necessitating other interventions. (Refer to CP: The Client at 4 Hours to 3 Days Postpartum, ND: Fluid Volume excess, high risk for.)

Encourage bedrest in flat-lying position, increase fluids, offer caffeinated beverage, assist as needed with client and infant care, and apply abdominal binder when client is upright, in presence of post-spinal headache. Notify physician or anesthesiologist, as indicated.

Reduces severity of headache by increasing fluid available for production of CSF and limiting position shifts of the brain. Severe headache may interfere with client's ability to carry out self-care and infant care. Ongoing headache may require more aggressive therapy.

Inspect breast and nipple tissue; assess for presence of engorgement and/or cracked nipples.

At 24 hours postpartum, breasts should be soft and nontender, with nipples free of cracks or reddened areas. Breast engorgement, nipple tenderness, or presence of cracks on nipple (if client is lactating) may occur 2–3 days postpartum and require prompt intervention to facilitate continuation of breastfeeding and prevent more serious complications.

ACTIONS/INTERVENTIONS

Independent

Encourage wearing of supportive bra.

Provide information to the lactating client about increasing the frequency of feedings, applying heat to breasts before feedings, proper positioning of the infant, and expressing milk manually. (Refer to CP: The Client at 4 Hours to 3 Days Postpartum, ND: Breastfeeding [specify].)

Suggest that client initiate feedings on nontender nipple for several feedings in succession if only one nipple is sore or cracked.

Apply ice to axillary area of breasts if the client is not planning to breastfeed. Provide tight compression with binder for 72 hours or use of well-fitting supportive bra. Avoid excess exposure of breasts to heat, or stimulation of breasts by infant, sexual partner, or client until suppression process is completed (approximately 1 wk).

Collaborative

Administer analgesics every 3–4 hr, progressing from i.v./intramuscular routes to oral route. Medicate lactating client 45–60 min before breastfeeding.

Review/monitor use of patient-controlled analgesia (PCA) as indicated.

Administer bromocriptine mesylate (Parlodel) twice daily with meals for 2–3 wk. Assess client for hypotension; remain with client during first ambulation. Provide information about the possibility of rebound breast engorgement or congestion when use of medication is discontinued.

Assist as needed with saline injection or administration of "blood patch" over site of dural puncture. Keep client in horizontal position following the procedure.

Provide rectal tube as indicated.

RATIONALE

Lifts breasts inward and upward, resulting in a more comfortable position and decreasing muscle fatigue.

These measures can help the lactating client stimulate the flow of milk and relieve stasis and engorgement. Use of "football hold" directs infant's feet away from abdomen. Pillow helps support infant and protects incision in sitting or side-lying position.

Initial suckling response is strong and may be painful. Starting feeding with unaffected breast and then proceeding to involved breast may be less painful and enhance healing.

Binding and ice prevent lactation by mechanical means and are the preferred method for suppression of lactation. Discomfort lasts approximately 48–72 hr, but eases or ceases with avoidance of nipple stimulation.

Promotes comfort, which improves psychologic status and enhances mobility. Judicious use of medication allows lactating mother to enjoy feeding without adverse effects on infant.

PCA provides rapid pain relief without excessive side effects/oversedation. Enhances sense of control, general well-being, and independence.

Bromocriptine acts to suppress secretion of prolactin, yet is a potent dopamine agonist receptor and can cause severe hypotension. Therefore, it should be initiated only after vital signs are stable and no sooner than 4 hr following delivery. Up to 40% of women experience problems of rebound congestion and engorgement.

Effective for relief of severe spinal headache. The blood patch procedure, which has a 90%–100% success rate, creates a blood clot, which produces pressure and seals the leak.

Relieves gas buildup.

NURSING DIAGNOSIS:	ANXIETY [SPECIFY LEVEL]
May be related to:	Situational crisis, threat to self-concept, interpersonal transmission/contagion, unmet needs.

Possibly evidenced by:	Increased tension, apprehension, feelings of inadequacy, sympathetic stimulation, sleeplessness.
DESIRED OUTCOMES— CLIENT WILL:	Verbalize awareness of feelings of anxiety.
	Identify ways of reducing or resolving anxiety.
	Report anxiety is reduced to a manageable level.
	Appear relaxed, able to sleep/rest appropriately.

ACTIONS/INTERVENTIONS	RATIONALE
Independent	
Encourage presence/participation of partner.	Provides emotional support; may encourage verbalization of concerns.
Determine client's level of anxiety and source of concern. Encourage client/couple to verbalize unmet needs and expectations. Provide information regarding the normalcy of such feelings.	Cesarean birth may be viewed by the client/couple as a failure at a life event and this may have a negative impact on the bonding/parenting process.
Assist client/couple in identifying usual coping mechanisms and developing new coping strategies if needed. (Refer to CP: The Client at 4 Hours to 3 Days Postpartum, ND: Coping, Individual, Ineffective, high risk for.)	Helps facilitate positive adaptation to new role; reduces feelings of anxiety.
Provide accurate information about client/infant status.	Fantasies caused by lack of information or misunderstanding may increase anxiety levels.
Initiate contact between client/couple and infant as soon as possible. If infant is sent to neonatal intensive care unit, establish line of communication between nursery staff and client/couple. Take pictures and allow for visits when client's physical status permits. (Refer to CP: The Parents of a Child with Special Needs.)	Reduces anxiety that may be associated with handling infant, fear of unknown, and/or assuming the worst regarding infant status.

NURSING DIAGNOSIS:	**SELF ESTEEM, SITUATIONAL LOW**
May be related to:	Perceived failure at a life event.
Possibly evidenced by:	Verbalization of negative feelings about self in situation (e.g., helplessness, shame/guilt).
DESIRED OUTCOMES— CLIENT/COUPLE WILL:	Discuss concerns related to her/his role in and perception of the birth experience.
	Verbalize understanding of individual factors that precipitated current situation.
	Express positive self-appraisal.

ACTIONS/INTERVENTIONS	RATIONALE
Independent	
Determine client's/couple's emotional response to cesarean birth.	Both members of the couple may have a negative emotional reaction to the cesarean delivery. An unplanned cesarean birth may have a negative effect on the client's self-esteem, leaving her feeling that she is inadequate and has failed as a woman. The father or partner, especially if he was unable to be present at the cesarean delivery, may feel that he abandoned his partner and did not fulfill his anticipated role as emotional supporter during the childbirth process. Even though a healthy baby may be the outcome, parents often grieve and feel a sense of loss at missing out on the anticipated vaginal delivery.
Review client's/couple's participation and role in birth experience. Identify positive behaviors during prenatal and antepartal process.	Grief response may be lessened if both mother and father were able to share in experience of delivery. Refocuses client's/couple's attention to help them view pregnancy in its totality and to see that their actions have contributed to an optimal outcome. May help to avoid guilt/placing of blame.
Emphasize similarities between vaginal and cesarean delivery. Convey positive attitude toward cesarean birth, and manage postpartal care as close as possible to care provided to clients following vaginal delivery.	Client may alter her perception of cesarean birth experience as well as her perception of her own wellness or illness based on the professional's attitudes. Similar care conveys the message that cesarean delivery is an acceptable alternative to vaginal delivery.
Collaborative	
Refer client/couple for professional counseling if reactions are maladaptive.	Client who is unable to resolve grief or negative feelings may need further professional help.

NURSING DIAGNOSIS:	INJURY, HIGH RISK FOR
Risk factors may include:	Biochemical or regulatory functions (e.g., orthostatic hypotension, development of PIH or eclampsia), effects of anesthesia, thromboembolism, abnormal blood profile (anemia/excessive blood loss, rubella sensitivity, Rh incompatibility), tissue trauma.
Possibly evidenced by:	[Not applicable; presence of signs/symptoms establishes an **actual** diagnosis.]
DESIRED OUTCOMES— CLIENT WILL:	Demonstrate behaviors to reduce risk factors and/or protect self.
	Be free of complications.

ACTIONS/INTERVENTIONS	RATIONALE

Independent

Review prenatal and intrapartal record for factors that predispose client to complications. Note Hb level and operative blood loss.	Presence of risk factors such as myometrial fatigue, uterine overdistention, prolonged oxytocin stimulation, general anesthesia, anemia/excessive blood loss, or prenatal thrombophlebitis renders the client more susceptible to postoperative complications.
Monitor BP, pulse, and temperature. Note cool, clammy skin; weak, thready pulse; behavior changes; delayed capillary refill; or cyanosis. (Refer to CP: Postpartal Hemorrhage.)	Elevated BP may indicate developing or continuing hypertension, necessitating magnesium sulfate ($MgSO_4$) or other antihypertensive treatment. Hypotension and tachycardia may reflect dehydration and hypovolemia but may not occur until circulating blood volume has decreased by 30%–50%, at which time signs of peripheral vasoconstriction may be noted. Pyrexia may indicate infection.
Inspect dressing for excessive bleeding. Outline, date drainage on dressings (if not changed). Notify physician of continued oozing.	Surgical wounds with a drain may saturate a dressing; however, oozing is usually not expected and may suggest developing complications.
Note character and amount of lochial flow and consistency of fundus.	Lochial flow should not be heavy or contain clots; fundus should remain firmly contracted at the umbilicus. A boggy uterus results in increased flow and blood loss.
Monitor fluid intake and urine output. Note appearance, color, concentration, and specific gravity of urine.	Kidney function is a key index to circulating blood volume. As output decreases, specific gravity increases, and vice versa. Bloody urine or urine containing clots signifies possible bladder trauma associated with surgical intervention.
Encourage early ambulation and exercise, except in client who received subarachnoid anesthesia, who may remain flat for 6–8 hr without use of pillow or raising head, as indicated by protocol and return of sensation/muscle control. (Refer to ND: Pain [acute]/Discomfort.)	Enhances circulation and venous return of lower extremities, reducing risk of thrombus formation, which is associated with stasis. Although recumbent position after subarachnoid anesthesia is controversial, it may aid in prevention of CSF leakage and resultant headache.
Assist client with initial ambulation. Provide adequate supervision in shower or sitz bath. Leave call bell within client's reach.	Orthostatic hypotension may occur when changing from supine to upright position on initial ambulation, or it may result from vasodilation caused by the heat of the shower or sitz bath.
Have client sit on floor or chair with head between legs, or have her lie down in a flat position, if she feels faint. Use ammonia capsule ("smelling salts").	Helps maintain or enhance circulation and delivery of oxygen to brain.
Assess for hyperreflexia, right upper quadrant pain, headache, or visual disturbances. Maintain seizure precautions, and provide quiet environment as indicated. (Refer to CP: The Client at 4 Hours to 3 Days Postpartum, ND: Fluid Volume excess, high risk for; Chapter 4, CP: Pregnancy-Induced Hypertension, ND: Injury, high risk for.)	Danger of eclampsia due to PIH exists for up to 72 hours postpartum, although literature suggests the convulsive state has occurred as late as the fifth day postpartum.

ACTIONS/INTERVENTIONS

Independent

Note effects of MgSO$_4$, if administered. Assess patellar response and monitor respiratory rate.

Inspect incision regularly; note signs of delayed or altered healing (e.g., lack of approximation).

Inspect lower extremities for signs of thrombophlebitis (e.g., redness, warmth, pain/tenderness). Note presence or absence of Homans' sign. (Refer to CP: Postpartal Thrombophlebitis.)

Encourage leg/ankle exercises and early ambulation.

Evaluate client's rubella status on prenatal chart (less than 1:10 titer indicates susceptibility). Assess client for allergies to eggs or feathers; if present, withhold vaccine. Provide written and oral information, and obtain informed consent for vaccination after reviewing side effects, risks, and the necessity to prevent conception for 2–3 months following the vaccination.

Collaborative

Replace fluid losses intravenously, as ordered.

Monitor postoperative Hb/Hct; compare with preoperative levels.

Increase oxytocin infusion if uterus is relaxed and/or lochia is heavy.

Administer MgSO$_4$ by infusion pump, as indicated.

RATIONALE

Absence of patellar reflex and respiratory rate below 12/min indicate toxicity and a need to reduce or discontinue drug therapy.

Excessive strain on the incision or delayed healing may render client prone to tissue separation and possible hemorrhage.

Elevated fibrin split products (possibly released from placental site), reduced mobility, trauma, sepsis, and extensive activation of blood clotting following delivery predispose the client to the development of thromboembolism. Homans' sign may be present with deep venous thrombus, but may be absent with superficial phlebitis. Plasma losses, elevated platelet counts, immobility, and relaxation of blood vessels from anesthesia place client at risk for thrombophlebitis.

Promotes venous return, prevents stasis/pooling in lower extremities, reducing risk of phlebitis.

Vaccination helps prevent teratogenic effects in subsequent pregnancies. Administration of vaccine in the immediate postpartal period may cause side effects of transient arthralgia, rash, and cold symptoms during incubation period of 14–21 days. Allergic anaphylactic or hypersensitivity response may occur, necessitating administration of epinephrine.

Average blood loss is usually 600–800 ml, but prenatal physiologic edema, which mobilizes postpartum, alleviates need for large fluid volume replacement. A total of 3 L of fluid infused intravenously in the intraoperative and early postoperative (24-hr) period is recommended.

Client with Hct of 33% or greater and increased plasma associated with pregnancy can tolerate actual blood loss of up to 1500 ml without difficulty. A significant change in volume may necessitate replacement with blood products, although iron replacement may be preferred.

Stimulates myometrial contractility and reduces blood loss. Oxytocin is usually added to infusion intraoperatively after delivery of the infant's shoulders and is maintained into the early postoperative period.

Helps reduce cerebral irritability in presence of PIH or eclampsia. (Refer to CP: The Client at 4 Hours to 3 Days Postpartum, ND: Fluid Volume excess, high risk for.)

ACTIONS/INTERVENTIONS	RATIONALE

Collaborative

Apply support hose or elastic wrap to legs when risk or symptoms of phlebitis are present.

Reduces venous stasis, enhancing venous return and reducing risk of thrombus formation.

Administer anticoagulant; evaluate coagulation factors, and note signs of failure to clot. (Refer to CP: Postpartal Thrombophlebitis.)

Although usually not required, may help prevent further development of thrombus.

Administer Rh$_0$(D) immune globulin (RhIgG) I.M. within 72 hr postpartum as indicated for Rh-negative mother who has not been previously sensitized and who delivers an Rh-positive infant with negative result on direct Coombs' test on cord blood. Obtain Betke-Kleihauer smear if significant fetal-maternal transfusion is suspected at delivery.

Dose of 300 μg is usually sufficient to promote lysis of fetal Rh-positive red blood cells that may have entered maternal circulation during delivery, and that may potentially cause sensitization and problems of Rh incompatibility in subsequent pregnancies. Presence of 20 ml or more of Rh-positive fetal blood in maternal circulation necessitates higher dose of RhIgG.

NURSING DIAGNOSIS:	**INFECTION, HIGH RISK FOR**
Risk factors may include:	Tissue trauma/broken skin, decreased Hb, invasive procedures and/or increased environmental exposure, prolonged rupture of amniotic membranes, malnutrition.
Possibly evidenced by:	[Not applicable; presence of signs/symptoms establishes an **actual** diagnosis.]
DESIRED OUTCOMES— CLIENT WILL:	Demonstrate techniques to reduce risks and/or promote healing.
	Display wound free of purulent drainage with initial signs of healing (i.e., approximation of wound edges), uterus soft/nontender, with normal lochial flow and character.
	Be free of infection, be afebrile, have no adventitious breath sounds, and void clear amber urine.

ACTIONS/INTERVENTIONS	RATIONALE

Independent

Encourage and use careful handwashing technique and appropriate disposal of soiled underpads, perineal pads, and contaminated linen. Discuss with client the importance of continuing these measures after discharge.

Helps prevent or retard spread of infection.

Review prenatal Hb/Hct; note presence of conditions that predispose client to postoperative infection.

Anemia, diabetes, and prolonged labor (especially with membranes ruptured) prior to cesarean delivery increase risk of infection and delayed healing.

Assess client's nutritional status. Note appearance of hair, fingernails, skin, and so forth. Note prepregnancy weight and prenatal weight gain.

Client who is 20% below normal weight, or who is anemic or malnourished, is more susceptible to postpartal infection and may have special dietary needs.

ACTIONS/INTERVENTIONS	RATIONALE
Independent	
Encourage oral fluids and diet high in protein, vitamin C, and iron.	Prevents dehydration; maximizes circulating volume and urine flow. Protein and vitamin C are needed for collagen formation; iron is needed for Hb synthesis.
Inspect abdominal dressing for exudate or oozing. Remove dressing as indicated.	A sterile dressing covering the wound in the first 24 hr following cesarean birth helps protect it from injury or contamination. Oozing may indicate hematoma, loss of suture approximation, or wound dehiscence, requiring further intervention. Removing the dressing allows incision to dry and promotes healing.
Note operative record for use of drain and nature of incision. Clean wound and change dressing when saturated.	Moist environment is an excellent medium for bacterial growth; bacteria can travel by capillary action through the wet dressing to the wound. (Note: Incision into the lower uterine segment heals more rapidly than classic incision and is less likely to rupture in subsequent pregnancies.)
Inspect incision for healing process, noting redness, edema, pain, exudate, or loss of approximation.	These signs indicate wound infection, usually caused by streptococci, staphylococci, or *Pseudomonas* species.
Assist as needed with removal of skin sutures or clips.	Incision is usually sufficiently healed to remove sutures on the fourth or fifth day following surgical procedure.
Encourage client to take warm showers daily.	Showers, usually allowed after the second day following cesarean birth, promote hygiene and may stimulate circulation and healing of wound.
Assess temperature, pulse, and white blood cell count.	Fever after the third postoperative day, leukocytosis, and tachycardia suggest infection. Elevation of temperature to 101°F (38.3°C) within the first 24 hr is highly indicative of infection; an elevation to 100.4°F (38.0°C) on any 2 of the first 10 days postpartum is significant.
Assess location and contractility of uterus; note involutional changes or presence of extreme uterine tenderness.	Following cesarean birth, the fundus remains at the level of the umbilicus for up to 5 days, when involution begins, accompanied by an increase in lochial flow. Delayed involution increases the risk of endometritis. Development of extreme tenderness signals possible retained placental tissue or infection.
Note amount and odor of lochial discharge or change in normal progression from rubra to serosa.	Lochia normally has a fleshy odor; however, in endometritis the discharge may be purulent and foul-smelling, and may fail to demonstrate normal progression from rubra to serosa to alba.
Maintain sterile closed urinary drainage system.	Prevents introduction of bacteria when indwelling cathether is used.
Provide perineal and catheter care, and frequent changes of peripads.	Helps eliminate medium of bacterial growth; promotes hygiene.

ACTIONS/INTERVENTIONS	RATIONALE

Independent

Maintain drainage bag in dependent position.

Note frequency/amount and characteristics of urine.

Promote rest and encourage use of semi-Fowler's position once anesthesia precautions are completed.

Assist client in splinting incision during lung exercises.

Inspect I.V. site for signs of erythema or tenderness.

Evaluate condition of nipples, noting presence of cracks, redness, or tenderness. Recommend routine examination of breasts. Review proper care and infant feeding techniques. (Refer to ND: Pain [acute]/Discomfort.)

Assess lung sounds and respiratory ease or effort. Note crackles/rhonchi, dyspnea, chest pain, fever, or mucopurulent sputum.

Institute turning, coughing, and deep-breathing routines with splinting of incision every 2–4 hr while awake. Note productive cough.

Collaborative

Administer oxytocin or ergot preparation. (Note: Oxytocin infusion is often ordered routinely for 4 hr following surgery.)

Monitor laboratory test results, such as blood urea nitrogen (BUN) and 24-hour urine for total protein, creatinine clearance, and uric acid as indicated.

Administer prophylactic antibiotic infusion, with first dose usually administered immediately after cord clamping and 2 more doses 6 hr apart.

Initiate use of incentive spirometer. Provide information as needed.

RATIONALE

Avoids urinary reflux, reducing risk of infection.

Urinary stasis increases the risk of infection. Cloudy or malodorous urine indicates presence of infection.

Rest reduces metabolic process, allowing oxygen and nutrients to be used for healing. Semi-Fowler's position promotes flow of lochia and reduces pooling in uterus, and maximizes respiratory function.

Helps prevent strain on incision and reduces likelihood of wound dehiscence.

Indicates local infection, requiring removal of catheter and possibly restarting the I.V. line in another site.

The development of nipple fissures/cracks potentiates risk of mastitis.

Rhonchi indicative of retained secretions should not be present, yet breath sounds may be diminished for the first 24 hr after surgery. Absence of lung sounds indicates consolidation or lack of air exchange, and possible atelectasis or pneumonia.

Improves depth of respirations and alveolar expansion; clears bronchial secretions that could block bronchioles. Productive cough indicates client is clearing bronchial secretions effectively.

Maintains myometrial contractility, thereby retarding bacterial spread through walls of uterus; aids in expulsion of clots/membranes.

In the client who has had PIH, kidney or vascular involvement may persist, or it may appear for the first time during the postpartal period. As steroid levels decrease following delivery, renal function, evidenced by BUN and creatinine clearance, begins to return to normal within 1 week; anatomic changes (e.g., dilation of ureters and renal pelvis) may take up to 1 month to return to normal.

Decreases likelihood of postpartal endometritis as well as complications such as incisional abscesses or pelvic thrombophlebitis.

Promotes sustained maximal respiration, inflates alveoli, and prevents atelectasis.

ACTIONS/INTERVENTIONS

Collaborative

Obtain sputum specimen as indicated by changes in color or odor of sputum, presence of congestion, and temperature elevation.

Review chest x-ray as indicated.

Obtain blood, vaginal, and urine cultures, if infection is suspected.

Administer specific antibiotic for identified infectious process.

RATIONALE

To identify specific pathogens and appropriate therapy.

Confirms presence of infiltrate(s) or atelectasis.

Bacteremia is more frequent in client whose membranes were ruptured for 6 hr or longer than in client whose membranes remained intact prior to cesarean delivery.

Necessary to eradicate organism.

NURSING DIAGNOSIS:	CONSTIPATION
May be related to:	Decreased muscle tone (diastasis recti, excess analgesia or anesthesia), effects of progesterone, dehydration, prelabor diarrhea, lack of intake, perineal/rectal pain.
Possibly evidenced by:	Reported abdominal/rectal fullness or pressure, nausea, less than usual amount of stool, straining at stool, decreased bowel sounds.
DESIRED OUTCOMES— CLIENT WILL:	Demonstrate return of intestinal motility as evidenced by active bowel sounds and the passing of flatus.
	Resume usual/optimal elimination pattern within 4 days postpartum.

ACTIONS/INTERVENTIONS

Independent

Auscultate for presence of bowel sounds in all 4 quadrants every 4 hr following cesarean birth.

Palpate abdomen, noting distention or discomfort.

Note passing of flatus or belching.

Encourage adequate oral fluids (e.g., 6 to 8 glasses/day) once oral intake resumes. Recommend increased dietary roughage and fruits and vegetables with seeds.

Encourage leg exercises and abdominal tightening; promote early ambulation.

RATIONALE

Determines readiness for oral feedings, and possible developing complication; e.g., ileus. Usually, bowel sounds are not heard on the first day after surgical procedure, are faint on the second day, and are active by the third day.

Indicates gas formation and accumulation or possible paralytic ileus.

Indicates return of motility.

Roughage (e.g., fruits and vegetables, especially with seeds and skins) and increased fluids provide bulk, stimulate elimination, and prevent constipated stool. (Note: Food or fluid offered prior to return of peristalsis may contribute to paralytic ileus.)

Leg exercises tighten abdominal muscles and improve abdominal motility. Progressive ambulation after 24 hr promotes peristalsis and gas expulsion, and alleviates or prevents gas pains.

ACTIONS/INTERVENTIONS

Independent

Identify those activities that client can use at home to stimulate bowel action.

Collaborative

Administer analgesics 30 min prior to ambulation.

Provide stool softener or mild cathartic.

Administer hypertonic or small soap suds enema.

Insert or maintain nasogastric tube as indicated.

RATIONALE

Helps in reestablishment of normal evacuation pattern and promotes independence.

Facilitates ability to ambulate; however, narcotics, if used, may reduce bowel activity.

Softens stool, stimulates peristalsis, and helps reestablish bowel function.

Promotes bowel evacuation and relieves gaseous distention.

May be necessary to decompress the stomach and relieve distention associated with paralytic ileus.

NURSING DIAGNOSIS:	KNOWLEDGE DEFICIT [LEARNING NEED], regarding physiologic changes, recovery period, self-care and infant care needs
May be related to:	Lack of exposure/recall, misinterpretation, unfamiliarity with resources.
Possibly evidenced by:	Verbalized concerns/misconceptions, hesitancy in or inadequate performance of activities, inappropriate behaviors (e.g., apathy).
DESIRED OUTCOMES— CLIENT WILL:	Verbalize understanding of physiologic changes, individual needs, expected outcomes.
	Perform necessary activities/procedures correctly and explain reasons for the actions.

ACTIONS/INTERVENTIONS

Independent

Assess client's readiness and motivation for learning. Assist client/couple in identifying needs.

Initiate written teaching plan using standardized format or checklist. Document information given and client's response.

RATIONALE

The postpartal period can be a positive experience if opportune teaching is provided to foster maternal growth, maturation, and competence. However, the client needs time to move from a "taking in" to a "taking hold" phase, in which her receptiveness and readiness is heightened and she is emotionally and physically ready for learning new information to facilitate mastery of her new role. By the second or third day postpartum, the client is usually receptive to learning.

Helps assure completeness of information parents receive from staff members and reduces client confusion caused by dissemination of conflicting advice or information.

ACTIONS/INTERVENTIONS	RATIONALE

Independent

Assess client's physical status. Plan group or individual sessions following administration of medication or when client is comfortable and rested.

Discomfort associated with incision or afterpains, or bowel/bladder discomfort, is usually less severe by the third postoperative day, allowing the client to concentrate more fully and be more receptive to learning.

Note psychologic state and response to cesarean birth and mothering role. (Refer to ND: Self Esteem, situational low.)

Anxiety related to ability to care for herself and her child, disappointment over the birth experience, or concerns regarding her separation from the infant may have a negative impact on client's learning abilities and readiness.

Provide information related to normal physiologic and psychologic changes associated with cesarean birth and needs associated with the postpartal period.

Helps client to recognize normal changes from abnormal responses that may require treatment. Client's emotional state may be somewhat labile at this time and often is influenced by physical well-being. Anticipating such changes may reduce the stress associated with this transition period that necessitates learning new roles and taking on new responsibilities.

Review self-care needs (e.g., perineal care, incisional care, hygiene, voiding). Encourage participation in self-care as client is able. Demonstrate method of getting out of a flat bed without the use of side rails.

Facilitates autonomy, helps prevent infection, and promotes healing. By turning on her side, using her arms to lift herself to a sitting position, and pushing with her hands to lift buttocks off the bed to a standing position, client can ease stress on incision.

Discuss appropriate exercise program, as prescribed.

A progressive exercise program can usually be started once abdominal discomfort has eased (by approximately 3–4 wk postpartum). Helps tone musculature, increases circulation, produces a trimmer figure, and enhances feelings of general well-being. Client should be advised not to lift objects heavier than the infant for approximately 2 wk, and to bend at knees when lifting baby.

Identify signs/symptoms requiring notification of healthcare provider (e.g., fever, dysuria, increase in amount of lochial flow or return to bright red lochial exudate, or separation of suture line).

Prompt evaluation and intervention may prevent/limit development of complications (e.g., hemorrhage, infection, delayed healing).

Demonstrate techniques of infant care. Observe return demonstration by client/couple. (Refer to Chapter 7, CP: The Infant at 2 Hours to 3 Days of Age, ND: Knowledge Deficit [Learning Need].)

Assists parents in mastery of new tasks.

Review information regarding appropriate choice for infant feeding (e.g., physiology of breastfeeding, positioning, breast and nipple care, diet, and removal of infant from breast; formula types/preparation and infant position during bottle feeding).

Promotes independence and optimal feeding experience. When bottle feeding, it is important to feed the infant alternately on the right and left side to promote eye development. Slight dehydration or physical or emotional trauma may delay onset of lactation for the client who has undergone a cesarean delivery.

ACTIONS/INTERVENTIONS	RATIONALE

Independent

Discuss plans for home management: assistance with housework, physical layout of house, infant sleeping arrangements.

Client who has undergone cesarean delivery may need more assistance when first home than the client who has given birth vaginally. Stairs and the use of low cradles or bassinets may cause difficulties for the postoperative client.

Provide numbers for appropriate telephone contacts. Identify available community resources; e.g., visiting nurse services, Public Health Service, Women, Infants, and Children (WIC) program, La Leche League, Mothers of Twins.

Provides ready resources to answer questions. Promotes independence and provides support for adaptation to multiple changes.

Discuss resumption of sexual intercourse and plans for contraception. Provide information about available methods, including advantages and disadvantages. (Refer to CP: Maternal Assessment: 1 Week Following Discharge, ND: Knowledge Deficit [Learning Need].)

Intercourse may be resumed as soon as it is comfortable for the client and healing has progressed, generally around 6 weeks postpartum. Couple may need clarification regarding available contraceptive methods and the fact that pregnancy could occur even prior to the 6-week visit.

Provide or reinforce information related to follow-up postpartal examination.

Postpartum evaluations for the client who has undergone cesarean delivery may be scheduled at 3 weeks rather than 6 weeks because of increased risk of infection and delayed healing.

NURSING DIAGNOSIS:	**URINARY ELIMINATION, ALTERED**
May be related to:	Mechanical trauma/diversion, hormonal effects (fluid shifts and/or increased renal plasma flow), effects of anesthesia.
Possibly evidenced by:	Increased bladder filling/distention, changes in amount/frequency of voiding.
DESIRED OUTCOMES—CLIENT WILL:	Resume usual/optimal voiding patterns following catheter removal.
	Empty bladder with each void.

ACTIONS/INTERVENTIONS	RATIONALE

Independent

Note and record amount, color, and concentration of urinary drainage.

Oliguria (output less than 30 ml/hr) may be caused by excess fluid loss, inadequate fluid replacement, or antidiuretic effects of infused oxytocin.

Test urine for albumin and acetone. Distinguish between proteinuria associated with PIH and that associated with normal processes. (Refer to CP: The Client at 4 Hours to 3 Days Postpartum, ND: Fluid Volume excess, high risk for.)

Catalytic process associated with uterine involution may result in normal proteinuria (1+) for the first 2 days postpartum. Acetone may indicate dehydration associated with prolonged labor and/or delivery.

Provide oral fluids; e.g., 6 to 8 glasses per day, as appropriate.

Fluids promote hydration and renal function, and help prevent bladder stasis.

ACTIONS/INTERVENTIONS	RATIONALE

Independent

Palpate bladder. Monitor fundal height and location and amount of lochial flow.

Renal plasma flow, which increases by 25%–50% during the prenatal period, remains elevated in the first week postpartum, resulting in increased bladder filling. Bladder distention can be assessed by degree of uterine displacement; causes increased uterine relaxation and lochial flow.

Note signs and symptoms of urinary tract infection (UTI) (e.g., cloudy color, foul odor, burning sensation, or frequency) following catheter removal.

Presence of indwelling catheter predisposes client to introduction of bacteria and UTI.

Use methods to facilitate voiding after catheter removal (e.g., run water in sink, pour warm water over perineum).

Client should void within 6–8 hr following catheter removal, yet may have difficulty emptying bladder completely.

Instruct client to perform Kegel exercise daily after effects of anesthesia have subsided.

Performing Kegel exercise 100 times per day increases circulation to perineum, aids in healing and recovery of tone of pubococcygeal muscle, and prevents or reduces stress incontinence.

Collaborative

Maintain intravenous infusion for 24 hr following surgery, as indicated. Increase infusion amount if output is 30 ml/hr or less.

Usually, 3 L of fluid, including lactated Ringer's solution, is adequate to replace losses and maintain renal flow/urine output.

Remove catheter per protocol/as indicated.

Generally, catheter may be safely removed between 6 to 12 hours postpartum; but for convenience it may remain in client until the morning after surgery.

Monitor laboratory test results, such as BUN and 24-hour urine for total protein, creatinine clearance, and uric acid as indicated.

In the client who has had PIH, kidney or vascular involvement may persist, or it may appear for the first time during the postpartal period. As steroid levels decrease following delivery, renal function, evidenced by BUN and creatinine clearance, begins to return to normal within 1 week; anatomic changes (e.g., dilation of ureters and renal pelvis) may take up to 1 month to return to normal.

NURSING DIAGNOSIS:	SELF CARE DEFICIT (specify)
May be related to:	Effects of anesthesia, decreased strength and endurance, physical discomfort.
Possibly evidenced by:	Verbalization of inability to participate at level desired.
DESIRED OUTCOMES— CLIENT WILL:	Demonstrate techniques to meet self-care needs.
	Identify/use available resources.

ACTIONS/INTERVENTIONS	RATIONALE
Independent	
Ascertain severity/duration of discomfort. Note presence of postspinal headache.	Intense pain affects emotional and behavioral responses, so that the client may be unable to focus on self-care activities until her physical needs for comfort are met. Intense headache associated with upright position requires modification of activities and additional assistance to meet individual needs.
Assess client's psychologic status.	Physical pain experience may be compounded by mental pain that interferes with client's desire and motivation to assume autonomy.
Determine type of anesthesia; note any orders or protocol regarding positioning.	Clients who have undergone spinal anesthesia may be directed to lie flat and without pillow for 6–8 hr following administration of anesthesia.
Reposition client every 1–2 hr; assist with pulmonary exercises, ambulation, and leg exercises.	Helps prevent surgical complications such as phlebitis or pneumonia, which can occur when discomfort levels interfere with client's normal repositioning/activity.
Offer assistance as needed with hygiene (e.g., mouth care, bathing, back rubs, and perineal care).	Improves self-esteem; increases feelings of well-being.
Offer choices when possible (e.g., selection of juices, scheduling of bath, destination during ambulation).	Allows some autonomy even though client depends on professional assistance.
Collaborative	
Administer analgesic agent every 3–4 hr, as needed.	Reduces discomfort, which could interfere with ability to engage in self-care.
Convert i.v. line to heparin lock as appropriate.	Permits unrestricted movement of extremities, thereby allowing client to function more independently, regardless of ongoing intermittent i.v. therapy (e.g., antibiotics).

Maternal Assessment: 24 Hours Following Early Discharge ___

This plan of care focuses on the client who is discharged within 24 hours of delivery. It is to be used in conjunction with CP: The Client at 4 Hours to 3 Days Postpartum.

CLIENT ASSESSMENT DATA BASE

CIRCULATION

Blood pressure remains at pregnant readings (slightly below baseline).

Pulse between 60 and 90 bpm.

Superficial varicosities may be visible in lower extremities.

EGO INTEGRITY

May feel isolated, anxious, depressed, or fatigued.

May report stressors (e.g., employment, financial, living situation), concerns about personal abilities and assumption of mothering role.

ELIMINATION

Voiding 100 ml or greater in amount, without suprapubic tenderness or retention.

Probably has not experienced a return of normal bowel habits.

Hemorrhoids varying in size and number may be present.

Abdominal musculature may be weak and of "bread dough" consistency.

FOOD/FLUID

Weight reduced by 10–12 lb following delivery.

Physiologic edema may still be present.

PAIN/DISCOMFORT

Discomforts associated with episiotomy, perineal trauma, hemorrhoids, or afterpains.

Contractions strong and regular in the first 24-hour period, diminishing daily in frequency and intensity.

SAFETY

Lochia rubra moderate in amount with fleshy odor, may increase during breastfeeding.

Striae may be present on abdomen, breasts, and thighs.

Perineum or site of episiotomy repair may be edematous with good approximation of wound edges.

SEXUALITY

Breasts soft, nontender, and free of masses.

Nipples soft and free of fissures or lesions.

Uterus firm, midline, and located at the umbilicus (uterus is larger in multipara or in client with overdistention).

SOCIAL INTERACTIONS

May report lack of/or inadequate support systems; concerns regarding roles of individual family members, role mastery, or disequilibrium (especially in blended family).

DIAGNOSTIC STUDIES

Routine assessment may include complete blood count, urinalysis, and culture and sensitivity, as indicated by physical finding.

NURSING PRIORITIES

1. Evaluate postpartum status of client.
2. Promote optimal physical and emotional well-being.
3. Facilitate client's/couple's positive adaptation to parenting roles, family growth, and autonomy.

NURSING DIAGNOSIS:	**PAIN [ACUTE]/DISCOMFORT***
May be related to:	Mechanical trauma, tissue edema/engorgement or distention, hormonal effects, excessive fatigue.
Possibly evidenced by:	Reports of cramping (afterpains) and perineal discomfort, guarding/distraction behaviors.
DESIRED OUTCOMES— CLIENT WILL:	Identify sources of discomfort.
	Take appropriate measures to reduce discomfort.
	*Authors' note: Currently there is no NANDA diagnostic label that addresses issues of comfort below the level of Pain [acute] or chronic. Although the label of **Discomfort** is not approved, we believe it speaks more directly to the identified problem.

ACTIONS/INTERVENTIONS	RATIONALE
Independent	
Inspect breast and nipple tissue; note presence of engorgement and/or cracked nipples.	Breast engorgement, nipple tenderness, or presence of cracks on nipple (in lactating client) may occur 2–3 days postpartum and result in severe discomfort.
Review appropriate interventions specific to lactating/nonlactating client. (Refer to CP: The Client at 4 Hours to 3 Days Postpartum, ND: Pain, [acute]/Discomfort.)	Reduces level of discomfort/pain and promotes self-care and sense of control.
Assess uterine tenderness; assess presence and frequency/intensity of afterpains.	Afterpains may continue for 2–3 days postpartum, although their frequency and intensity lessen with time. Factors intensifying afterpains include multiparity, uterine overdistension, and breastfeeding.

ACTIONS/INTERVENTIONS	RATIONALE
Independent	
Ascertain frequency/amount of voidings. Instruct client in use of Kegel exercise. (Refer to ND: Urinary Elimination, altered, high risk for.)	Return of normal bladder function may take 4–7 days, and overdistention of bladder may create feelings of urgency and discomfort. Kegel exercise aids in healing and recovery of tone of pubococcygeal muscle to limit urinary stress incontinence.
Inspect condition of perineum or site of episiotomy repair. Note edema, ecchymosis, lacerations, or discomfort. Recommend that client inspect area daily.	Identifies potential sources of pain and discomfort. Routine monitoring may prevent or lessen development of complications.
Recommend use of ice, sprays, topical ointments, creams, sitting with gluteal muscles contracted over site of episiotomy repair, and warm sitz (tub) baths.	Ice or other cold application in the first 24 hours postpartum reduces edema and provides localized anesthesia. Heat promotes vasodilation and perineal healing. Topical medications contain local anesthetics and reduce discomfort. Use of gluteal tightening while sitting reduces stress and direct pressure on perineum.
Inspect perineum for hemorrhoids. Suggest reinsertion of hemorrhoid with lubricated finger cot or rubber glove.	Aids in regression of hemorrhoids, reduces vulvar varicosities, and promotes return to normal bowel functioning.
Provide information about needs for sleep and rest; assess emotional state and well-being.	Overwhelming fatigue and negative feelings may magnify discomfort associated with normal healing and regeneration in the postpartal period.
Encourage client to adopt progressive level of ambulation and activity. Assess cultural impact on activity.	Early, progressive ambulation facilitates bladder and bowel functioning and enhances circulation, thereby reducing edema and promoting healing. Various cultural groups believe in restricting activity (e.g., some Southeast Asians may believe that the mother should remain in bed close to a fireplace for 30 days after delivery).
Collaborative	
Suggest use of mild analgesics as recommended or prescribed by physician or healthcare provider. Emphasize need to avoid products containing aspirin. For lactating client, medications should be taken 30–60 min prior to breastfeeding.	Promotes comfort without side effects of acetylsalicylic acid (reduced prothrombin synthesis may possibly increase lochial discharge). Analgesics reduce discomfort associated with oxytocin stimulation of myometrium during lactation.
Suggest use of gentle laxative (milk of magnesia) or stool softeners.	Enhances bowel elimination, reducing discomfort of constipation and associated hemorrhoids. (Refer to CP: The Client at 4 Hours to 3 Days Postpartum, ND: Constipation.)

NURSING DIAGNOSIS:	**INFECTION, HIGH RISK FOR**
Risk factors may include:	Tissue trauma and/or broken skin, decreased hemoglobin (Hb), invasive procedures and/or increased environmental exposure.

Possibly evidenced by:	[Not applicable; presence of signs/symptoms establishes an **actual** diagnosis.]
DESIRED OUTCOMES— CLIENT WILL:	Identify techniques to reduce risks and/or promote healing.
	Display wound free of purulent drainage.
	Be free of infection, be afebrile, and have normal lochial flow and character.

ACTIONS/INTERVENTIONS	RATIONALE
Independent	
Assess client's temperature, pulse, and respirations.	Elevation of vital signs may reflect developing infection.
Recommend medical asepsis for pad changes, and application of topical sprays, ointments, or witch hazel compresses.	Helps prevent rectal contaminants from entering vagina or urethra.
Encourage client to take warm sitz baths 3 to 4 times daily for 20 min, especially if signs of localized infection are present.	Promotes localized vasodilation, and increased oxygenation of tissues, enhancing healing.
Reiterate instructions regarding massage of fundus (i.e., gently 4 to 5 times daily with cupped hand, using second hand for support above symphysis pubis several times per day).	Enhances uterine contractility. Uterus involutes approximately 1 to 2 cm (1 fingerbreadth) per day from the level of the umbilicus. Delayed involution may suggest infection.
Note amount and odor of lochial discharge. Review normal progression from rubra to serosa to alba.	Lochia normally has a fleshy odor; however, in endometritis, the discharge may be purulent and foul-smelling, and may fail to demonstrate normal progression.
Evaluate condition of nipples.	The development of nipple fissures/cracks potentiates risk of mastitis.
Recommend routine examination of breasts and perineum.	Early detection of developing problems allows for intervention, thereby reducing the risk of serious complications.
Provide information about urinary tract infection (UTI) and evaluate client for signs and symptoms, including dysuria, frequency, urgency, and pain. Note any tenderness of suprapubic or costovertebral angle.	Stasis, poor hygiene, overdistention, or bacteria introduced during labor and delivery may predispose client to development of UTI.
Review importance of nutrition, fluid intake, and adequate rest.	Promotes healing and general well-being, reducing risk of infection.
Collaborative	
Obtain "clean catch" urine specimen for culture; if signs or symptoms present, notify healthcare provider.	Verifies presence and type of infection, and appropriate treatment needs.
Discuss rationale and protocol for administration of antibiotic therapy if UTI is present.	Antibiotic therapy eradicates pathogenic organisms.

ACTIONS/INTERVENTIONS

Collaborative

Discuss findings suggestive of endometritis with physician or nurse midwife. Help family arrange for transportation to health center or hospital emergency room for further assessment.

Initiate use of home I.V. service or visiting nurse services if antibiotic by parenteral infusion is ordered. (Refer to CP: Puerperal Infection.)

RATIONALE

Findings need to be confirmed by healthcare provider and by laboratory culture.

Allows client to remain at home while receiving treatment to eradicate infection.

NURSING DIAGNOSIS:	FLUID VOLUME DEFICIT, HIGH RISK FOR
Risk factors may include:	Reduced intake and/or inadequate replacement, increased urine output, hemorrhage.
Possibly evidenced by:	[Not applicable; presence of signs/symptoms establishes an **actual** diagnosis.]
DESIRED OUTCOMES— CLIENT WILL:	Display blood pressure (BP) and pulse within normal limits, firm uterus at the umbilicus, with moderate flow of lochia rubra.

ACTIONS/INTERVENTIONS

Independent

Assess BP and pulse.

Reinforce the use of uterine massage and fundal monitoring.

Discuss normal involutionary changes and signs of subinvolution.

Assess client's understanding of normal lochial changes.

Assist client using a mirror to assess own episiotomy/laceration repair.

Discuss needs for fluid replacement and signs of dehydration, especially in lactating client.

Assess voiding frequency and amounts.

RATIONALE

Risk of postpartal hemorrhage exists up to 28 days following delivery. Possible causes of hemorrhage include inadequate myometrial contractions (uterine atony), retention of placental tissue, and birth canal lacerations. Hypotension and tachycardia may reflect hypovolemia.

Promotes uterine contactility, reducing risk of atony and hemorrhage.

Client should be able to identify signs of hemorrhage and institute appropriate interventions if excessive bleeding occurs. (Refer to CP: Postpartal Hemorrhage.)

Briskly flowing, bright red lochia with clots is abnormal and indicates possible hemorrhage. Multiparas or clients with overdistention of the uterus tend to have more lochia than primiparas. Breastfeeding clients have a large amount of lochia during or just after feedings.

Lacerations of the birth canal constitute the second leading cause of postdelivery hemorrhage.

Client should consume at least 8 glasses or more of fluid per day to replace losses and to provide sufficient fluid for milk production.

Kidney function is an indicator of circulating blood volume.

ACTIONS/INTERVENTIONS

Collaborative

Notify physician or healthcare provider if fundus remains boggy or fails to contract with massage.

Prepare client and her family for transfer to physician's office or hospital setting if necessary.

Provide information about use of ergot preparation. Assess BP prior to administration. (Note: Ergot is contraindicated in lactating client.)

RATIONALE

Medication may be required to maintain continued myometrial contraction. Client may need to be evaluated by physician.

Situation may warrant additional evaluation/intervention, use of hospital emergency equipment, or treatment for stabilization purposes.

Ergot preparation may be necessary to maintain myometrial contractility; however, it causes generalized vasoconstriction, possibly leading to hypertension.

NURSING DIAGNOSIS:	KNOWLEDGE DEFICIT [LEARNING NEED], regarding progression of condition, self-care needs, and possible complications.
May be related to:	Unfamiliarity with information resources, lack of recall/incomplete information presented, misinterpretation.
Possibly evidenced by:	Verbalizations of concerns/misconceptions, hesitancy in or inadequate performance of activities.
DESIRED OUTCOMES— CLIENT WILL:	Verbalize understanding of physiologic changes, individual needs, expected outcomes.
	Perform necessary activities/procedures correctly and explain reasons for actions.

ACTIONS/INTERVENTIONS

Independent

Assess client's knowledge, understanding, and ability to apply concepts related to self-care.

Identify client's perception of learning needs regarding self-care and of needs related to anticipated physical and emotional changes.

Provide information related to normal uterine involutional and lochial changes and the benefits of fundal massage.

Review nutritional status and prenatal and postdelivery Hb and Hct levels. Provide appropriate information about dietary and fluid needs. (Refer to CP: Maternal Assessment: 1 Week Following Discharge, ND: Nutrition, altered, less than body requirements, high risk for.)

RATIONALE

Usually, some information is presented during hospitalization; however, fatigue, anxiety, or time limitations may have a negative impact on learning at that time. Reinforcement may therefore be needed.

Collaborative plan based on client's perceived needs reduces anxiety, promotes self-responsibility, and optimizes learning.

Self-massage stimulates uterine contractility, reduces lochial flow, and promotes involution.

Helps determine needs for further learning.

ACTIONS/INTERVENTIONS	RATIONALE
Independent	
Provide information about breast care for nonlactating client, including discussion of the need for support, application of ice, and protocol for use of oral lactation suppressants; for example, the ingestion of bromocriptine mesylate (Parlodel) with meals.	Mechanical means of lactation suppression through use of binder and ice are recommended over lactation suppressants, which have a high rate of rebound engorgement.
Provide information for lactating client, including nipple and breast care, physiology of lactation, concept of demand feedings, infant positioning, dietary and fluid needs, and the need to avoid taking medications without first consulting healthcare provider.	Helps promote successful lactation, enhances milk supply, and reduces possible trauma to nipples. Some drugs are contraindicated and should be used with caution during lactation because of possible effects in newborn.
Discuss need for sleep and rest.	Extra sleep and rest are needed to overcome sleep deficit and fatigue and facilitate coping.
Provide information regarding hygiene and perineal care.	Helps facilitate autonomy, prevent infection, and aid healing.
Discuss importance of progressive postpartal exercise program.	Beneficial in toning musculature; increases circulation, and enhances feelings of general well-being.
Review importance of preventing venous stasis and signs/symptoms of complications (e.g., warmth, redness, tenderness, presence of positive Homans' sign).	Plasma losses, increased platelets, and persistent vasodilation from progesterone increase likelihood of venous stasis (e.g., visible varicosities) and thrombophlebitis.
Discuss relationship between parenting role, use of effective coping mechanisms, and physical and emotional factors (e.g., adequate rest, nutrition, and support).	Provides information to assist client in making decisions regarding routine activities that foster positive physical and emotional adaptation.
Review symptoms/normalcy of transitory depression (postpartal blues).	As many as 80% of mothers experience a transitory depression, which usually resolves spontaneously within a week or so. Persistence of mood swings and emotional lability indicate need for further evaluation.
Provide number of 24-hour telephone resource contact.	Promotes reassurance that assistance is available if needed.
Reinforce importance of 6-week postpartal examination by healthcare provider.	Follow-up visit is necessary to evaluate recovery of reproductive organs, healing of incision/episiotomy repair, general well-being, and adaptation to life changes.
Refer family to community resource groups or for follow-up with social services or home healthcare agency.	Provides information and emotional support; reduces possibility of negative outcome for infant and family.

NURSING DIAGNOSIS:	SLEEP PATTERN DISTURBANCE
May be related to:	Hormonal and psychologic responses (intense exhilaration, anxiety, excitement), pain/discomfort, exhausting process of labor/delivery, needs/demands of family members.
Possibly evidenced by:	Verbal reports of difficulty falling asleep/not feeling well rested, irritability, dark circles under eyes, frequent yawning.
DESIRED OUTCOMES— CLIENT WILL:	Identify adjustments to accommodate changes required by demands of new family member.
	Attain at least 8 hr of sleep per night and nap daily.
	Report feeling rested.

ACTIONS/INTERVENTIONS	RATIONALE
Independent	
Assess client's perception of fatigue, needs for sleep, and sleep deficits.	Identifies client's perception of the problem.
Assess home environment, family size and situation, routine, and available help.	The client who is discharged early may believe that she has to take on sole responsibility for infant care tasks, as well as immediately assuming her former roles associated with household management and mothering tasks. Such a situation results in excess fatigue, intensifying a sleep deficit. Examination of household pattern allows realistic appraisal of available times for resting and sleeping.
Assist client in planning rest/sleep periods during day, realistically, within schedule of family members.	
Discuss need to retire earlier than usual while infant is waking for night feedings.	
Provide information related to positive aspects of sleep and rest.	Sleep and inactivity reduce basal metabolic rate and allow oxygen and nutrients to be used for healing.
Encourage client to take a vitamin and iron tablet daily, and to select appropriate diet.	Helps restore Hb levels needed to transport oxygen and promote healing; helps overcome nutritional deficiencies, which contribute to feelings of excess fatigue and inadequate energy levels.
Encourage limitation of number and length of visiting sessions.	Overexhaustion may result from time spent with frequent visitors and well-meaning friends.
Collaborative	
Compare prenatal and postpartal Hb/Hct levels.	Low Hb/Hct levels increase feelings of fatigue, weakness, and faintness.

NURSING DIAGNOSIS:	URINARY ELIMINATION, ALTERED, HIGH RISK FOR
Risk factors may include:	Hormonal effects (fluid shifts and/or increased renal plasma flow), mechanical trauma, tissue edema.

Possibly evidenced by:	[Not applicable; presence of signs/symptoms establishes an **actual** diagnosis.]
DESIRED OUTCOMES— CLIENT WILL:	Empty bladder with each void.

ACTIONS/INTERVENTIONS	RATIONALE

Independent

Assess urinary functioning, noting frequency and amount of voidings per day and feelings of urine retention or bladder fullness.	Voidings should be moderate in amount (100 ml) to be considered sufficient, although client does not measure them at home. Client should empty her bladder 5 to 7 times per day, depending on amount of prenatal fluid retention and degree of diuresis. Retention may occur, possibly leading to infection or overdistention, which may cause nerve damage.
Assess fundal height and location before and after voiding. Note displacement to the right of umbilicus.	A full bladder displaces the fundus and may interfere with contraction or involution of uterus.
Discuss normal fluid needs and replacement.	Six to 8 glasses of fluid per day help prevent stasis and dehydration and replace fluid lost at delivery.
Note prenatal and intrapartal history of episodes of UTI, catheterizations, or bladder trauma.	These factors may contribute to infection with consequent alteration in pattern of elimination.
Instruct client to use Kegel exercise 50 to 100 times daily.	Increases circulation to perineum and helps treat stress incontinence.
Encourage client to sit in warm bath or take a warm shower if she has difficulty voiding.	Warm water running over the body or relaxation of the perineum and urethra facilitates voiding.

NURSING DIAGNOSIS:	**SELF CARE DEFICIT, HIGH RISK FOR**
Risk factors may include:	Fatigue, decreased endurance, pain/discomfort.
Possibly evidenced by:	[Not applicable; presence of signs/symptoms establishes an **actual** diagnosis.]
DESIRED OUTCOMES— CLIENT WILL:	Demonstrate interest in learning concepts of self-care.
	Assume increasing responsibility for own care.

ACTIONS/INTERVENTIONS	RATIONALE

Independent

Assess client's physical and psychologic well-being.	Any alteration in physical or emotional well-being may retard assumption of autonomous role in self-care. Until client moves from a "taking in" to a "taking hold" phase, she may require assistance with self-care and infant care.

ACTIONS/INTERVENTIONS	RATIONALE
Independent	
Assess client's fatigue level, length of labor, time of delivery (i.e., day or night), and sleep deficit. (Refer to ND: Sleep Pattern disturbance.)	Physical need for sleep must be met before client can begin to assume self-care.
Note degree of autonomy and self-responsibility.	Client begins to assume increasing responsibility for her own care as her condition improves.
Evaluate client's understanding of self-care and self-responsibility. Provide information as needed.	Knowledge base determines amount of information necessary to facilitate assuming self-care role.
Evaluate plans for home assistance during post-partal recovery period.	Help in the home, especially for the first several days following discharge, is critical to assist the client and her family with household management and meal preparation, and to provide care as needed for client and infant.
Discuss available community resources (e.g., visiting nurse services, home care aide).	Visiting nurse can assess health status of client. Home care aide, now an integral part of many hospital early discharge programs, assists in home management and provides specific infant/client care as necessary.

Maternal Assessment: 1 Week Following Discharge _____

CLIENT ASSESSMENT DATA BASE

CIRCULATION

Vital signs within normal limits.

EGO INTEGRITY

Emotional tone and responses may vary from one of delight to a sense of overwhelming disorganization or anxiety, especially in first-time mother.

ELIMINATION

May report voiding difficulty or stress incontinence.

May report difficulty with bowel evacuation, with decreased frequency, hard-formed stool.

PAIN/DISCOMFORT

May report continued discomfort associated with afterpains.

Engorgement may be present in lactating client.

SAFETY

Episiotomy or cesarean incision free of edema, indurated areas, redness, and exudate; tissue edges approximated.

SEXUALITY

Uterus nontender, palpable at symphysis pubis.

Lochial flow scant and pinkish-brown in color (serosa) and of 4 to 10 days' duration.

Breasts in lactating client increased in size and with increased milk supply.

Nipples free of redness, cracks, and fissures.

Engorgement may be present in lactating client, subsiding in nonlactating client.

DIAGNOSTIC STUDIES

Urine: Negative for albumin/glucose.
Additional testing: As indicated; e.g., urinalysis, culture and sensitivity, complete blood count to include white blood cell (WBC) count, hemoglobin/hematocrit (Hb/Hct).

NURSING PRIORITIES

1. Promote maternal/infant well-being.
2. Foster optimal adaptation to physical and emotional changes.
3. Provide anticipatory guidance for optimal integration of new family member and adaptation to role changes.

ACTIONS/INTERVENTIONS	RATIONALE
Independent	
Discuss signs of excess physical and emotional fatigue.	Lack of energy, deep circles under the eyes, and statements indicating extreme fatigue indicate inadequate sleep and rest. Self-monitoring and awareness of developing problem allows for timely intervention.
Review intrapartal and early postpartal events.	Cumulative sleep loss must be overcome as soon as possible to facilitate psychologic and physiologic recuperation.
Determine infant's sleep-wake cycles. Suggest ongoing efforts to modify the infant's behaviors to promote more wakeful periods during the daytime.	Helps infant to maintain progressively longer wakeful periods during the day and to sleep longer stretches at night. (Note: Approximately 5 weeks are needed to regulate the infant's cycle.)
Encourage restriction or lessening of outside activities. Limit number of visitors.	Helps prevent overexhaustion.
Provide information about daily iron and vitamin intake and the need for balanced diet.	Helps restore Hb levels needed for oxygen transport, promotes healing, and overcomes nutritional deficiencies, which may contribute to feelings of excess fatigue and inadequate energy levels.
Determine family structure and number of members. Assess work capabilities and responsibilities of each member.	Household tasks should be shared so that division of labor reduces amount of responsibility that client assumes and allows client to conserve energy.
Review family's daily routine.	Assists client in creative problem-solving to identify times available for resting and napping throughout the day.
Assess availability/use of support systems.	Identifies needs and means of physical and emotional assistance.
Encourage client to establish a quiet, relaxing routine prior to retiring (e.g., reading a book or having a glass of warm milk or wine).	Aids in relaxation; promotes sleep.

NURSING DIAGNOSIS:	KNOWLEDGE DEFICIT [LEARNING NEED], regarding self-care and infant care
May be related to:	Lack of exposure/recall, misinterpretation, unfamiliarity with resources.
Possibly evidenced by:	Verbalization of concerns/misconceptions, hesitancy in or inadequate performance of activities, inappropriate behaviors (e.g., crying).
DESIRED OUTCOMES— CLIENT WILL:	Identify individual learning needs.
	Perform necessary activities/procedures correctly and explain reasons for the actions.
	Verbalize understanding of physiologic changes, individual and infant needs
	Modify behaviors when appropriate.

ACTIONS/INTERVENTIONS	RATIONALE

Independent

Determine client's perception of problems and needs.	Establishes individual needs and allows for optimal information sharing.
Ascertain understanding of normal physical changes at 1 week following discharge. Provide information about appropriate measures to take should a problem arise.	Identifies normal and abnormal physical findings, and encourages anticipatory planning, enhancing independence.
Identify emotional concerns at this time, and discuss normalcy of these feelings.	Most mothers, especially first-time mothers, verbalize a sense of disorganization and feelings of an emotional letdown in the early postpartal period. Such feelings are intensified by fatigue and by crying infant.
Provide information as needed about signs and symptoms associated with endometritis, mastitis, incisional and urinary tract infection (UTI), and the need to notify healthcare provider.	Identifies potential problems necessitating intervention by healthcare provider.
Provide information regarding resumption of menstrual cycle/ovulation and sexual intercourse.	Among nonlactating women, 40% menstruate by 2 weeks postpartum; of these, 50% do not ovulate during the first menstrual cycle. Among lactating women, 15% resume menstrual cycle by 6 weeks postpartum, and 80% of the first menstrual cycles are anovulatory. Couple can resume sexual activity when client is comfortable and lochial flow has ceased (usually 3–4 wk after vaginal delivery). Client who underwent cesarean delivery should delay intercourse until 6 weeks postpartum.
Discuss plans for contraceptive usage.	Conception could occur prior to the 6-week checkup, and studies indicate increased risk of complications or untoward outcomes for pregnancies spaced close together. Couple needs to select and use a temporary or permanent method of family planning.

377

ACTIONS/INTERVENTIONS	RATIONALE

Independent

Provide information about physiologic changes in sexual response postpartum. (Refer to CP: Maternal Assessment: 4 to 6 Weeks Following Delivery, ND: Sexuality Patterns, altered.)	Reduction in rapidity and intensity of sexual response is normal. Continued low estrogen levels result in vaginal dryness, possibly necessitating use of water-soluble jelly, cocoa butter, or contraceptive creams or jellies for lubrication. Size of orgasmic platform and strength of orgasmic contraction are reduced, and vasoconstriction of labia minora and labia majora is delayed.
Reinforce information, as appropriate, for lactating client regarding physiology of lactation, dietary concerns, measures to reduce discomfort of engorgement, and nipple/breast care. Recommend books and other written materials and support groups.	Facilitates positive adaptation to breastfeeding role.
Review nutritional needs for lactating or nonlactating client; include information on caloric needs, protein, iron, and vitamin C. (Refer to ND: Nutrition, altered, less than body requirements.)	Helps client meet nutritional needs necessary for recuperation, restoration, and healing in postpartal period.
Emphasize need to prevent venous stasis, and review signs of phlebitis formation; e.g. warmth, redness, tenderness, calf pain.	Changes in circulating volume or cellular components and alterations in mobility enhance risk of thrombophlebitis.
Instruct client in appropriate muscle-tightening exercises, e.g., Kegel exercise.	Helps strengthen and tone perineal urethral muscles to improve control of urine flow.
Discuss/evaluate ongoing exercise program. Provide information about importance of adhering to prescribed program.	Exercise helps tone muscles and restore body contours.
Provide information for client with cesarean delivery regarding activity level and exercise and the need to avoid strenuous lifting/stretching.	Lifting any object heavier than the baby for 2 weeks after delivery may contribute to stress on healing tissues and result in wound dehiscence.
Reinforce need for evaluation by healthcare provider at 4–6 weeks after delivery.	Necessary to ensure that physiologic/emotional homeostasis has been reestablished.
Identify community resources; e.g., breastfeeding support groups, parenting classes.	Helps meet continued educational needs of client/couple.

NURSING DIAGNOSIS:	**PARENTING, ALTERED, HIGH RISK FOR**
Risk factors may include:	Lack of support between/from significant others, multiple demands of home/family, excess fatigue, unrealistic expectations for self/infant/partner, presence of stressors (e.g., financial, housing, employment, use of outside helper/extended family members).
Possibly evidenced by:	[Not applicable; presence of signs/symptoms establishes an **actual** diagnosis.]
DESIRED OUTCOMES— CLIENT/COUPLE WILL:	Identify concerns related to parenting.
	Discuss parenting role realistically.
	Demonstrate appropriate bonding behaviors.
	Identify available resources.

ACTIONS/INTERVENTIONS	RATIONALE
Independent	
Assess client's/couple's interaction with infant. Document verbal and nonverbal responses and presence of positive or negative behaviors.	In American culture, attachment is considered positive if the parent makes eye contact with the infant, calls the infant by name, uses an en face position, talks in a high-pitched voice, and holds the baby close.
Note impact of culture on interaction.	Different cultures have different values/beliefs about what constitutes positive attachment behaviors.
Assess client's/couple's strengths and weaknesses, maturity level, reaction to conception, and preparation for parenting.	Directly impacts on ability/desire to gain comfort/skill in parenting.
Determine client's/couple's perception of infant behaviors.	Client/couple with unrealistic perception of infant behaviors or who voices displeasure with specific caretaking tasks (e.g., diapering/feeding) will need closer monitoring and more extensive support.
Develop plan for subsequent visits, highlighting areas of particular concern.	Helps promote positive adaptation to new role; helps client focus on possible problems.
Collaborative	
Refer family to social services home healthcare agency follow-up, or to community resource groups.	Provides support and reduces possible negative outcomes for infant/family.

NURSING DIAGNOSIS:	**PAIN/DISCOMFORT*, HIGH RISK FOR**
Risk factors may include:	Tissue edema/engorgement, mechanical trauma, excessive fatigue.
Possibly evidenced by:	[Not applicable; presence of signs/symptoms establishes an **actual** diagnosis.]
DESIRED OUTCOMES— CLIENT WILL:	Use appropriate measures to promote comfort.
	Verbalize relief of pain/discomfort.
	*Authors' note: Currently there is no NANDA diagnostic label that addresses issues of comfort below the level of Pain [acute] or chronic. Although the label of **Discomfort** is not approved, we believe it speaks more directly to the identified problem.

ACTIONS/INTERVENTIONS	RATIONALE
Independent	
Determine location/nature of discomfort.	Identifies individual needs.
Review sleep/rest pattern; note feelings of excess fatigue.	Fatigue can negatively affect lactation and increase discomforts associated with engorgement, as well as impair coping and client's response to pain.

ACTIONS/INTERVENTIONS	RATIONALE
Independent	
Inspect breasts for degree of engorgement.	Helps determine severity of problem. Engorgement is usually more severe in primipara than in multipara.
Encourage use of supportive bra.	Supports and uplifts, alleviating pain and tenderness caused by heavy, engorged breasts.
Recommend application of ice or cool compresses for 20–30 min 3 to 4 times daily, for nonlactating client; apply breast binder. Advise client to avoid breast stimulation or milk expression.	Provides vasoconstriction of blood vessels; promotes local anesthesia and comfort. Prevents or reduces milk production and engorgement.
Provide nonlactating client with information about possible rebound congestion, which is especially likely to occur after 14-day administration of bromocriptine mesylate (Parlodel).	Up to 40% of women experience rebound congestion and engorgement related to stopping of lactation suppressants such as bromocriptine mesylate (Parlodel).
Encourage use of creams, air-drying of nipples for 20 min after feedings, avoidance of soaps, and avoidance of plastic liners inside nursing pads. Instruct client to change pads when wet or moist.	Helps toughen nipples and prevent cracking. By allowing nipples to remain in a moist environment, plastic liners promote bacterial growth and may cause skin breakdown.
Note frequency and length of feedings in lactating client.	Engorgement may interfere with breastfeeding, because it makes the breast and nipple hard, making it difficult for the infant to suckle. Increasing frequency of feedings during engorgement promotes comfort and helps to empty breasts to ensure an adequate milk supply.
Suggest warm compresses before feedings for lactating client.	Aids in let-down reflex to promote easier emptying during feeding.
Instruct lactating client in removal of milk through manual expression or use of breast pump.	Removal of milk from breast of provides relief from engorgement; however, removal of too much milk increases the milk supply, possibly causing further engorgement.
Inspect nipples for any areas of indurated masses, cracks, fissures, or redness.	Sore or cracked nipples can create intense discomfort during lactation, especially at the beginning of the feeding when the infant is most hungry and sucking is most intense.
Limit feedings to 5 min on each breast when nipple is cracked, gradually increasing feedings by 2 min each day. Initiate feeding on nontender nipple for several feedings in succession if only one nipple is sore or cracked.	Helps limit exposure to trauma; however, limiting sucking for too long reduces milk supply and promotes engorgement. Baby suckles most intensely in the first 5 min of the feeding, creating greater pressure on the initial breast.
Note fundal height; assess for rigidity or guarding on examination. Note presence of foul-smelling lochia.	Uterine discomfort should have disappeared by 1 wk following discharge. Continued tenderness may signify infection.
Inspect site of episiotomy repair or cesarean incision.	Continued discomfort, tenderness, edema, or loss of tissue approximation indicates need for further evaluation by healthcare provider.
Suggest continued sitz baths 3 to 4 times daily for 20 min if site of episiotomy is uncomfortable, or if third- to fourth-degree lacerations were present at delivery.	Promotes vasodilation and increased tissue oxygenation/nutrition, enhancing healing.

ACTIONS/INTERVENTIONS

Collaborative

Suggest use of mild nonaspirin analgesics if necessary, especially 30–60 min before breastfeeding.

Refer to healthcare provider if uterine or wound discomfort is excessive.

RATIONALE

Reduces discomfort and promotes relaxation during feeding; facilitates the let-down reflex in lactating client.

Further evaluation is needed to determine the cause of discomfort and appropriate interventions.

NURSING DIAGNOSIS:	FAMILY COPING: POTENTIAL FOR GROWTH
May be related to:	Sufficiently meeting individual needs and adaptive tasks, enabling goals of self-actualization to surface.
Possibly evidenced by:	Family member(s) moving in direction of health-promoting and enriching lifestyle.
DESIRED OUTCOMES— CLIENT/FAMILY WILL:	Verbalize gradual improvement and smooth transition of new family member into home situation.
	Identify tasks leading to desired changes.
	Express feelings of self-confidence and satisfaction with progress and adaptation being made.

ACTIONS/INTERVENTIONS

Independent

Evaluate situational support and home assistance (e.g., husband, relatives, friends, private duty nurses, home care service).

Determine past successful coping mechanisms.

Encourage client to rest and to assume only the responsibilities directly related to care of herself and of the newborn. Encourage client to allow others to take on responsibilities related to upkeep of the house and meals.

Discuss client's/couple's perceptions of adjustment to the infant and to parenting roles and responsibilities. Provide information about normalcy of feelings of inadequacy, stress, and disequilibrium associated with role transition, especially for first-time parents. Document areas of concern for future assessments.

Evaluate family structure and situation, relationships of individual members to one another, and cultural background.

RATIONALE

Home assistance is an essential element in facilitating postpartal adaptation.

Building on strengths promotes self-esteem and enhances ability to deal with current situation.

Allows client to focus energy on interaction between infant and herself; allows client to conserve energy for physical and emotional recuperation.

First-time parents have been known to experience varying degrees of stress and crisis associated with adjustment to their child and integration of this child into the family. The challenge of the crisis can serve as a catalyst to growth and enhanced adaptive capacity.

Blended family resulting from remarriage may require a longer period of adaptation and present a more complex situation than a nuclear family. Extended families may provide added physical and emotional support.

ACTIONS/INTERVENTIONS

Independent

Provide anticipatory guidance related to the time needed to adjust to the new situation and family member.

Collaborative

Discuss need for family counseling; make appropriate referrals when indicated.

RATIONALE

Crisis associated with the birth of a newborn is often resolved in 4–6 wk. However, because of the potentially overwhelming transition required, the crisis may last as long as 3 months.

May be necessary to help members resolve changes and to continue positive adjustment to new roles.

NURSING DIAGNOSIS:	**NUTRITION, ALTERED, LESS THAN BODY REQUIREMENTS, HIGH RISK FOR**
Risk factors may include:	Intake insufficient to meet metabolic demands/correct existing deficiencies (e.g., lactation, anemia/excessive blood loss, infection/excessive tissue trauma, desire to regain prenatal weight).
Possibly evidenced by:	[Not applicable; presence of signs/symptoms establishes an **actual** diagnosis.]
DESIRED OUTCOMES— CLIENT WILL:	Report dietary intake that meets needs for lactation (as appropriate) and tissue healing/general physical restoration. Continue to take daily vitamin preparation as needed.

ACTIONS/INTERVENTIONS

Independent

Determine dietary intake for past 24 hr, history of dietary habits prior to and during pregnancy, and cultural beliefs/background.

Provide information regarding the basic food groups to correct deficiencies and inadequacies within constraints of family budget and cultural preferences. Stress need for increased amounts (and food sources) of dietary protein, calories, and vitamin C.

Review prenatal Hb and Hct and the amount of blood loss at delivery. Note signs of anemia (e.g., dizziness, excess fatigue, and pallor).

Provide information about need for daily intake of vitamin and iron preparation, as indicated.

Suggest temporary use of ready-made convenience foods or having meals prepared by relatives, friends, or significant other(s).

RATIONALE

Identifies usual eating habits/deficiencies and individual needs.

Protein is needed to promote tissue growth, healing, and regeneration and to offset catabolic process. Calories are necessary for normal metabolic processes, especially for the underweight client; vitamin C is necessary for cell wall synthesis. Financial needs may necessitate use of protein sources other than meat.

Preexisting anemic state or excessive blood loss may result in pallor and listlessness. Reduced Hb levels may retard healing process.

Iron and vitamin intake for 4 to 6 weeks postpartum can overcome dietary deficiencies, ensure nutritious milk supply, and aid in tissue healing.

Demands of caring for newborn, leave little time for preparation of balanced meals.

382

ACTIONS/INTERVENTIONS	RATIONALE

Independent

Weigh client. Establish desired weight, and compare with prepregnancy and initial postpartum weight.

Average weight loss at delivery is 12 lb, mainly attributable to infant and products of conception. An additional loss of approximately 5 lb usually follows over the next 2 wk.

Determine caloric requirements for nonlactating client and possible weight reduction diet.

Caloric requirements return to prepregnancy levels unless client was severely underweight. Desired weight can be obtained by reducing caloric intake by 300 kcal/day and establishing an appropriate exercise program.

Discuss dietary needs for the lactating client. Identify foods that may have allergic or other adverse effects on infant, and discuss ways of assessing infant's discomfort.

Intake needs to be increased by 500–800 kcal/day to provide adequate milk production and infant nourishment. Protein needs are 10 g less than they were during pregnancy. Needs for iron, calcium, thiamine, ascorbic acid, and vitamin D are similar to those during pregnancy; the need for vitamin A, niacin, and riboflavin increase. Some foods are passed through the mother's milk and may cause discomfort or allergic reaction in the infant.

Review fluid needs for lactating client.

Fluid intake should be 2500–3000 ml/day.

Provide information regarding progressive postpartal exercise program. Provide illustrations.

Exercise increases metabolic rate and improves utilization of calories while enhancing muscle tone.

Collaborative

Consult with dietitian as needed.

May be necessary to plan and restructure diet.

NURSING DIAGNOSIS:	INFECTION, HIGH RISK FOR
Risk factors may include:	Tissue trauma and/or broken skin, decreased Hb, invasive procedures and/or increased environmental exposure, malnutrition.
Possibly evidenced by:	[Not applicable; presence of signs/symptoms establishes an **actual** diagnosis.]
DESIRED OUTCOMES— CLIENT WILL:	Relate techniques to reduce risks and promote healing.
	Display signs of wound healing and be free of purulent drainage.
	Be free of infection.

ACTIONS/INTERVENTIONS	RATIONALE

Independent

Check vital signs; assess client's general physical status.

Temperature greater than 100.4°F (38°C), general malaise, anorexia, and chills suggest infection.

ACTIONS/INTERVENTIONS	RATIONALE
Independent	
Review intrapartal and postpartal events, noting prolonged labor, premature rupture of membranes, excessive blood loss, or retained/adherent placenta.	These factors increase risk of endometritis or other infectious process.
Determine whether infant was colonized with staphylococci in the nursery.	Increases risk of cross-contamination, especially to lactating clients.
Evaluate client's hygiene practices. Stress need for washing hands before and after perineal pad changes and before handling breasts or infant.	Identifies practices that could contribute to development of infection.
Assess height of fundus. Note color, amount, and character of lochial flow.	Endometritis may be associated with subinvolution or with presence of foul-smelling or purulent lochial flow.
Inspect site of episiotomy repair or cesarean incision. Note redness, exudate, or loss of tissue approximation.	These signs indicate infection.
Assess nipples for cracks or fissures. Provide or reinforce information regarding breast and nipple care. Discuss use of creams, air-drying of nipples, and the need to avoid use of plastic-lined nursing pads.	Identifies potential source of infection. Breast care measures help toughen nipples, prevent skin breakdown and cracking, and limit presence of moisture, reducing risk of infection.
Discuss dietary practices. Stress need for increased amounts of food rich in protein, calories, iron, and vitamin C.	Protein helps in tissue growth and healing; calories are necessary to spare proteins. Vitamin C is needed for cell wall synthesis; iron is used for Hb synthesis.
Note presence of risk factors such as delivery trauma, malnutrition, diabetes, previous UTI/renal problems, or use of indwelling catheter.	These factors may predispose the client to UTI following delivery.
Assess for and review signs and symptoms of UTI (e.g., dysuria, hematuria, frequency, urgency, retention, fever, and pain in suprapubic region or costovertebral angle).	UTI requires prompt evaluation and intervention to prevent further involvement and complications.
Note reports of stress incontinence.	May indicate cystocele and the need for further evaluation or surgical repair.
Instruct in use of appropriate muscle-tightening exercises (e.g., Kegel exercise).	Exercise strengthens and tones perineal and urethral muscles to improve control of urine flow and reduce risk of infection.
Test urine pH.	Alkaline urine increases potential for bacterial growth.
Encourage client to increase fluid intake, especially with cranberry or orange juice.	Helps prevent urinary stasis; produces more acidic urine.
Collaborative	
Assess lab results, especially WBC count.	Leukocytosis during initial 10 to 12 days postpartum is a normal protective mechanism associated with an increase in neutrophils and a shift to the left and must be distinguished from an abnormal finding indicating infection.

ACTIONS/INTERVENTIONS

Collaborative

Obtain cultures of lochia, nipple discharge, wound drainage, or urine as indicated.

Discuss antibiotic administration, as appropriate.

Refer for urologic consultation, as indicated.

RATIONALE

Confirms presence of infection and identifies type.

Antimicrobial agent whose selection is based on culture and sensitivity findings helps eradicate pathogenic bacteria.

May be needed for persistent symptoms, cystocele, or failure to respond to antimicrobial agents.

NURSING DIAGNOSIS:	**ROLE PERFORMANCE, ALTERED**
May be related to:	Situational crisis (addition and demands of new family member, changes in responsibilities of family members).
Possibly evidenced by:	Change in usual patterns or responsibility, conflict in roles.
DESIRED OUTCOMES— CLIENT WILL:	Verbalize awareness of role expectations and potential problems.
	Begin to set realistic goals.
	Talk with family members about situation and changes that have occurred.

ACTIONS/INTERVENTIONS

Independent

Determine family structure and individual expectations.

Evaluate individual and family goals and client's perception of new family situation. Encourage open communication and sharing of feelings and concerns among family members.

Aid client in setting realistic goals and expectations for herself.

RATIONALE

The ease with which each family member adapts to the new role and accommodates the new member may be influenced by the size, stability, and complexity of the family. For example, the blended family may create special concerns whereby the newborn is a half-brother or half-sister. Although all members of the family are to some extent influenced by the transition, the client herself often suffers the greatest impact in terms of personal and professional responsibilities and must make the most significant accommodations and sacrifices in terms of her time and energy.

Client who feels cheated, disappointed, or unfulfilled with the mothering role may have difficulty adapting, as may the mother who is forced to return to work for economic reasons but would prefer to remain at home. Identification of problems can be helpful in reaching solutions that are compatible for all concerned.

Too much activity and unrealistic goals compound fatigue and reduce energy levels needed for coping and role integration.

ACTIONS/INTERVENTIONS

Independent

Assist client in acquiring skill and comfort in feeding and bathing infant.

Reinforce client's successes at mothering and specific accomplishments of individual family members.

Discuss concerns; provide information about potential sources and ways of evaluating child care providers.

Collaborative

Refer client to visiting nurse services or community support groups (e.g., La Leche League, stepfamily organizations).

Refer for professional counseling.

RATIONALE

Client who is having difficulty or feels awkward providing care may believe that she is failing in her mothering skills.

Client's self-confidence may be tenuous; she may need constant assurance that she is performing well. Recognition of efforts of those involved supports ongoing change and participation in problem-solving.

Sufficient time is required to select safe and appropriate resources that will meet individual needs and allow client to return to personal and professional activities.

Client may need additional assistance in home adjustment. Four weeks may be required for families to integrate infant care into their patterns of daily living.

Further intervention may be needed to promote positive individual and family adjustment.

NURSING DIAGNOSIS:	BODY IMAGE DISTURBANCE
May be related to:	Unrealistic expectations of postpartum recovery, permanency of some changes.
Possibly evidenced by:	Verbalization of negative feelings about body, feelings of helplessness, preoccupation with change, focus on past appearance, fear of rejection/reaction by others.
DESIRED OUTCOMES— CLIENT WILL:	Verbalize realistic perceptions of new body contours.
	Report acceptance of self as she is at this moment.
	Dress comfortably.
	Set realistic goals for change.
	Initiate progressive, ongoing prescribed exercise program.

ACTIONS/INTERVENTIONS

Independent

Determine perception of new body image and of actual or imagined changes that pregnancy and childbirth created.

RATIONALE

Client's self-esteem and adaptation to body image are influenced by her perceptions. The client who has fantasized or imagined that she would resume her prepregnancy appearance and body contours following delivery may be depressed or disappointed when this has not occurred. The client may actually grieve the loss of her prepregnancy appearance. A potential crisis exists, particularly

ACTIONS/INTERVENTIONS	RATIONALE
Independent	
	for the emotionally immature client who places much emphasis on appearance. The adolescent, whose primary focus may be dating or re-entry into a heterosexual relationship, may experience even greater difficulty adapting to and coping with a new body image.
Provide information honestly regarding integumentary and musculoskeletal changes.	Chloasma, nevi, palmar erythema, fine hair growth, changes in condition of hair and fingernails, and joint hypermobility usually disappear or return to prepregnancy state. Coarse hair, areolar hyperpigmentation, linea nigra, increased foot growth, and spider nevi may not regress completely post partum. Approximately 6 wk is required for abdominal wall and uterus to return to prepregnancy state.
Discuss ways of dressing attractively and the importance of taking time for personal appearance with application of cosmetics, trips to the hairdresser, and so forth.	Attractive, loose-fitting, nonmaternity clothes and new hair-style enhance self-esteem and feelings of attractiveness.
Evaluate client's normal physical activity level and participation in sports or exercise program.	Involvement in physical activities aids client in regaining both a positive self-image and her prepregnancy shape.
Provide information about postpartal exercises (e.g., lifting hips off bed or sleeping on abdomen).	Regular exercise program that is specific for each day up to 1 week post partum is continued thereafter, as indicated, to trim figure and increase muscle tone.
Weigh client, review ideal weight, and discuss proper nutrition as the key to losing weight. Discourage dieting in the lactating client until she stops breastfeeding.	The client retains approximately 60% of weight gained in excess of 24 lb (11 kg), which must be lost through proper diet and exercise. Restriction of calories in the lactating mother results in inadequate milk production.
Ascertain male partner's perception of client's physical appearance. Recommend avoidance of jokes or negative comments regarding her weight and appearance. Encourage male to express caring through increased time and attention or small gifts such as flowers and cards.	Helping male partner become aware of the client's emotional feelings may prevent him from making comments about her body that could reinforce negative feelings. Client may misinterpret the male's focus on the newborn as lack of interest in her, which may enhance her feelings of unattractiveness.
Collaborative	
Refer for counseling, support groups, or follow-up with community resources as needed.	May be necessary to resolve conflicts of self-esteem and poor body image.

NURSING DIAGNOSIS:	**CONSTIPATION, HIGH RISK FOR**
Risk factors may include:	Inadequate fluid/fiber intake, decreased physical activity, pain on defecation.

387

ACTIONS/INTERVENTIONS	RATIONALE
Independent	
Discuss normal evacuation pattern. Determine presence of hemorrhoids, perineal trauma, or third-degree lacerations.	A history of problems with evacuation or constipation may contribute to problems following delivery, especially after the dilating and relaxing effects of progesterone experienced during the prenatal period.
Review role of client's current intake and the role of fluid and diet in stool formation and evacuation.	Lack of roughage and inadequate fluid intake reduce peristaltic motion of fecal matter through intestine, thereby increasing water reabsorption, resulting in dry, hard stools.
Encourage adequate fluid intake (including lactation needs as appropriate) and diet high in roughage, fruits, and vegetables.	Use of warm beverages (hot water, coffee, tea), fruits/juices, and roughage promotes soft formed stool, eases evacuation, and supports client self-care.
Assess healing of episiotomy or lacerations. Provide information regarding the use of sitz baths 3 to 4 times daily.	Warmth from sitz bath helps relax anal sphincter, promotes healing, encourages general relaxation, and reduces discomfort associated with evacuation.
Recommend regular exercise, including daily walking program.	Activity enhances muscle tone, stimulates peristalsis, and enhances sense of well-being. (Note: Some cultures limit activity following delivery for a prescribed period of time.)
Collaborative	
Encourage continued use of stool softener, if appropriate.	Helps prevent straining and reduces pain associated with evacuation.
Provide information regarding use of laxatives, enemas, or suppositories.	May be necessary to stimulate peristalsis, promote evacuation, and prevent fecal impaction.

ACTIONS/INTERVENTIONS	RATIONALE

Independent

Ascertain frequency of voiding and character of urine. Note condition of skin, lips, and mucous membranes.	Declining frequency/amount, presence of dark/strong urine, dry lips/mucous membranes, and poor skin turgor suggest inadequate fluid intake in relation to fluid needs.
Note reports of excessive fatigue or dizziness.	Hypovolemia may result in orthostatic changes.
Assess blood pressure (BP) and pulse.	Decrease in BP and increase in pulse may reflect hypovolemia.
Note fundal height.	Failure of the fundus to involute properly (should be located at the symphysis pubis) is associated with increased vaginal flow.
Assess character and amount of lochial flow.	A return to bright red bleeding is abnormal. Brisk, heavy flow indicates late postpartal hemorrhage secondary to retained placental fragments. (Refer to CP: Postpartal Hemorrhage.)
Review client's activity level.	Slight increase in flow may be secondary to inadequate rest associated with periods of increased activity.
Assess condition of perineum or cesarean incision; note healing.	To identify delayed healing and the potential for hemorrhage or dehiscence.

Collaborative

Review postpartal Hb/Hct levels obtained prior to discharge; compare with present levels if available.	Provides comparative readings to assess severity of blood loss. Hb/Hct should return to normal within 3 days postpartum. Hb should not drop more than 2 g/100 ml unless blood loss is excessive. (Each milliliter of blood lost contains 0.5 mg of Hb.)
Notify healthcare provider and prepare client for additional evaluation/intervention as necessary.	Repeat laboratory studies or more invasive procedure such as surgical dilatation and curettage (D and C) may be necessary to determine severity of condition, or to diagnose/correct problem.
Provide information regarding medications such as ergot (0.2 mg every 4 hr for 2–4 days) as needed.	Used to promote uterine contractility, which may foster passage of retained placental tissue.

NURSING DIAGNOSIS:	FAMILY COPING, INEFFECTIVE: COMPROMISED, HIGH RISK FOR
Risk factors may include:	Situational/developmental changes, temporary family disorganization and role changes, little support provided by client for partner/family members.
Possibly evidenced by:	[Not applicable; presence of signs/symptoms establishes an **actual** diagnosis.]
DESIRED OUTCOMES— CLIENT/FAMILY WILL:	Identify individual stressors.
	Set realistic goals and expectations.

DESIRED OUTCOMES—CLIENT/FAMILY WILL:	Verbalize resources within themselves to deal with the transition.
	Recognize need for and use outside support appropriately.

ACTIONS/INTERVENTIONS	RATIONALE
Independent	
Evaluate client's actual and perceived physiologic state.	Negative feelings, especially in the primipara, may be manifested by real or imagined physiologic symptoms. First-time parents, perhaps owing to unrealistic perceptions, tend to experience the greatest degree of crisis, disintegration, and problems with adjustment.
Assess psychologic status and discuss normalcy of negative feelings in the client/couple.	The fourth trimester, a transitional period lasting approximately 3 months following birth, is a difficult period, because the client is vulnerable to negative feelings during crisis resolution and adaptation to stress. Negative feelings of anxiety, depression, and isolation are common, and awareness of the normalcy of these feelings may offset excessive self-concern or self-preoccupation.
Determine individual stressors for client/couple. Note strengths, weaknesses, coping mechanisms, and presence of realistic problem-solving capabilities.	The degree of individual and family stress depends on realistic perception of events, available coping mechanisms, and situational support. Crisis "balancing" factors help facilitate quick resolution of problems, positive adaptation, and growth for client/couple and family. Lack of balancing factors results in continued state of disorganization and persistence of crisis state.
Assist couple with identification of anticipated and unanticipated stressors and formulation of realistic problem-solving.	Emotional disorganization associated with crisis is often accompanied by distortion of cognitive perceptions and the ability to respond appropriately to stressors.
Assess available means of assistance with housework and meal preparation.	Assistance with physical labor needed for household maintenance frees the client to devote her psychologic energies to herself and infant.
Assess for maladaptive behaviors or ineffective coping.	Potential for maladaptation, disequilibrium, and continued crisis exists, necessitating immediate intervention, especially if existing support systems are inadequate for the postpartal mother.
Provide telephone contact number for 24-hour access.	New mothers (regardless whether first or fifth child) need access to healthcare resources early in the postpartal period and thereafter to facilitate adaptation.
Collaborative	
Refer client to appropriate community agency, counselor, or social services.	May need additional assistance if existing support systems are inadequate or not available.

Maternal Assessment: 4 to 6 Weeks Following Delivery ———

CLIENT ASSESSMENT DATA BASE

ACTIVITY/REST

Lack of energy, fatigue, inability to maintain usual/expected routines.

CIRCULATION

Vital signs have returned to normal prepregnancy levels.

EGO INTEGRITY

Emotional response may include irritability, anxiety, or feeling emotionally overwhelmed.

ELIMINATION

Bowel sounds are active in all quadrants; usual elimination pattern resumes.

Abdominal muscle tone improving; some degree of flaccidity may persist.

Dipstick urinalysis for albumin, ketones, and glucose should be negative.

FOOD/FLUID

Return to prepregnancy weight, with retention of approximately 60% of weight gain in excess of 24 lb.

SAFETY

Cesarean incision, perineal laceration/repair should be healed.

Striae and linea nigra beginning to fade.

SEXUALITY

Lochial flow is absent.

Menstruation may resume beginning 4–5 wk postpartum, especially in nonlactating client.

Libido may be decreased.

Intercourse may be painful (dyspareunia).

Breasts in nonlactating client are soft, nontender, and of prepregnancy size; breasts in lactating client are full, free of nipple cracks and fissures, and lactation is well established.

Uterus not palpable, having returned to near prepregnancy size.

Pelvic examination, if performed, shows restored muscle tone, with cervix healed and closed, appearing as transverse slit.

SOCIAL INTERACTION

May be planning on returning to/seeking employment, or involvement in activities outside the home.

DIAGNOSTIC STUDIES

Dependent on assessment findings, individual client needs.
Hemoglobin/hematocrit (Hb/Hct): 12 g and 37%
Papanicolaou smear: Negative.
Culture/sensitivity of drainage/urine.

NURSING PRIORITIES

1. Promote maternal/infant well-being.
2. Provide/reinforce health teaching.
3. Foster positive client and family adaptation to newborn.

DISCHARGE GOALS

1. Maternal/infant physiologic/psychologic needs being met.
2. Current health care behaviors and ongoing needs understood.
3. Satisfactory adaptation to parenting roles reported/observed.

NURSING DIAGNOSIS:	**FAMILY COPING: POTENTIAL FOR GROWTH**
May be related to:	Sufficiently meeting individual needs and adaptive tasks, enabling goals of self-actualization to surface.
Possibly evidenced by:	Family member(s) moving in direction of health-promoting and enriching lifestyle.
DESIRED OUTCOMES— CLIENT/COUPLE WILL:	Verbalize continued improvement with transition of new family member into home situation.
	Undertake tasks leading to change.
	Express feelings of self-confidence and satisfaction with progress and adaptation being made.

ACTIONS/INTERVENTIONS	RATIONALE
Independent	
Assess client's/couple's self-esteem and adaptation to parenting.	Parents need to learn to be flexible and adapt positively to changing circumstances rather than adhere to rigid schedules.
Determine parents' perception of family growth, mastery of infant care activities, and satisfaction or dissatisfaction with maternal/paternal role.	Parents should recognize that required skills change with the child's mental and physical growth. Increased self-esteem is associated with mastery of infant care tasks and satisfaction with parental role.
Discuss client's/couple's ability to modify or accept infant's behaviors. Provide appropriate anticipatory guidance.	Helps foster mutual capacity for behavior modification in parents and infant. To facilitate growth, parents need to learn to respond to the infant's needs while not neglecting the needs of other family members, to accept both successes and failures in attempts to modify the infant's behavior, and to make necessary adaptations based on needs of individual family members.
Evaluate ongoing educational and maturational progress and adjustment in sibling(s). Assess quality of interaction of sibling(s) with other children.	Helps identify actual or potential problems with family integration. Hostile-aggressive interaction of sibling(s) with other children signals inappropriate method of coping.

392

ACTIONS/INTERVENTIONS

Independent

Provide bibliography list for parents and children. Encourage client/couple to spend time alone with each child, and allow opportunity for ongoing verbalization of feelings.

Assess parental response to positive or negative feedback from spouse or others (e.g., mother, mother-in-law, other family member, healthcare providers).

Collaborative

Refer to social service, visiting nurse services, or professional counselor, as appropriate.

RATIONALE

Helps parents to assist siblings with positive role adaptation; allows incorporation of newborn into family structure.

Mastery of parental tasks and growing self-esteem fosters independence, continued growth, and reduces excessive need for support of others.

May be needed to support desires for learning of new tasks/roles and continued growth.

NURSING DIAGNOSIS:	NUTRITION, ALTERED, LESS THAN BODY REQUIREMENTS, HIGH RISK FOR
Risk factors may include:	Inadequate caloric intake/increased caloric needs (lactation).
Possibly evidenced by:	[Not applicable; presence of signs/symptoms establishes an **actual** diagnosis.]
DESIRED OUTCOMES— CLIENT WILL:	Identify individual needs and appropriate goal weight.
	Eat a well-balanced diet.
	Maintain/demonstrate progress toward desired weight.

ACTIONS/INTERVENTIONS

Independent

Weigh client. Compare current weight with prepregnancy and ideal weight. Evaluate weight changes since delivery.

Determine dietary habits using 24-hour recall. Provide information and encourage use of all food groups for a balanced diet.

Review Hb and Hct. Note behaviors associated with low Hb (e.g., fatigue, dizziness). Discuss dietary intake/use of sources rich in iron if Hb levels are low.

Reinforce individual dietary needs in relation to type of infant feeding (i.e., breast or bottle).

RATIONALE

Weight generally returns to prepregnancy level by 6 weeks postpartum, with approximately 60% retention of weight gain in excess of 24 lb.

Helps identify and correct inadequacies of protein, vitamin, or mineral intake.

Hb levels should be 12 g/100 ml; Hct 37% (plus or minus 5%). Reduction of activity may be necessary if Hb is low. Ingestion of iron-rich or fortified foods helps restore low iron levels, but supplements (such as prenatal vitamins with iron) may be needed for as long as 2 months to correct iron deficiency.

Lactating client requires 500–800 cal/day more than the usual 2000 cal/day for the nonlactating client. Fluid intake should be increased by 500 ml/day for adequate milk production. Lactating client should not begin weight reduction diet while breastfeeding.

ACTIONS/INTERVENTIONS

Independent

Provide information regarding iron and vitamin supplements and appropriate measures to facilitate absorption of iron (e.g., taking iron tablets between meals with fruit juice) as indicated.

RATIONALE

Supplements may be required to correct vitamin and iron deficiencies. Iron is best absorbed in acidic medium; taking iron with milk or meals impedes absorption.

NURSING DIAGNOSIS:	**KNOWLEDGE DEFICIT [LEARNING NEED], regarding recuperation, self-care, infant needs**
May be related to:	Information misinterpretation, lack of recall.
Possibly evidenced by:	Verbalization of concerns/misconceptions, inaccurate follow-through of instructions, development of preventable complications.
DESIRED OUTCOMES— CLIENT WILL:	Verbalize understanding of appropriate healthcare behaviors related to current situation.
	Seek appropriate postpartal follow-up.

ACTIONS/INTERVENTIONS

Independent

Review client's understanding of physiologic recovery for this time period.

Review client's understanding of information received during prenatal, intrapartal, and postpartal periods, and provide information and/or clarify misconceptions as necessary.

Reinforce information regarding infant care, immunization needs, feeding, and normal/anticipated growth and development. Provide pamphlets and identify other resources.

Discuss client's expectations regarding employment, family, and her own needs.

Assist in developing realistic plans, identifying resources, and setting goals.

RATIONALE

By the end of the puerperium, involution should be complete (with the uterus returning to normal size and cessation of lochia) and incisions should be healed. However, the body may not have resumed its prepregnancy state. The client may still be 10 or more lb over her usual weight; she may note sore nipples and contour changes such as widening of her hips, breast enlargement/sagging, and decreased abdominal muscle tone with protruding stomach.

In many cases, material presented during these previous periods is not incorporated or valued and/or is misinterpreted because of such other factors as pain and fatigue. Repetition of information is helpful at this time and provides an opportunity for discussion of ideas and concerns.

Aids in meeting physical, psychologic, and nutritional needs of infant. Availability of written materials and other resources increases likelihood that client can find answers to questions as they arise, enhancing independence and responsibility.

Balancing multiple demands may be overwhelming, especially if the client's/family's expectations are unrealistic.

Sharing of duties and responsibilities helps reduce individual fatigue, enhances adaptation to changes, and promote general well-being.

ACTIONS/INTERVENTIONS

Independent

Encourage client to involve other family members in this process.

Determine client's/couple's plans for contraceptive use. Provide information and review options as indicated.

Assess client's understanding and practice of breast self-examination. Provide information/visual aids as needed.

Provide information to lactating client regarding breastfeeding in relation to professional or working demands. Review options of using breast pump, manual expression, and gradual weaning.

Provide information about need for follow-up medical care.

RATIONALE

Involvement in the problem-solving process promotes willingness to follow through on solutions. In addition, changes in sexual response, family demands, and ongoing fatigue affect the client's level of functioning and well-being.

Helps prevent unwanted or unplanned pregnancies; fosters adoption of family planning method. Studies suggest that closely spaced pregnancies (less than 9 months apart) have increased risks for both mother and infant.

Helps client understand the importance of health promotion and of early detection of abnormalities.

Assists client with identifying problems and making decisions to meet infant's and her own needs during times of separation.

Reevaluation at 6 months postpartum provides opportunity to assess client's well-being and identify any unresolved/developing problems.

NURSING DIAGNOSIS:	SEXUALITY PATTERNS, ALTERED
May be related to:	Individual response to health-related transition, altered body functioning (including lactation), lack of privacy, fear of pregnancy.
Possibly evidenced by:	Reported difficulties, changes in sexual behaviors/activities.
DESIRED OUTCOMES—CLIENT/COUPLE WILL:	Discuss nature of current sexual relationship in comparison to before and during pregnancy.
	Identify potential problems during the early post delivery period.
	Resume sexual relationship as desired.
	Adopt a mutually agreeable method of contraception.

ACTIONS/INTERVENTIONS

Independent

Discuss client's/couple's sexual relationship prior to pregnancy and the effects that newborn has had on client's/couple's physiologic and psychologic energy levels.

RATIONALE

Nature of sexual relationship prior to pregnancy affects resumption of sexual activity more than any other factor. However, fatigue, physical discomforts, stress of new roles/responsibilities, depression, and individual self-perceptions may delay this process. In addition, presence of baby may have negative influence on lovemaking, leaving one or both members of the couple frustrated and unsatisfied.

ACTIONS/INTERVENTIONS	RATIONALE

Independent

Determine client's body image and her feelings of physical attractiveness following delivery. Note views of significant other(s).

Much of sexual response and desire is psychologically based, so that a negative body image may reduce sexual urges. Partner may not find mate as sexually attractive if she is lactating or has not regained her prepregnancy weight and body contours.

Provide information about physiologic changes in sexual response for first 3 months following delivery.

Reduction in rapidity/intensity of response is normal. Continued low estrogen levels result in vaginal dryness. Size of orgasmic platform and strength of orgasmic contraction are reduced; vasoconstriction of labia minora and labia majora is delayed.

Prepare couple for possibility of a temporary difficulty with achieving erection or arousal.

Fatigue and heightened expectations may increase or decrease libido, altering sexual response.

Ascertain whether couple has resumed sexual relationship.

Most couples can safely resume intercourse 3–4 wk after vaginal delivery or following 6-week checkup after cesarean delivery.

Assess degree of pleasure or displeasure associated with resumption of sexual activity. Suggest use of water-soluble jelly, cocoa butter, or contraceptive creams or jellies for lubrication; and side-by-side or female superior positions.

Vaginal dryness may cause pain/dyspareunia, necessitating use of lubrication. Female superior or side-by-side position allows client to control the rate and degree of penile penetration, thereby gradually distending tissues and reducing discomfort.

Discuss alternatives to penile penetration to achieve orgasm (e.g., masturbation, lubricated stroking of genital area, or cunnilingus).

Helps client achieve sexual gratification while avoiding possible discomfort associated with penile penetration. (Note: Some couples might not find such alternatives mutually acceptable.)

Encourage verbalization of concerns.

May stimulate identification of problems and foster creative problem-solving.

Encourage couple to share intimate thoughts.

Helps create open communication; increases psychologic readiness for sexual relationship.

Discuss effects of lactation on sexual response and interest level. Suggest planning lovemaking so that it occurs just after or midway between feedings.

Lactating women often have a greater interest in resuming sexual activity than nonlactating women and may report higher levels of postdelivery eroticism. Orgasm may stimulate the let-down reflex; breastfeeding itself may evoke sexual arousal, possibly to the point of reaching plateau/orgasmic levels. Intercourse may be more enjoyable just after or midway between feedings when breasts are not as full or leaking and infant is not likely to be hungry.

Discuss client's/couple's choice of contraception method. Reinforce information and provide new oral and written information as needed regarding method, effectiveness, proper usage, expense, availability, advantages/disadvantages, and contraindications. Assess plan for future offspring and desired family size.

Pregnancy is possible before onset of regular menses. Cooperation with contraceptive method is enhanced if client/couple participates in decision-making process. Couple may elect to adopt temporary means of contraception (foams, condom, or gel) until postpartal examination by healthcare provider, or couple may elect surgical

ACTIONS/INTERVENTIONS

Independent

RATIONALE

method (vasectomy or tubal ligation). Although oral contraceptives may be the most practical and effective method for the sexually active adolescent, they are contraindicated for breastfeeding clients and for clients with diabetes, hypertension, kidney or cardiac problems, or history of phlebitis. Because of the risk of infection, intrauterine device is not usually advised for the diabetic client. (Note: Client should be refitted for a diaphragm following birth of infant or a weight change of 10 lb or more.)

Collaborative

Refer for counseling as indicated.

Couple unable to achieve mutual sexual satisfaction may need help in analyzing causative factors and in initiating open communication and problem-solving with each other.

NURSING DIAGNOSIS:	**PARENTING, ALTERED, HIGH RISK FOR**
Risk factors may include:	Lack of/or ineffective role model, lack of support between/from significant other(s), unrealistic expectation for self/infant/partner, presence of stress (addition of new family member, financial concerns).
Possibly evidenced by:	[Not applicable; presence of signs/symptoms establishes an **actual** diagnosis.]
DESIRED OUTCOMES— CLIENT/COUPLE WILL:	Demonstrate responsiveness to infant cues.
	Verbalize positive resolution of feelings regarding change in lifestyle, addition of new family member.
	Report satisfaction with parenting roles.

ACTIONS/INTERVENTIONS

Independent

Assess strength of parent-infant attachment.

Review cultural factors and expectations.

Note progress toward recovery and stabilization of lifestyle.

RATIONALE

Attachment bond should be strong 4–6 wk postpartum. Little or no reciprocal interaction requires immediate intervention.

Cultural beliefs affect parent-child interaction (e.g., types of behaviors observed and the degree of attachment noted).

Failure to progress and/or continuation of postpartal depression have a negative impact on attachment and indicate need for further evaluation/intervention.

ACTIONS/INTERVENTIONS

Independent

Assess resolution of grief associated with assumption of new role and loss of former lifestyle.

Discuss client's use and adequacy of current/available resources.

Discuss client's/couple's concerns regarding infant behaviors and parenting skills. Reinforce previous information.

Administer Neonatal Perception Inventory as indicated.

Note presence of problems and evidence of possible neglect or abuse. Notify authorities as indicated.

Collaborative

Refer client/couple to peer support group, postpartal parenting group, or classes, such as Parent Effectiveness Training.

Refer to community health nurse, social services, or professional counselor.

RATIONALE

Adaptation to the new parenting role and integration of the infant into the family involve some grieving over the loss of former life patterns and the need to reduce or alter career pursuits or social roles.

Without effective support, the difficult process of integrating a new member into the family may be more difficult.

Assists in relieving anxiety, provides opportunity for positive reinforcement for efforts, and promotes growth.

Assesses adaptive potential of mother-infant pair and provides a statistically significant relationship between the findings at 1 month and the emotional development of the child at age $4^1/2$, and later at age 10 to 11.

Index of suspicion requires further evaluation to determine necessary interventions.

Sharing of concerns may increase parent's knowledge of childrearing and child development and provide supportive atmosphere during role acquisition and transition.

May be necessary to assist parents in adopting effective parenting skills.

NURSING DIAGNOSIS:	INFECTION, HIGH RISK FOR
Risk factors may include:	Broken skin and/or traumatized tissues, retained placental fragments, invasive procedures, exposure to pathogens.
Possibly evidenced by:	[Not applicable; presence of signs/symptoms establishes an **actual** diagnosis.]
DESIRED OUTCOMES— CLIENT WILL:	Display complete involution, with lochial flow absent, and vital signs within normal limits.
	Be free of signs of mastitis, with nipples free of cracks and fissures and breasts nontender.
	Achieve timely healing of incisions/lacerations.

ACTIONS/INTERVENTIONS

Independent

Review type of delivery and prenatal or intrapartal events that might have predisposed client to infection or excessive trauma.

RATIONALE

Provides clues to increased risk for postpartal complications.

ACTIONS/INTERVENTIONS	RATIONALE

Independent

Assess client for any vaginal discharge or persistence/return of lochial flow. Note odor of drainage.	Although lochial flow should have ceased by this time, the client may have resumed her menstrual cycle or may have failed to complete involution. The presence of foul-smelling discharge is indicative of infection and requires further evaluation.
Note status of perineum, incisions/lacerations, uterus, and cervix.	Wound should be well approximated without inflammation or drainage. Uterus should return to near prepregnancy state by 4–6 wk postpartum, with closure of the cervix completed. Relaxed or tender uterus, and opening of the cervix suggests infection.
Note fever, chills, tachycardia, headache, malaise, vomiting, diarrhea, and abdominal tenderness.	These general signs and symptoms suggest endometritis.
Assess nipples for redness, cracks, or fissures. If present, suggest use of localized heat, starting feedings on unaffected nipple, limiting infant suckling, and air-drying nipples for 20–30 min after each feeding.	Helps prevent clogged nipples and lobes, which can lead to mastitis. Limiting feeding on affected breast and initiating feeding on unaffected breast help reduce trauma to nipple and allow healing to occur.
Encourage breast support and application of local heat.	Facilitates circulation/lymph drainage and increases oxygen/nutrients to affected area to promote healing.
Assess breasts for marked tenderness, redness, palpable mass(es), or areas of induration. Suggest increased rest and fluids, localized heat, and frequent emptying of breasts if inflammation is present. Instruct in use of manual expression or breast pump.	Induration or mass(es) may indicate full milk duct, possible tumor, or mastitis. Rest, fluids, heat, and frequent emptying of breasts help reduce discomfort associated with full breasts and relieve stasis and engorgement, especially if breastfeeding is contraindicated during antibiotic therapy for mastitis.
Instruct client to discontinue breastfeeding if fever is present prior to antibiotic administration or if indicated by antibiotic therapy selected.	Breast milk may become purulent; antibiotic may cross into the breast milk. Stopping breastfeeding helps conserve energy for healing.
Note reports of dysuria, frequency, foul/cloudy urine, dragging back pain.	Indicative of urinary tract infection, which requires further evaluation to rule out cystocele.
Recommend increased fluid intake.	Promotes urine output, reducing urinary stasis and risk of infection or reinfection.

Collaborative

Refer to healthcare provider as indicated.	Promotes diagnosis/treatment; may prevent progression and/or limit severity of problem.
Culture lochia/drainage as indicated.	Identifies infectious organism and appropriate treatment.
Review appropriate use of analgesics/antipyretics.	Analgesics promote comfort; antipyretics reduce/control fever. (Note: Drugs may be contraindicated until diagnosis is made.)
Initiate/provide information about antibiotic therapy.	Vancomycin and cephalosporins are particularly effective against staphylococcal infections.

ACTIONS/INTERVENTIONS

Collaborative

Provide information about ergot preparations if prescribed (0.2 mg every 4 hr for 2–3 days).

Assist as needed with incision/drainage/care of wound. Carry out sterile dressing changes as needed.

Prepare client/family for follow-up procedures such as dilatation and curettage (D and C), as indicated.

RATIONALE

Promotes myometrial contractility, which may result in passage of tissue causing infection.

May be necessary if abscess develops, although such progression can usually be prevented with prompt diagnosis and treatment.

Surgical removal of placental fragments through D and C may be necessary.

NURSING DIAGNOSIS:	COPING, INDIVIDUAL/FAMILY, INEFFECTIVE, (specify) HIGH RISK FOR
Risk factors may include:	Situational/developmental changes, temporary family disorganization and role changes, little support provided for client by partner/family members.
Possibly evidenced by:	[Not applicable; presence of signs/symptoms establishes an **actual** diagnosis.]
DESIRED OUTCOMES— CLIENT WILL:	Report assistance from significant other(s) and effective use of resources.
	Verbalize sense of competence and not feeling overwhelmed with infant care.
	Plan activities outside of house for client/couple, the baby, and siblings.
	Demonstrate initial progress toward realistic goals.

ACTIONS/INTERVENTIONS

Independent

Assess past and present coping skills; explore available coping strategies, relationships between individual and family members, and support systems.

Determine client's perception of stressors and events of past 6 wk and of her own adaptability. Note competency in organizing activities associated with infant care and parental responsibilities.

RATIONALE

Past coping skills may be effective in the current situation, or client may need to develop new coping strategies. Positive coping mechanisms involve open communication of fears and wishes among family members, empathy, competency in role playing and role reversal, and negotiation within the family structure to the mutual satisfaction of each member.

Accurate perception of problems and adaptability to changing or new situations are factors that promote positive coping during times of increased stress/crisis. Persistent feelings of being overwhelmed by activities associated with child care, persistent depression or exhaustion, or persistent low self-esteem indicates negative coping.

ACTIONS/INTERVENTIONS	RATIONALE
Independent	
Allow client opportunity to cry or to express her concerns freely. Use "self-disclosure" if appropriate.	Provides opportunity for emotional catharsis and relief of tension. Self-disclosure—i.e., the sharing of one's own experiences with client—may be effective in stimulating client to talk, providing that the disclosure is client- rather than nurse-centered.
Identify and discuss apparent strengths of client/couple. Avoid criticism.	Promotes self-awareness and fosters positive self-esteem and coping.
Assess response of siblings to new baby. Provide anticipatory guidance regarding typical sibling reactions. Recommend appropriate children's books and other reading matter.	All siblings are somewhat resentful of the diminished parental attention that occurs when the new baby arrives, and acting-out behaviors may reflect normal feelings of frustration.
Encourage client to develop creative solutions and to rearrange schedule to spend time alone with her other child(ren).	Individual attention to sibling(s) reduces feelings of threat that the new baby creates, allows sibling(s) to feel secure in the child-parent relationship, and helps foster coping.
Suggest that client plan activities outside of home with baby and sibling(s).	Provides stimulation and change of daily routine for mother, baby, and sibling(s).
Help client/couple set priorities for tasks and to accept help from friends and relatives for tasks related to housework and cooking.	Allows client to focus on her infant and family. Excessive concerns about housework and cooking detract from time and energy devoted to the baby and family.
Provide information about increased needs for sleep and rest.	Excessive fatigue can have a negative effect on coping skills, especially those needed for 24-hour responsibility associated with infant care.
Determine client's opportunities for recreation and relaxation. Encourage client to participate in appropriate activities.	Provides positive outlet for release of stress, and enhances feelings of wellness and self-esteem.
Encourage client/couple to arrange for time together away from newborn.	Allows time for needed growth/reflection; helps achieve a sense of equilibrium.
Assess amount of support client receives from significant other(s) or family members, and the demands placed on her by each individual.	Lack of effective support and assistance may impair client's ability to cope and increase risk of postpartal depression, especially if husband expects to receive the same amount of attention following delivery as before delivery.
Discuss client's/couple's plans for the future, especially if client expects to return to work. Review plans for child care.	Return to employment and/or addition of outside responsibilities will affect all family members and requires sharing of duties/household tasks. Confidence in child care arrangements eases or reduces parent's anxiety/guilt regarding separation from infant.
Collaborative	
Recommend peer support group or parenting group.	Mutual sharing of successes and failures associated with parenting helps foster coping and helps client to recognize normalcy of her situation and feelings.

ACTIONS/INTERVENTIONS	RATIONALE

Collaborative

Reinforce availability of healthcare resources.

Relieves parents of feeling solely responsible for health of new baby; provides needed information regarding sources of healthcare.

Refer to community health nurse, social service, or professional counselor, as appropriate.

Negative coping manifested by excessive feelings of failure, depression, self-accusatory thoughts, excess use of drugs (such as alcohol), or a sense of being overwhelmed with child care suggests postpartal psychosis, which tends to peak at 6 weeks postpartum and indicates need for further evaluation and follow-up.

NURSING DIAGNOSIS:	CONSTIPATION, HIGH RISK FOR; BOWEL INCONTINENCE, HIGH RISK FOR
Risk factors may include:	Decreased muscle tone, inadequate fluid/dietary intake, reduced physical activity, pain on defecation.
Possibly evidenced by:	[Not applicable; presence of signs/symptoms establishes an **actual** diagnosis.]
DESIRED OUTCOMES— CLIENT WILL:	Identify/use appropriate interventions related to specific situation.
	Reestablish optimal bowel pattern.

ACTIONS/INTERVENTIONS	RATIONALE

Independent

Review usual evacuation pattern prior to pregnancy.

Provides useful information for setting goals. Problems may be new, or they may be longstanding and aggravated by pregnancy.

Evaluate nature and severity of problems associated with evacuation.

Helps in determining individual needs and selecting specific interventions.

Determine methods used to correct constipation.

Every effort should be made to use diet and exercise to promote bowel functioning and to reduce dependence on laxatives, if used.

Review dietary and fluid intake and exercise level. Recommend increased intake of fluids, whole grains, fruits, and vegetables, as well as daily exercise as appropriate.

Stimulates peristalsis, reducing excessive water absorption from fecal matter, thus promoting a softer stool.

Note presence of hemorrhoids/bleeding. Suggest reinsertion of hemorrhoid with lubricated glove or finger cot.

Painful or bleeding hemorrhoids may increase likelihood that client will postpone evacuation, which would contribute to further constipation and dry stool as more fluid is absorbed from the stool.

Assess intrapartal record for possible third- or fourth-degree laceration.

Lacerations extending into the anal sphincter may cause client to postpone evacuation, which increases constipation.

ACTIONS/INTERVENTIONS

Collaborative

Refer for evaluation of rectocele or fecal incontinence.

RATIONALE

May require surgical intervention. Incontinence may be associated with nerve damage to anal sphincter occurring with fourth-degree laceration.

Postpartal Hemorrhage _____

Postpartal hemorrhage is usually defined as the loss of more than 500 ml of blood during and/or after delivery. It is one of the leading causes of maternal mortality. Hemorrhage may occur early, within the first 24 hours after delivery, or late, up to 28 days postpartum (the end of the puerperium).

CLIENT ASSESSMENT DATA BASE: GENERAL FINDINGS

ACTIVITY/REST

May report excessive fatigue.

CIRCULATION

Blood loss at delivery generally 400–500 ml (vaginal delivery), 600–800 ml (cesarean delivery), although research suggests blood loss is often underestimated.

History of chronic anemia, congenital/incidental coagulation defects, idiopathic thrombocytopenia purpura.

EGO INTEGRITY

May be anxious, fearful, apprehensive.

SEXUALITY

Labor may have been prolonged/augmented or induced, precipitous/traumatic; use of forceps, general anesthesia, tocolytic therapy.

Difficult or manual delivery of placenta.

Examination of placenta following birth may have revealed missing placental fragments, tears, or evidence of torn blood vessels.

Vaginal birth after cesarean (VABC).

TEACHING/LEARNING

Previous postpartal hemorrhage, pregnancy-induced hypertension (PIH), uterine or cervical tumors, grand multiparity.

Ongoing/excess aspirin ingestion.

EARLY POSTPARTAL HEMORRHAGE (UP TO 24 HR FOLLOWING DELIVERY)

CIRCULATION

Changes in blood pressure (BP) and pulse (may not occur until blood loss is significant).

Delayed capillary refill.

Pallor; cold/clammy skin.

Dark, venous bleeding from uterus externally evident (retained placenta).

May have excessive vaginal bleeding, or oozing from cesarean incision or episiotomy; oozing from intravenous catheter, sites of intramuscular injections, or urinary catheter; bleeding gums (signs of disseminated intravascular coagulation [DIC]).

Profuse hemorrhage or symptoms of shock out of proportion to the amount of blood lost (inversion of uterus).

ELIMINATION

Difficulty voiding may reflect hematoma of the upper portion of the vagina.

PAIN/DISCOMFORT

Painful burning/tearing sensations (lacerations), severe vulvar/vaginal/pelvic/back pain (hematoma), lateral uterine pain, flank pain (hematoma into the broad ligament), abdominal tenderness (uterine atony, retained placental fragments), severe uterine and abdominal pain (uterine inversion).

SAFETY

Lacerations of the birth canal: persistent trickle of bright red blood (may be profuse) with firm, well-contracted uterus; visible tears in labia majora/labia minora, from vaginal introitus to perineum; extended tears from episiotomy, extension of episiotomy into vaginal vault, or tears in cervix.

Hematomas: unilateral, tense fluctuant bulging mass at vaginal introitus or encompassing labia majora; firm, painful to touch; unilateral bluish or reddish discoloration of skin of perineum or buttocks. (Abdominal hematoma following cesarean delivery may be asymptomatic except for changes in vital signs.)

SEXUALITY

Soft, boggy, or enlarging uterus, difficult to palpate; bright red bleeding from vagina (slow or profuse); large clots expressed on massage of uterus (uterine atony).

Uterus firm, well-contracted or partially contracted, and slightly boggy (retained placental fragments).

Fundus of uterus inverted; comes into close contact with, or may protrude through, the external os (uterine inversion).

Current pregnancy may have involved uterine overdistention (multiple gestation, polyhydramnios, macrosomia), abruptio placentae, placenta previa.

LATE POSTPARTAL HEMORRHAGE (24 TO 28 DAYS FOLLOWING DELIVERY)

CIRCULATION

Continued oozing or sudden bleeding.

May appear pale, anemic.

PAIN/DISCOMFORT

Uterine tenderness (retained placental fragments).

Vaginal/pelvic discomfort, backache (hematoma).

SAFETY

Foul-smelling lochial discharge (infection).

Premature rupture of membranes.

SEXUALITY

Fundal height or uterine body fails to return to prepregnancy size and function (subinvolution).

Leukorrhea may be present.

Continues to pass tissue.

DIAGNOSTIC STUDIES

Blood typing: Determines Rh, ABO group, and cross-match.

Complete blood count: Reveals decreased hemoglobin/hematocrit (Hb/Hct) and/or elevated white blood cell (WBC) count (shift to the left, and increased sedimentation rate suggests infection).

Uterine and vaginal culture: Rules out postpartal infection.

Urinalysis: Ascertains damage to bladder.

Coagulation profile: Elevated fibrin degradation product/fibrin split product (FDP/FSP) levels, decreased fibrinogen levels; activated partial thromboplastin time/partial thromboplastin time (APTT/PTT), pro-thrombin time prolonged in presence of DIC.

Sonography: Determines presence of retained placental tissue.

NURSING PRIORITIES

1. Maintain or restore circulating volume/tissue perfusion.
2. Prevent complications.
3. Provide information and appropriate support for client/couple.

DISCHARGE GOALS

1. Tissue perfusion/organ function within normal limits (WNL).
2. Complications prevented/resolving.
3. Clinical situation and treatment needs understood.

NURSING DIAGNOSIS:	**FLUID VOLUME DEFICIT [ACTIVE LOSS]**
May be related to:	Excessive vascular loss.
Possibly evidenced by:	Hypotension, increased pulse, changes in mentation, decreased/concentrated urine, dry skin/mucous membranes, delayed capillary refill.
DESIRED OUTCOMES— CLIENT WILL:	Demonstrate stabilization/improvement in fluid balance as evidenced by stable vital signs, prompt capillary refill, appropriate sensorium, and individually adequate urine output and specific gravity.

ACTIONS/INTERVENTIONS	RATIONALE
Independent	
Review records of pregnancy and labor/delivery, noting causative factors or those contributing to hemorrhagic situation (e.g., lacerations, retained placental fragments, sepsis, abruptio placentae, amniotic fluid emboli, or retention of dead fetus for more than 5 wk).	Aids in establishing appropriate plan of care and provides opportunity to prevent or limit developing complications.
Assess and record amount, type, and site of bleeding; weigh and count pads; save clots and tissue for evaluation by physician.	Estimate of blood loss, venous versus arterial, and presence of clots helps to make a differential diagnosis and determines replacement needs. (Note: One gram of increased pad weight is equal to approximately 1 ml of blood loss.)

ACTIONS/INTERVENTIONS	RATIONALE
Independent	

Assess location of uterus and degree of uterine contractility. Gently massage boggy uterus with one hand while placing second hand just above the symphysis pubis.

Degree of uterine contractility aids in differential diagnosis. Increasing myometrial contractility may decrease blood loss. Placing one hand above symphysis pubis prevents possible uterine inversion during massage.

Note hypotension or tachycardia, delayed capillary refill, or cyanosis of nail beds, mucous membranes, and lips.

These signs reflect hypovolemia and developing shock. Changes in BP are not detectable until fluid volume has decreased by 30%–50%. Cyanosis is a late sign of hypoxia. (Refer to ND: Tissue Perfusion, altered.)

Monitor hemodynamic parameters, such as central venous pressure or pulmonary artery wedge pressure, if available.

Provides more direct measurement of circulating volume and replacement needs.

Institute bed rest with legs elevated 20 to 30 degrees and trunk horizontal.

Bleeding may decrease or cease with reduction in activity. Proper positioning increases venous return, ensuring greater availability of blood to brain and other vital organs.

Maintain NPO (nothing by mouth) regimen while determining client status/needs.

Prevents aspiration of gastric contents in the event that sensorium is altered and/or surgical intervention is required.

Monitor intake and output; note urine specific gravity.

Useful in estimating extent/significance of fluid loss. Adequate perfusion/circulating volume is reflected by output 30–50 ml/hr or greater.

Avoid repeat/use caution when performing vaginal and/or rectal examinations.

May increase hemorrhage if cervical, vaginal, or perineal lacerations or hematomas are present. (Note: Careful examination may be required to monitor status of hematomas.)

Provide quiet environment and psychologic support.

Promotes relaxation; reduces anxiety and metabolic demand.

Assess for persistent perineal pain or feeling of vaginal fullness. Apply counterpressure on labial or perineal lacerations.

Hematomas often result from continued bleeding birth canal lacerations.

Monitor clients with placenta accreta (slight penetration of myometrium by placental tissue), PIH, or abruptio placentae for signs of DIC. (Refer to Chapter 4, CP: Prenatal Hemorrhage, ND: Injury, high risk for, maternal.)

Thromboplastin released during attempts at manual removal of the placenta may result in coagulopathy.

Collaborative

Start 1 or 2 I.V. infusion(s) of isotonic or electrolyte fluids with 18-gauge catheter or via central venous line. Administer whole blood or blood products (e.g., plasma, cryoprecipitate, platelets) as indicated.

Necessary for rapid or multiple infusions of fluid or blood products to increase circulating volume and enhance clotting.

Administer medications as indicated:

Oxytocin, methylergononovine maleate, prostaglandin $F_2\alpha$.

Increases contractility of boggy uterus and myometrium, closes off exposed venous sinuses, and stops hemorrhage in presence of atony.

ACTIONS/INTERVENTIONS	RATIONALE
Collaborative	
Magnesium sulfate ($MgSO_4$).	Some studies report use of $MgSO_4$ to facilitate uterine relaxation during manual examination.
Heparin.	If other means fail, heparin may be used cautiously to stop the clotting cycle.
Antibiotic therapy (based on culture and sensitivity of lochia).	Antibiotics act prophylactically to prevent infection or may be needed for infection that caused or contributed to uterine subinvolution or hemorrhage.
Sodium bicarbonate.	May be necessary to correct acidosis.
Monitor laboratory studies as indicated:	
Hb and Hct.	Helps in determining amount of blood loss. Each ml of blood carries 0.5 mg of Hb.
Serum pH levels.	With prolonged shock, tissue hypoxia and acidosis may occur in response to anaerobic metabolism.
Platelets, FDP, fibrinogen, and APTT.	Helps determine severity of problem and effects of therapy.
Insert indwelling urinary catheter.	Provides more accurate assessment of renal function and perfusion relative to fluid volume.
Assist with procedures as indicated:	
Manual separation and removal of placenta.	Hemorrhage stops once placental fragments are removed and uterus contracts, closing venous sinuses.
Insertion of large indwelling catheter into cervical canal.	Some studies have reported success in controlling hemorrhage caused by implantation of placenta into noncontractile cervical segment by placing an indwelling catheter in the cervical canal and filling the balloon with 60 ml of saline solution to act as a tamponade.
Uterine replacement or packing if inversion seems about to recur.	Replacement of uterus allows uterus to contract, closing venous sinuses and controlling bleeding.
Prepare for surgical intervention as indicated; e.g., exploration/repair to close tear, laceration, or episiotomy extension; evacuation of hematoma; dilatation and curretage (D and C); bilateral ligation of hypogastric arteries, supracervical hysterectomy, or immediate abdominal hysterectomy.	Surgical repair of lacerations/episiotomy, incision/evacuation of hematomas, and removal of retained tissues will stop bleeding. Immediate abdominal hysterectomy is indicated for abnormally adherent placenta. (Note: D and C may be contraindicated if there is concern the procedure may traumatize the implantation site and increase bleeding.)

NURSING DIAGNOSIS:	**TISSUE PERFUSION, ALTERED**
May be related to:	Hypovolemia.

Possibly evidenced by:	Diminished arterial pulsations, cold extremities, changes in vital signs, delayed capillary refill, changes in sensorium, decreased milk production.
DESIRED OUTCOMES— CLIENT WILL:	Display BP, pulse, arterial blood gases, and Hb/Hct WNL.
	Demonstrate normal hormonal functioning by adequate milk supply for lactation and resumption of normal menses.

ACTIONS/INTERVENTIONS	RATIONALE
Independent	
Note Hb/Hct prior to and following blood loss. Assess nutritional state, height, and weight.	Comparative values help determine severity of blood losses. Preexisting state of poor health increases extent of injury from oxygen deficits.
Monitor vital signs; record degree and duration of hypovolemic episode.	Extent of pituitary involvement may be related to degree and duration of hypotension. Increased respiratory rate may reflect an effort to combat metabolic acidosis.
Note level of consciousness and any behavior changes.	Changes in sensorium are early indicators of hypoxia. Cyanosis, a later sign, may not appear until P_{O_2} levels fall below 50 mm Hg.
Assess color of nail beds, buccal mucosa, gums, and tongue; note skin temperature.	With compensatory vasoconstriction and shunting to vital organs, circulation in peripheral blood vessels is reduced, with resulting cyanosis and cool skin temperatures.
Assess breasts daily, noting presence or absence of lactation and changes in breast size.	Anterior pituitary damage or involvement (Sheehan's syndrome) reduces prolactin levels, resulting in absence of milk production and eventually a decrease in breast tissue.
Collaborative	
Monitor ABGs and pH level.	Helps in diagnosing degree of tissue hypoxia or acidosis resulting from lactic acid buildup from anaerobic metabolism.
Administer oxygen therapy as needed.	Maximizes available oxygen for circulatory transport to tissues.
Insert airway; suction as indicated.	Facilitates oxygen administration.

NURSING DIAGNOSIS:	ANXIETY [SPECIFY LEVEL]
May be related to:	Situational crisis, threat of change in health status or death, interpersonal transmission/contagion, physiologic response (release of catecholamines).
Possibly evidenced by:	Increased tension, apprehension, feelings of inadequacy/helplessness, sympathetic stimulation, focus on self, restlessness.

<table>
<tr>
<td>DESIRED OUTCOMES—
CLIENT WILL:</td>
<td>Verbalize awareness of feelings and causes of anxiety (postpartal hemorrhage is perceived as a threat to her physical integrity).

Identify healthy ways to deal with feelings.

Report anxiety is lessened.

Appear relaxed, able to sleep/rest appropriately.</td>
</tr>
</table>

ACTIONS/INTERVENTIONS	RATIONALE
Independent	
Evaluate client's psychologic response to postpartal hemorrhage and perception of events. Clarify misconceptions.	Aids in formulation of plan of care. Client's perception of the event may be distorted, intensifying her anxiety.
Evaluate physiologic response to postpartal hemorrhage; e.g., tachycardia, tachypnea, restlessness, or irritability.	Although changes in vital signs may be due to physiologic responses, they may be intensified or complicated by psychologic factors.
Convey calm, empathic, supportive attitude.	Can help client maintain emotional control in response to changing physiologic status. Aids in reducing interpersonal transmission of anxiety.
Provide information about treatment modalities and effectiveness of interventions.	Accurate information can reduce anxiety and fear of the unknown.
Assist client in identifying feelings of anxiety; provide opportunity for client to verbalize feelings.	Verbalization provides an opportunity to clarify information, correct misconceptions, and gain perspective, facilitating the problem-solving process.
Assess coping strategies and long-term implications of hemorrhagic episode. (Refer to ND: Parenting, altered, high risk for.)	Prolonged or excessive anxiety may be anticipated if complications are permanent (such as with anterior pituitary necrosis).
Collaborative	
Refer client/couple for counseling or to a community support group such as COPE (Coping with Overall Pregnancy Experience).	Helps reduce anxiety through peer or professional support and interaction.

<table>
<tr>
<td>NURSING DIAGNOSIS:</td>
<td>FLUID VOLUME EXCESS, HIGH RISK FOR</td>
</tr>
<tr>
<td>Risk factors may include:</td>
<td>Excessive/rapid replacement of fluid losses, intravascular fluid shifts (PIH).</td>
</tr>
<tr>
<td>Possibly evidenced by:</td>
<td>[Not applicable; presence of signs/symptoms establishes an actual diagnosis.]</td>
</tr>
<tr>
<td>DESIRED OUTCOMES—
CLIENT WILL:</td>
<td>Display BP, pulse, urine specific gravity, and neurologic signs WNL, without respiratory difficulties.</td>
</tr>
</table>

ACTIONS/INTERVENTIONS	RATIONALE
Independent	
Monitor for increasing BP and pulse; note respiratory signs of dyspnea, stridor, moist crackles, or rhonchi.	If fluid replacement is excessive, symptoms of circulatory overload and respiratory difficulties (e.g., pulmonary edema) may occur.
Monitor infusion rate manually or electronically (preferable). Record intake/output. Measure urine specific gravity.	Intake should approximate output with stabilization of fluid levels. Specific gravity readings change inversely to output, so that as kidney function improves, specific gravity readings decrease, and vice versa. (Note: Output may be diminished in the client with glomerular spasms due to PIH until extracellular fluids return to general circulation.)
Assess neurologic status, noting behavior changes and increasing irritability.	Behavioral changes may be an early sign of cerebral edema owing to fluid retention.
Collaborative	
Monitor Hct level.	As plasma volume is restored, the Hct level drops.

NURSING DIAGNOSIS:	INFECTION, HIGH RISK FOR
Risk factors may include:	Traumatized tissue, stasis of body fluids (lochia), decreased Hb, invasive procedures.
Possibly evidenced by:	[Not applicable; presence of signs/symptoms establishes an **actual** diagnosis.]
DESIRED OUTCOMES— CLIENT WILL:	Verbalize understanding of individual causative/risk factors.
	Display WBC count and vital signs WNL, lochia free of odor.

ACTIONS/INTERVENTIONS	RATIONALE
Independent	
Demonstrate proper handwashing and self-care techniques. Review appropriate handling and disposal of contaminated materials (e.g., peripads, tissues, dressings).	Prevents cross-contamination/spread of infectious organisms.
Note alterations in vital signs or WBC count.	Temperature elevations of 100.4°F (38°C) on 2 consecutive days (not counting the first 24 hours postpartum), tachycardia, or leukocytosis with shift to the left signifies infection.
Note symptoms of malaise, chills, anorexia, uterine tenderness, or pelvic pain.	These symptoms indicate systemic involvement, possibly leading to bacteremia, shock, or death if not treated.
Monitor rate of uterine involution and nature and amount of lochial discharge. (Refer to CP: Puerperal Infection.)	Uterine infection delays involution and prolongs lochial flow.

ACTIONS/INTERVENTIONS

Independent

Investigate other potential sources of infection, such as respiratory (changes in breath sounds, productive cough, purulent sputum), mastitis (swelling, erythema, pain), or urinary tract infection (cloudy, odoriferous urine; urgency, frequency, pain).

Collaborative

Assess Hb/Hct levels. Administer iron supplement, as indicated.

Obtain Gram stain or bacterial culture if lochia is foul-smelling or profuse.

Administer intravenous antibiotics, as indicated.

Assist as necessary with surgical procedures (e.g., D and C, hysterectomy).

RATIONALE

Differential diagnosis is critical for effective treatment.

Anemia often accompanies infection, delays healing, and impairs the immune system.

Gram stain identifies type of infection; cultures identify specific pathogen.

Broad-spectrum antibiotic may be ordered until results from culture and sensitivity studies are available, at which time organism-specific antibiotic may be started.

D and C may be necessary to remove any remaining placental fragments; hysterectomy may be necessary in septic shock.

NURSING DIAGNOSIS:	**PAIN, HIGH RISK FOR**
Risk factors may include:	Tissue trauma/distention.
Possibly evidenced by:	[Not applicable; presence of signs/symptoms establishes an **actual** diagnosis.]
DESIRED OUTCOMES— CLIENT WILL:	Identify individually appropriate methods to promote comfort.
	Verbalize relief of pain and discomfort.

ACTIONS/INTERVENTIONS

Independent

Determine characteristics, type, location, and duration of pain. Assess client for persistent perineal pain, feeling of fullness in vagina, uterine contractions, or abdominal tenderness.

Assess possible psychologic causes of discomfort.

RATIONALE

Aids in differential diagnosis and selection of treatment methods. Discomfort associated with hematomas is due to pressure from concealed hemorrhage into vaginal or perineal tissues. Abdominal tenderness may result from uterine atony or retained pieces of placenta. Severe pain, both uterine and abdominal, may occur with inversion of the uterus. Lacerations may result in painful burning or tearing sensations.

Emergency situation may precipitate fear and anxiety, which intensity perception of discomfort. (Refer to ND: Anxiety [specify level].)

ACTIONS/INTERVENTIONS	RATIONALE

Independent

Instruct client in relaxation techniques; provide diversional activities as appropriate.

Educating client in physiologic and psychologic methods of pain control decreases anxiety and perception of discomfort.

Provide comfort measures, such as application of ice to perineum or heat lamp to episiotomy extension.

Cold applications minimize edema and reduce hematoma and pain sensation; heat promotes vasodilation, which facilitates resorption of hematoma.

Collaborative

Administer analgesics, narcotics, or sedatives as indicated.

Decreases pain and anxiety; promotes relaxation.

NURSING DIAGNOSIS:	KNOWLEDGE DEFICIT [LEARNING NEED], regarding condition, prognosis, and treatment needs
May be related to:	Lack of exposure to, and unfamiliarity with, information resources.
Possibly evidenced by:	Request for information, statement of misconceptions, inappropriate or exaggerated behaviors.
DESIRED OUTCOMES— CLIENT WILL:	Verbalize in simple terms the pathophysiology and implications of her clinical situation.

ACTIONS/INTERVENTIONS	RATIONALE

Independent

Explain predisposing or causative factors and treatment specific to the cause of hemorrhage.

Provides information to help client/couple understand and cope with situation.

Assess client's/couple's level of knowledge, readiness, and ability to learn. Listen, talk calmly, and allow time for questions and review of material.

Provides information necessary to develop individual plan of care. Reduces anxiety and stress, which can block learning, and provides clarification and repetition to enhance understanding.

Discuss short-term implications of postpartal hemorrhage, such as delay or interruption in process of maternal-infant attachment (client is unable to assume care of self and infant as soon as she desires).

Reduces anxiety and provides realistic time frame for resumption of bonding and infant care activities.

Discuss long-term implications of postpartal hemorrhage as appropriate; e.g., risk of postpartal hemorrhage in subsequent pregnancies, uterine atony, or the inability to bear children in the future if hysterectomy is performed.

Permits client to make informed decisions and to begin to resolve feelings about current and past events.

Instruct client to report failure to lactate, fatigue, loss of pubic or axillary hair, amenorrhea, genital atrophy, premature aging (cachexia).

These signs suggest Sheehan's syndrome, which occurs in 15% of survivors of severe postpartal hemorrhage; causes partial or total loss of thyroid, adrenocortical, and gonadal functions and requires long-term treatment with estrogen, thyroid,

413

ACTIONS/INTERVENTIONS

Independent

RATIONALE

or cortisone replacement therapy. (Note: Sheehan's syndrome often results in irreversible infertility, reduced resistance to infection, premature aging, and increased risk of shock.)

Refer to support group(s) if appropriate.

Specific groups, such as a hysterectomy support group, may provide ongoing information to facilitate positive adaptation.

NURSING DIAGNOSIS:	PARENTING, ALTERED, HIGH RISK FOR
Risk factors may include:	Interruption in bonding process, physical condition, perceived threat to own survival.
Possibly evidenced by:	[Not applicable; presence of signs/symptoms establishes an **actual** diagnosis.]
DESIRED OUTCOMES— CLIENT WILL:	Demonstrate appropriate behaviors associated with positive attachment to infant.
	Assume responsibility for physical and emotional care of the newborn, as able.
	Express comfort with parenting role.

ACTIONS/INTERVENTIONS

Independent

Explain factors resulting from postpartal hemorrhage that necessitate separation of mother and infant.

Provide opportunity for client/couple to express their fears and anger at the situation.

Discuss client's perceptions of infant care responsibilities and parenting role.

Encourage contact with infant (verbal reports, photos, information from significant other who has seen baby) until client can see and begin to care for the infant.

Evaluate attachment process, bonding behaviors, and parenting abilities once client assumes care of her infant.

Provide client/couple with information on community resources and with follow-up healthcare referrals, including parenting classes, child care facilities, and well-baby clinics.

RATIONALE

Reduces anxiety and feelings of frustration and helplessness related to client's inability to assume caregiving role with infant.

Promotes acceptance of physiologic and psychologic constraints, which reduces anxiety.

Provides information about how client views these role changes; identifies areas of learning need.

Reassures mother of infant's health status and of proper care being given to the infant.

Provides information on psychologic and physiologic capabilities related to parenting; identifies client's needs.

Reinforces positive information previously given by health team. Reduces anxiety; promotes independence and personal growth.

Postpartal Diabetes Mellitus

_____

(To be used in conjunction with customary postpartal plans of care.)

CLIENT ASSESSMENT DATA BASE

(Refer to Chapter 4, CP: Diabetes Mellitus: Prepregnancy/Gestational; and Chapter 5, CP: Intrapartal Diabetes Mellitus.)

ACTIVITY/REST

Fatigue, especially when labor was long or difficult; increasing glucose needs.

CIRCULATION

May have elevated blood pressure (BP), edema (signs of pregnancy-induced hypertension [PIH]) that developed during prenatal, intrapartal, or postpartal period.

History of vascular changes associated with diabetes that impair circulation/kidney functioning; venous thrombosis.

FOOD/FLUID

Polydipsia, polyphagia.

Nausea/vomiting.

Ketonuria, elevated serum glucose.

May report episodes of hypoglycemia, glycosuria.

Type of infant feeding planned affects caloric needs and insulin requirements.

SAFETY

Healing of episiotomy or cesarean incision may be delayed.

May report visual disturbances.

SEXUALITY

Uterus may be relaxed/boggy, and lochia may be heavy with clots present.

Current pregnancy may have involved uterine overdistention (macrosomia or polyhydramnios).

Labor may have been prolonged/augmented or induced.

Preterm, large-for-gestational age, or low-birth-weight infant.

TEACHING/LEARNING

Change in stability of diabetes, adjustment of insulin therapy.

DIAGNOSTIC STUDIES

Fasting (daily) or random blood sugars: Assesses control (increased risk of hypoglycemia).
Hemoglobin/hematocrit: Baseline studies.
Glycosylated hemoglobin (HbA$_{1c}$): May be elevated (greater than 8.5%), indicating inadequate control of serum glucose levels.
Urinalysis: May show glucose, ketones, or protein.

NURSING PRIORITIES

1. Maintain normoglycemia.
2. Prevent or minimize complications.
3. Promote parent-infant bonding.
4. Provide information concerning postpartal changes and diabetic management.

NURSING DIAGNOSIS:	**NUTRITION, ALTERED, LESS THAN BODY REQUIRE-MENTS, HIGH RISK FOR**
Risk factors may include:	Inability to ingest/utilize nutrients appropriately.
Possibly evidenced by:	[Not applicable; presence of signs/symptoms establishes an **actual** diagnosis.]
DESIRED OUTCOMES— CLIENT WILL:	Maintain serum glucose levels within individually determined parameters.
	Verbalize understanding of and participate in self-monitoring and individual treatment regimen.

ACTIONS/INTERVENTIONS	RATIONALE
Independent	
Review onset of diabetes (prepregnancy versus gestational) and type of infant feeding planned.	The client with gestational diabetes mellitus usually requires no further insulin after delivery; the client with prepregnancy onset must be re-regulated based on fasting blood sugar and 1-hour postprandial blood glucose levels. Additionally, breastfeeding has an antidiabetogenic effect because carbohydrates are utilized in milk production.
Assess for hypoglycemic or hyperglycemic reactions. Note changes in mentation and behavior, visual disturbances, nausea or vomiting, tachycardia, slurred speech, or Kussmaul's respirations.	Since the half-life of human placental lactogen is 20–30 min, most of this insulin antagonist has disappeared within 2 to 3 hours postpartum, rendering the client susceptible to hypoglycemia if insulin dosages are not accurately recalculated.
Monitor urine for glucose and ketones.	The presence of ketones indicates inadequate carbohydrate intake and fat breakdown and may necessitate modifying diet or discontinuing breastfeeding.
Advise GDM client to avoid obesity and to lose weight during postpartal period if she is not lactating.	Helps reduce risk of developing insulin-dependent diabetes (type I), although 70% of individuals who develop GDM develop type II diabetes later in life, often within 10 years.
Collaborative	
Monitor serum glucose levels by fingerstick per protocol and as indicated.	Insulin requirements decrease in the first 48–96 hr postpartum following removal of the placenta with its anti-insulin hormones. Such a change results in a glucose-insulin imbalance. Frequent assessment (e.g., every 2 hr) is continued until serum

ACTIONS/INTERVENTIONS	RATIONALE
Collaborative	
	glucose levels stabilize and carbohydrate hemostasis occurs. Hypoglycemia is common during the first 24 hr following delivery. Hyperglycemia may compromise wound healing, and poor control is associated with increased morbidity and infection.
Discontinue insulin infusion following vaginal delivery, as indicated; continue infusion of glucose until oral feedings are started.	Insulin requirements quickly decline following delivery of the placenta. Glucose infusion helps prevent hypoglycemic response. (Note: I.V. infusion of 5% dextrose with insulin at 1 unit/hr via pump may be used to maintain normoglycemic control in early postpartal period.)
Continue insulin infusion following cesarean birth until client has resumed eating.	Surgical procedure/stress may increase insulin needs.
Administer insulin subcutaneously or monitor self-administration of insulin for client with prepregnancy diabetes.	During first 1 or 2 days postpartum, insulin dosage is usually equal to one half to two thirds of prepregnancy levels with the resumption of a "regular" diet.
Adjust diet to increase calories by 600–800 kcal/day if client is breastfeeding.	Inadequate caloric intake with resulting hypoglycemia negatively affects milk supply and letdown reflex.
Reevaluate serum glucose levels at 6-week checkup or when breastfeeding stops. Institute new dietary insulin control if fasting plasma glucose is greater than 140 mg/dl, or if 2-hour oral glucose tolerance test (GTT) is 140–200 mg/dl and at least one other value is greater than 200 mg/dl.	Although temporary remission of diabetes may occur, necessitating lowering insulin needs, return to prepregnancy doses are usually required by 6 weeks postpartum or when weaning occurs.

NURSING DIAGNOSIS:	**INJURY, HIGH RISK FOR, multiple factors**
Risk factors may include:	Biochemical or regulatory complications (e.g, uterine atony/hemorrhage, hypertension [PIH], hyperglycemia).
Possibly evidenced by:	[Not applicable; presence of signs/symptoms establishes an **actual** diagnosis.]
DESIRED OUTCOMES— CLIENT WILL:	Display vital signs, reflex response, lochial discharge, and white blood cell (WBC) count within normal limits, with uterus well contracted.

ACTIONS/INTERVENTIONS	RATIONALE
Independent	
Monitor contractility and location of uterus.	Uterine atony and hemorrhage may occur, owing to overdistention associated with a large (macrosomic) infant, polyhydramnios, or oxytocin stimulation.

417

ACTIONS/INTERVENTIONS	RATIONALE

Independent

Gently massage uterus as indicated.	Increases uterine tone and myometrial contractility, reducing risk of hemorrhage.
Assess amount and type of lochia flow with each check of the fundus. (Refer to CP: Postpartal Hemorrhage, ND: Fluid Volume deficit, high risk for.)	Increased or heavy flow may indicate developing complication.
Assess bladder fullness; encourage voiding within 6–8 hr following delivery. Monitor intake and output.	Polyuria (increased urine output) associated with diabetes occurs as a means of excreting excess glucose and retained fluids. A full bladder may interfere with uterine involution.
Monitor BP and pulse. Note location and extent of edema and presence of proteinuria, visual disturbances, hyperreflexia, or right upper quadrant pain. Institute seizure precautions. (Refer to Chapter 4, CP: Pregnancy-Induced Hypertension.)	With hemorrhage, BP decreases and pulse increases. Elevated BP, proteinuria, and extensive edema may indicate PIH or potential eclampsia. Danger of eclampsia exists for up to 72 hours postpartum, but can actually occur for up to a week postpartum, depending on severity of hypertension, fluid retention, and organ involvement.
Monitor temperature and WBC count. Assess lochia and episiotomy or abdominal incision. Note progressive rate of uterine involution. (Refer to CP: Puerperal Infection.)	Infection is indicated by elevated temperature and WBC count; redness, erythema, or exudate at site of episiotomy or abdominal incision; and foul-smelling lochia. Infection may occur in diabetic client owing to poor healing associated with vascular involvement and hyperglycemia.

NURSING DIAGNOSIS:	**KNOWLEDGE DEFICIT [LEARNING NEED], regarding condition, prognosis, and treatment needs**
May be related to:	Lack of exposure/recall, misinterpretation, unfamiliarity with resources.
Possibly evidenced by:	Verbalization of concerns/misconceptions, inadequate performance of procedures, development of preventable complications.
DESIRED OUTCOMES— CLIENT/COUPLE WILL:	Verbalize understanding of physiologic changes, individual needs, possible outcomes.
	Perform necessary activities/procedures correctly and explain reasons for actions.
	Select family planning method prior to discharge.

ACTIONS/INTERVENTIONS	RATIONALE

Independent

Discuss dietary needs based on individual weight gain and choice of infant feeding.	Calorie needs will be determined by desired weight goal and whether client is breastfeeding.

ACTIONS/INTERVENTIONS	RATIONALE
Independent	
Stress importance of home monitoring of condition and maintenance of log of dietary intake, medication, exercise, and signs/symptoms of serum glucose fluctuation.	Although the demands of pregnancy are concluded, postpartal demands of healing/return to nonpregnant state and needs of infant and family will affect diabetic control. Keeping a log provides insight to individual needs/responses to therapy.
Provide information for Class A diabetic client (White's classification) about the need to return for a 3-hour GTT at 6-week postpartal visit or at cessation of breastfeeding. If test results are normal, annual follow-up testing is required.	About 18% of Class A diabetic clients manifest carbohydrate intolerance at 6 weeks postpartum. Greater than 70% of clients with GDM eventually develop type II diabetes, many within 10 years following delivery.
Identify signs/symptoms requiring notification of healthcare provider; e.g., continued oozing or lack of progression of lochia, fever, or foul-smelling urine/vaginal drainage.	Prompt evaluation and intervention may prevent or limit development of complications such as hemorrhage and infection.
Discuss client's/couple's plans for future pregnancies and the impact of diabetes on fertility. Review the critical importance of obtaining metabolic control of diabetes prior to conception.	Diabetes, if well controlled, does not alter or reduce fertility rate. Uncontrolled diabetes and elevated HbA_{1c} levels during organogenesis greatly increase incidence of malformations. Good metabolic control started before conception and continued during these critical weeks may prevent such malformations.
Determine client's/couple's plans for selecting a contraceptive method.	Choosing a method of contraception involves some compromise between benefits and risks, especially with the diabetic. Risk of using oral contraceptives or the intrauterine device (IUD) in diabetic clients must be weighed against the risk of pregnancy with other forms of contraception.
Provide information and review side effects associated with contraceptive choices:	
Oral contraceptives.	Side effects include elevated BP and acceleration of blood vessel disease (thrombophlebitis, vascular complications). Estrogen increases the production of cholesterol and triglycerides, and progesterone interferes with insulin activity, accelerating the subclinical diabetic process and creating deterioration in the diabetic state. (Note: Progestin-only or triphasic products are considered safer than combined oral contraceptives.)
IUD.	Some studies indicate an increased risk of pelvic salpingitis (especially during first 20 days following insertion).
Barrier methods (i.e., condom, diaphragm, cervical caps, sponges, or spermicidal creams).	No side effects or contraindications of these methods are specific for diabetic client, although these methods are not as effective in preventing unwanted pregnancies, due in part to inconsistent use. When a device such as the diaphragm is used in conjunction with a spermicidal cream, effectiveness is significantly increased.

ACTIONS/INTERVENTIONS	RATIONALE

Independent

Tubal ligation.	May be desirable for diabetic client with complications of nephropathy, retinopathy, or vascular disease, rather than risk the possibility of future pregnancies with negative maternal/fetal outcomes.
Provide information about effects of diabetes on future offspring.	Heredity contributes to the risk of diabetes. Type I (insulin-dependent) diabetes mellitus appears to be transmitted less frequently to offspring of diabetic women than to offspring of diabetic men, although this phenomenon may be due to perinatal loss of affected offspring by diabetic mothers. If a parent develops type II diabetes mellitus, the children are at a greater risk than the general population for developing this type of diabetes.

(Refer to CP: The Client at 4 Hours to 3 Days Postpartum, ND: Knowledge Deficit [Learning Need], for additional actions.)

NURSING DIAGNOSIS:	PARENTING, ALTERED, HIGH RISK FOR
Risk factors may include:	Interruption in bonding process, physical illness/changes in physical abilities.
Possibly evidenced by:	[Not applicable; presence of signs/symptoms establishes an **actual** diagnosis.]
DESIRED OUTCOMES— CLIENT/COUPLE WILL:	Verbalize fears and concerns about infant's condition.
	Participate optimally in infant contact and care.
	Demonstrate positive attachment behaviors.

ACTIONS/INTERVENTIONS	RATIONALE

Independent

Determine current status of infant.	The special needs of the infant of the diabetic mother include hypoglycemia, hypocalcemia, prematurity, and respiratory distress syndrome, possibly necessitating a short- or long-term stay in the neonatal intensive care unit (NICU). Such separation, with diminished physical contact coupled with excessive parental anxiety, may interfere with positive bonding and may create a high-risk parenting situation.
Provide information concerning condition of infant.	Information helps to reduce fears and to emphasize the reality of the infant's presence.
Determine client's/couple's feelings concerning infant. Observe contact with infant. (Refer to CP: The Parents of a Child with Special Needs.)	Provides baseline for future comparison; identifies needs and potential concerns.
Assess effectiveness/use of support systems by client/couple.	Strong system of support from family/friends or community facilitates positive adaptation to stress.

ACTIONS/INTERVENTIONS	RATIONALE

Independent

Encourage frequent interaction with infant and participation in infant care tasks as client's/infant's condition allows.

Couple may be extremely anxious if infant is in NICU and may be fearful of touching or holding the infant.

Facilitate communication between couple and nursery staff. Point out normal and positive aspects of infant.

Staff can reduce fears, act as role models, and facilitate bonding, especially in caring for preterm infant.

Refer parents to other couples who have had similar experiences with their newborn infants or to the appropriate support groups.

Increases parents' sense of support and helps them to feel that they are not alone. Provides opportunity for creative problem-solving.

Assess client's eyesight and ability to provide infant care in client with longstanding diabetes.

Retinopathy may progress during the prenatal period and negatively affect client's independence, requiring additional teaching and support.

Collaborative

Refer to visiting nurse services or parenting classes, as indicated.

Client/couple may need additional assistance to promote family integration.

(Refer to CP: Maternal Assessment: 4 to 6 Weeks Following Delivery, ND: Parenting, altered, high risk for.)

Puerperal Infection

Puerperal infection is an infection of the reproductive tract occurring within 28 days following childbirth or abortion. It is one of the major causes of maternal death (ranking second to postpartal hemorrhage) and includes localized infectious processes as well as more progressive processes that may result in metritis, endometritis, peritonitis, or pelvic cellulitis (parametritis).

CLIENT ASSESSMENT DATA BASE

ACTIVITY/REST

Malaise, lethargy.

Exhaustion and/or ongoing fatigue (prolonged labor, multiple postpartal stressors).

CIRCULATION

Tachycardia of varying severity.

ELIMINATION

Diarrhea may be present.

Bowel sounds may be absent if paralytic ileus occurs.

EGO INTEGRITY

Marked anxiety (peritonitis).

FOOD/FLUID

Anorexia, nausea/vomiting.

Thirst, dry mucous membranes.

Abdominal distention, rigidity, rebound tenderness (peritonitis).

NEUROSENSORY

Headache.

PAIN/DISCOMFORT

Localized pain, dysuria, abdominal discomfort.

Severe or prolonged afterpains, lower abdominal or uterine pain and tenderness with guarding (endometritis).

Unilateral/bilateral abdominal pain/rigidity (salpingitis/oophoritis, parametritis).

RESPIRATION

Rapid/shallow respirations (severe/systemic process).

SAFETY

Temperature: 100.4°F (38.0°C) or higher occurring on any 2 successive days, excluding the first 24 hours postpartum, is indicative of infection; however, temperature greater than 101°F (38.9°C) in the first 24 hours is highly indicative of ensuing infection.

Low-grade fever of less than 101°F suggests incisional infection; fever greater than 102°F (38.9°C) is indicative or more extensive infection (e.g., salpingitis, parametritis, peritonitis).

Chills may occur; severe/recurrent chills (often lasting 30–40 min), with temperature spikes to 104°F, suggest pelvic infections, thrombophlebitis or peritonitis.

Report of internal monitoring, frequent intrapartal vaginal examinations, lapses in aseptic technique.

Traumatic delivery and/or lacerations of reproductive tract, operative procedures/incisions.

Preexisting infections, including human immunodeficiency virus.

Environmental exposure.

SEXUALITY

Premature or prolonged rupture of membranes, prolonged labor (24 hours or more).

Retention of products of conception, uterine exploration/manual removal of placenta, or postpartal hemorrhage.

Incision edges may be reddened, edematous, firm, tender, or separated, with drainage of purulent or sanguineous liquid.

Uterine subinvolution may be present.

Lochia may be foul-smelling, odorless (as in infection by beta-hemolytic streptococci), scant, or profuse.

SOCIAL INTERACTION

Low socioeconomic status with corresponding stressors.

TEACHING/LEARNING

Lack of prenatal care.

Lack of or inadequate perineal care.

Chronic conditions; e.g., malnutrition, anemia, diabetes.

DIAGNOSTIC STUDIES

White blood cell (WBC) count: Normal or elevated with differential shifted to the left.
Erythrocyte sedimentation rate (ESR), and red blood cell (RBC) count: Markedly increased in presence of infection.
Hemoglobin/hematocrit (Hb/Hct), RBC count: Decreased in presence of anemia.
Cultures (aerobic/anaerobic) of intrauterine or intracervical material or wound drainge, or Gram stain of lochia, cervix, and uterus: Identify causative organism(s).
Urinalysis and culture: Rule out urinary tract infection.
Ultrasonography: Determines presence of retained placental fragments; locates peritoneal abscess.
Bimanual examination: Determines nature and location of pelvic pain, mass or abscess formation, or presence of thrombosed veins.

NURSING PRIORITIES

1. Control spread of infection.
2. Promote healing.
3. Support ongoing process of family acquaintance.

DISCHARGE GOALS

1. Infection resolving.
2. Involution progressing, sense of well-being expressed.
3. Attachment/bonding demonstrated and care of infant resumed.

NURSING DIAGNOSIS:	INFECTION, HIGH RISK FOR, spread/sepsis
Risk factors may include:	Presence of infection, broken skin and/or traumatized tissues, high vascularity of involved area, invasive procedures and/or increased environmental exposure, chronic disease (e.g., diabetes), anemia, malnutrition, immunosuppression and/or untoward effect of medication (e.g., opportunistic/secondary infections).
Possibly evidenced by:	[Not applicable: presence of signs/symptoms established an **actual** diagnosis.]
DESIRED OUTCOMES— CLIENT WILL:	Verbalize understanding of individual causative risk factors. Initiate behaviors to limit spread of infection as appropriate, reduce risk of complications. Achieve timely healing, free of additional complications.

ACTIONS/INTERVENTIONS

Independent

Review prenatal, intrapartal, and postpartal record.

Maintain strict handwashing policy for staff, client, and visitors.

Provide for and instruct client in proper disposal of contaminated linens, dressings, chux, and peripads. Implement setup of isolation, if indicated.

Demonstrate/encourage correct perineal cleaning after voiding and defecation, and frequent changing of peripads.

Demonstrate proper fundal massage. Review importance and timing of procedure.

Monitor temperature, pulse, and respirations. Note presence of chills or reports of anorexia or malaise.

Observe/record other signs of infection (e.g., foul-smelling lochia or drainage; subinvolution of uterus; extreme uterine tenderness; or incisional redness, edema, drainage, or separation).

Monitor oral/parenteral intake, stressing the need for at least 2000 ml fluid per day. Note urine output, degree of hydration, and presence of nausea, vomiting, or diarrhea.

Encourage semi-Fowler's position.

RATIONALE

Identifies factors that place client in high-risk category for development/spread of postpartal infection.

Helps to prevent cross-contamination.

Prevents spread of infection.

Cleaning removes urinary/fecal contaminants. Changing pad removes moist medium that favors bacterial growth.

Enhances uterine contractility; promotes involution and passage of any retained placental fragments.

Elevations in vital signs accompany infection; fluctuations, or changes in symptoms, suggest alterations in client status. (Note: Persistent fever unresponsive to antibiotic therapy may indicate pelvic thrombophlebitis.)

Allows early identification and treatment; promotes resolution of infection. (Note: Although localized infections are usually not severe, progression to necrotizing fasciitis can be life-threatening.)

Increased intake replaces losses and enhances circulating volume, preventing dehydration and aiding in fever reduction.

Enhances flow of lochia and uterine/pelvic drainage.

ACTIONS/INTERVENTIONS	RATIONALE

Independent

Promote early ambulation, balanced with adequate rest.

Increases circulation; promotes clearing of respiratory secretions and lochial drainage; enhances healing and general well-being. (Note: Presence of pelvic/femoral thrombophlebitis may require strict bedrest.)

Investigate reports of leg or chest pain. Note pallor, swelling, or stiffness of lower extremity. (Refer to CP: Postpartal Thrombophlebitis.)

These signs and symptoms are suggestive of septic thrombus formation. (Note: Embolic sequelae, especially pulmonary embolism, may be initial indicator of thrombophlebitis.)

Recommend that breastfeeding mother periodically check infant's mouth for presence of white patches.

Oral thrush in the newborn is a common side effect of maternal antibiotic therapy.

Collaborative

Encourage application of moist heat in the form of sitz baths and of dry heat in the form of perineal lights for 15 min 2 to 4 times daily.

Water promotes cleansing. Heat dilates perineal blood vessels, increasing localized blood flow and promoting healing.

Demonstrate perineal application of antibiotic creams, as appropriate.

Eradicates local infectious organisms, reducing risk of spreading of infection

Monitor laboratory studies, as indicated:

Culture(s)/sensitivity.

Identifies infectious process, causative organism, and appropriate antimicrobial agents.

Complete blood count, WBC count, differential, and ESR.

Aids in tracking resolution of infectious or inflammatory process. Identifies degree of blood loss and determines presence of anemia.

Partial thromboplastin time/prothrombin time (PTT/PT), clotting times.

Helps in identifying alterations in clotting associated with development of emboli. Aids in determining effectiveness of anticoagulation therapy.

Renal/hepatic function studies.

Hepatic insufficiency and decreased renal function may develop, altering drug half-life and increasing risks of toxicity.

Administer medications as indicated:

Antibiotics, initially broad-spectrum, then organism specific as indicated by results of cultures/sensitivity.

Combats pathogenic organisms, helping to prevent infection from spreading to surrounding tissues and bloodstream. (Note: Parenteral route is preferred for parametritis, peritonitis, and, on occasion, endometritis.)

Oxytocics, such as methylergonovine maleate (Methergine) or ergonovine maleate (Ergotrate).

Promotes myometrial contractility to retard the spread of bacteria through the uterine walls, and aids in the expulsion of clots and retained placental fragments.

Anticoagulants (e.g., heparin).

In presence of pelvic thrombophlebitis, anticoagulants prevent or reduce additional thrombi formation and limit spread of septic emboli.

ACTIONS/INTERVENTIONS

Collaborative

Assist with procedures, such as incision and drainage, or dilatation and curettage (D and C), as necessary.

Administer whole blood/packed RBCs, if needed.

Provide supplemental oxygen when necessary.

Arrange for transfer to intensive care setting as appropriate.

RATIONALE

Draining/cleaning the infected area promotes healing and reduces risk of rupture into peritoneal cavity. D and C may be needed to remove retained products of conception and/or placental fragments.

Replaces blood losses and increases oxygen-carrying capacity in presence of severe anemia/hemorrhage.

Promotes healing and tissue regeneration, especially in presence of anemia; may enhance oxygenation when pulmonary emboli are present.

May be necessary for client with severe infection (e.g., peritonitis, sepsis) or pulmonary emboli to provide appropriate care leading to optimal recovery.

NURSING DIAGNOSIS:	NUTRITION, ALTERED, LESS THAN BODY REQUIREMENTS
May be related to:	Intake insufficient to meet metabolic demands (anorexia, nausea/vomiting, medical restrictions).
Possibly evidenced by:	Aversion to eating, decreased oral intake or lack of oral intake, unanticipated weight loss.
DESIRED OUTCOMES— CLIENT WILL:	Meet nutritional needs as evidenced by timely wound healing, appropriate energy level, weight loss, and Hb/Hct within normal postpartal expectations.

ACTIONS/INTERVENTIONS

Independent

Encourage choice of foods high in protein, iron, and vitamin C when oral intake permitted.

Promote intake of at least 2000 ml/day of juices, soups, and other nutritious fluids.

Encourage adequate sleep/rest.

Collaborative

Administer parenteral fluids/nutrition, as indicated.

Administer iron preparations and/or vitamins, as indicated.

RATIONALE

Protein helps promote healing and regeneration of new tissue. Iron is necessary for Hb synthesis. Vitamin C facilitates iron absorption and is necessary for cell wall synthesis.

Provides calories and other nutrients to meet metabolic needs and replaces fluid losses, thereby increasing circulating fluid volume.

Reduces metabolic rate, allowing nutrients and oxygen to be used for healing process.

May be necessary to combat dehydration, replace fluid losses, and provide necessary nutrients when oral intake is limited/restricted.

Useful in correcting anemia or deficiencies when present.

ACTIONS/INTERVENTIONS

Collaborative

Assist with placement of nasogastric or Miller-Abbott tube.

RATIONALE

May be necessary for gastrointestinal decompression in presence of abdominal distention or peritonitis.

NURSING DIAGNOSIS:	PAIN [ACUTE]
May be related to:	Body response to infective agent, properties of infection (e.g., skin/tissue edema, erythema).
Possibly evidenced by:	Verbalizations, restlessness, guarding behavior, self-focusing, autonomic responses.
DESIRED OUTCOMES— CLIENT WILL:	Identify/use individually appropriate comfort measures. Report discomfort is relieved/controlled.

ACTIONS/INTERVENTIONS

Independent

Assess location and nature of discomfort or pain.

Provide instruction regarding, and assist with, maintenance of cleanliness and warmth.

Change client's position frequently. Provide comfort measures; e.g., back rubs, linen changes.

Instruct client in relaxation techniques; provide diversionary activities such as radio, television, or reading.

Encourage continuation of breastfeeding as client's condition permits. Otherwise suggest and provide instruction in use of manual or electric breast pump.

Collaborative

Administer analgesics or antipyretics.

Apply local heat using heat lamp or sitz bath as indicated.

RATIONALE

Aids in differential diagnosis of tissue involvement in infectious process.

Promotes general well-being and healing. Alleviates discomfort associated with chills.

Reduces muscle fatigue, promotes relaxation and comfort.

Refocuses client's attention, promotes positive attitude, and enhances comfort.

Prevents discomfort of engorgement; promotes adequacy of milk supply in breastfeeding client.

Reduces associated discomforts of infection.

Heat promotes vasodilation, increasing circulation to the affected area and promoting localized comfort.

NURSING DIAGNOSIS:	PARENTING, ALTERED, HIGH RISK FOR
Risk factors may include:	Interruption in bonding process, physical illness, perceived threat to own survival.
Possibly evidenced by:	[Not applicable; presence of signs/symptoms establishes an **actual** diagnosis.]

DESIRED OUTCOMES—CLIENT WILL:	Exhibit ongoing attachment behaviors during parent-infant interactions.
	Maintain/assume responsibility for physical and emotional care of the newborn, as able.
	Express comfort with parenting role.

ACTIONS/INTERVENTIONS

Independent

Provide opportunities for maternal-infant contact whenever possible. Place pictures of infant at client's bedside, especially if hospital policy requires separation of infant from mother during febrile period.

Monitor client's emotional responses to illness and separation from infant, such as depression and anger.

Encourage client to feed infant if possible and to increase her participation in infant care as the infection resolves.

Observe maternal-infant interactions.

Encourage father/other family members to care for and interact with the infant.

Collaborative

Make arrangements for appropriate follow-up evaluation of mother-infant interactions/responses.

Identify individual support systems; refer to home care agencies as indicated.

RATIONALE

Facilitates attachment, prevents client from engaging in self-preoccupation to the exclusion of the infant.

Normal expectations are of an uncomplicated postpartal period with the family unit intact. Illness due to infection alters the situation and may result in separation of client from family or newborn, which can contribute to feelings of isolation and depression.

Success in accomplishing infant care tasks enhances client's outlook and promotes her attachment with infant. (Note: Dependent on type of infection, bottle-fed infants may need to be separated from mother for longer period because they do not receive protective advantages of breastfeeding.)

Provides information regarding status of bonding process and client needs.

May be encouraging to mother to know that family is caring for the infant and providing emotional support.

Provides resources and support to client; useful in identifying specific needs and problem-solving.

Client may require assistance with home maintenance and activities of daily living while following discharge instructions for rest and recuperation.

Postpartal Thrombophlebitis _____

Superficial thrombophlebitis is seen more often in the postpartal period than during pregnancy and is more common in women with preexisting varices. Postpartal deep vein thrombosis (DVT) and superficial thrombophlebitis have been attributed to trauma to pelvic veins from pressure of the presenting fetal part, sluggish circulation caused by mechanical edema, and alterations in coagulation related to large amounts of estrogens produced during pregancy. Thrombosis that involves only the superficial veins of the leg or thigh is unlikely to generate pulmonary emboli.

CLIENT ASSESSMENT DATA BASE

ACTIVITY/REST

History of prolonged sitting, either work-related or as a result of activity restrictions.

Immobility associated with bedrest and anesthesia.

CIRCULATION

Varicose veins.

Slight elevation of pulse rate (superficial).

History of previous venous thrombosis, heart problems, hemorrhage, pregnancy-induced hypertension, hypercoagulability in early puerperium.

Peripheral pulses diminished, positive Homans' sign may or may not be noted (indicators of DVT).

Lower extremity (calf/thigh) may be warm and pinkish-red in color, or affected limb may be cool, pale, edematous.

FOOD/FLUID

Excessive weight gain/obesity.

Milk supply may occasionally be reduced in lactating client.

PAIN/DISCOMFORT

Tenderness and pain in affected area (e.g., calf or thigh).

Thrombosis may be palpable, bumpy/knotty.

SAFETY

Presence of postpartal endometritis or pelvic cellulitis.

Temperature may be slightly elevated; progression to marked elevation and chills (signs of DVT).

SEXUALITY

Multiparity.

Prolonged labor associated with fetal head pressure on pelvic veins, use of stirrups or faulty positioning of extremities during intrapartal phase, or operative delivery, including cesarean birth.

TEACHING/LEARNING

Use of oral contraceptives.

Use of estrogen for suppression of lactation.

429

DIAGNOSTIC STUDIES

Doppler ultrasonography: Reveals increased circumference of affected extremity.

Impedance plethysmography: Detects venous obstruction.

Contrast venography: Confirms diagnosis of DVT.

Hemoglobin/hematocrit: Identify hemoconcentration.

Coagulation studies: Reveal hypercoagulability.

NURSING PRIORITIES

1. Facilitate resolution of thrombus.
2. Promote optimal comfort.
3. Prevent complications.
4. Provide information and emotional support.

DISCHARGE GOALS

1. Tissue perfusion improved in affected limb/area.
2. Pain/discomfort relieved.
3. Complications prevented/resolved.
4. Disease process/prognosis and therapeutic needs understood.

NURSING DIAGNOSIS:	TISSUE PERFUSION, ALTERED
May be related to:	Interruption of venous flow.
Possibly evidenced by:	Edema of affected extremity; erythema (superficial thrombophlebitis) or pallor and coolness (DVT), diminished peripheral pulses.
DESIRED OUTCOMES— CLIENT WILL:	Demonstrate improved circulation of involved extremity with palpable peripheral pulses of good quality, adequate capillary refill, and decreased edema and erythema.

ACTIONS/INTERVENTIONS	RATIONALE
Independent	
Encourage bedrest.	Minimizes the possibility of dislodging thrombus and creating emboli.
Observe extremity for color; inspect from groin to foot for edema. Note asymmetry; measure and record calf circumference of both legs.	Symptoms help distinguish between superficial thrombophlebitis and DVT. Redness, heat, tenderness, and localized edema are characteristic of superficial involvement. Pallor and coolness of extremity are characteristic of DVT. Calf vein involvement of DVT is associated with absence of edema; femoral vein involvement is associated with mild to moderate edema; ileofemoral vein thrombosis will be characterized by severe edema.

ACTIONS/INTERVENTIONS	RATIONALE

Independent

Assess capillary refill, and check for Homans' sign.

Diminished capillary refill and positive Homans' sign indicate DVT. (Note: Homan's sign may be absent in presence of DVT.)

Encourage elevation of feet and lower legs above heart level.

Rapidly empties superficial and tibial veins and keeps veins collapsed, thereby increasing venous return.

Caution client not to cross legs or wear constrictive clothing.

Physical restriction of circulation impairs blood flow, thus increasing venous stasis, pain, and trauma.

Instruct client to avoid rubbing and massaging the affected extremity.

To prevent dislodging thrombus, which could lead to embolism.

Encourage deep-breathing exercises.

Produces increased negative pressure in thorax, which assists in emptying large veins.

Assess respiratory ease and lung sounds, noting crackles or friction rub. Note reports of chest pain and feelings of anxiety.

Sharp substernal chest pain, sudden apprehension, dyspnea, tachypnea, and hemoptysis are indicative of pulmonary emboli, especially in DVT. (Note: Client may remain symptom-free and undiagnosed.)

Initiate progressive ambulation following acute phase.

Increases venous return; helps prevent stasis.

Collaborative

Apply warm, moist compresses to affected extremity.

Increases circulation to area; promotes vasodilation, venous return, and resolution of edema.

Administer anticoagulation therapy, using heparin (via continuous intravenous drip, intermittent administration using heparin lock, or subcutaneous administration) or coumarin derivatives.

Heparin is usually preferred initially, owing to its prompt and predictable antagonistic action toward thrombin formation and to its prevention of further clot formation. Because of its large molecular size, heparin does not pass through to breast milk as coumarin derivatives do; however, coumarin, which blocks formation of prothrombin from vitamin K, may be used for long-term therapy following discharge.

Apply elastic support hose to legs with care to avoid any tourniquet effect.

Useful in superficial thrombosis because they exert a sustained, evenly distributed pressure over the entire surface of calves and thighs, reducing caliber of superficial veins, increasing blood flow to deep veins, and reducing stasis.

Monitor laboratory studies:

Prothrombin time, partial thromboplastin time/activated partial thromboplastin time.

Monitors effectiveness of anticoagulant therapy.

Hb/Hct.

Hemoconcentration and dehydration can potentiate clot formation.

AST (SGOT), lactate dehydrogenase (LDH).

Elevated levels may indicate emboli.

NURSING DIAGNOSIS:	PAIN [ACUTE]
May be related to:	Presence of inflammatory process, vascular spasms, accumulation of lactic acid.
Possibly evidenced by:	Verbalizations, restlessness, guarding behavior, self-focus, autonomic responses.
DESIRED OUTCOMES— CLIENT WILL:	Participate in behaviors/techniques to promote comfort.
	Report pain is relieved/controlled.
	Appear relaxed and sleep/rest appropriately.

ACTIONS/INTERVENTIONS	RATIONALE
Independent	
Assess degree of discomfort or pain; palpate leg with caution. Note guarding of extremity.	Degree of pain is directly related to extent of arterial involvement, degree of hypoxia, and extent of edema associated with thrombus development in inflamed venous wall. Client may guard or immobilize affected extremity to decrease painful sensations associated with muscle movement.
Maintain bedrest as appropriate.	Reduces discomfort associated with muscle contraction and movement. Minimizes possibility of dislodging thrombus.
Monitor vital signs, noting elevated temperature or pulse.	Elevation of vital signs may indicate increasing pain; fever may contribute to general discomfort.
Elevate affected extremity; provide foot cradle.	Encourages venous return, facilitates circulation. Foot cradle keeps pressure of bedclothes off of the affected leg, thereby reducing pain.
Encourage change of position, keeping extremity elevated.	Decreases or prevents fatigue, helps minimize muscle spasm, and increases venous return.
Explain procedures, treatments, and nursing interventions.	Involving the client in the nursing care increases her sense of control and decreases her level of anxiety. (Note: Anxiety/fear can result in muscle tension and increased perceptions of pain.)
Investigate reports of sudden and/or sharp chest pain, dyspnea, tachycardia, or apprehension.	These signs and symptoms suggest pulmonary emboli as a complication of DVT.
Collaborative	
Administer medications as indicated:	
Analgesics (narcotic/nonnarcotic).	Relieve pain and decrease muscle tension.
Antipyretics, anti-inflammatory agents (e.g., aspirin, phenylbutazone).	Reduce fever and inflammation.
Apply moist heat to extremity.	Causes vasodilatation, which increases circulation, relaxes muscles, and may stimulate release of endorphins.

NURSING DIAGNOSIS:	ANXIETY [SPECIFY LEVEL]
May be related to:	Change in health status, perceived or actual threat to self, situational crisis, interpersonal transmission of anxiety from family members.
Possibly evidenced by:	Increased tension, apprehension, restlessness, sympathetic stimulation.
DESIRED OUTCOMES—CLIENT WILL:	Verbalize awareness of feelings of anxiety.
	Report anxiety reduced to a manageable level.
	Exhibit a decrease in behavioral signs such as restlessness and irritability.

ACTIONS/INTERVENTIONS

Independent

Explain procedures, treatments, and nursing interventions.

Encourage measures to reduce emotional tension, such as relaxation techniques and verbalization of concerns.

Monitor vital signs and behavioral signs such as restlessness, irritability, and crying.

Assist client in caring for herself and infant.

Involve client/significant other(s) in development of plan of care; review instructions and restrictions.

Encourage contact, by telephone or in person, with spouse and children if client is hospitalized. Encourage visits/contact with newborn.

RATIONALE

Reduces fear of the unknown; promotes client's learning and involvement in treatment.

Energy-release techniques and verbalization of concerns lessen anxiety. Relaxation prevents muscle fatigue and allows client to rest.

May reflect change in level of anxiety; may indicate client's ability to cope with events.

Client's anxiety may lessen when she finds that her needs are met and that she is able to cope and engage in self-care and infant care tasks.

Provides information and helps the client and significant other understand the need for the interventions and restrictions; provides them with a sense of control over the situation.

Helps to reduce feelings of separation and isolation.

NURSING DIAGNOSIS:	KNOWLEDGE DEFICIT [LEARNING NEED], regarding condition, treatment needs, and prognosis
May be related to:	Lack of exposure/recall, misinterpretation.
Possibly evidenced by:	Verbalizations, inaccurate follow-through of instructions, development of preventable complications.
DESIRED OUTCOMES—CLIENT WILL:	Verbalize understanding of condition, treatment, and restrictions. Initiate necessary behavioral changes.

ACTIONS/INTERVENTIONS	RATIONALE

Independent

Assess client's knowledge and understanding of disease process. Provide information and correct misconceptions as needed.

Helps in determining specific needs and clarifying previous information.

Provide information about management and diagnostic tests. Identify signs and symptoms requiring notification of healthcare provider; e.g., coolness or pallor of extremity, tenderness in affected area, or edema.

Can increase understanding and decrease anxiety associated with condition and home management. Progression of condition and/or development of bleeding requires prompt evaluation and possible changes in therapy to prevent serious complications.

Review purposes of bedrest and antiembolic stocking if worn. Encourage removal of elastic stockings for brief intervals at least twice daily.

Continuous constriction may alter or reduce surface perfusion, leading to muscle fatigue. Removal of elastic stockings allows for detection of further vascular involvement or inflammation.

Discuss possible interactions between oral anticoagulant therapy and other medications (e.g., salicylates, vitamins, antibiotics, barbiturates, and alcohol).

Oral anticoagulant therapy may last 3–4 months and may cause problems or require alterations in drug dosage if it is allowed to interact with other medications. Salicylates and excess alcohol decrease prothrombin activity; vitamin K in multivitamins increases prothrombin activity; antibiotics alter intestinal flora and may interfere with vitamin K synthesis; barbiturates increase metabolism of coumarin drugs.

Recommend safety measures to avoid trauma, such as use of a soft toothbrush and use of electric razors for shaving. Report any bleeding.

Alterations in coagulation process may result in increased tendency to bleed, which may indicate a need to alter anticoagulant therapy.

The Parents of a Child With Special Needs _____

The birth of a child with special needs, regardless of whether the condition is temporary or permanent, creates unique concerns for the family, who mourns the loss of a normal healthy child. Conditions range from prematurity, growth deviations, and infections to gross anomalies. Although each case is individual and varies in degree of involvement, many similarities are observed in the parents' responses to their child.

CLIENT ASSESSMENT DATA BASE

(Refer to Client Assessment Data Base in CPs: The Client at 4 Hours to 3 Days Postpartum; 24 Hours Following Early Discharge; 1 Week Following Discharge; and 4 to 6 Weeks Following Delivery as appropriate.)

EGO INTEGRITY

Varied emotional responses (e.g., calm, withdrawal, irritability, restlessness, weeping, anger).

History of postpartal depression or psychosis.

SAFETY

History of exposure to teratogenic factors.

Presence of infectious agents, premature rupture of membranes.

SEXUALITY

Intrapartal event (e.g., dysfunctional labor, hemorrhage).

History of birth of a child with special needs and/or perinatal loss.

DIAGNOSTIC STUDIES

Genetic studies/chromosomal analysis: Helps determine presence of syndromes/inherited disorders, general prognosis, and future expectations.
Other testing: Dependent on specific findings and individual risk factors.

NURSING PRIORITIES

1. Facilitate grieving and positive coping.
2. Provide appropriate information related to short- and long-term implications of child's illness or anomaly.
3. Facilitate learning of parenting role and participation in infant care tasks.

NURSING DIAGNOSIS:	GRIEVING [expected]
May be related to:	Perceived loss of the perfect child/pregnancy/delivery, alterations of future expectations.
Possibly evidenced by:	Expression of distress at loss, sorrow, guilt, anger; choked feelings; reliving of pregnancy events; interference with life activities; crying.
DESIRED OUTCOMES— CLIENT/COUPLE WILL:	Verbalize feelings freely/effectively.
	Demonstrate expected grief responses.
	Look forward/plan for future one day at a time.

ACTIONS/INTERVENTIONS	RATIONALE

Independent

Promote trusting relationship with parents and significant other(s). Encourage verbalization of feelings through listening and an unhurried attitude.	Facilitates sharing of feelings, fears, and concerns. Helps parents to focus on reality of the situation and examine their emotional responses. Grieving for the loss of the perfect child must be completed before parents can establish a positive relationship with their offspring. Staff needs to remain available even if client seems self-sufficient or withdrawn.
Facilitate the grief process even if the newborn's problem is temporary or surgically correctable.	The amount of grief the parents experience is independent of the severity/permanency of the infant's problem.
Determine parents' religious orientation, and contact appropriate support if they desire it.	Many couples lean heavily on their faith as a source of strength during crisis resolution. (Note: Perception of situation/condition and individual's response will also be affected by religious beliefs.)
Assess for usual grieving responses (i.e., initial shock, disbelief, and denial, then anger, guilt, sadness, and negative self-evaluation/questioning, followed by acceptance). Let parents know that these responses are normal.	Grief is the anticipated, healthy emotional response to the profound experience of giving birth to a special needs child, and it involves mourning the loss of the idealized perfect newborn.
Note the stage of grief being expressed. Discuss the individual nature of movement through the stages of grief; let parents know that delays in the grief process or relapses of grief are normal	The process of grieving is not usually a fluid progression through the stages to resolution; more often the individual fluctuates between the stages, possibly skipping one or more. Understanding that grieving is individual helps the couple to let each other grieve at his or her own pace.
Accept use of defense mechanisms (e.g., denial, anger, or silence). Encourage expression of angry feelings, setting limits on unacceptable acting-out behavior.	Use of defense mechanisms at this time may be the best way for parents to deal productively with the situation. However, continued use of defense mechanisms may impair resolution of grief. Additionally, preventing destructive behavior is important to the maintenance of the client's self-esteem.
Provide information about extreme mood swings, which may be hormonally induced in the postpartal period.	Usual hormonal adjustments of postpartal period can trigger labile responses and may require further evaluation/treatment.
Offer objective feedback, without judgment, on how behavior is being perceived.	When behavior is unacceptable, gentle statements about angry or withdrawn actions can help the individual cope more effectively with the situation.
Avoid "personalizing" statements made by the parents.	Parents may use the nurse as a sounding board and means of ventilating their feelings. Their statements, although spoken to the individual nurse, are usually directed at the situation in general.
Ascertain parents' perceptions of infant's special needs and condition.	The parents' emotional responses are associated with the perceived loss of the perfect child, in addition to concerns about the infant's well-being/life expectancy. They may occur regardless of

ACTIONS/INTERVENTIONS	RATIONALE

Independent

	whether the defect appears to healthcare professionals to be relatively minor and/or reparable, or major and life-threatening.
Ask parents what helps them most in dealing with the affected child. Observe nonverbal signals such as anguished tone of voice, looking down, or crying.	Parents may have a hard time handling the crisis and may have difficulty identifying means of facilitating coping.
Encourage parents to see, hold, and help care for the child.	Interacting with the child as he/she is helps parents to work toward the acceptance phase of the grief process.
Instruct parents in caring for the infant. (Refer to ND: Knowledge Deficit [Learning Need].)	Grieving may increase the parents' fear of caring for the child; in many cases, they feel overwhelmed initially.
Prepare parents for/role-play difficult situations such as discharge from the hospital and other people's thoughtless comments, questions, and stares.	Parents can develop plan of action before actual confrontation with difficult situations.
Evaluate parents for abnormal grief responses, such as inappropriate humor, lack of interest in infant, continued denial of or failure to recognize infant's problem, poor eye contact, continual crying, excessive or vague complaints, inability to carry out self-care activities, or use of distancing in interactions with child (e.g., holding child at arm's length instead of cuddling).	Inappropriate initial responses may result in long-term emotional dysfunction and lack of resolution of grief. Thus, the grief process may be left open-ended, and the parents' unresolved feelings continually resurface. Early identification of problems and prompt intervention facilitates individual growth and coping abilities. (Note: Parents may be afraid of becoming emotionally attached if they believe that the child might die.)

Collaborative

Refer for appropriate individual or family counseling.	Counseling may be necessary for resolution of grief and maintenance of family unity.

NURSING DIAGNOSIS:	PARENTING, ALTERED, HIGH RISK FOR
Risk factors may include:	Delay/interruption in bonding process, perceived threat to infant's survival, presence of stress (financial, family needs), lack of appropriate response of newborn, lack of support between/from significant other(s).
Possibly evidenced by:	[Not applicable; presence of signs/symptoms establishes an **actual** diagnosis.]
DESIRED OUTCOMES— PARENT(S) WILL:	Demonstrate beginning attachment behaviors. Verbalize acceptance of situation. Develop realistic plans for care of the infant.

437

ACTIONS/INTERVENTIONS	RATIONALE

Independent

Provide information honestly about newborn's appearance and condition at birth, encouraging an optimistic perspective (e.g., let parents know the potential for survival or recovery). Describe appearance and show pictures of newborn if initial interaction is delayed or following surgery.

Helps to prepare parents psychologically for interaction with newborn and reduces the shock associated with initial viewing of infant. The child's appearance may be incongruent with the parents' idealized picture of the perfect infant. Aids in developing parents' trust and giving them accurate information with which to make decisions. Optimistic perspective helps encourage parents to develop an attachment, although the infant may be unable to participate actively in the interactional process because of illness and/or need for technologic assistance.

Facilitate communication between parents and nursery staff through use of telephone and letters, especially if infant is transferred to a high-risk facility. Suggest that parents provide tapes, photographs, and personal items for use in infant's environment.

Maintains open channel for exchange of information and clarification of concerns. Fosters continued acquaintance process; helps parents to feel an integral part of infant care and growth. Parents can talk, sing, or tell stories into tape recorder, which can be played for infant, providing audio stimulation and voice recognition of parents.

Encourage verbalization of feelings regarding prenatal/intrapartal and postpartal periods and perceptions of the financial and emotional burdens created by the birth of special needs infant.

Unresolved anticipatory anger and excessive threats to self-esteem and to financial status may predispose parents to subconscious or overt rejection of infant.

Discuss normalcy of feelings related to the grief response (e.g., shock, disbelief, anger, guilt, and sadness).

Parents need to identify and cope with their own grief response before they can begin to bond emotionally with the newborn.

Provide anticipatory and ongoing emotional support to client/couple.

Helps couple whose infant's prognosis is grave to bond with and then let go of infant if death ensues. Parental anticipatory grieving, which begins during the intrapartal period and lasts until the infant dies or shows signs of improvement, may result in a withdrawal from bonding as a protective mechanism. (Refer to CP: Perinatal Loss.)

Determine parents' understanding of infant's condition and needs. Review and clarify questions, and provide opportunity for discussion about the condition and its short- and long-term implications as early as possible following birth.

Initial denial, shock, and disbelief may interfere with understanding and processing of information. Parents may cling to unrealistic expectations or goals if they are not psychologically ready to accept the situation. Review of information helps to dispel fantasies, initiate the grief process, and mobilize internal and external support.

Provide information regarding physical and personality characteristics appropriate for gestational age when child is preterm, rather than the characteristics of a full-term infant.

Allows appropriate comparisons for helping parents to identify parenting behaviors and activities appropriate for their infant.

Assist parents in identifying familial characteristics, personality traits, positive attributes, and normal behaviors in the infant.

Emphasizes the infant's value as a person and facilitates recognition of individual capabilities and personality traits. Initiates process of attachment and bonding, and allows parents to see similarities between their infant and a normal newborn.

438

ACTIONS/INTERVENTIONS	RATIONALE
Independent	
	(Note: Some parents, regardless of how minor the defect is, may have difficulty accepting a baby who is not "perfect".)
Promote early parent-infant interaction. Assess parents' perception of infant.	Helps couple to acknowledge the reality of the situation and to begin to work through appropriate psychologic tasks; determines parents' readiness for involvement in infant care tasks.
Provide privacy for parents to interact with baby.	Parents may want to talk or sing to infant, but may not feel comfortable with an "audience."
Review couple's parenting experience and preparation, and previous coping skills. (Refer to ND: Family Coping, ineffective: compromised, high risk for.)	Provides indications of emotional readiness to adopt parenting roles and responsibilities. Such readiness varies considerably, depending on coping skills and past experiences.
Assess parents for development of attachment behaviors while in the hospital (e.g., talking to, holding, and naming infant; asking appropriate questions regarding infant's condition and needs).	Indicates development of positive parent-infant ties, which help foster optimal growth and development of infant.
Note parental cues indicating readiness for involvement in infant's care and future planning. Encourage parental involvement in planning care and making decisions.	Readiness for parental involvement indicates that client/couple is attaching emotionally to infant, is becoming increasingly concerned for the infant's welfare, and is feeling emotionally able to begin to assume responsibility for infant's care. Parental involvement may enhance feelings of control, promote self-esteem, and reduce anxiety.
Demonstrate special infant care techniques, positions for holding and feeding infant, and ways of talking to infant. Assess parents' need to have staff remain with them or to be left alone with infant.	The nurse acts as a role model in caring for the infant at a time when the parents are acutely aware of others' responses and identify with those responses. Anxiety associated with a new parenting role may be minimized by participation in newborn care.
Encourage appropriate parental participation in infant care.	Reduces anxiety, improves parental self-esteem, and facilitates development of positive parent-infant attachment, which helps to assure appropriate continuity of physical and emotional care necessary for the infant's optimal development.
Identify newborn's responses and behavioral cues.	Aids parents in determining when to interact with infant, what behaviors are appropriate, and when to modify their approach based on infant's tolerance for stimulation.
Provide positive feedback as parents accomplish tasks. Inform staff of parents' capabilities.	Increases sense of self-worth and self-confidence in providing infant's care. Staff coordination provides consistency in approach and helps prevent misunderstandings.
Arrange for meeting with other parents who have faced the same or a similar problem.	May aid couple in realistically identifying infant's specific needs and abilities.

ACTIONS/INTERVENTIONS

Independent

Note client's/couple's behaviors following client's discharge; e.g., continued visits or telephone calls, and preparation for infant's discharge, or lack of physical contact, failure to name infant or change of name from original choice, negative comments about infant, expressed concerns about adequacy in caring for infant, and failure to visit or communicate with professionals.

Evaluate appropriateness of discharge planning/preparation.

Discuss alternatives to taking baby home (e.g., foster care, institutionalization, adoption) as indicated. Be supportive of final decision; assist parents in evaluating long-term implications of decision.

Collaborative

Schedule team conference. Identify acute care and community resources for infant and parents (e.g., public health nurse, home care agencies, charitable organizations [such as Easter Seals], and support groups).

Refer for counseling or parenting classes, as indicated.

RATIONALE

Involved behaviors demonstrate continued concern for child's comfort and indicate increasing strength of attachment. Although withdrawal behaviors may represent a normal response to prevent attachment to an infant who may not survive, they may also indicate potential problems, including high-risk parenting (emotional or physical abuse) following discharge, so that further evaluation and/or interventions may be needed.

Realistic preparation indicates client's readiness for parenting following infant's discharge.

Parents who choose not to cope with the long-term commitment of raising a child with special needs may need to seek alternative care.

Coordinated multidisciplinary planning for discharge can ease the transition from hospital to home and reduce anxiety associated with increased parental responsibilities following discharge.

May be necessary if attachment behaviors are incomplete or absent.

NURSING DIAGNOSIS:	FAMILY COPING, INEFFECTIVE: COMPROMISED, HIGH RISK FOR
Risk factors may include:	Situational crises, temporary preoccupation by a significant person who is trying to manage emotional conflicts and personal suffering and is unable to perceive or act effectively in regard to client's needs, temporary family disorganization/role changes.
Possibly evidenced by:	[Not applicable; presence of signs/symptoms establishes an **actual** diagnosis.]
DESIRED OUTCOMES— FAMILY WILL:	Participate in problem-solving and use resources appropriately.
	Demonstrate integration of infant into family unit.

ACTIONS/INTERVENTIONS

Independent

Evaluate normal family coping mechanisms and relationships between family members.

RATIONALE

Helps in identifying strengths and weaknesses and availability of support systems.

ACTIONS/INTERVENTIONS	RATIONALE
Independent	
Provide calm supportive environment and role-modeling for parents.	External stressors may interfere with incorporation of therapeutic interventions by parents. Psychosocial needs of parents may be met through positive role-modeling by healthcare providers.
Provide emotional support by allowing time, privacy, and opportunity for open discussion. Provide information honestly; keep client/couple informed regarding infant's condition.	Helps client/couple to identify and clarify fears and concerns, and to correct misconceptions.
Determine parental concerns, emotions, and degree of anxiety. Assess past experiences with stress and past coping mechanisms and support systems.	Past experience with stress or crisis influences current stress response and management, resulting in either functional or dysfunctional behavior.
Encourage verbalization of fears, and initiate discussion of opportunities.	Parents may be hesitant to share concerns with staff. Fears may go unaddressed unless staff conscientiously creates opportunities for discussion during their client/infant care activities.
Provide parents with realistic responses and reinforcement, giving consideration to their capacity to process information and their knowledge of the situation.	Lack of knowledge contributes to increased anxiety, which interferes with the ability to cope. However, anxiety needs to be minimized in order for parents to process information. Repetition of explanations enhances understanding.
Encourage parents to express their own dependency needs and to focus on themselves and their own discomfort.	Both parents may need to devote time and energy to understanding and dealing with their own feelings prior to directing their concern to the infant.
Assess individual and collective responses of family members to infant's condition/appearance. Encourage family to verbalize their perceptions of the impact of the infant's illness or condition on the family.	Parental feelings toward the infant are critical, because feelings that are related to physical appearance and capabilities are internalized in the infant as development occurs.
Use role-playing techniques or play therapy with siblings. Demonstrate these techniques for parents to use. Provide information about age-appropriate discussions with siblings.	Helps young children express feelings about infant. Using words and expressions appropriate to the age of the other children helps the parents in talking with them about the new baby.
Evaluate and help parents recognize signs of ineffective family coping in siblings (e.g., interpersonal problems, excessive quarreling, psychosomatic illnesses, school problems, regressive behaviors).	Early recognition allows the family to take steps to correct these problems and to seek professional help if necessary.
Encourage client/couple to arrange sibling visits and to allow older siblings the opportunity to participate in infant care, if possible.	Helps siblings to realize that they are in important part of infant care, which may eliminate feelings of abandonment and increase feelings of self-worth.
Place family photos in isolette or crib; encourage siblings to talk to infant, to make tape recordings, or to give gifts (e.g., pick out a small toy, draw a picture).	Provides sense of family unity and includes siblings in activities.
Recommend that client/couple spend special time alone with siblings.	Caring for an infant with special needs is so time-consuming that little time is left for siblings, who may feel abandoned, replaced, ignored, angry, and jealous.

ACTIONS/INTERVENTIONS	RATIONALE

Independent

Offer opportunity for contact with couples facing similar problems.	Provides peer support helpful in nurturing the couple; promotes positive behaviors and provides opportunity for sharing ideas and interventions that have been successful.
Initiate follow-up phone calls and/or home visits.	Provides continuity of care and a continued source of emotional support.
Be supportive of couple's decision to take infant home or to use institutional help or assistance. Help couple to look at long-term effects of decision. Note cultural meaning of condition/birth anomaly.	Such decisions are difficult and may have cultural implications. To avoid increasing their guilt and confusion, make the parents aware of options, give support for their decision without judgment, and let them know that they may change their minds.
Encourage parents to maintain or reestablish good communication between themselves and to take time out from child care for time alone together. Encourage use of resources such as respite care.	Facilitates rapport between parents, helps maintain healthy relationship, and fosters coping and family growth.
Encourage each partner to allow time for himself or herself, apart from the other.	Helps foster individual coping mechanisms, which can ultimately foster a stronger family.
Refer to community or social services, as appropriate. Identify available respite services. Provide additional referrals, including clergy, psychiatric services, and parent support groups, as indicated.	A coordinated and consistent network of multidisciplinary support enhances management of parental anxiety and assists in development of effective coping skills required by the short- and long-term complications related to the child's special needs.
Encourage couple to seek genetic counseling if appropriate. (Refer to Chapter 4, CP: Genetic Counseling.)	Thorough evaluation of genetic factors may provide answers to some of the couple's questions.
Suggest that couple attend marital support group or seek marital counseling, as indicated.	May help couple cope with a crisis that can potentially strengthen or destroy the relationship. Family disintegration is often a consequence of the birth of an infant with a disorder or anomaly. Such disintegration is a direct response to the intense emotional and physical demands created by the infant's long-term health problems.

NURSING DIAGNOSIS:	**KNOWLEDGE DEFICIT [LEARNING NEED], regarding infant care**
May be related to:	Lack of/unfamiliarity with information resources, misinterpretation, lack of recall.
Possibly evidenced by:	Verbalization of problem/concerns/misconceptions, inaccurate follow-through of instructions, hesitancy or inadequate performance of activities, inappropriate/aggravated behaviors (e.g., agitated, apathetic).

<table>
<tr><td>DESIRED OUTCOMES—
CLIENT/COUPLE WILL:</td><td>Verbalize understanding of infant's behaviors, physical status, and care needs.

Participate in infant's care.

Demonstrate mastery of infant care/treatment activities.

Plan appropriately for discharge, home management, and use of available resources.</td></tr>
</table>

ACTIONS/INTERVENTIONS	RATIONALE

Independent

Keep parents informed about changes in infant's physiologic status.	Helps parents to acknowledge possible positive or negative outcomes regarding infant's potential for survival and growth.
Explain plan of care for infant, including rationale for associated tests, procedures, and treatment. Discuss infant's response to treatment. Let parents know when tests are to be performed.	Promotes understanding, clarifies misconceptions, and reduces anxiety. Parents may choose not to visit infant when testing is scheduled.
Review normal behavior for infant's gestational age based on Dubowitz examination.	Provides information to promote understanding of behaviors and motor characteristics typical for gestational age.
Discuss infant's personality traits and individual differences noted from comparison with other infants of same gestational age. Provide information about appropriate stimulation for infant.	Allows couple to gain skill in recognizing responses of infant, acknowledging individual differences, and developing methods for dealing with them.
Introduce client/couple to parent of a baby (in the nursery if possible) with the same or similar special need.	Sharing concerns with another parent can foster acceptance of the situation.
Encourage optimal participation in infant care. Reinforce the idea that infant belongs to the parents, not the nursery. Talk about the infant by name, noting attractive features and other attributes.	Fosters attachment process. Allows parents to demonstrate newly learned behaviors, increasing comfort in handling and caring for the infant. Reminds parents that child is a living being, not a disease or condition.
Encourage questions, provide answers clearly and concisely, and reinforce information as needed. Assess parents' readiness to receive information. Encourage parents to verbalize concerns.	Helps to identify learning needs and to clarify misconceptions. Denial used initially as a coping mechanism may interfere with learning. Repetition enhances comprehension. Verbalization of concerns promotes atmosphere of trust and is conducive to learning.
Set short-term, measurable goals with parents.	Learning to adjust to problems step by step, one day at a time, helps parents to see that progress is being made and reduces the overwhelming stress of the total situation.
Provide encouragement for each task accomplished.	Increases parents' self-confidence in their ability to care for infant.
Review assessment of gestational age, expected potential, immediate and long-term prognosis, and discharge of infant. Be realistic but positive.	Parents need to know the expectations they can have of their child. Infant may be at risk for neuromuscular disorders, developmental delays, be-

ACTIONS/INTERVENTIONS	RATIONALE

Independent

Keep parents informed, be honest, and let parents know whether answers are available.	havior problems, or learning disabilities that may be directly associated with gestational age at birth. Honesty maintains trust between nurse and parents and promotes realistic hope.
Discuss results of ophthalmologic examination when performed prior to infant discharge. Provide information to parents about importance of scheduling reevaluations.	In the preterm infant, retinal scar tissue formation may persist for as long as 5 months, resulting in varying degrees of visual impairment.
Review results of other routine tests, such as hearing testing and B-mode ultrasonography of the head.	These tests are performed for early identification of significant problems (presence and extent of hearing loss, intraventricular hemorrhage) and for provision of appropriate interventions.
Provide information related to home care of infant. Encourage family to read available literature.	Helps parents to gain competence and comfort in caring for infant after discharge.
Discuss purpose and availability of early intervention programs and community resources.	Provides guidance for long-term planning to optimize affective, cognitive, and social development of infant.
Encourage other members of family to learn to care for infant.	Eases the parents' burden of caring for infant and promotes a sense of family unity.
Recommend parents contact other parents of children with similar needs (e.g., Down syndrome, muscular dystrophy, or cerebral palsy groups; or Parents Encouraging Parents).	Provides support and promotes the realization that parents are not alone in their struggle.
Refer to social service agencies or community resources, including national foundations (e.g., Easter Seal centers, Shriners for orthopedic defects), public assistance groups, and Medicaid, as appropriate. Discuss need to notify insurance company immediately following birth.	Couple may be unaware of available financial assistance or free services and may be overwhelmed by incurred or future expenses. Referrals help ensure continuation of support from healthcare agencies. Clarification of available insurance coverage may affect choice of treatment options. (Note: Infant may not be covered by insurance if notification is not made within time period specified by third-party payor.)
Make follow-up phone calls and/or home visits.	Aids in adjustment of care for home environment. Lets couple know that someone cares and is available should difficulties arise.

NURSING DIAGNOSIS:	**SOCIAL ISOLATION, HIGH RISK FOR**
Risk factors may include:	Perceived situational crisis, assuming sole/full-time responsibility for infant's care, lack of resources or inappropriate use of resources.
Possibly evidenced by:	[Not applicable; presence of signs/symptoms establishes an **actual** diagnosis.]
DESIRED OUTCOMES— CLIENT/COUPLE WILL:	Verbalize awareness of potential problems.
	Identify resources available for assistance.
	Develop plans to resume social activities.

ACTIONS/INTERVENTIONS	RATIONALE

Independent

Discuss situation with couple and determine their perceptions of how they will manage care.

Identifies problem areas and helps with planning interventions for appropriate care. After discharge, the parents quickly become consumed, both emotionally and physically, in child's care, and they may withdraw from usual social interactions and activities.

Listen to parents' expressions of feelings of inadequacy or guilt that may accompany the birth of a child with special needs. Help the couple cope with feelings that are expressed. (Refer to ND: Family Coping, ineffective: compromised, high risk for.)

Parents may withdraw from society or social interaction because of feelings of shame or a sense of failure as parents. They may also have fears that the child will die or will receive substandard care from others. Unresolved guilt may be responsible for overindulgent behaviors and unwillingness to let others care for the child. Resolution of guilt may promote development of effective parenting skills.

Assist couple with plans for responsible, skilled adults to care for child. Such adults may be relatives, friends, or trained caregivers, such as "mother's helpers."

The couple needs time away from child's constant demands to maintain their own relationship and to keep the situation in perspective. Reduces risk of developing impaired ability to perform family caregiver role.

Discuss plans for resumption of activities engaged in before the birth (e.g., hobbies, employment) if possible.

Returning to normal routines fosters self-esteem and sense of self-worth; however, child's condition may significantly alter the family's previous patterns so that reduction or elimination of outside work or some leisure activities may be necessary. (Note: Support from parents sharing similar situation provides opportunity for creative problem-solving and continuation of activities.)

Prepare parents for/role-play responses to possible reactions by the public.

Preparation helps couple to identify possible actions or ways of managing uncomfortable social situations and eliminates the need for isolating themselves from social contacts as a protective mechanism.

Encourage parents to plan family outings such as trips to beach, picnics, walks, and movies.

Helps meet individual and collective needs for social experiences.

Collaborative

Provide social service and public health referrals before discharge.

Maintains continuity of support network from the hospital to the home.

Assist couple in contacting support groups.

A support group serves as a social outlet, provides role models, and may be a resource for sharing child care.

Perinatal Loss _____

Perinatal loss may occur anytime during gestation or the neonatal period. Usually when pregnancy culminates in the death of a fetus or neonate, the loss is both unexpected and devastating for the client/couple. The loss of a child that is wanted can be as traumatic (or even more traumatic) as the loss of a close adult family member or friend. This plan of care focuses on the emotional needs of the postpartal client who must cope with the death of a child (to be used in conjunction with routine postpartal plans of care).

CLIENT ASSESSMENT DATA BASE

CIRCULATION

History of essential hypertension, vascular disease.

EGO INTEGRITY

Emotionally labile; anxiety, fear, shock, disbelief, depression.

ELIMINATION

Chronic nephritis.

FOOD/FLUID

Poor maternal nutritional status.

SAFETY

Exposure to toxic/teratogenic agents.

History of traumatic event(s).

Presence of pelvic inflammatory disease, sexually transmitted diseases, or exposure to contagious diseases such as rubella, cytomegalovirus, active herpes.

Premature rupture of membranes.

Abnormalities of placenta/cord noted at delivery.

ABO incompatibility.

SEXUALITY

Bicornate or septate uterus, uterine fibroid tumors (leiomyoma), or other abnormalities of the maternal reproductive organs.

Occurrence of traumatic delivery, intrapartal complications.

TEACHING/LEARNING

May report medication, drug/alcohol use or abuse.

Family history of genetic conditions.

DIAGNOSTIC STUDIES

(Refer to Chapter 4, CP: Genetic Counseling.)

NURSING PRIORITIES

1. Facilitate the grieving process.
2. Provide information regarding events surrounding the loss and future implications.

DISCHARGE GOALS

1. Supports identified and in place.
2. Plans made for disposition of infant's body.

NURSING DIAGNOSIS:	GRIEVING [expected]
Related to:	Death of fetus/infant.
Possibly evidenced by:	Verbal expression of distress, anger, loss, guilt; crying; alteration in eating habits or sleep pattern.
DESIRED OUTCOMES— CLIENT/COUPLE WILL:	Verbalize stage of the grief process being experienced.
	Express feelings appropriately.
	Identify problems of the grieving process (e.g., physical problems of eating, sleeping) and seek appropriate help.

ACTIONS/INTERVENTIONS	RATIONALE

Independent

Code patient's chart, room door, and/or head of bed, as indicated.	Alerts hospital staff and volunteers so they are aware of patient's loss.
Provide a private room if client desires it, with frequent contact by the nurse. Encourage unlimited visiting by family and friends.	A place where family and friends can talk or cry without restriction promotes ventilation of feelings and family sharing. (Note: Client may prefer carefully screened roommate(s), who can provide contact and comfort when family and friends are not available.)
Include partner in planning care. Provide opportunity for partner to be seen individually. Encourage discussion of concerns.	Participation in planning and decision-making acknowledges that partner has also lost a child and may need time to express feelings of loss and receive support without having to be supportive of client and others.
Assess client's/couple's knowledge and interpretation of events surrounding the death of the fetus or infant. Provide information and correct misconceptions based on couple's readiness and ability to listen effectively.	Often, after the death of a child, parents respond with shock, denial, or disbelief. These emotional reactions may hinder the couple's ability to process information and interpret the significance of events. Concrete thinking patterns (literal interpretation) may be the only available means of coping with information at this time.
Determine significance of the loss for both members of the couple. Note how strongly couple desired this pregnancy.	Extent and duration of the grief response may depend on the significance of the loss (e.g., whether pregnancy was planned, whether couple has lost other pregnancies, length of time associated with trying to conceive). In addition, parents may feel the loss throughout their lives, mourning for the child they will never know or watch grow up.

447

ACTIONS/INTERVENTIONS	RATIONALE

Independent

Identify stage of grief being expressed; e.g., denial, anger, bargaining, depression, acceptance. Use therapeutic communication skills (e.g., Active-listening, acknowledgment), respecting client's desire/request not to talk.

When a child dies in utero, is stillborn, or dies after birth, grief is felt, regardless of whether the child was wanted or unwanted. If the work of grieving is not completed, grief may become dysfunctional, resulting in behaviors that are detrimental to personal safety and to the future of the family and marriage/relationship.

Discuss the individual nature of movement through the stages of grief; tell client/couple that delays in the grief process or relapses of grief are normal.

The process of grieving is not usually a fluid progression through the stages to resolution but rather fluctuation between stages and possibly the skipping of stages. Understanding that grieving is individual helps the couple to let each other grieve at his or her own pace.

Note communication patterns between members of the couple and support systems.

In many cases, anger and blame may be shown toward one another. Anger may stem from fear of losing another child or a threat to self-esteem.

Encourage family's expression of feelings, and listen (remaining silent or commenting as appropriate). Note body language. Promote relaxed atmosphere.

Verbal and nonverbal cues provide information about family's degree of sadness, guilt, and fear. Grieving families need repeated opportunities to verbalize their experience. Time is needed to develop a therapeutic milieu. Active-listening conveys caring, which communicates an awareness of the unique meaning of the loss to the client.

Acknowledge what has happened as often as necessary, reinforcing the reality of the situation and encouraging discussion by the client.

Many families have no previous experience coping with the death of a young person and have few role models to whom they can refer. The nurse can act as an educator and facilitator regarding ways to act and talk about the event and can clarify misconceptions.

Take pictures of the child wrapped in newborn attire. Encourage couple to see or hold the child if appropriate. Offer the couple footprints, hospital bracelets, or lock of hair if desired.

Pictures and touching or holding infant can be helpful and may initiate acceptance of the reality of the loss. (Note: Couple may not be ready to cope with the loss. Remembrances of the infant, if not taken by the parents, should be filed with the chart, so that they are available if couple requests them at a later time.)

Note client's activity level, sleep pattern, appetite, and personal hygiene.

These areas may be neglected because of the process of grieving and degree of depression. Sleep patterns may be disrupted, leading to fatigue and further inability to cope with distress. Client may need assistance in meeting physical needs and may need assurance that it is acceptable to continue with usual activities.

Provide physical care (e.g., bath, back rub, nourishment) as needed.

Demonstrates caring and nurturing and helps client conserve energy needed to meet the demands of the grieving process.

Discuss anticipated physical and emotional responses to loss. Evaluate coping skills. Note religious beliefs and ethnic background.

Helps couple to recognize normalcy of their initial and subsequent responses. Grieving is individual, and the extent and nature of the response is influenced by personality traits, past coping skills, religious beliefs, and ethnic background.

ACTIONS/INTERVENTIONS	RATIONALE

Independent

Review role changes and plans to deal with loss. Note presence of siblings.

Most families anticipate a healthy pregnancy and positive outcome and are not prepared to focus on funeral arrangements, what to do with the nursery, how to carry on their lives, and how to plan for the care of the other children.

Discuss ways for parents to talk with siblings. Stress importance of words that are used, as when the word "sleep" is substituted for "death." Encourage parents to give simple, honest explanations, using correct words, at the level of the child's understanding.

Provides parents with ideas for handling difficult new experience. Siblings' sleeping patterns may be disturbed by their belief that they may also die. Siblings may feel guilt or responsible for the death, especially if they had negative thoughts about the pregnancy or infant.

Assess severity of depression.

Client/couple may isolate themselves and have difficulty making decisions.

Review the client's/couple's verbal cues regularly. Note signs of developing or increasing somatic complaints, preoccupation with the death, loss of normal behavior patterns, overactivity with no apparent sense of loss, excessive hostility, or agitated depression.

May indicate change in client's/couple's manner of coping with the situation. Guilt, failure, and depression may be more pronounced in couples who have had previous child loss(es). Other signs may suggest dysfunctional grieving.

Collaborative

Refer to or contact clergy, according to family's wishes.

The family may want to speak to a minister or spiritual advisor to provide baptism, last rites, and/or counseling.

Assist with making requests and obtaining signatures for performance of autopsy if appropriate. Review benefits and limitations of autopsy.

Families may want or need explanation of cause of death, which may not be possible.

Provide information about disposition of infant's body. Contact mortician of family's choice if assistance is required.

Bodies of children, like those of adults, must be removed from hospitals to mortuary facilities or other disposition, usually within 24 hr of death.

Refer to or contact social services if necessary.

Family may need assistance in planning for cost of funeral and other necessities.

Schedule follow-up meetings or phone calls, as appropriate. Refer to community resources (e.g., visiting nurse services, Compassionate Friends).

Provides client/couple with opportunity for discussion and asking questions. Assists client/couple at critical moments in the grief process.

Refer for counseling or psychiatric therapy if necessary.

Counseling or therapy may be necessary in cases of pathologic grief to help individual(s) identify possible causes of the abnormal reaction and to achieve resolution of the grieving process.

NURSING DIAGNOSIS: **FAMILY PROCESSES, ALTERED, HIGH RISK FOR; ROLE PERFORMANCE, ALTERED, HIGH RISK FOR**

Risk factors may include: Situational crisis (death of child).

449

Possibly evidenced by:	[Not applicable; presence of signs/symptoms establishes an **actual** diagnosis.]
DESIRED OUTCOMES— FAMILY WILL:	Express feelings freely and appropriately.
	Demonstrate individual involvement in problem-solving process directed at resolution of crisis.
	Verbalize understanding of role expectations/obligations.
	Identify needs and resources to nurture roles/family ties.

ACTIONS/INTERVENTIONS	RATIONALE
Independent	
Evaluate current family situation and psychosocial status (e.g., other children, extended family, support systems).	Family members may provide support for one another. Disbelief, anger, and denial, however, may temporarily impair parenting skills, and other children may be ignored or treated differently than they had been prior to the death of the infant.
Review family's strengths, resources, and coping skills.	Family members may be depressed, may feel totally inadequate, and may need to review what has happened and what their purpose in life may be.
Encourage discussion of feelings and listen for verbal cues indicating feelings of failure, guilt, or anger. Discuss normalcy of feelings.	Verbalization of feelings may trigger recognition of their causes and can be used to verify the acceptability of these feelings. Parents may be afraid to describe negative feelings that they believe are abnormal. Realization that feelings of grief, guilt, and anger are normal may help to alleviate the parents' sense of failure.
Discuss situation in terms of activities that need to be completed or continued and the available resources.	In many cases, grief causes immobilization, resulting in dysfunctional parental patterns so that normal household routines are disrupted and outside assistance is required.
Identify expected role changes required by the loss.	Anticipated changes include period of disorientation or breakdown in normal patterns of conduct, followed by a period of reorganization, in which energy is appropriately invested in new people and activities.
Provide information and assist parent(s) to deal with situation, balancing self-care and grief needs and parenting responsibilities.	Death of a child requires unanticipated changes in parental roles. With death of a first child, the only parental function that occurs is grief. If there are other children, however, parents may express concern about their parenting abilities. Feelings of failure or guilt may lead to a sense of ultimate inadequacy.
Offer client simple choices of activities, with the opportunity to do more as she progresses.	The client needs to receive the message that she is seen as a functional, capable person even though she may not feel competent.

ACTIONS/INTERVENTIONS	RATIONALE

Collaborative

Refer to resources such as social services, visiting nurse services, and other agencies.

May be necessary to assist family members or to replace them when they are not available to help (because of distance and/or their own lack of coping skills). Fosters growth and individuation of family members.

Refer to parent support groups (e.g., Compassionate Friends).

Reviewing the situation with others who have gone through the same process can reaffirm normalcy of parents' feelings and responses. (Note: Referral is best made when the client/couple is experiencing depression and shock. It is more difficult to refer the client/couple during the stages of denial and anger.)

Refer for psychiatric counseling or psychotherapy if indicated.

Additional support in coping with grief may be needed. Psychotherapy may be helpful in cases of pathologic grief or overprotectiveness, which can negatively affect normal parenting and integration of loss into usual activities.

Administer medications judiciously, as needed (e.g., sedatives, antianxiety/antidepressants).

May help client obtain sleep/rest (e.g., following difficult or exhausting delivery or cesarean birth). (Note: Inappropriate use of medications can cloud emotional responses and inhibit the grieving process.)

NURSING DIAGNOSIS:	**SELF ESTEEM, SITUATIONAL LOW**
May be related to:	Perceived failure at a life event.
Possibly evidenced by:	Negative self-appraisal in response to life event in a person with a previous positive self-evaluation, verbalization of negative feelings about the self (helplessness, uselessness), difficulty making decisions.
DESIRED OUTCOMES— CLIENT/COUPLE WILL:	Identify strengths and resources available.
	Express positive self-appraisal.
	Demonstrate adaptation to death of infant and integration of loss into daily life by planning for the future.

ACTIONS/INTERVENTIONS	RATIONALE

Independent

Determine couple's self-perceptions as individuals and parents. Evaluate family's response to loss, noting blame placed by family members.

Giving birth provides opportunities for giving love, being loved, building self-esteem, feeling proud and accomplished, establishing a reason for living, and creating a bridge to the future. Loss of the pregnancy and newborn is therefore frequently associated with feelings of inadequacy, powerlessness, and inferiority, directly affecting sense of self and possibly shattering one's self-

ACTIONS/INTERVENTIONS	RATIONALE
Independent	esteem as a parent. Expression of anger or blame by other family members may further reduce self-esteem. (Note: Sense of loss/failure may be exacerbated in cases of repeated miscarriages or serial fetal/neonatal deaths.)
Discuss with parent(s) what has occurred and how they perceive the death.	Anger among family members may be transferred to client/couple, resulting in a distortion of actual events.
Discuss destructive behaviors, differentiating the responses of others from self-elicited responses (e.g., expressions of blame and/or guilt).	Destructive behaviors may be apparent during the phases of anger, isolation, and depression. Denial may be used as protection against loss of self-esteem. Guilt may be verbalized, especially if the loss is related to a genetic problem, uterine trauma (e.g., car accident or fall), or teratogens from environmental exposure or drug ingestion.
Provide opportunity for verbalization, venting of emotions, and crying.	Sharing of loss provides opportunity for needed acceptance, helps parents to sort through feelings, and validates parents' normal feelings of powerlessness and inadequacy.
Discuss parenting needs of other children as appropriate.	Continuing to care and to feel needed assists in preserving client's/couple's identity as worthwhile parent(s).
Provide positive reinforcement for identifying needs and concerns.	Aids in coping with sadness of situation. Helps parents to accept themselves as worthy human beings.
Collaborative	
Assist with referrals for counseling and coordination of appointments (e.g., with social services or support groups).	Client's/couple's ability to coordinate and perform tasks may be compromised. Referrals help provide support and assistance, which can facilitate integration of loss into daily life and enhance self-esteem.

NURSING DIAGNOSIS:	SPIRITUAL DISTRESS, (DISTRESS OF THE HUMAN SPIRIT), HIGH RISK FOR
Risk factors may include:	Need to adhere to personal religious beliefs/practices; blame for loss directed at self or God.
Possibly evidenced by:	[Not applicable; presence of signs/symptoms establishes an **actual** diagnosis.]
DESIRED OUTCOMES— CLIENT/COUPLE WILL:	Discuss beliefs/values about spiritual issues.
	Verbalize acceptance of situation and hope for the future.
	Demonstrate ability to help self and/or participate in usual activities.

ACTIONS/INTERVENTIONS

Independent

Discuss the loss with client/couple. (Refer to ND: Knowledge Deficit [Learning Need].)

Establish supportive relationships and resources to use following discharge (e.g., extended family, friends, or religious affiliations).

Encourage discussions of perceptions of unfairness. Identify such perceptions as part of grief process. Maintain a nonjudgmental attitude while providing opportunity for client/couple to express anger.

Collaborative

Refer to hospital chaplain, rabbi, or appropriate spiritual advisor. Work with mortician, as appropriate, in assisting family with plans for funeral.

RATIONALE

Grieving and trying to make sense out of the loss and to find meaning in life without the baby may cause the couple to question their religious beliefs and to feel cheated or angry. Discussion of objective findings can help the client/couple begin to cope appropriately with feelings of distress.

Use of a support system is a constructive means of coping with grief and maintaining perspective.

Families suffering perinatal loss often question their religious beliefs and are concerned about the purpose of life and death. Anger related to powerlessness may result in placing blame on oneself or someone else, or at God for "selecting them to suffer."

Specialists in spiritual beliefs and ritual may be needed to help in making decisions related to burial and loss. Symbolism and ritual can provide comfort and connect family members with their spiritual beliefs.

NURSING DIAGNOSIS:	KNOWLEDGE DEFICIT [LEARNING NEED], regarding perinatal loss, future expectations
May be related to:	Lack of exposure to or unfamiliarity with information resources, misinterpretation of information.
Possibly evidenced by:	Request for information, statement of misconception.
DESIRED OUTCOMES— CLIENT WILL:	Differentiate between causes of death that are controllable and those that are uncontrollable.
	Verbalize understanding of reasons for loss, when known.
	Discuss possible short- and long-term effects of the loss.

ACTIONS/INTERVENTIONS

Independent

Assess family's readiness and ability to understand and retain information.

RATIONALE

Emotional responses may interfere with the ability to hear and process information. The stage of denial is not the best time for the individual to attempt to process information, and repetition of information may be needed because of the individual's uncertainty about and lack of control of the situation. Simple reinforcement of reality may be all that family members are receptive to at the moment.

ACTIONS/INTERVENTIONS	RATIONALE

Independent

Provide information about possible short- and long-term physical and emotional effects of grief, including somatic symptoms, sleeplessness, nightmares, dreams of the infant or the pregnancy, emptiness, fatigue, altered sexual response, and loss of appetite.

In many cases, parents do not know why their child died and may have a fear of future pregnancies. Causes of intrauterine death, stillbirth, or perinatal death are sometimes uncertain even after autopsy, and families may feel guilty about the cause of death. Providing information about these factors can be helpful in resolving the grief of these individuals. Helps prepare couple for normal changes and difficulties associated with usual activities of daily living, and helps couple recognize extent of loss.

Review sequence of events and diagnostic tests performed, using pictures if available and appropriate.

During the severe stress that follows the loss, the client/couple understands and retains information more easily if it is presented in a concrete manner. Symbols such as footprints or pictures of the infant may be important.

Identify family's priorities when providing information.

Families have different needs for information, depending on the stage of family development and on whether death was intrauterine, due to external causes, or due to genetic problems.

Allow client to introduce the subject of another pregnancy.

Individuals determine their own readiness to think about and discuss this possibility. The usual recommendation is to avoid considering pregnancy until grief has been resolved, or until at least 6 months after the loss.

Identify client's/couple's perceptions of events, and correct misunderstandings, as indicated.

Inaccurate perceptions need to be assessed on a continual basis and valid information reiterated.

Prepare parents for reactions of friends and family; role-play responses.

Family members and friends often do not appreciate the intensity of the parents' grief. Role-playing can prepare parents for varied responses from friends and relatives, who may avoid talking about the loss, mistakenly believing that avoiding the topic is therapeutic.

Refer to chaplain and community support groups. (Refer to ND: Spiritual Distress, high risk for.)

In many cases, the parents do not trust information until they have heard it from multiple sources.

Review information provided by referal agencies/ groups.

Support groups provide information and assistance from people who have experienced similar losses and provide reassurance of normalcy of physical and emotional responses.

Discuss appropriateness of genetic counseling as indicated.

Genetic counseling may be suggested if the parents fear reoccurrence of the problem, even if the problem is not thought to be genetic. The terms congenital, teratogenic, and trauma should be defined and differentiated so that parents can comprehend risk factors.

CHAPTER **7**
NEWBORN CONCEPTS

Neonatal Assessment Tool _____

As in the maternal assessment tools, the newborn assessment tool has been constructed using a nursing focus instead of the familiar "head-to-toe" or medical approach of "review of systems." This tool is not divided into subjective/objective sections because the information recorded here is objectively obtained from physical assessment of the newborn and review of maternal, intrapartal, and delivery records. However, specific subjective questions may be indicated based on individual physical findings. Assessment components may be deleted or added, depending on the individual practitioner's capabilities and hospital policies. On occasion, information may be recorded more than once when it has implications for multiple diagnostic divisions. In addition, some tests (e.g., the Brazelton Neonatal Assessment Scale) may not be completed initially because of the length of time they require and because of shortened hospital stays. These tests should be performed or completed during follow-up examinations or home visits, as appropriate. Because the assessment is an ongoing process, it is essential to note infant age whenever material is added to the data base.

Although the divisions are alphabetized for ease of presentation, they can be prioritized or rearranged to meet individual needs.

NEWBORN ASSESSMENT TOOL

Name: _____ Sex: _____ Race: _____
Mother's name: _____ Father's name: _____
Birth date: _____ Time: _____ Apgar scores: _____
Time of exam: _____ Infant age: _____ Gestational age: _____

ACTIVITY/REST

Spontaneous activity: _____
Waking states noted:
   Drowsy: _____ Active alert: _____
   Quiet alert: _____ Crying: _____
Sleep states noted: Deep sleep: _____
   Light sleep (REM): _____

CIRCULATION

BP: _____ Apical pulse: _____ PMI: _____
Heart sounds: _____ Murmur: _____

Location: _____ Loudness: _____ Intensity: _____
Pulse: Brachial: _____ Femoral: _____ Dorsalis pedis: _____
Skin color: Ruddy: _____ Mottled: _____
   Harlequin: _____ Gray: _____
   Cyanosis: Location: _____ Effect of crying: _____
Hb: _____ Hct: _____

EGO INTEGRITY

Brazelton Neonatal Assessment Scale: _____
General areas of concern:
   Attention to stimuli: Visual: _____
     Auditory: _____
   Habituation to stimuli: _____
   Social behaviors/willingness to be cuddled: _____
   Consolability: _____ Self-consolation: _____

ELIMINATION

Bowel sounds: Present: _____ Character: _____
Abdomen: Intact: _____ Soft: _____ Mass: _____
   Protuberant: _____ Distended: _____ Scaphoid: _____
   Liver palpable: _____ Spleen palpable: _____
   Kidney palpable: R: _____ L: _____
   Absence of musculature: _____
Anus: Patent: _____ Fissures: _____ Pilonidal cyst: _____
Meconium passed: _____ Time: _____
Bladder: Palpable: _____
Urine: Time of first voiding: _____ Amount/frequency (24 hours): _____
   Color: _____ Urates present: _____
Generalized edema: Present: _____
   Resolved: _____
Male meatal opening: Normal: _____
   Hypospadias: _____ Phimosis: _____
   Epispadias: _____ Circumcision: _____

FOOD/FLUID

Birth weight: _____ Current weight: _____ Length: _____
Skin: Moist/dry: _____ Turgor: _____
Edema: General: _____ Localized: _____
Fontanels: Normal: _____ Depressed: _____
Mouth: Symmetric movement of lips and mouth: _____
   Lip/palate intact: _____
   Labial tubercle: _____
   Sucking pads: _____
   Epstein's pearls: _____ Thrush: _____
   Tongue: Size: _____ Moves freely: _____ Midline: _____
   Mucus: Amount: _____ Character: _____
   Teeth present: _____
   Micrognathia: _____
   Drooling: _____ Character: _____
Strength of reflexes: Rooting: _____ Sucking: _____
   Swallowing: _____ Gag: _____
   Feeding vigor: _____
Regurgitation: Amount: _____ Frequency: _____
Vomiting: Character: _____ Projectile: _____

Behavior: Irritable: _____   Jittery: _____
Hb: _____   Hct: _____

HYGIENE

Infant is unable to care for self and is totally dependent (Level 4).

NEUROSENSORY

Level of consciousness: _____
Response to stimuli: _____
Spontaneous alertness: _____
Cry: Strength: _____   Character: _____
Head: Appearance: _____   Circumference: _____ cm
   Overriding of sutures: _____   Molding: _____
   Caput succedaneum: _____   Craniotabes: _____   Cephalhematoma: _____
Fontanels (anterior/posterior): Palpable: _____
   Depressed: _____   Bulging: _____
Hair texture: _____   Distribution: _____
Facial appearance: _____
   Movement: Symmetric: _____   Paralysis: _____
Eyes: Parallel plane: _____   Hypertelorism: _____
   Agenesia: _____   Color: _____
   Blink response: _____   Nystagmus: _____
   Strabismus: Transient: _____   Constant: _____
   Subconjunctival hemorrhage: R: _____   L: _____
   Brushfield spots: _____   Epicanthic folds: _____
   Conjunctivitis: Chemical: _____ Infectious: _____
   Tears: Present: _____   Stagnant: _____
   Eyelids: Edema: _____   Inflammation: _____
   Setting sun: _____   Ptosis: _____
Pupil: Size: R: _____   L: _____   Red reflex: _____
   Reaction to light: R: _____   L: _____
Cornea: Clear: _____   Hazy: _____   Cloudy: _____
   Reflex present: _____
Sclera color: _____
Visual response: Gazes at object: _____
   Follows object: _____
Ears: Amount of cartilage: _____   Tympanic membrane: _____
   Preauricular skin tabs: _____
   Position on plane with angle of eye: _____   Low-set: _____
Nose: Appearance: _____   Septum intact: _____
Neck/head moves freely: _____   Rigidity/torticollis: _____
Hearing: Response to sound: _____
Muscle tone: Strong flexor: _____
   Hypotonicity: _____   Hypertonicity: _____
   Comparative movement: Arms: _____   Legs: _____
   Posture: Symmetric: _____
Reflexes: Ciliary: _____   Doll's eyes: _____
   Rooting: _____   Sucking: _____
   Moro: Bilateral: _____   Unilateral: _____
   Palmar grasp: _____   Plantar grasp: _____
   Babinski's: _____   Tonic neck: _____
   Traction: _____   Stepping: _____
   Prone crawl: _____   Trunk incurvation: _____
Muscle tremors: Fine/rapid: _____

Coarse with activity: _____ At rest: _____
Stiffening/rigidity: _____Deviation of eyes: _____

PAIN/DISCOMFORT

Observe (not test for) response to painful stimuli: Restlessness: _____
   Irritability: _____
   Constant cry: _____
   Withdrawal: _____

RESPIRATION

Apgar score: 1 minute: _____ 5 minutes: _____
Resuscitative measures/oxygen: _____ Time: _____
Respiratory rate: _____ Apnea (duration): _____
   Response to stimulation: _____
Chest: Appearance: _____ Circumference: _____ Cm
Chest-abdominal movement: Symmetric: _____ Synchronized: _____
   Inspiratory lag: _____ Paradoxical breathing: _____
   Diaphragmatic respirations: _____
Chest: Hyperexpansion: _____ Hypoexpansion: _____
Retractions: Intercostal: _____ Subcostal: _____
   Substernal: _____
Air passage through both nares: _____
Flaring of nostrils (mild/marked): _____
Grunting: _____
Breath sounds: _____
   Crackles: _____ Rhonchi: _____
Percussion: _____
Tracheal position: _____
Cyanosis: Location: _____ Effect of crying: _____
Mucus: Amount: _____ Character: _____
Hb: _____ ABGs: _____

SAFETY

Type of delivery: _____
Temperature: Rectal: _____ Axillary/skin: _____
Skin: Texture: _____ Moist/dry: _____ Color: _____
   Vernix caseosa: _____ Lanugo: _____
   Contusions: _____ Lacerations: _____ Abrasions: _____
   Milia: _____ Petechiae: _____
   Erythema toxicum neonatorum: _____
   Impetigo: _____ Moles: _____
   Meconium staining: _____
Pigment: Café au lait spots: _____ Mongolian spots: _____
   Telangiectatic nevi: _____ Nevus flammeus (port-wine stain): _____
   Nevus vascularis (strawberry hemangioma): _____ Cavernous hemangioma: _____
Umbilical cord: Number of vessels: _____ Color: _____
   Bleeding: _____ Exudate: _____
   Hernia: _____ Cutis navel: _____
   Granulation tissue present: _____
Clavicle: Intact: _____ Knot/crepitus/location: _____
Extremities: Comparative use: Arms: _____ Legs: _____
   Equal length :Arms: _____ Legs: _____
   Number of fingers: _____ Number of toes: _____
   Syndactylism: _____ Simian crease: _____ Sole creases: _____

Gluteal folds: Equal: _____ Ortolani's maneuver: _____
Talipes equinovarus (clubfoot): _____
Talipes calcaneus: _____
Spine: Straight: _____ Curved: _____
Vertebrae present: _____
Dermal sinus: _____ Nevus pilosus: _____
Coombs' test: _____ WBC count: _____

SEXUALITY

Breasts: Distance between: _____ cm Areolar diameter: _____ cm
Enlargement: _____ Discharge: _____
Supernumerary nipples: _____
Female genitalia:
Labia majora larger than labia minora (Y/N): _____
Reddened: _____ Swollen: _____
Vaginal/hymenal tag: _____ Vaginal discharge: _____
Smegma: _____ Bleeding (amount): _____
Male genitalia:
Scrotum: Rugae present: _____ Swelling: _____
Testicles descended/size: R: _____ cm L: _____ cm
Hydrocele: _____
Ambiguous genitalia: _____

SOCIAL INTERACTIONS

Parent-infant interaction: Maternal/paternal (M/P) response:
Facial expression: _____
Verbal response: To infant: _____
To spouse/significant other(s): _____
Use of infant's name: _____
Behaviors: Eye contact: _____ Touching: _____
Kissing: _____ Cuddling: _____
Examining: _____ Identifying familial characteristics: _____
Other: _____
Interaction with other family members/siblings: _____
Pregnancy planned: _____
Prenatal care (date begun): _____
Classes: _____

TEACHING/LEARNING

Gestational age: _____
Tool used (e.g., Dubowitz, Ballard, Brazelton, Lubchenco): _____

Discharge Plan Considerations:

Date/time information obtained: _____
Anticipated date/time of discharge: _____
Resources available: Persons: _____
Approved car seat: _____

The primary focus at this time is the transition from intrauterine to extrauterine life with introduction to family members as the neonate's condition warrants.

NEONATAL ASSESSMENT DATA BASE (Full-Term)

CIRCULATION

Apical pulse may fluctuate from 110 to 180 bpm.

Blood pressure 60 to 80 mm Hg (systolic), 40 to 45 mm Hg (diastolic).

Heart sounds: Located in mediastinum with point of maximal intensity just to the left of the midsternum at third or fourth intercostal space.

Murmurs common during the first few hours of life.

Umbilical cord white and gelatinous, contains two arteries and one vein.

ELIMINATION

May void at birth.

FOOD/FLUID

Weight: 2500 to 4000 g (5 lb 8 oz to 8 lb 13 oz).

Length: 44 to 55 cm (18 to 22 inches).

Skin turgor elastic (varies according to gestational age).

NEUROSENSORY

Muscle tone: Hypertonic flexion of all extremities.

Awake and active, demonstrates sucking reflex for first 30 min following birth (first period of reactivity).

Asymmetric appearance (molding, edema, hematoma).

Cry strong, lusty, medium pitch (high-pitched cry suggests genetic abnormality, hypoglycemia, or prolonged narcotic effect).

RESPIRATION

Apgar score: 1 minute: _____ 5 minutes: _____. Optimal score should be between 7 to 10.

Rate ranges from 30 to 60/min; periodic pattern may be noted.

Breath sounds bilateral, occasional crackles common initially.

Thorax cylindric; prominent xiphoid cartilage common.

SAFETY

Temperature ranges from 36.5°C to 37.5°C (97.7°F to 99.4°F).

Some vernix present (amount and distribution dependent on gestational age).

Skin: Smooth, flexible; peeling of hands/feet may be noted; pink-tinged or ruddy color; may be mottled, display minor bruising (e.g., forceps delivery), or harlequin color changes; petechiae on head/face (may reflect increased pressure associated with delivery or nuchal cord); port-wine stains, telangiectatic nevi (eyelids, between brows, or on occiput), or mongolian spots (primarily lower back and buttocks) may be noted.

Scalp abrasion may be present (internal electrode placement).

DIAGNOSTIC STUDIES

Cord pH: Levels of 7.20 to 7.24 reflect a preacidotic state; lower levels indicate significant asphyxia.
Hemoglobin/hematocrit (Hb/Hct): Hb level of 15–20 g and Hct of 43%–61%.
Direct Coombs' test on cord blood: Determines presence of antigen-antibody complexes on red blood cell membrane, reflecting hemolytic condition.

NURSING PRIORITIES

1. Promote effective cardiopulmonary effort.
2. Provide a thermoneutral environment, and maintain body temperature.
3. Prevent injury or complications.
4. Promote parent-infant attachment.

NURSING DIAGNOSIS:	**GAS EXCHANGE, IMPAIRED, HIGH RISK FOR**
Risk factors may include:	Prenatal or intrapartal stressors, excess production of mucus, and cold stress.
Possibly evidenced by:	[Not applicable; presence of signs/symptoms establishes an **actual** diagnosis.]
DESIRED OUTCOMES— NEONATE WILL:	Maintain patent airway with respiratory and heart rates within normal limits (WNL); generalized cyanosis absent.
	Be free of signs of respiratory distress.

ACTIONS/INTERVENTIONS	RATIONALE

Independent

Measure Apgar score at 1 and 5 min following delivery.	Helps determine need for immediate intervention (e.g., suctioning, oxygen). A total score of 0 to 3 represents severe asphyxia or possible dysfunction in neurologic and/or chemical control of respiration. Scores of 4 to 6 signify moderate difficulty adapting to extrauterine life. Scores of 7 to 10 indicate no difficulty adapting to extrauterine life.
Note prenatal complications affecting placental and/or fetal status (e.g., cardiac or kidney disorders, pregnancy-induced hypertension, or diabetes).	Such complications may result in chronic hypoxia and acidosis, increasing risk of central nervous system damage and requiring correction after delivery.
Review intrapartal fetal status, including fetal heart rate (FHR), periodic changes in FHR, beat-to-beat variability, scalp pH level, and color and amount of amniotic fluid.	As in prenatal complications, intrapartal events may create fetal distress and hypoxia that persist into the immediate postdelivery period, resulting in depressed or ineffective respiratory effort. Fetus with scalp pH level less than 7.20; prolonged, variable, or late decelerations, and reduced FHR variability; oligohydramnios; or meconium-stained amniotic fluid will require greater efforts to achieve stabilization following birth than fetus with no sign of hypoxia or distress.

ACTIONS/INTERVENTIONS	RATIONALE
Independent	
Note duration of labor and type of delivery.	Thoracic compression during passage through the birth canal aids in clearing the lungs of approximately 80–110 ml of fluid. An infant delivered following percipitous labor (of less than 3 hours) or delivered by cesarean section has excessive mucus because of inadequate thoracic compression.
Note times at which medications (e.g., magnesium sulfate or meperidine hydrochloride [Demerol]) were administered to mother.	Medications may depress newborn's respiratory efforts and reduce the newborn's ability to oxygenate tissues.
Assess initial respiratory rate and effort.	The first breath, which is the most difficult, establishes a functional residual capacity (FRC), so that 30%–40% of lung tissue remains fully expanded provided that adequate surfactant levels are present. Failure to achieve an FRC makes each subsequent breath as tiring and difficult as the initial breath. Tachypnea (respiratory rate greater than 60/min) is usually associated with normal anticipated changes in the first period of reactivity (30 min following birth), but may also represent an attempt to eliminate excess carbon dioxide.
Note presence of nasal flaring, chest retractions, expiratory grunting, crackles, or rhonchi.	These signs are normal and transient in the first period of reactivity, but may indicate respiratory distress if they persist. Crackles may be heard until fluid is reabsorbed from lungs. Rhonchi indicate aspiration of oral secretions.
Clear airway; gently suction nasopharynx, as needed, using a bulb syringe or DeLee mucus-trap catheter (preferably while neonate's head is on maternal perineum if meconium-stained amniotic fluid is present). Monitor apical pulse during suctioning.	Helps remove accumulated fluid, facilitates respiratory effort, and helps prevent aspiration. Suctioning of the oropharynx causes vagal stimulation leading to bradycardia.
Dry infant with warm blankets, place stockinette cap on head, and place either in parent's arms or in prewarmed heating unit.	Reduces effects of cold stress (i.e., increased oxygen needs) and associated hypoxia, which can further depress respiratory efforts and result in acidosis as infant resorts to anaerobic metabolism with lactic acid end products. (Refer to ND: Body Temperature, altered, high risk for.)
Place infant in modified Trendelenburg position at a 10-degree angle.	Facilitates drainage of mucus from nasopharynx and trachea by means of gravity.
Note pitch and intensity of cry.	Initially, a lusty, strong cry increases alveolar P_{O_2} and produces the necessary chemical changes to convert fetal to neonatal circulation, so that the heart rate increases to 175–180 bpm and then usually returns to normal within the next 4–6 hr.
Note apical pulse.	A heart rate less than 100 bpm indicates severe asphyxia and the need for immediate resuscitation. Tachycardia (heart rate greater than 160 bpm) may indicate recent asphyxia or a normal response associated with the first period of reactivity.

ACTIONS/INTERVENTIONS	RATIONALE

Independent

Provide appropriate tactile and sensory stimulation.

Stimulates respiratory effort and may increase inspired oxygen.

Note presence of wide-eyed stare.

Indicates chronic intrauterine hypoxia, which is possibly associated with acidosis and requires resuscitative measures.

Observe skin color for location and extent of cyanosis. Assess muscle tone.

Acrocyanosis, suggesting sluggish peripheral circulation, occurs normally in 85% of newborns during the first hour; however, generalized cyanosis and flaccidity indicate inadequate tissue oxygenation.

Suction gastric contents if amniotic fluid was meconium-stained.

Helps reduce incidence of aspiration pneumonia in early neonatal period.

Collaborative

Administer warmed oxygen via mask at 4–7 L/min if indicated.

Provides additional oxygen and supports respiratory effort if marked pallor or generalized cyanosis is present. In cases of prolonged hypoxia, fetal circulation may persist, because elevated Po_2 levels are necessary to reduce pulmonary vascular resistance, increase blood flow to the lungs, and increase pressure on the left side of the heart, which closes the ductus arteriosus and the foramen ovale.

Assist with drawing of cord blood.

If there is indication of respiratory distress in the newborn, a cord pH level may be obtained to confirm presence and duration of prenatal asphyxia.

Perform deep suctioning if infant shows evidence of respiratory depression that does not respond to gentle suction or to gentle tactile stimulation.

Promotes patent airway. If meconium staining is present, deep suctioning, in conjunction with suctioning while infant's head is on perineum, is necessary to prevent meconium aspiration.

Administer medications, as indicated (e.g., Naloxone [Narcan], administered intravenously or through umbilical vessel catheter).

Narcan is a fast-acting narcotic antagonist that counteracts respiratory depression caused by exposure to maternal anesthetics or narcotics.

Provide resuscitative measures, and prepare for transfer of infant to a neonatal intensive care unit (NICU) or level III/IV facility, as indicated.

Infants requiring extensive resuscitative efforts must be observed and cared for by personnel who have been specifically trained to care for sick newborns.

NURSING DIAGNOSIS: **BODY TEMPERATURE, ALTERED, HIGH RISK FOR**

Risk factors may include: Extreme of age (inability to shiver, large body surface in relation to mass, limited amounts of insulating subcutaneous fat, nonrenewable sources of brown fat and few white fat stores, thin epidermis with close proximity of blood vessels to the skin).

Possibly evidenced by: [Not applicable; presence of signs/symptoms establishes an **actual** diagnosis.]

ACTIONS/INTERVENTIONS	RATIONALE
Independent	
Ascertain medications mother received during prenatal and intrapartal periods. Note presence of fetal distress or hypoxia.	Fetal hypoxia or maternal use of Demerol alters fetal metabolism of brown fat, often causing significant drop in neonate's temperature. Magnesium sulfate can cause vasodilation and interfere with infant's ability to retain heat.
Dry newborn's head and body, place stockinette cap on head; and wrap in warm blankets.	Reduces evaporative and conductive heat loss, protects moist infant from drafts or cooling air currents, and limits stress of movement from a warm uterine environment to a much cooler environment (possibly 15°F [9°C] lower than intrauterine temperatures). (Note: Due to the relatively large surface area of the newborn head in relation to that of the body, an infant may experience dramatic heat loss from a moist, uncovered head.)
Place newborn in prewarmed environment or in parent's arms. Warm objects coming in contact with infant (e.g., scales, stethoscopes, examination tables, and hands).	Prevents heat loss by conduction, whereby heat is transferred from the newborn to objects or surfaces cooler than the newborn. Being held close to the parent's body and skin-to-skin contact reduce the newborn's heat loss.
Note environmental temperature. Eliminate drafts and minimize use of air conditioners; warm oxygen if it is administered via mask.	A decrease in the environmental temperature of 2°C (3.6°F) is sufficient to double the oxygen consumption of a term neonate. Heat loss by convection occurs when infant loses heat to cooler air currents. Loss by radiation occurs when heat is transferred from the newborn to objects or surfaces not in direct contact with newborn (e.g., incubator sides or walls).
Assess neonate's core temperature; monitor skin temperature continually with skin probe as appropriate.	Skin temperature should be maintained close to 36.5°C (97.6°F). Core temperature (rectal) is usually 0.5°C (0.9°F) higher than skin temperature, yet continuous transfer from core to skin occurs, so that the greater the difference between core and skin temperature, the more rapid the transfer and the faster the core temperature cools.
Provide gradual warming for cold-stressed infant, keeping air temperature 1.5°C (2.7°F) warmer than body temperature.	Too-rapid increase in temperature may result in apnea in cold-stressed infant.
Observe infant for signs of cold stress (e.g., drop in skin temperature, increased activity, flexion of extremities, pallor and/or mottling, and cool skin, hands, and feet).	When the environmental temperature falls below the thermoneutral zone, the infant increases activity levels (increasing metabolic rate and oxygen consumption), flexes extremities to reduce amount of body surface exposed, and releases adrenal

ACTIONS/INTERVENTIONS

Independent

Note signs of respiratory distress (e.g., apnea, generalized cyanosis, bradycardia, and severe grunting, retraction of respiratory muscles, and nasal flaring). Provide support as needed.

Collaborative

Provide metabolic support (glucose or buffer), as indicated.

Consider admission to NICU.

RATIONALE

catecholamines, which promote heat release from stored brown fat and cause vasoconstriction, further cooling the skin.

These signs indicate negative effects of prolonged cold stress, which necessitate close monitoring. Peripheral vasoconstriction leads to metabolic acidosis; pulmonary vasoconstriction results in respiratory compromise and persistence of fetal circulation with failure of ductus arteriosus and foramen ovale to close.

Side effects of prolonged hypothermia (cold stress) may include increased oxygen consumption leading to hypoxia, acidosis, and respiratory compromise; increased metabolic rate and glucose consumption, resulting in hypoglycemia; as well as release of free fatty acids in the bloodstream, which compete with bilirubin binding sites on albumin, therefore increasing the risk of jaundice and kernicterus. Administration of glucose or bicarbonate can correct hypoglycemia, acidosis, and/or asphyxia.

Permits close observation and use of aggressive care methods in cases of severe neonatal cold stress with secondary symptoms.

NURSING DIAGNOSIS:	FAMILY PROCESSES, ALTERED, bonding
May be related to:	Developmental transition and/or gain of a family member.
Possibly evidenced by:	Hesitance of parent(s) to hold/interact with infant, verbalization of concerns.
DESIRED OUTCOMES— PARENT(S) WILL:	Initiate attachment process in ways that are meaningful to family members.
	Properly identify infant to assure correct family association.

ACTIONS/INTERVENTIONS

Independent

Inform parents of neonate's immediate needs and of care being provided.

RATIONALE

Alleviates parents' anxiety regarding condition of their newborn. Helps parents to understand rationale for interventions in initial newborn period.

ACTIONS/INTERVENTIONS

Independent

Place infant in mother's/father's arms as soon as neonatal condition permits.

Encourage parent(s) to stroke and speak to newborn; encourage mother to breastfeed infant if desired.

Share information gained from initial physical assessment of newborn.

Discuss infant's capabilities for interaction. (Refer to Chapter 6, CP: Stage IV (First 4 Hours Following Delivery of the Placenta), ND: Family Processes, altered, bonding.)

Using legally acceptable identification system, place arm or leg bands on infant and one wrist band on mother. Take infant's footprints and mother's fingerprint (index finger).

Provide appropriate information in the event of unanticipated complications or the need for transfer to NICU.

RATIONALE

The first hour of an infant's life is an especially significant time for family interaction in that it can promote initial attachment between parents and infant and acceptance of the newborn as a new family member.

Provides opportunity for parents and newborn to initiate acquaintance and attachment process.

Helps parents to view infant as a separate person with unique physical characteristics.

Helps facilitate parent-infant interaction.

Establishes family unit and prevents confusion regarding identification of infant. A more accurate method of identification, DNA fingerprinting, is being used and may supplant traditional footprinting and fingerprinting.

Keeping parents informed about infant's change in status, and actual or potential actions to be instituted, helps to assure them that everything possible is being done to care for infant and promotes parental cooperation with emergency measures.

NURSING DIAGNOSIS:	INJURY, HIGH RISK FOR, multiple factors
Risk factors may include:	Undetected or untreated congenital anomalies, exposure to infectious agents.
Possibly evidenced by:	[Not applicable; presence of signs/symptoms establishes an **actual** diagnosis.]
DESIRED OUTCOMES—NEONATE WILL:	Be free of injury/complications.

ACTIONS/INTERVENTIONS

Independent

Perform routine physical assessment of newborn, noting number of cord vessels and presence of anomalies.

Bathe newborn immediately after delivery if exposure to infectious agents has occurred.

RATIONALE

Helps detect abnormalities and neurologic defects, establishes gestational age, and identifies the need for closer monitoring and more intensive care. Cord should contain three vessels. Presence of only one artery is associated with genitourinary abnormalities.

Prevents newborn from contracting hepatitis B virus or from becoming a chronic carrier when exposed to maternal serum blood products at delivery.

ACTIONS/INTERVENTIONS	RATIONALE
Independent	
Describe to parents the appropriate rationale for actions taken to prevent injury (e.g., prophylactic administration of eye ointment and vitamin K).	Reduces parental anxiety created by a lack of understanding of the need to protect neonate against eye infection and hemorrhagic diseases.
Collaborative	
Clamp newborn's umbilical cord approximately $1/2$ to 1 inch from abdomen within 30 sec after birth, while infant is at the level of the mother's introitus.	Holding infant below the level of the introitus or delaying cord clamping accounts for transfer of 50–100 ml of blood from the placenta, possibly contributing to polycythemia and hyperbilirubinemia in the neonatal period.
Administer eye prophylaxis in the form of erythromycin ointment (Ilotycin) approximately 1 hr after birth (after period of parent-infant interaction).	Helps prevent ophthalmia neonatorum caused by *Neisseria gonorrhoeae*, which may be present in the mother's birth canal. Erythromycin effectively eradicates both gonorrheal and chlamydial organisms. Eye prophylaxis clouds infant's vision, reducing infant's ability to interact with parents.
Administer hepatitis B immune globulin (HBIG) and hepatitis B vaccine if mother's serum contains hepatitis B surface antigen (HB_sAg), hepatitis B core antigen (HB_cAg), or e antigen (HB_eAg).	Reduces risk of newborn's contracting hepatitis B or becoming a chronic carrier.

NEONATAL ASSESSMENT DATA BASE (Full Term)

(Refer to CP: The First Hour of Life.)

ACTIVITY/REST

Wakeful state may be as little as 2–3 hr first several days.

Infant appears semi-comatose while in deep sleep; grimacing or smiling is evident in rapid-eye-movement (REM) sleep; averages 20 hr of sleep per day.

CIRCULATION

Apical pulse averages 120–160 bpm (115 bpm at 4–6 hr, rising to 120 bpm at 12–24 hr after birth); may fluctuate from 70–100 bpm (sleeping) to 180 bpm (crying).

Peripheral pulses may be weak (bounding pulses suggest patent ductus arteriosus); brachial and radial pulses are more easily palpated than femoral pulses (absence of femoral and dorsalis pedis pulses suggests coarctation of the aorta).

Heart murmur often present during transition periods.

Blood pressure (BP) ranges from 60 to 80 mm Hg (systolic)/40 to 45 mm Hg (diastolic), average resting pressure approximately 74/46 mm Hg; BP lowest at 3 hr of age.

Umbilical cord clamped securely with no oozing of blood noted; shows signs of drying within 1–2 hr of birth, shriveled and blackened by day 2 or 3.

ELIMINATION

Abdomen soft without distention; active bowel sounds present several hours after birth.

Urine colorless or pale yellow, with 6 to 10 wet diapers per 24 hours.

Passage of meconium stool within 24–48 hr of birth.

FOOD/FLUID

Mean weight 2500 to 4000 g (5 lb 8 oz to 8 lb 13 oz); less than 2500 g suggests small for gestational age (SGA) (e.g., prematurity, rubella syndrome, or multiple gestation), greater than 4000 g suggests large for gestational age (LGA) (e.g., maternal diabetes; or may be associated with heredity). (Refer to CPs: The Preterm Infant; Newborn: Deviations in Growth Patterns.)

Weight loss 5%–10% initially.

Mouth: Scant saliva; Epstein's pearls (epithelial cysts) and sucking blisters are normal on hard palate/gum margins, precocious teeth may be present.

NEUROSENSORY

Head circumference 32–37 cm; anterior and posterior fontanels are soft and flat.

Caput succedaneum and/or molding may persist for 3–4 days; overriding of cranial sutures may be noted, slightly obliterating anterior fontanel (2–3 cm in width) and posterior fontanel (0.5–1.0 cm in width).

Eyes and eyelids may be edematous; subconjunctival or retinal hemorrhage may be noted; chemical conjunctivitis lasting 1–2 days may develop following instillation of therapeutic ophthalmic drops.

Strabismus and doll's eye phenomenon often present.

Top of ear aligns with inner and outer canthi of eye (low-set ears suggest genetic or kidney abnormalities).

Neurologic examination: Presence of Moro, plantar, palmar grasp, and Babinski's reflexes; reflex responses are bilateral/equal (unilateral Moro reflex may indicate fractured clavicle or brachial plexus injury); transient crawling movements may be seen.

Absence of jitteriness, lethargy, hypotonia, and paresis.

RESPIRATION

Transient tachypnea may be noted, especially following cesarean or breech delivery.

Breathing pattern: Diaphragmatic and abdominal with synchronous movement of chest and abdomen (inspiratory lag or alternating seesaw movements of the chest and abdomen reflect respiratory distress); slight or occasional nasal flaring may be noted; marked nasal flaring, expiratory grunting, or marked retraction of intercostal, substernal, or subcostal muscles indicates respiratory distress; inspiratory crackles may persist for first few hours after birth (rhonchi on inspiration or expiration may indicate aspiration).

Chest circumference approximately 30–35 cm (1–2 cm smaller than circumference of head).

SAFETY

Skin color: Acrocyanosis may be present for several days during transition period (general ruddiness may indicate polycythemia); reddened or ecchymotic areas may appear over cheeks or on lower jaw or parietal areas as a result of forceps application at delivery.

Cephalhematoma may appear day after delivery, increasing in size by 2 to 3 days of age, then be reabsorbed slowly over 1 to 6 months.

Extremities: Normal range of motion in all, mild degree of bowing or medial rotation of lower extremities; good muscle tone.

SEXUALITY

Female genitalia: Vaginal labia may be slightly reddened or edematous, vaginal/hymenal tag may be noted; white mucous discharge (smegma) or slight bloody discharge (pseudomenstruation) may be present.

Male genitalia: Testes descended, scrotum covered with rugae, phimosis common (opening of prepuce narrowed, preventing retraction of foreskin over the glans).

TEACHING/LEARNING

Gestational age between 38 and 42 weeks based on Dubowitz criteria.

DIAGNOSTIC STUDIES

White blood cell (WBC) count: 18,000/mm^3, neutrophils increase to 23,000–24,000/mm^3 the first day after birth (decline occurs in sepsis).
Hemoglobin (Hb): 15–20 g/dl (lower levels associated with anemia or excessive hemolysis).
Hematocrit (Hct): 43%–61% (elevation to 65% or over indicates polycythemia; decreased levels reflect anemia or prenatal/perinatal hemorrhage).
Guthrie inhibition assay: Tests for presence of phenylalanine metabolites, indicating phenylketonuria (PKU).
Total bilirubin: 6 mg/dl on first day of life, 8 mg/dl at 1 to 2 days, and 12 mg/dl at 3 to 5 days.
Dextrostix: Initial glucose drop during first 4–6 hr after birth averages 40 to 50 mg/dl, raising to 60 to 70 mg/dl by day 3.

NURSING PRIORITIES

1. Facilitate adaptation to extrauterine life.
2. Maintain thermoneutrality.

3. Prevent complications.
4. Promote parent-infant attachment.
5. Provide information and anticipatory guidance to parent(s).

DISCHARGE GOALS

1. Newborn adapting effectively to extrauterine life.
2. Free of complications.
3. Parent-infant attachment is initiated.
4. Parent(s) express confidence regarding infant care.

NURSING DIAGNOSIS:	BODY TEMPERATURE, ALTERED, HIGH RISK FOR
Risk factors may include:	Extreme of age (inability to shiver, larger body surface in relation to mass, limited amounts of insulating subcutaneous fat, nonrenewable sources of brown fat and few white fat stores, thin epidermis with close proximity of blood vessels to the skin).
Possibly evidenced by:	[Not applicable; presence of signs/symptoms establishes an **actual** diagnosis.]
DESIRED OUTCOMES— NEONATE WILL:	Maintain temperature within normal limits. Be free of signs of cold stress or hyperthermia.

ACTIONS/INTERVENTIONS	RATIONALE

Independent

Maintain ambient temperature within established thermoneutral zone (TNZ) considering neonate's weight, gestational age, and usual clothing provided.

In response to lower environmental temperature, full-term infants increase their body temperature by crying or increasing motor activity, thereby possibly consuming more energy (stored glucose) and increasing their oxygen needs. Conversely, failure to maintain the environmental temperature within the upper limits of the TNZ may result in increased oxygen consumption, dehydration, hypotension, seizures, and apnea associated with hyperthermia.

Monitor infant's axillary, skin (abdominal), or tympanic and environmental temperature at least every 30–60 min during stabilization period, or more frequently per protocol.

Temperature stabilization may not occur until 8–12 hr following birth. Rates of oxygen consumption and metabolism are minimal when skin temperature (a reliable indicator of energy exchanges between infant and environment) is maintained above 36.5°C (97.7°F). Skin temperature measured over the abdomen (away from bony area) is an earlier, more reliable indicator of cold stress, because it drops in response to peripheral vasoconstriction. Axillary temperature readings may be misleading, because friction in the armpit, where brown fat stores are located, can cause false elevations. Core body temperature, as assessed by rectal temperatures, may remain misleadingly high, especially in the cold-stressed infant, as a

ACTIONS/INTERVENTIONS

Independent

RATIONALE

result of vasoconstriction and metabolism of brown fat stores. Core temperature may fall only after the infant has exhausted compensatory mechanisms and has markedly increased oxygen consumption. (Note: Rectal perforation may occur with insertion of rectal thermometer, and its occurrence is associated with 70% mortality.)

Assess respiratory rate; note tachypnea (rate greater than 60/minute).

Infant becomes tachypneic in response to increased oxygen needs associated with cold stress and attempts to eliminate excess carbon dioxide to reduce respiratory acidosis.

Postpone initial bath until body temperature is stable and reaches 36.5°C (97.7°F).

Helps prevent further heat losses due to evaporation. Larger appropriate-for-gestational age (AGA) infants tend to maintain body temperature more easily than the SGA infant.

Avoid cooling infant during bath by working rapidly, exposing only a portion of the body at a time, and drying each part immediately. Ensure that environment is free of drafts.

Reduces possible heat loss through evaporation and convection; helps conserve energy.

Note secondary signs of cold stress (e.g., irritability, pallor, mottling, respiratory distress, tremors, jitteriness, lethargy, and cool skin).

Hypothermia, which increases the utilization rate of oxygen and glucose, is often accompanied by hypoglycemia and respiratory distress. Cooling also results in peripheral vasoconstriction, with a drop in skin temperature observed as pallor or mottling. Irritability and apnea may be associated with hypoxia. Untreated or undetected cold stress may progress to metabolic acidosis associated with anaerobic glycolysis; pulmonary vasoconstriction or persistent fetal circulation; inhibition of lecithin formation and increased severity of respiratory distress; and release of fatty acids into bloodstream, where they compete for bilirubin binding sites on albumin molecules.

Maintain thermoneutral environment through use of automatically controlled or manually adjustable heating equipment. Maintain controlled heat source at 37°C (98.6°F). Position crib or incubator away from heat sources such as sunlight, heaters, or bilirubin lights. Promote gradual warming of infant as needed (1°C per hour). Adjust clothing as indicated.

Prevents heat imbalance or losses. Gradual warming of hypothermic infant helps avoid possible apneic spells, hypotension, seizures, or dehydration associated with too-rapid warming and hyperthermia.

Assess for behavioral signs associated with hyperthermia (e.g., increased restlessness, perspiration that begins on head or face and proceeds to chest, apnea, seizure, and hypotension activity).

Heat dissipation occurs through peripheral vasodilation and through augmentation of cooling by evaporation and by increase in insensible water loss. Apnea, seizures, and hypotension may be related to peripheral vasodilation, which causes increased evaporative water losses, cerebral ischemia, and dehydration.

ACTIONS/INTERVENTIONS

Independent

Note signs of dehydration (e.g., poor skin turgor, delayed voiding, dry mucous membranes, elevated temperature, sunken fontanels).

Initiate early oral feeding.

Assess infant for other disease processes, such as infection, if temperature deviates more than 1°C (1.8°F) from one reading to next.

Collaborative

Make arrangements for transfer to neonatal intensive care unit (NICU) if indicated.

Obtain cultures as indicated.

Administer seizure-control medication (e.g, phenobarbital), as needed.

RATIONALE

Axillary temperature greater than 37.5°C (99.5°F) is considered hyperthermic and may result in overheating infant. Dehydration may develop in relation to a threefold to fourfold increase in insensible water loss.

For every 1°C (1.8°F) increase in body temperature, metabolism and fluid needs increase approximately 10%. Failure to replace fluid losses further contributes to dehydrated state.

Temperature instability or subnormal temperature may indicate infection. In addition, central nervous system (CNS) disorders and dehydration may cause hyperthermia.

If temperature remains low regardless of appropriate intervention related to thermoregulation, transfer of infant may be necessary for closer observation and treatment.

Determines presence and type of bacteria and the appropriate treatment.

Acts directly on cerebrum to quiet excessive motor activity.

NURSING DIAGNOSIS:	GAS EXCHANGE, IMPAIRED, HIGH RISK FOR
Risk factors may include:	Prenatal/intrapartal stressors, excess production of mucus, and fluctuations of body temperature.
Possibly evidenced by:	[Not applicable; presence of signs/symptoms establishes an **actual** diagnosis.]
DESIRED OUTCOMES— NEONATE WILL:	Maintain patent airway with respiratory rate within normal limits (WNL) (between 30 and 60/min). Be free of signs of respiratory distress.

ACTIONS/INTERVENTIONS

Independent

Estimate gestational age using Dubowitz criteria.

RATIONALE

Surfactant system develops as gestation progresses. Once fetus reaches 35 weeks' gestation, the presence of phosphatidylglycerol (a component of the surfactant complex, that indicates fetal lung maturity) markedly decreases the incidence of respiratory distress syndrome (RDS). Infants of diabetic mothers who have been exposed to prolonged hyperinsulinemia in response to maternal hyperglycemia may have depressed surfactant production and greater respiratory distress even though they are beyond 35 weeks' gestation at birth.

ACTIONS/INTERVENTIONS	RATIONALE
Independent	
Review prenatal and intrapartal events, noting risk factors that could have contributed to excess lung fluid or aspiration of amniotic fluid (e.g., maternal diabetes, cesarean birth or breech delivery, maternal bleeding, intrapartal asphyxia, maternal oversedation).	Such events contribute to the infant's inability to clear airway of excess fluid, mucus, and aspirated material, and to the collection of excess fluid in lungs, resulting in type II RDS, which usually resolves within 6 hours.
Assess respiratory rate and effort. Differentiate periodic breathing patterns from apneic episodes.	Normal respiratory rate is 30–60/min. Periodic breathing that is of no physiologic significance is manifested by apneic periods lasting 5–15 sec occurring during REM sleep and periods of motor activity. It is easily converted to a normal breathing pattern by increasing inspired oxygen through tactile and sensory stimulation. Apneic episodes last longer than 20–30 sec, may be associated with changes in heart rate and skin color, and require further assessment and intervention.
Suction nasopharynx as needed. Note color, amount, and character of regurgitated mucus.	Ensures clearance of airway, which is critical to neonate, who is an obligatory nose breather and may not learn to open the mouth in response to nasal obstruction until 3 to 4 weeks of age. Regurgitation of mucus associated with an episode of gagging often occurs in the second period of reactivity (2–6 hours after delivery).
Position infant on side with rolled towel for support at back.	Facilitates drainage of mucus.
Auscultate breath sounds and record equality and clarity. Note presence of crackles or rhonchi.	Breath sounds should be equal bilaterally. Inspiratory crackles may be present in the first few hours following delivery until lung fluid is absorbed from distal bronchioles. Persistent crackles may indicate RDS or pneumonia. Rhonchi heard on inspiration or expiration, caused by air moving through passages that have been narrowed by secretions or swelling, may indicate retained secretions/aspiration.
Review delivery records for presence of meconium at birth or meconium-stained amniotic fluid; determine whether appropriate suctioning of oropharynx was performed while infant's head was still on perineum.	When meconium is present, inappropriate suctioning before the initial breath predisposes infant to development of meconium-aspiration pneumonia.
Observe and record signs of respiratory distress (e.g., grunting, retraction of respiratory muscles, nasal flaring, and tachypnea).	These signs represent compensatory mechanisms to overcome hypoxia. Expiratory grunting occurs as an attempt to maintain alveolar expansion and to retain air. Retraction of respiratory muscles increases tidal volume, nasal flaring increases the diameter of the nares, and tachypnea occurs in an attempt to eliminate excess carbon dioxide.
Assess infant for presence, location, and degree of cyanosis and its relationship to activity.	Peripheral cyanosis (acrocyanosis) associated with vasomotor instability, hypothermia, or local venous or arterial obstruction may persist through the transition period. Mild cyanosis and mottling may occur in second period of reactivity in associ-

ACTIONS/INTERVENTIONS

Independent

Assess relationship between infant's skin temperature and ambient air temperature.

Monitor infant for signs of hypothermia or hyperthermia. (Refer to ND: Body Temperature, altered, high risk for.)

Note symmetry of chest movement.

Auscultate heart sounds; note presence of murmurs.

Collaborative

Administer supplemental oxygen, as indicated by newborn's condition.

Record use and results of mechanical monitoring and support.

Assess Hb and Hct levels. Note results of Betke-Kleihauer test. Monitor arterial blood gases.

RATIONALE

ation with fluctuations in cardiac and respiratory rates. Cyanosis that worsens with crying suggests cardiac problems rather than respiratory problems, in which cyanosis is usually improved with crying.

Oxygen consumption is minimal when the difference between skin temperature and ambient air temperature is less than 1.5°C (2.7°F).

Hypothermia and hyperthermia increase metabolic rate and oxygen consumption, causing a possible cycle of metabolic acidosis and hypoxia that perpetuates fetal circulation, reduces surfactant levels, and increases respiratory distress. A drop in skin temperature to 35.9°C (96.6°F) increases oxygen consumption by 10%. Too-rapid warming of infant may lead to hyperthermia, which increases oxygen consumption by 6%.

Asymmetry may indicate pneumothorax associated with previous resuscitative measures.

Transient cardiac murmurs (usually systolic) may exist in the early newborn period because of persistence or reopening of fetal structures in response to hypoxia and crying. Patent ductus arteriosus often occurs with hypoxia, pulmonary vasoconstriction, right-to-left shunting, and congestive heart failure, or more significantly with prenatal or birth asphyxia, hyperviscosity, polycythemia, aspiration syndrome, and hypoglycemia. Foramen ovale normally closes at 1 to 2 hours following delivery; ductus arteriosus closes at 3 to 4 days of age. Inadequate lung perfusion and poorly ventilated lung tissue promote airway constriction and respiratory compromise.

Persistent uninterrupted oxygen depletion increases hypoxic state, resulting in metabolic acidosis secondary to anaerobic metabolism.

Unmonitored use of oxygen therapy can result in oxygen toxicity. Transcutaneous monitoring helps prevent hypoxic states and evaluates therapeutic effectiveness.

The infant whose Hb level is lower than normal has reduced oxygen-carrying capacity and possibly severe hypoxia. Hb levels less than 15 g/dl may be due to blood loss, hemolysis, or decreased red blood cell (RBC) production. Clinical signs of cyanosis may not appear until Hb levels are decreased by slightly more than 3 g/dl in central arterial blood or 4–6 g/dl in capillary blood. Betke-Kleihauer test identifies fetal bleeding in utero.

ACTIONS/INTERVENTIONS

Collaborative

Note Rh factor and ABO blood group of infant and mother; note results of Coombs' test. (Refer to CP: Newborn: Hyperbilirubinemia.)

Review chest x-ray.

RATIONALE

Identifies possible antigen–antibody reaction to Rh or ABO incompatibility, which contributes to lowered Hb levels and oxygen-carrying capacity.

May be necessary to diagnose pneumothorax.

NURSING DIAGNOSIS:	NUTRITION, ALTERED, LESS THAN BODY REQUIRE-MENTS, HIGH RISK FOR
Risk factors may include:	Increased metabolic rate, high caloric requirement, fatigue, minimal nutritional stores.
Possibly evidenced by:	[Not applicable; presence of signs/symptoms establishes an **actual** diagnosis.]
DESIRED OUTCOMES— NEONATE WILL:	Be free of signs of hypoglycemia, with blood glucose level WNL.
	Display weight loss equal to or less than 5%–10% of birth weight by time of discharge.

ACTIONS/INTERVENTIONS

Independent

Review mother's prenatal history for possible stressors impacting on neonatal glucose stores, such as diabetes, pregnancy-induced hypertension (PIH), or cardiac or renal disorders. Note results of tests related to fetal growth and placental/fetal well-being.

Note Apgar scores, condition at birth, type/timing of infant feeding, and initial temperature on admission to the nursery.

Reduce physical stressors such as cold stress, physical exertion, and excessive exposure to radiant warmers.

RATIONALE

Full-term infants who are especially susceptible to hypoglycemia are those who are chronically stressed in utero, are exposed to high glucose levels in utero, are SGA or LGA, or are acutely ill. The infant has unique nutritional needs related to a rapid metabolic rate, high caloric requirement, potential loss of fluid and electrolytes due to increased insensible water losses through pulmonary and cutaneous routes, and a potential for inadequate or depleted glucose stores.

Birth stressors and cold stress increase metabolic rate and rapidly deplete glucose stores, possibly using as many as 200 calories/kg/min in the delivery room prior to admission to the nursery. First feeding may occur in delivery room for clients choosing to breastfeed; bottle-fed infants usually have their first feeding during the second period of reactivity.

Hypothermia increases energy consumption and use of nonrenewable brown fat stores. Respiratory distress and/or ambient temperatures above TNZ increase metabolic rate and activity level as well as insensible water losses. For every 1°C increase in body temperature, metabolism and fluid needs increase approximately 10%.

ACTIONS/INTERVENTIONS	RATIONALE

Independent

Weigh infant on admission to nursery and daily thereafter. Note presence of postmaturity syndrome or wasting.

Establishes caloric and fluid needs according to baseline weight, which normally drops by 5%–10% within the first 3 to 4 days of life because of limited oral intake and loss of excess extracellular fluid. Infant with postmaturity syndrome has increased metabolic and caloric needs in early newborn period.

Screen for hypoglycemia using Dextrostix at 1 hour of age, and more frequently as indicated for high-risk or symptomatic infant.

Newborns may maintain maternal glucose level for up to 1 hr following birth, but after this time, glucose consumption may exceed intake and production, resulting in hypoglycemia. A history of intrauterine or postdelivery stress or hypoxia markedly increases the risk of hypoglycemia.

Observe infant for tremors, irritability, tachypnea, diaphoresis, cyanosis, pallor, and seizure activity.

Indicates hypoglycemia associated with blood glucose levels less than 45 mg/dl.

Monitor newborn for ruddiness; note elevated Hb/Hct levels (Hb greater than 20 g/dl, Hct greater than 60%).

RBCs are high consumers of glucose, predisposing the polycythemic infant to hypoglycemia.

Auscultate bowel sounds. Note absence of abdominal distention, presence of lusty cry that quiets when oral stimulus is provided, and rooting/sucking behaviors.

Indicators showing that neonate is hungry/ready for feeding.

Initiate early oral feeding with 5–15 ml of sterile water, then dextrose and water, according to hospital protocol, progressing to formula for bottle-fed infants.

Initial feeding for breastfed infants usually occurs in the delivery room. Otherwise, water may be offered in the nursery to assess effectiveness of sucking, swallowing, gag reflexes, and patency of esophagus. If aspirated, sterile water is easily absorbed by pulmonary tissues. Early feedings help meet caloric and fluid needs, especially in an infant whose metabolic rate uses 100–120 calories/kg of body weight every 24 hr. Human milk or formula has a greater sustained effect on glucose levels and reduces risk of rebound hypoglycemia associated with bolus feeding of D_5W and $D_{10}W$.

Note frequency and amount/length of feedings. Encourage demand feedings instead of "scheduled" feedings. Note frequency, amount, and appearance of regurgitation. (Refer to ND: Knowledge Deficit [Learning Need]; and Chapter 6, CP: The Client at 4 Hours to 3 Days Postpartum, ND: Breastfeeding [specify].)

Infant hunger and length of time between feedings vary from feeding to feeding. Six feedings of approximately 3 oz (an average of 17 oz of formula in 24 hours) usually meet nutritional and fluid requirements of a 6-lb infant. Excessive regurgitation contributes to fluid loss and dehydration, increasing replacement needs.

Evaluate maternal/infant satisfaction following feedings.

Provides opportunity to answer client questions, offer encouragement for efforts, identify needs, and problem-solve solutions.

Monitor color, concentration, and frequency of voidings.

Fluid requirements range from 140 to 160 ml/kg per 24 hours because the newborn has proportionately less fluid reserve and higher water needs than the older child or adult. Loss of fluid and lack of oral intake rapidly deplete extracellular fluid and result in reduced urine output.

ACTIONS/INTERVENTIONS

Independent

Observe infant for indications of feeding problems (e.g., recurrent or bile-colored regurgitation, abdominal distention, abnormal stools, excessive mucus production, choking, or refusal to feed).

Collaborative

Obtain immediate blood glucose if Dextrostix level is less than 45 mg/dl.

Administer glucose immediately, orally or intravenously.

Follow up glucose administration with Dextrostix every 30 min–2 hr, based on severity of hypoglycemia, infant's symptoms, and hospital protocol.

Avoid oral feedings for distressed infants, or infants with polycythemia and hyperviscosity, or infants with gastrointestinal (GI) anomalies. Institute I.V. therapy of $D_{10}W$, with infusion rate of 80–120 ml/kg/day.

Administer glucagon or hydrocortisone if I.V. $D_{10}W$ therapy is not effective in resolving hypoglycemia.

RATIONALE

These problems may indicate intestinal obstruction, cystic fibrosis, or tracheoesophageal fistula.

Blood glucose measurement confirms Dextrostix findings and the need for intervention.

Infant may need supplemental glucose to raise serum levels.

Enhances the finding and facilitates the treatment of rebound hypoglycemia. Rebound hypo-gly-cemia is especially common following bolus feedings or bolus infusions of glucose or glucagon that are not followed by continuous glucose infusions.

Polycythemia and hyperviscosity potentially diminish circulation and availability of oxygen to digestive structures, so that introducing feedings may predispose infant to development of necrotizing enterocolitis.

Glucagon stimulates liver to break down stored glycogen. Steroids stimulate gluconeogenesis in the liver, thereby increasing blood glucose level.

NURSING DIAGNOSIS:	INFECTION, HIGH RISK FOR
Risk factors may include:	Broken skin, traumatized tissue, environmental exposure, inadequate acquired immunity.
Possibly evidenced by:	[Not applicable; presence of signs/symptoms establishes an **actual** diagnosis.]
DESIRED OUTCOMES— NEONATE WILL:	Be free from signs of infection. Display timely healing of cord stump and circumcision site, free of drainage or erythema.

ACTIONS/INTERVENTIONS

Independent

Review maternal risk factors that predispose infant to infection, which may be acquired transplacentally, via the ascending route, or at delivery. (Refer to Chapter 4, CP: Prenatal Infection; Chapter 6, CP: Puerperal Infection.)

RATIONALE

Maternal fever during the week prior to birth, prolonged rupture of membranes (greater than 24 hr), prolonged labor, foul-smelling amniotic fluid, and presence of infectious disease, such as gonorrhea, chlamydial infection, group B streptococcal infection, or TORCH group of viruses (toxoplasmosis, other viruses, rubella, cytomegalovirus, and herpes simplex viruses), all predispose infant to infection.

ACTIONS/INTERVENTIONS	RATIONALE

Independent

Determine newborn's gestational age.	Transfer of immunoglobulin E and G (IgE and IgG) antibodies via the placenta increases significantly in the last trimester, providing passive immunity to gram-positive cocci (pneumococci, streptococci, and meningococci), *Hemophilus influenzae*, viruses, and toxins (diphtheria and tetanus bacilli). However, the newborn is normally deficient in immunoglobulin M (IgM), which is stimulated by infectious agents (antibodies to blood group antigens, gram-negative enteroorganisms, and some viruses), and lacking in immunoglobulin A (IgA), which possibly provides protection on the secretory surfaces of the respiratory, urinary, and gastrointestinal tracts.
Scrub hands and arms with iodophor preparation prior to entering nursery, after contact with contaminated material, and after handling each infant. Teach parents and siblings proper handwashing technique to use before handling infant.	Proper handwashing is the most important single factor in protecting newborns from infection. Iodophor preparation is effective against both gram-positive and gram-negative organisms.
Monitor personnel, parents, and visitors for infectious illnesses, skin lesions, fever, or herpes. Limit contact with infant appropriately.	Helps prevent spread of infection to newborn.
Maintain individual equipment and supplies for each infant.	Helps prevent cross-contamination of infants through direct contact or droplet infection.
Inspect skin daily for rashes or interruptions in skin integrity. Use mild soaps, and gently pat skin dry after bathing; avoid excessive rubbing.	Skin is a nonspecific immunity barrier preventing invasion of pathogens. The likelihood of infection is increased by a significant number of potential portals of entry for infectious organisms, such as umbilical vessels, site of circumcision, and skin breaks associated with forceps or internal scalp electrode application. Chemicals and perfumes in soaps may predispose skin to rashes and breakdowns, vigorous rubbing may traumatize delicate skin.
Apply Eucerin Creme to identified dry areas, especially at ankles and wrists.	Helps prevent skin cracking and breakdown, especially in infant with dry skin due to excessive weight loss, dysmaturity, or prolonged exposure to phototherapy or radiant heat.
Encourage early breastfeeding, as appropriate.	Colostrum and breast milk contain high amounts of secretory IgA, which provides a form of passive immunity as well as macrophages and lymphocytes that foster local inflammatory response.
Assess cord and skin area at base of cord daily for redness, odor, or discharge. Facilitate drying through exposure to air by folding diaper below, and T-shirt above, the cord stump.	Promotes drying and healing, enhances normal necrosis and sloughing, and eliminates moist medium for bacterial growth.
Inspect infant's mouth for white plaque on oral mucosa, gums, and tongue. Distinguish between white patches of thrush and milk curds.	White patches that cannot be removed and that tend to bleed when touched are caused by *Candida albicans*, resulting from direct contact with contaminated birth canal, hands, or breast. (Note: Use of improperly cleaned nipple/breast shields or breast pump may result in colonization of the breasts.)

ACTIONS/INTERVENTIONS	RATIONALE

Independent

Note presence of lethargy, poor weight gain, restlessness, lowered temperature, jaundice, respiratory symptoms, or visible lesions. Isolate infant, as indicated; notify physician.

These signs indicate possible infection. Transplacentally acquired infections tend to affect liver and CNS function; ascending route infections, in many cases, result in bacteremia or pneumonia.

Collaborative

Monitor laboratory studies, as indicated:

WBC count.

Deficiency of neutrophils, which participate in the early phagocytic response, and deficiencies of specific immunoglobulins predispose the full-term infant to infection, particularly in the first 4 to 6 weeks of life. Normal WBC count of $18,000/mm^3$ does not increase in the newborn in response to infection, and it often drops during sepsis.

Serum levels of IgE, IgM, and IgA.

Elevated IgM levels at birth may occur in response to an infectious organism in utero. IgE levels are increased in the third trimester and provide infant with passive immunity to some organisms. IgA is found in colostrum and provides some passive immunity until the infant begins to produce IgA at approximately 4 weeks of age.

Cultures of lesions, pustules, or drainage when present (distinguish between possible infectious rashes and erythema toxium neonatorum).

Identifies possible pathogens. Vesicles or lesions of erythema toxium neonatorum (thought to be a local inflammatory response) contain eosinophils and are of no clinical significance.

Blood cultures.

Diagnose presence of bacteremia or sepsis and identify causative agents.

Administer topical, oral, or parenteral antibiotics.

Eradicates pathogenic organisms.

Apply nystatin (Mycostatin) to mouth; swab over oral mucosa, gums, and tongue. Wash mouth with sterile water prior to application.

Eradicates *Candida albicans*, the causative organism for thrush and mycotic stomatitis.

NURSING DIAGNOSIS:	INJURY, HIGH RISK FOR, multiple factors
Risk factors may include:	Birth trauma, aspiration, abnormal blood profile, congenital anomalies, drug effects.
Possibly evidenced by:	[Not applicable; presence of signs/symptoms establishes an **actual** diagnosis.]
DESIRED OUTCOMES— NEONATE WILL:	Be free of injury or aspiration.
	Display bilirubin levels below 18 mg/dl.
PARENT(S) WILL:	Identify individual risks.
	Demonstrate behaviors to protect newborn from environmental injury.

ACTIONS/INTERVENTIONS	RATIONALE
Independent	
Perform thorough newborn assessment for possible abnormal findings. Note crepitus, interruption in clavicle, abnormal Moro reflex, skull depression, or absence of movement of extremities.	Helps detect possible birth injuries, such as fractures of the clavicle, skull, or extremities.
Assess infant for congenital anomalies, especially cleft lip or palate, spina bifida, club foot, congenital hip dislocation, hypospadias, or epispadias.	Identifies conditions requiring immediate intervention. (Note: Extra gluteal folds, unequal extremities, resistance to abduction, and Ortolani's sign [audible click on rotation] indicate congenital hip dislocation).
Position newborn on abdomen or side with rolled blanket at back. Monitor infant for difficulty in handling mucus.	Helps prevent aspiration. During second period of reactivity, increased mucus production and gagging may predispose infant to airway obstruction, which can lead to asphyxia and death if it is undetected or untreated.
Never leave infant unattended in room or on unenclosed surface.	Reduces risk of injury due to undetected regurgitation or falls.
Assess infant for evidence of jaundice; note levels of direct and indirect bilirubin, behavior changes, and CNS signs associated with kernicterus. (Refer to CP: Newborn: Hyperbilirubinemia.)	Increasing jaundice may indicate Rh or ABO incompatibility or breast milk-induced jaundice, with possible outcome of kernicterus if condition is left untreated.
Assess infant for CNS, gastric, vasomotor, and respiratory signs of drug effect/withdrawal. (Refer to CP: The Infant of an Addicted Mother.)	Onset of withdrawal often occurs 24 hours after delivery. (Note: As many as one third of infants who have withdrawal signs can be managed without additional medical treatment.)
Collaborative	
Administer vitamin K (AquaMEPHYTON) intramuscularly.	Because the newborn's intestinal tract is sterile at birth, and because feedings may be delayed, infant does not have the intestinal flora needed to promote coagulation by activation of factors II, VII, IX, and X.
Schedule heel-stick testing for PKU, preferably within 72 hr after initiating intake of normal amounts of protein.	Identifies elevated serum levels of phenylpyruvic acid, which occur when phenylalanine is not converted to tyrosine because of absence of the liver enzyme phenylalanine hydroxylase. Excessive levels of the acid can result in CNS involvement, mental retardation, seizure activity, growth retardation, and absence of melanin.
Monitor x-ray studies; assist with diagnostic testing, as indicated.	Confirms presence of congenital abnormalities, such as hip dysplasia.

NURSING DIAGNOSIS:	**FLUID VOLUME DEFICIT, HIGH RISK FOR**
Risk factors may include:	Delayed feedings, limited oral intake, excessive regurgitation, increased insensible water losses.
Possibly evidenced by:	[Not applicable; presence of signs/symptoms establishes an **actual** diagnosis.]

480

DESIRED OUTCOMES— NEONATE WILL:	Void 2 to 6 times daily with output of 15–60 ml/kg/day by the second day of life.
	Produce urine free of uric acid crystals and urates.

ACTIONS/INTERVENTIONS	RATIONALE

Independent

Record initial and subsequent voidings.	Following birth, vascular resistance within renal vessels lessens and blood flow increases, but normal functioning may not be established until 24 hours following delivery. Urine output is usually limited and voiding scanty until fluid intake is adequate. During the first 2 days of life, the newborn usually voids 2 to 6 times daily. Thereafter, newborn usually voids 6 to 10 times daily, with output of 15–60 ml/kg/24 hours.
Initiate oral feedings; note amount ingested and regurgitated.	Oral fluid requirements range from 140 to 160 ml/kg/day by the third to fourth day of life (average is 105 ml/kg/day, or 5 oz/kg/day). Appropriate fluid ingestion helps promote hydration and offset kidney's inability to concentrate urine and to conserve fluid during periods of high insensible losses and fluid and electrolytic stress.
Monitor fluid intake and output. Note color and concentration of urine and the presence of peach-colored crystals on diaper.	Bladder usually empties when it contains between 15 and 40 ml of urine. Excessive drooling and mucus production, regurgitation, and poor fluid intake contribute to dehydration and scanty urine output. Urates and uric acid crystals reflect the need for increased fluid intake.
Note presence of blood in urine.	Bloody urine usually suggests pseudomenstruation in female infant or circumcision-related problems in male infant, but may also indicate renal injury, possibly associated with birth asphyxia, renal vein thrombosis, or infection.
Note presence of edema; assess infant's hydration level (e.g., indicated by skin turgor and presence of mucus).	Edematous or well-hydrated infant voids earlier after birth than dehydrated infant and has increased urine output.
Reduce cold stressors; optimize respiratory effort and thermoregulation.	Limited tubular reabsorption and low renal threshold reduce reabsorption of bicarbonate (HCO_3), predisposing infant to metabolic acidosis associated with reduced buffering capacity to offset respiratory imbalances.
Palpate for bladder distention, restlessness, discomfort, or bladder pressure if infant fails to void within 24 hours after birth.	Helps in determining presence of urine; may suggest problem related to bladder or anomalies of urethra that may prevent voiding.

Collaborative

Assist with suprapubic bladder aspiration if indicated.	May be used to ascertain the presence or absence of urine if voiding has not occurred.

<table>
<tr><td>NURSING DIAGNOSIS:</td><td>CONSTIPATION, HIGH RISK FOR</td></tr>
<tr><td>Risk factors may
include</td><td>Inadequate fluid intake, intestinal obstruction.</td></tr>
<tr><td>Possibly evidenced by:</td><td>[Not applicable; presence of signs/symptoms establishes an actual diagnosis.</td></tr>
<tr><td>DESIRED OUTCOMES—
NEONATE WILL:</td><td>Pass meconium stool within 48 hours after birth.</td></tr>
</table>

ACTIONS/INTERVENTIONS	RATIONALE

Independent

Review intrapartal record for indications of passage of meconium.

Relaxation of anal sphincter may occur in response to vagal stimulation related to hypoxia, causing meconium passage in utero or at delivery.

Note maternal complications negatively affecting meconium passage.

Stressors such as cesarean delivery or PIH delay initial meconium passage and possibly contribute to development of hyperbilirubinemia.

Auscultate bowel sounds.

Air ingestion into the GI tract normally stimulates onset of bowel sounds within 1 to 2 hours after delivery.

Take rectal temperature or insert soft rubber catheter into anus with caution.

Easy passage indicates patency of anus (rules out imperforate anus).

Monitor frequency and amount/length of feeding, frequency of voiding, skin turgor and status of fontanels, and weight. Encourage early feeding; provide extra water as indicated. (Refer to ND: Fluid Volume deficit, high risk for.)

Inadequate oral intake, as evidenced by decreased urine output, changes in skin turgor, sunken fontanels, and excessive weight loss, can lead to constipation.

Note passage of first meconium:

Once the infant wakens and the first feeding is initiated, passage of meconium usually follows, establishing patency of lower GI tract. Approximately 6% of healthy infants do not defecate by 24 hours after birth. Failure to pass stool by 48 hours usually indicates intestinal obstruction.

Record frequency, color, consistency, and odor of stools.

Number, consistency, and color of stools vary, depending on ingestion of human milk or formula.

Note deviations from normal stool cycle (meconium stools for 3–4 days followed by transitional stools, which are greenish-brown and may last for 3–6 days, followed by formed or loose yellow stools).

Thick, puttylike meconium suggests meconium ileus or possible cystic fibrosis; a small putty-like stool may indicate bowel stenosis or atresia. Loose green or diarrheal stool may indicate infection or gastroenteritis, or may be a normal result of high bilirubin content occurring while infant undergoes phototherapy.

Assess abdomen for constant or intermittent distention. Note persistent vomiting and presence of bile in vomitus.

Abdominal distention and persistent vomiting suggest obstruction. Obstruction that is high or complete is associated with vomiting soon after birth; more distal lesions are associated with later vomiting. Bile-stained gastric contents suggest duode-

ACTIONS/INTERVENTIONS

Independent

Observe for motility disturbance associated with constipation, vomiting, and fluid and electrolytic imbalances.

Note cluster of GI signs such as abdominal distention and tenderness, poor feeding, vomiting, presence of blood in stool (positive result on Hematest), or presence of reducing substances in blood.

Collaborative

Assist with diagnostic studies (e.g., abdominal x-rays, contrast studies, and upper GI barium series or enema).

Transfer infant to acute care setting (NICU) if indicated.

RATIONALE

nal obstruction. Paralytic ileus or partial obstruction is characterized by intermittent distention. Intestinal obstruction is the most frequent GI emergency requiring surgery in the neonatal period.

These signs may indicate aganglionic megacolon (Hirschsprung's disease), whereby absence of parasympathetic nerve cells in both the muscles and submucosa of the rectosigmoid colon inhibits passage of fecal material.

These signs may indicate necrotizing enterocolitis, the onset of which ranges from the first day to the first month of life. Necrotizing enterocolitis is associated with ischemia of intestines precipitated by systemic shock and hypoxia.

Helps in determining degree and location of obstruction and in diagnosing possible malrotation.

May be needed for intermittent gastric suctioning, surgical repair, or initiation of total parenteral nutrition.

NURSING DIAGNOSIS:	KNOWLEDGE DEFICIT [LEARNING NEED], regarding growth/development and infant care
May be related to:	Lack of exposure, misinterpretation, unfamiliarity with information resources.
Possibly evidenced by:	Verbalization of questions/misconceptions, hesitancy to perform care activities, inaccurate follow-through of instructions.
DESIRED OUTCOMES— PARENT(S) WILL:	Verbalize understanding of newborn's individual needs. Demonstrate appropriate behaviors to meet physiologic and emotional needs of newborn. Identify signs/symptoms requiring medical intervention.

ACTIONS/INTERVENTIONS

Independent

Appraise level of parents' understanding of infant's physiologic needs and adaptation to extrauterine life associated with maintenance of body temperature, nutrition, respiratory needs, and bowel and bladder functioning. Provide information and correct misconceptions, as appropriate; encourage discussion and questions.

RATIONALE

Identifies areas of concern/need requiring additional information and/or demonstration of care activities.

ACTIONS/INTERVENTIONS	RATIONALE

Independent

Discuss newborn behaviors after the first and during the second periods of reactivity.

Promotes understanding of infant behaviors. After first period of reactivity, infant usually falls into a deep sleep, followed by the second period of reactivity, which involves wakefulness, mucus regurgitation, gagging, and often passage of first meconium stool.

Perform newborn physical assessment in presence of parents. Provide information about normal variations and characteristics, such as pseudomenstruation, breast enlargement, physiologic jaundice, caput succedaneum, cephalhematoma, and milia.

Helps parents to recognize normal variations, and may reduce anxiety.

Discuss and demonstrate normal newborn reflexes; review ages at which each reflex disappears.

Encourages early detection of CNS abnormalities associated with prolonged presence of reflexes.

Provide information about newborn interactional capabilities, states of consciousness, and means of stimulating cognitive development. (Refer to Chapter 6, CP: The Client at 4 Hours to 3 Days Postpartum, ND: Parenting, altered, high risk for.)

Helps parents recognize and respond to infant cues during interactional process; fosters optimal interaction, attachment behaviors, and cognitive development in infant. The state of consciousness can be divided into the sleep and wake states, involving separate and predictable behavioral characteristics.

Discuss different types of cries that the neonate may use in communication and the means to assess significance of each. Demonstrate consoling measures.

Crying does not necessarily indicate hunger. Other causes include the need to be held, burped, or changed, or just a need to express irritability, as all babies tend to have a particular part of the day (often suppertime) when irritability increases. Parents' success or failure at consoling the newborn has a tremendous impact on their feelings of competence. Crying episodes usually vary in length from 3–7 min after initiation of consoling measures.

Provide information related to thermoregulatory mechanisms of the newborn, types of heat loss, and ways to minimize or prevent excessive heat loss or overheating.

Reduces risk of possible complications associated with hypothermia and hyperthermia.

Provide information about infant's normal sleep patterns and ways of promoting sleep.

The infant usually requires at least 17 hr of sleep per day for normal growth.

Demonstrate and supervise infant care activities related to feeding and holding; bathing, diapering, and clothing; care of circumcised male infant; and care of umbilical cord stump. Provide written information for parents to refer to after discharge.

Promotes understanding of principles and techniques of newborn care; fosters parents' skills as caregivers.

Discuss infant's nutritional needs, variability in infant appetite from one feeding to the next, and means of assessing adequate hydration and nutrition.

Alleviates potential concern that may result if infant's intake varies from feeding to feeding. Helps to ensure adequate nutritional and fluid intake.

Discuss types of formula preparations available, economics of each method, and necessary preparation and storage of formula.

Helps ensure proper preparation and administration of formula.

ACTIONS/INTERVENTIONS

Independent

Identify dangers associated with bottle propping.

Instruct parents regarding positioning of newborn after feedings and use of bulb syringe. Note infant's gag reflex.

Instruct parents regarding special care of diapers, recognition of rashes, and appropriate treatment.

Discuss nail care in newborn, including peeling of soft nails or nail trimming with manicure scissors or special infant nail scissors during infant's sound sleep.

Emphasize newborn's need for follow-up evaluation by healthcare provider.

Provide information about routine laboratory testing, as indicated.

Discuss manifestations of illness and infection and the times at which a healthcare provider should be contacted. Demonstrate proper technique for taking temperature and administering oral medications as required.

RATIONALE

Bottle propping robs infant of needed skin-to-skin contact with parents and may cause blockage of air passage if nipple lodges against back of infant's throat, or aspiration if infant regurgitates. Bottle propping may also cause otitis media associated with drainage of nasal mucus or occlusion of duct when eustachian tube orifice opens during swallowing.

Weak gag reflex predisposes newborn to aspiration. Positioning newborn on the abdomen or side with rolled towel at back allows external drainage of mucus or vomitus, reducing risk of aspiration. When infant is placed on back in carrier seat or carriage, head should be elevated 30 to 45 degrees. Syringe removes secretions from nasopharynx, clearing air passages.

Prevents diaper rash.

Prevents infant's scratching with long nails and injury associated with movement during the cutting process.

Ongoing evaluation is important for monitoring growth and development.

Increases likelihood of parents following through with urine and blood testing for genetic disorders, such as PKU and congenital hypothyroidism, which if undetected can cause mental and physical retardation.

Early recognition of illness and prompt use of healthcare facilitate treatment and positive outcome. To obtain an axillary temperature appropriately, thermometer should be held in place in the center of the axilla. Use of a rectal thermometer is not recommended until infant is older. Improper administration of medication increases risk of aspiration.

Neonatal Assessment: 24 Hours Following Early Discharge

This plan of care is intended to be used in conjunction with CP: The Neonate at 2 Hours to 3 Days of Age, which covers the time frame in which the early discharge visit normally occurs. The home assessment at 24 hours following discharge involves evaluation of the newborn's ability to adapt positively to extrauterine life.

NEONATAL ASSESSMENT DATA BASE

To meet the stringent criteria for early discharge, the newborn must be a normal, healthy infant as determined by thorough physical examination: Gestational age 38 to 42 weeks, birth weight 2500 to 4000 g, vital signs and temperature stable, Apgar score greater than 7 at 1 and 5 min, normal elimination pattern, successful feeding. (Refer to CP: The Neonate at 2 Hours to 3 Days of Age.)

DIAGNOSTIC STUDIES

Hematocrit (Hct): 40%–61%.

Coombs' test: Negative.

Screening tests, such as phenylketonuria (PKU) and thyroid tests completed.

NURSING PRIORITIES

1. Support transition of newborn to extrauterine life.
2. Promote positive parent-infant interaction.
3. Provide support and information regarding home care of infant.

NURSING DIAGNOSIS:	NUTRITION, ALTERED, LESS THAN BODY REQUIREMENTS
May be related to:	Inability to ingest adequate nutrients (due to fatigue, excessive oropharyngeal secretions).
Possibly evidenced by:	Weight loss, decreased urine output, dry mucous membranes, poor skin turgor, sunken fontanels.
DESIRED OUTCOMES— NEONATE WILL:	Be adequately hydrated with normal urine output.
	Display weight loss less than 10% of birth weight.

ACTIONS/INTERVENTIONS	RATIONALE
Independent	
Weigh infant. Compare weight with birth weight and discharge weight.	Nutrient needs are based on body weight. Weight gains or losses indicate adequacy of intake. Neonates need 100–120 kcal/kg (54 calories/lb) each day. Only breast milk or formula should be given. Feedings should be provided approximately every 3 hr (six to eight times a day) or on demand. Average fluid requirements are 5 oz/kg/24 hr.

ACTIONS/INTERVENTIONS

Independent

Observe infant for possible signs of regurgitation. Encourage parents to establish relaxed mood during feedings and to place infant on right side after feeding.

Assess infant's hydration level, noting condition of fontanels, skin turgor, amount of mucus production, and color and quantity of urine. Observe infant for jitteriness or lethargy.

Note frequency, amount, and appearance of stool and urine. Palpate abdomen for softness.

Review parents' feeding practices and knowledge, noting how often baby is nursing or feeding, how many minutes infant nurses on each breast, and whether infants takes additional water or formula during a 24-hour period. If possible, observe parents and infant during feeding.

Assess reflexes associated with feeding, and note presence of oropharyngeal secretions.

Determine neonate's current sleep-wake pattern.

Collaborative

Review Dextrostix results. If infant appears jittery or lethargic, provide feeding of dextrose solution and continue to observe.

RATIONALE

During the transitional period, neonates may normally regurgitate feedings. Calmness and self-assurance of parents helps infant relax during feeding; proper positioning facilitates gastric emptying into intestines.

Depressed fontanels, poor skin turgor, reduced urine output, and dry mucous membranes suggest dehydration. Jitteriness may indicate hypoglycemia.

Evaluates adequacy of oral intake. Neonates should void at least twice in the first 24 hours after discharge, advancing to approximately 7 times per 24 hours. Presence of urates in urine indicates need for additional fluid intake. The neonate may pass stool 2 to 7 times per 24 hours. Stool is initially meconium and changes in accordance with diet.

Knowledgeable parents are better prepared to alter schedules and respond to feeding needs and changes. Anticipatory guidance increases their self-confidence and helps avoid problems. Excessive parental anxiety may interfere with mother's let-down reflex, increase infant's anxiety, and result in poor oral intake. (Note: In addition, milk supply is not yet well-established for specific needs of neonate.)

Poor sucking and swallowing reflexes or excessive secretions may negatively affect intake.

At 24 hours of age, a healthy neonate has not yet established a sleep-wake pattern and may be excessively tired as a result of birth stress.

Normal glucose levels are between 45 and 130 g/dl; levels less than 45 g/dl indicate hypoglycemia. Administration of dextrose solution should correct hypoglycemia.

NURSING DIAGNOSIS: **BODY TEMPERATURE, ALTERED, HIGH RISK FOR**

Risk factors may include: Extreme of age (immature regulatory mechanisms [hypothalamus], ineffective shivering mechanism, reduced subcutaneous fat, proximity of blood vessels to the skin surface, and large ratio of body surface to mass).

Possibly evidenced by: [Not applicable; presence of signs/symptoms establishes an **actual** diagnosis.]

DESIRED OUTCOMES— NEONATE WILL:	Maintain axillary temperature between 36.2° and 36.8°C (97° and 98°F) when in an open crib with one blanket.
PARENT(S) WILL:	Identify/use individually appropriate measures to protect neonate.

ACTIONS/INTERVENTIONS

Independent

Discuss importance of thermoregulation in the newborn and possible negative effects of excess chilling.

Demonstrate proper technique for assessing axillary temperature.

Note signs of increased irritability, pallor, mottling, or lethargy; note restlessness and perspiration on head or face.

Assess environment for thermal loss through conduction, convection, radiation, or evaporation (e.g., cool or drafty room, inadequate clothing on infant, or absence of head covering) or for thermal excess (e.g., crib in sunlight or near heaters).

Assist parents in learning appropriate actions to maintain infant's temperature, such as appropriately bundling infant and covering head if axillary temperature is lower than 36.1°C (97°F) and rechecking temperature 1 hr later.

RATIONALE

A thermoneutral home environment is needed to assist the infant's own thermoregulatory ability. Temperature fluctuations in the newborn require use of calories to regain balance at the cost of growth. In addition, chilling increases the risk of newborn jaundice because the affinity of serum albumin for bilirubin is diminished.

Improper technique may lead to inaccurate results.

Indicates hypothermia or hyperthermia.

Body temperature of newborn fluctuates quickly as the environmental temperature changes.

Information helps parents create an optimal environment for their infant. Wrapping infant and putting cap on head helps retain body heat. Axillary temperature evaluates effectiveness of the interventions. (Note: Informing parents that infant's hands may remain cool even though body temperature is within normal limits [WNL] reduces anxiety.)

NURSING DIAGNOSIS:	INJURY, HIGH RISK FOR, central nervous system damage
Risk factors may include:	Biochemical or regulatory function (inability to break down red blood cells quickly enough during the transition period). The primary complication is kernicterus associated with deposition of unconjugated bilirubin in the basal ganglia of the brain.
Possibly evidenced by:	[Not applicable; presence of signs/symptoms establishes an **actual** diagnosis.]
DESIRED OUTCOMES— NEONATE WILL:	Maintain bilirubin level WNL.
PARENT(S) WILL:	Identify signs of increasing jaundice.
	Verbalize understanding of treatment needs.

ACTIONS/INTERVENTIONS

Independent

Assess neonate's buccal membranes, sclera, and skin for jaundice. Instruct parents to observe infant for passage of meconium stool.

Review proper care of jaundiced neonate, providing anticipatory guidance. (Refer to CP: Newborn: Hyperbilirubinemia.)

Collaborative

Obtain blood specimen as indicated if jaundice is noted.

Arrange for medical follow-up regarding hyperbilirubinemia.

RATIONALE

Yellowing sclera is the first sign of jaundice and is followed by yellowed skin tone on blanching; jaundice progresses in a cephalocaudal direction.

Information is essential for parents to manage care appropriately and to identify changes in condition that warrant further assessment and treatment.

Determines bilirubin level in presence of jaundice. Decisions regarding treatment are based on serial serum bilirubin levels. Physiologic jaundice becomes pathologic at level above 12.8 mg/dl.

Prompt, responsible follow-up and treatment are necessary to avert serious complications.

NURSING DIAGNOSIS:	PARENTING, ALTERED, HIGH RISK FOR
Risk factors may include:	Lack of support between/from significant other(s), lack of knowledge, ineffective or no available role model, unrealistic expectations for self/infant/partner, unmet social/emotional maturation needs of client/partner, presence of stressor (e.g., financial, housing).
Possibly evidenced by:	[Not applicable; presence of signs/symptoms establishes an **actual** diagnosis.]
DESIRED OUTCOMES— PARENT(S) WILL:	Verbalize realistic expectations of infant's needs. Identify individual methods and resources for meeting infant needs.

ACTIONS/INTERVENTIONS

Independent

Reassess risk factors that may have been identified during prenatal or intrapartal periods (e.g., unwanted pregnancy, previous abortion, or lack of support systems).

Observe parent-infant interaction. Talk with parents about their perceptions of and feelings toward the infant. Reinforce positive bonding efforts.

RATIONALE

Follow-up of risk factors is important to evaluate progress or areas of need. Early discharge is ideal for many families, but some clients who are at high risk for child abuse may also be included within the early discharge population.

Because of their dependent state, infants are vulnerable to negative parental behaviors, inadequate nurturing, and abuse. The "taking-in" phase, during which the mother is still trying to assimilate the details of labor and delivery, lasts 2 to 3 days. Stress and inadequate help in the home during this early period may negatively affect transition to the childrearing phase, interfering with proper nurturing, with possible failure of the newborn to thrive or to develop a sense of trust during infancy.

ACTIONS/INTERVENTIONS	RATIONALE

Independent

Assist parents to identify the resources available to them; e.g., community or support services, home health aide, or mother's helper.

Enables parents to anticipate availability and appropriateness of resources. Mother normally needs additional assistance to meet the needs of her infant, her family, and herself and to cope with unanticipated stress during the initial postpartal period.

Make arrangements for follow-up phone calls or visits.

Provides support and the opportunity to note progress. Frequency of calls or visits depends on needs of the individual situation; 3 visits in the first week is desirable.

Provide parents with a contact phone number they can use to ask questions, discuss concerns, or seek assistance.

Knowing that someone is available to help if needed may lessen parents' stress.

Collaborative

Refer for professional mental health counseling if indicated.

Postpartal stress may trigger depression, which is more likely to resolve quickly and not progress to more severe depression if the mother obtains help from skilled professionals.

NURSING DIAGNOSIS:	GAS EXCHANGE, IMPAIRED, HIGH RISK FOR
Risk factors may include:	Excessive production of mucus and/or amniotic fluid remaining in the lungs, decreased hemoglobin levels.
Possibly evidenced by:	[Not applicable; presence of signs/symptoms establishes an **actual** diagnosis.]
DESIRED OUTCOMES— NEONATE WILL:	Maintain patent airway with unlabored breathing at 30 to 60/min.
PARENT(S) WILL:	Be free of signs of respiratory distress.
	List signs reflecting respiratory distress and appropriate actions.

ACTIONS/INTERVENTIONS	RATIONALE

Independent

Auscultate breath sounds bilaterally to assess respiratory rate and quality.

Neonate should breathe 30 to 60 times per minute without signs and symptoms of respiratory distress or congestion. Absence of lung sounds or persistence of crackles or rhonchi indicates possible aspiration of amniotic fluid or persistent fluid in lung tissue.

Encourage parent(s) to position neonate on abdomen or right side; demonstrate clearing of nares, as needed, with bulb syringe.

Enhances air movement and reduces risk of aspiration.

ACTIONS/INTERVENTIONS

Independent

Assist parent(s) in learning signs of neonatal distress (e.g., grunting, retractions, nasal flaring, or tachypnea), noting when they should call healthcare provider.

Collaborative

Obtain heel-stick Hct, as indicated.

Provide healthcare referral if respiratory rate is not within normal range.

RATIONALE

Reduces anxiety and provides guidelines for parents so they know the appropriate times at which to seek help.

May be required routinely or if respiratory distress is noted. Hct below the normal range of 43–61% reduces oxygen-carrying capacity and may compromise respiratory function.

Immediate care may be needed to prevent development of serious respiratory problems.

NURSING DIAGNOSIS:	KNOWLEDGE DEFICIT [LEARNING NEED], regarding infant care
May be related to:	Lack of recall and/or incomplete information presented, misinterpretation.
Possibly evidenced by:	Verbalizations of concerns/misconceptions, hesitancy in/or inadequate performance of activities.
DESIRED OUTCOMES— PARENT(S) WILL:	Carry out infant care tasks appropriately.
	Assume responsibility for own learning.
	Verbalize the rationale for specific actions.

ACTIONS/INTERVENTIONS

Independent

Encourage parents to voice concerns. Provide explanations and answer questions as physical assessment is performed.

Provide oral and written information, as needed, about home management and care of the neonate, and indications for notifying healthcare provider.

Evaluate home environment for presence of heat, running water, cleanliness, electricity, number of persons in household, size of home, and facilities, crib, and clothing for the baby.

Provide appropriate information related to infant safety. (Refer to CP: The Neonate at 2 Hours to 3 Days of Age, ND: Injury, high risk for, multiple factors.)

RATIONALE

Helps determine parents' ability to care appropriately for newborn. The first 24 hours after delivery is one of great transition for parents, especially for mothers, who must now recall and apply information related to newborn care as learned in prenatal classes or during the brief hospital stay. New unexpected areas of needed information may arise as parents actually assume their caregiving roles.

Decreases anxiety, increases self-confidence, and promotes quality care for the neonate; helps ensure prompt treatment of problems.

Identifies necessary items that are lacking or conditions that present safety/health concerns.

Helps reduce incidence of accidental injury or trauma.

ACTIONS/INTERVENTIONS

Independent

Assess parents' understanding of physiologic aspects of breastfeeding, as appropriate.

Discuss plans for follow-up appointments for tests, such as PKU or thyroid screening tests, as indicated.

Assist parents in scheduling first appointment with healthcare provider.

Refer to other healthcare providers, community agencies, or support groups (e.g., La Leche League).

RATIONALE

Identifies need for further information.

Determines parent's awareness of the need for further testing. PKU testing is performed after milk stool is noted in breastfed infants, or within 72 hours after feeding is begun in bottle-fed infants.

Establishes importance of checkup for the infant and provides parents with opportunity to have their questions answered.

Helps to promote high-level wellness and family independence. Parents are more likely to use services that are familiar or recommended to them.

NURSING DIAGNOSIS:	INFECTION, HIGH RISK FOR
Risk factors may include:	Thin, permeable skin and extra portals of entry (umbilical cord, circumcision); immature immunologic system; lack of normal intestinal flora.
Possibly evidenced by:	[Not applicable; presence of signs/symptoms establishes an **actual** diagnosis.]
DESIRED OUTCOMES— NEONATE WILL:	Be free of signs of infection.
PARENT(S) WILL:	Identify individual risk factors and appropriate actions.

ACTIONS/INTERVENTIONS

Independent

Wash hands, and instruct parents to do so before handling infant.

Observe infant for skin abnormalities (e.g., blisters, petechiae, pustules, plethora, or pallor).

Discuss skin care, including bathing every other day, or less often, as indicated, and using mild antibacterial soap. Recommend sponge bathing until umbilical cord detaches.

Inspect umbilical cord.

Review appropriate cord care. Ensure that clothes and diaper do not cover stump. Provide information regarding the normal progression of cord resolution.

RATIONALE

Minimizes introduction of bacteria and spread of infection.

These abnormalities may be signs of infection. (Refer to CP: The Neonate at 2 Hours to 3 Days of Age, ND: Infection, high risk for.)

Guidelines for parents help them protect fragile skin of infant from excessive drying or damage.

The umbilical cord is an open site susceptible to infection. It should show evidence of beginning dryness, and no bleeding, exudate, odor, or oozing should be present by the second day of life.

Reduces likelihood of infection; promotes drying. Cord should fall off by the second week of life. (Note: Knowing it does not hurt the baby when the cord detaches provides reassurance to parents.)

492

ACTIONS/INTERVENTIONS	RATIONALE

Independent

Inspect site of circumcision if performed. Note undue bleeding, oozing, or swelling. (Refer to CP: Circumcision.)

Complete healing of circumcision does not occur until 7 to 10 days after the procedure.

Observe for/discuss signs of infection. Assess axillary temperature as indicated.

Infection in the neonate may be manifested by pallor, irritability, lethargy, poor feeding, vomiting, diarrhea, loose stools, oliguria, or temperature instability. Parental awareness promotes early recognition and increases likelihood of prompt medical attention.

Recommend avoiding contact with family members or visitors who have infections or have recently been exposed to infectious processes.

Because the neonate is more susceptible when exposed to some infections, visitors should be screened. (Note: Communicability is usually highest during the incubation period of many diseases.)

Neonatal Assessment: 1 Week Following Discharge _____

At 1 week of age, the newborn continues to adapt to extrauterine life, both physiologically and behaviorally. Within this adaptation period are many normal variations. Review prior assessments for risk factors or deviations from expected norms.

CLIENT ASSESSMENT DATA BASE

ACTIVITY/REST

May be wakeful/fussy between feedings.

May sleep more or less than the customary 17 hr/day.

CIRCULATION

Heart rate ranges from 110 to 160 bpm, is strong and regular.

EGO INTEGRITY (parents)

May verbalize unrealistic expectations of themselves and of neonate.

May express feelings of ineptness or inadequate knowledge.

ELIMINATION

Urine pale and straw-colored, with output of 6 to 10 wet diapers per day.

Abdomen soft with bowel sounds in all 4 quadrants.

Defecation pattern varies; stool formed, yellow/brown, and passed 2 to 3 times per day in neonate fed cow's milk formula; mustard-colored, loose, and passed initially with each feeding, then possibly every few days, in breastfed neonate.

FOOD/FLUID

May have difficulty adjusting to breastfeeding or bottle feeding; oral intake may be inadequate or excessive.

Weight gain averaging 1 oz/day.

NEUROSENSORY

Facial expression symmetric.

Reflexes associated with feeding (sucking, swallowing, gag, and rooting) present and strong.

Moro, grasp, and stepping reflexes present with strong, symmetric response.

Uncoordinated motor and reflex activity present (continued development of the neurologic system).

Muscle tone good; head lag present.

PAIN/DISCOMFORT

Irritability, crying associated with colic may occur.

RESPIRATION

Respiratory rate 30–60/min with no signs of difficulty (e.g., grunting, retraction, or nasal flaring).

Normal alternation between rapid and slow rate occurs in response to stimuli.

Cry strong, lusty, demanding, and purposeful.

Lungs bilaterally clear; breath sounds equal.

SAFETY

Skin pink and warm to the touch, with good skin turgor; free of rashes; transitory color change or mottling may appear in response to cold.

Skin may appear slightly dry or peeling in folds.

Slight jaundice involving only upper body or upper extremities may be present, peaking at day 4 or 5, subsiding within 7 days of onset.

Temperature stable: axillary, 36.5° to 37°C (97.6° to 98.6°F); rectal, 36.6° to 37.2°C (97.8° to 99°F).

Umbilical cord stump drying, with no evidence of inflammation; slight bleeding may be noted with detachment 7–14 days after birth.

SEXUALITY

Circumcised penis well-healed and free of exudate.

DIAGNOSTIC STUDIES

Tests dependent on individual findings/concerns.

Screening repeated at 7 to 14 days of age to detect inborn errors of metabolism.

NURSING PRIORITIES

1. Facilitate newborn's continued physiologic and behavioral adaptation to extrauterine life.
2. Promote adequate fluid and nutritional intake.
3. Provide information to parent(s) about newborn's safety, developmental needs, and interactional capabilities.
4. Encourage parental use of support systems.

NURSING DIAGNOSIS:	NUTRITION, ALTERED, LESS THAN BODY REQUIREMENTS, HIGH RISK FOR
Risk factors may include:	Inability to ingest adequate nutrients (fatigue, excessive oropharyngeal secretions, increased metabolic rate).
Possibly evidenced by:	[Not applicable; presence of signs/symptoms establishes an **actual** diagnosis.]
DESIRED OUTCOMES— NEONATE WILL:	Gain 1 oz/day after initial weight loss.
	Remain well hydrated as evidenced by adequate urine output, good skin tugor, etc.
PARENT(S) WILL:	Demonstrate proper, and comfort with, infant feeding techniques.

ACTIONS/INTERVENTIONS	RATIONALE

Independent

Weigh newborn. Compare current weight with birth weight. Note weight lost and regained.

Growth is individual, but most full-term, average-for-gestational age infants regain birth weight within 10 to 14 days of birth. Large infants lose proportionately more weight than small infants. Insufficient gains indicate nutritional risks or possible malnutrition.

Emphasize importance of weighing breastfed infant at 2 weeks of age.

Evaluation at 2 weeks of age is critical to detect possible failure to thrive or slow weight gains.

Assess hydration level (e.g., status of fontanels, skin turgor, mucous membranes, and urine output).

Sunken fontanels, poor skin turgor, decreased production of mucus, and decreased urine output indicate inadequate fluid intake. Well-hydrated tissue may indicate adequate nutrition and fluid balance.

Review parents' knowledge of infant's feeding needs. Observe feeding, evaluating parents' technique (e.g., positioning, burping, and length of feeding). Discuss importance of alternating infant's position (e.g., alternating right and left for bottle-fed baby to simulate breastfeeding).

Normal feeding should take 20–30 min. Improper positioning of infant at the breast, or improper technique of holding the bottle, may contribute to inadequate compression of maternal milk ducts or excessive air ingestion. Alternating infant's position provides stimulation and assists in development of eye muscles.

Discuss emotional needs of infant in relation to feedings (e.g., the need for holding and cuddling and for a quiet, nondistracting environment).

Skin-to-skin contact allows infant to focus on feeding, fosters optimal emotional interaction between parents and infant, and provides tactile stimulation, which is critical to the total process of acquiring infant's trust. Delayed gratification of hunger needs may lead to mistrust and lack of synchrony needed for the mutual gratification of mother and infant.

Observe infant during feeding, noting presence or development of feeding reflexes (i.e., rooting, sucking, swallowing, and gag).

A deviation in any of the feeding reflexes may lead to inadequate intake of nutrients.

Note frequency and amounts of feeding.

Breastfed infant may initially want to nurse every 2–3 hr with 1 or 2 night feedings, because breast milk is rapidly digested. Formula-fed infant is usually satisfied with feedings provided every 3–4 hr. Intake is considered adequate for formula-fed infant if 6 to 10 feedings of approximately 2–3 oz each are ingested in a 24-hour period.

Ascertain number of voidings per day and color of urine.

Infant is adequately hydrated if voidings occur 6 to 10 times per day and urine is pale or straw-colored.

Review infant's sleeping and waking habits.

Nutritional satisfaction is indicated if infant sleeps soundly between feedings and wakes every 2–5 hr for feedings, and if feedings cause infant to stop crying.

Identify cues suggesting newborn fatigue (e.g., loss of eye contact [turning away from or closing of eyes], decreased muscle tone, and reduced activity of extremities/neck).

Recognition of these cues may promote intervention to prevent undue fatigue and associated complications. Excessive handling/overstimulation can elevate newborn's metabolic rate and thereby increase caloric use in place of promoting growth.

ACTIONS/INTERVENTIONS	RATIONALE

Independent

Determine mother's perception of her success or failure related to infant feedings.

Feelings of success or failure regarding feedings influence the mother's self-esteem. Negative self-esteem associated with the newborn's poor oral intake may establish a vicious cycle whereby mother's anxiety increases at mealtime and infant becomes anxious in response to maternal anxiety and feeds poorly. Negative patterns at mealtime may persist throughout infancy and childhood, affecting mother-child interactions.

Auscultate bowel sounds. Note color, consistency, and odor of stools.

Hyperactivity or hypoactivity of the gastrointestinal tract leads to inadequate utilization of food. Elimination pattern is individual and is influenced by therapy (e.g., bilirubin phototherapy) and by amount and type of feedings (e.g., breast or bottle). Green or loose stool may indicate infection or passage of excess bilirubin. Constipated stool may indicate dehydration.

Assess infant's temperature and pulse. (Refer to ND: Infection, high risk for, multiple factors.)

Infection interferes with weight gain by increasing metabolic rate and negatively affecting oral intake.

Using 24-hour recall, evaluate adequacy of maternal diet in mothers who breastfeed their infants. Note amount of calories and fluids, and the use of a variety of foods from all the basic food groups.

Good nutrition in the mother enhances the nutrition of the breastfed newborn and helps mother maintain adequate energy level.

Assess adequacy of maternal milk supply and let-down reflex. Discuss ways to increase milk supply and promote the let-down reflex. Review effects of smoking.

Maternal milk production may not be adequate to meet newborn's growth needs. Maternal caloric intake should be 500–800 kcal more than the level during pregnancy, with 2–3 qts of fluid consumed per 24 hours. Adequate rest is necessary for milk production. Using relaxation techniques or drinking several ounces of dark beer each day may reduce anxiety and facilitate the let-down reflex. (Note: Smoking interferes with the let-down reflex, and nicotine is passed through breast milk to the infant.)

Review the preparation, sterilization, and availability of different types of formula.

Enhances proper use of commercially prepared formula. Dilution of ready-to-feed formula has been linked to failures of infant growth (height and weight).

Measure specific gravity of urine.

Increased specific gravity (above 1.008) in the absence of other complications may indicate the need for additional fluid intake.

Test stool for glucose.

Increased glucose in stool may indicate an intolerance to formula or an error in metabolism.

Reinforce instructions regarding the need to obtain urine from diaper for phenylketonuria (PKU) screening between 2 and 4 weeks after birth, or to bring child to laboratory for Guthrie test or heelstick method of PKU testing.

Helps ensure that infant is screened for PKU, an autosomal recessive disorder in which absence of a liver enzyme inhibits the conversion of phenylalanine to tyrosine, with a resultant increase in phenylpyruvic acid and possible development of mental retardation.

497

ACTIONS/INTERVENTIONS

Collaborative

Refer to community agency, visiting nurse services, or Women, Infants, and Children (WIC) program.

Obtain dietary consultation for breastfeeding mother as indicated.

Refer lactating mother to local support groups such as La Leche League.

RATIONALE

Nutritional problems identified in the newborn may necessitate close or frequent monitoring and support.

May be necessary to identify and meet individual nutritional needs.

Assists with problem solving related to breastfeeding.

NURSING DIAGNOSIS:	KNOWLEDGE DEFICIT [LEARNING NEED], regarding newborn needs/care
May be related to:	Lack of recall/incomplete information presented, misinterpretation.
Possibly evidenced by:	Verbalizations of concerns/misconceptions, hesitancy in or inadequate performance of activities, development of preventable complications.
DESIRED OUTCOMES— PARENT(S) WILL:	Verbalize understanding of infant's needs. Adopt safe child care practices.

ACTIONS/INTERVENTIONS

Independent

Assess parents' comfort and skill with infant care tasks (e.g., bathing, feeding, diapering, and recognizing infant's nutritional and physiologic needs). Demonstrate, supervise, and/or reinforce skills, as needed.

Review proper technique for preparation, sterilization, and storage of formula and bottles.

Discuss normal patterns of newborn growth and development, behaviors, and physical and social capabilities. Provide information about newborn's temperament and about appropriate parental responses to personality. Share with parents the Brazelton assessment process.

RATIONALE

Determines ability to provide appropriate care and identifies individual needs. Recognition of strengths and efforts enhances parent's sense of competence.

Faulty technique in formula preparation may lead to enteric infection. Bacterial growth can be controlled by discarding unfinished formula or by refrigerating prepared formula and discarding any unused portion after 24 hours. Unopened commercially prepared formula may be stored at room temperature. Overdilution of formula can lead to alterations in electrolyte balance and to inadequate caloric intake. Underdilution of formula can increase renal solute load, causing dehydration.

Assists parents in monitoring infant's physical and cognitive growth and optimizing infant's developmental potential. By observing and understanding newborn's personality traits, parents learn to respond appropriately to individual needs of their newborn. Parents need to realize that newborn's behaviors are individually determined and not entirely a reflection of their parenting abilities.

ACTIONS/INTERVENTIONS	RATIONALE

Independent

Note family history of possible neurologic or sensory deficits.

Family history of such problems may identify a genetic disorder related to seizure activity, deafness, blindness, retardation, cerebral palsy, or muscular weakness. Information may heighten parents' awareness of the need for further assessment or follow-up to determine the presence/extent of the problem and the appropriate treatment.

Discuss newborn's ability to become habituated to stimuli.

The ability of newborn infants to lessen their responses to repeated stimuli allows them to sleep while family members carry out normal household activities. Some newborns may not become habituated to stimuli as easily as others and need a quiet environment for sleeping.

Provide information about home management of the common cold in infant. Discuss recognition of signs such as nasal congestion, coughing, sneezing, low-grade fever, and swallowing difficulty (indicating sore throat).

Promotes parental comfort in managing mild illnesses at home.

Recommend offering extra sterile water, reducing feeding amounts, using upright position for feeding and sleeping (elevating mattress to a 30-degree angle), nasal/oral suctioning, using a cool-mist humidifier, and medicating infant only with physician's orders.

Promotes comfort. Smaller feedings help prevent overtiring of infant. Extra fluids and use of humidifier help liquefy secretions; upright positioning of head and chest promotes optimal lung expansion.

Identify signs of illness necessitating medical attention, and inform parents of availability of community agencies. Place list of emergency numbers next to telephone.

Prepares parents to seek prompt medical attention and to act quickly in an emergency.

Discuss plans for follow-up appointments for tests, such as PKU screening.

Screening tests are usually repeated in 1 to 2 weeks.

NURSING DIAGNOSIS:	INJURY, HIGH RISK FOR, multiple factors
Risk factors may include:	Physical (hyperbilirubinemia), environmental (inadequate safety precautions), chemical (drugs in breast milk), psychologic (inappropriate parental stimulation or interaction).
Possibly evidenced by:	[Not applicable; presence of signs/symptoms establishes an **actual** diagnosis.]
DESIRED OUTCOMES— NEONATE WILL:	Be free of injury.
PARENT(S) WILL:	Identify individual risk factors/concerns.
	Adopt behaviors that provide safe growth-promoting environment.

ACTIONS/INTERVENTIONS	RATIONALE

Independent

Evaluate skin color from head to toe and color return on blanching of sternum. Note behavior changes (e.g., lethargy, reduced Moro reflex, poor feeding, and listlessness). (Refer to CP: Newborn: Hyperbilirubinemia.)

Hyperbilirubinemia due to elevated levels of unconjugated bilirubin can result in kernicterus, which is associated with deposition of excess bile pigments in the basal ganglia of the brain.

Note presence/resolution of cephalhematoma.

Large cephalhematoma may contribute to increased bilirubin levels during reabsorption of blood.

Determine parental knowledge of infant safety (e.g., use of car seats, proper restraints, and protected surfaces; proper assessment of bath water and formula temperature).

Most common injuries in the newborn are related to accidental falls from unprotected surfaces. Bath water or formula should be comfortably warm to the inside of the wrist. Infant needs to be in approved car seat at all times when riding in any vehicle.

Ascertain mother's use of drugs (prescription/over-the-counter/street), especially if she is breastfeeding. Discuss potentially harmful effects of specific and commonly ingested drugs, and the need to avoid taking medication until after discussion with healthcare provider.

Many drugs are passed to infant through breast milk. Nicotine, caffeine, alcohol, cocaine, marijuana, and other drugs tend to reach levels in newborn that are directly related to maternal intake. Caffeine (equivalent to more than 1 or 2 cups of coffee/tea per day) may cause restlessness, sleeplessness, and significant diuresis. Excessive alcohol may increase circulating cortisol levels. Insulin, aspirin, most antibiotics, epinephrine, and antidiarrheal agents are usually viewed as safe if used in moderation.

Collaborative

Refer family to social service or to protective services if potential for abuse, or possible safety or risk factors, are identified.

May be necessary for further evaluation of newborn's well-being and parents' child care practices.

NURSING DIAGNOSIS:	BODY TEMPERATURE, ALTERED, HIGH RISK FOR
Risk factors may include:	Extreme of age (immaturity of the hypothalamus, inability to shiver or perspire adequately).
Possibly evidenced by:	[Not applicable; presence of signs/symptoms establishes an **actual** diagnosis.]
DESIRED OUTCOMES— NEONATE WILL:	Maintain temperature within normal limits.
PARENT(S) WILL:	Verbalize understanding of the influence of heat, cold, and dehydration on the newborn's temperature.
	Demonstrate appropriate regulation of newborn's environment and clothing.

ACTIONS/INTERVENTIONS	RATIONALE

Independent

Assess newborn's temperature. Note diaphoresis (over-heating) or pallor, cyanosis, or coolness associated with hypothermia.

Detects deviations from normal range: rectal, 36.6°C to 37.2°C (97.8°F to 99.0°F); axillary, 36.5°C to 37.0°C (97.6°F to 98.6°F). Thin skin and the proximity of blood vessels to skin surface result in rapid circulatory changes with cooling.

Review thermoregulatory needs of newborn.

Assist parents in recognizing importance of heat regulation; helps protect newborn from harm caused by temperature extremes. (Note: Body temperature fluctuations require expenditure of calories to regain balance, decreasing reserves available for growth. In addition, chilling increases the risk of newborn jaundice as the affinity of serum albumin for bilirubin is diminished.)

Assess environmental temperature and infant's dress and coverings in relation to parental attire. Provide guidelines for dressing and bundling newborn, controlling environmental temperature, and evaluating infant for overheating or underheating.

Infant is usually comfortable when dressed in the same number of clothing layers as parents. Overdressing in warm temperatures causes discomfort and prickly heat. Underdressing in cold temperatures results in discomfort and possible frostbite of cheeks, fingers, and toes. Informed parents can lessen the risks of such complications.

Suggest use of hat in all temperatures.

Protects infant's scalp from sunburn and shades eyes in summer; minimizes heat loss in cool environment.

Have parents check temperature of bath water.

Water temperature should feel warm to inside of wrist or elbow to avoid chilling or scalding newborn.

NURSING DIAGNOSIS:	CONSTIPATION, HIGH RISK FOR; DIARRHEA, HIGH RISK FOR
Risk factors may include:	Type and amount of oral intake; medications or dietary intake of the lactating mother; presence of allergies, infection.
Possibly evidenced by:	[Not applicable; presence of signs/symptoms establishes an **actual** diagnosis.]
DESIRED OUTCOMES— NEONATE WILL:	Evacuate with ease stool that is yellow-brown or golden-yellow and soft, with frequency appropriate for type of feeding.
PARENT(S) WILL:	Adjust specific contributing factors to promote optimal bowel pattern.

ACTIONS/INTERVENTIONS	RATIONALE

Independent

Determine frequency, amount, character, and odor of stool.	Newborn's elimination pattern is individual. Stool of newborns fed on cow's milk is pale yellow and formed, and is usually passed one to two times per day. Stool of newborns who are breastfed is golden or mustard-colored, and initially may be passed with every feeding, then may only be passed every few days. Diarrhea may be caused by overfeeding or enteric infection, constipation may be caused by dehydration or inappropriate lactating diet.
Evaluate total fluid intake and number of wet diapers over 24 hours. Assess hydration status. Obtain urinary specific gravity and Labstix results.	Alterations in hydration status may be associated with or cause altered bowel function. Less than five voidings per day indicates the need for increased fluid intake.
Auscultate bowel sounds.	An area of absent or diminished bowel sounds may signify blockage at a proximal segment of the bowel. Hyperactive bowel sounds indicate irritability.
Palpate for abdominal distention or tenderness.	Gas accumulation is associated with constipation or enteric infection and can cause varying degrees of discomfort.
Inspect perianal area for irritation, discharge, or rectal fissures.	Improper technique in formula preparation may result in bacterial growth, diarrhea, and resultant skin irritation.
Encourage positioning of newborn on right side after feedings.	Allows swallowed air to rise above fluid and exit through esophagus, and permits ingested formula or breast milk to flow toward pyloric sphincter.
Review fluid intake and diet of lactating mother, using 24-hour recall. Encourage client to increase frequency of feedings and infant's intake of water between feedings. Note infant's behavior in response to mother's ingested foods; counsel mother to avoid problem foods.	Inadequate fluid intake promotes constipation. In addition, certain foods ingested by lactating mother can alter newborn's elimination pattern and result in excess gas accumulation and constipation or diarrhea. Avoidance of these foods usually eliminates the problem.
Assess drug use in lactating client.	Use of cathartics may cause loose stools in infant.

Collaborative

Instruct parent(s) in proper technique of administering glycerin suppository.	Glycerin suppository aids in the passage of hard stool. Promotes parental management of infant's needs.
Refer parent(s) to healthcare provider for severe or protracted problems, or for suspected enteric infections.	May be necessary to determine exact cause of problem and to bring about resolution. Antispasmodics or antidiarrheal medications may be necessary.

502

NURSING DIAGNOSIS:	SKIN INTEGRITY, IMPAIRED, HIGH RISK FOR
Risk factors may include:	Excretions (ammonia formation from urea), chemical irritation from laundry detergent or diapering material, mechanical factors (long fingernails).
Possibly evidenced by:	[Not applicable; presence of signs/symptoms establishes an **actual** diagnosis.]
DESIRED OUTCOMES— NEONATE WILL:	Be free of diaper dermatitis/dermal injury.
PARENT(S) WILL:	Identify and adopt measures to maintain skin integrity.

ACTIONS/INTERVENTIONS

Independent

Assess diaper area for presence of rash that may be eroded, tender, indurated, or encrusted.

Recommend diaper changes, thorough cleaning and drying of area after each voiding and stool, exposure of area to air or heat, and application of a thin coat of petroleum jelly or A and D Ointment over the diaper area. Stress importance of not applying ointments before exposure to heat source, or use of cornstarch/powders.

Encourage parents to change brand of detergent and fabric softener or diaper (e.g., brand of disposable diaper, or cloth versus disposable) if rash develops or fails to clear.

Review proper/safe nail cutting techniques; e.g., cutting nails straight across with blunt-ended infant scissors/clippers while newborn sleeps.

Collaborative

Recommend contacting healthcare provider for severe or persistent diaper rash.

Demonstrate application of medicated topical creams, and explain treatment schedule.

RATIONALE

Early diagnosis and intervention may prevent spread of dermatitis to entire buttock area.

Prevention of diaper rash maintains perineal skin integrity. Exposure to heat aids in drying and healing. Use of 25-watt bulb placed 61 cm (24 inches) from affected area is preferable to use of sunlight through window, which may cause sunburn. Infant may need to be gently restrained to prevent possible contact with heat source and should not be left unattended. Petroleum jelly or A and D Ointment acts as a barrier to protect the skin, but may intensify effects of heat resulting in a burn. Powders tend to cake with urine and irritate buttocks; use of cornstarch may lead to a fungal infection.

Eliminates possible causes of rash.

At about 1 week of age, the tips of the newborn's nails separate from the underlying skin. Uncoordinated activity of the upper extremities creates the risk of dermal trauma.

May need additional help and further treatment or stronger therapeutic agents.

Eradicates organisms causing dermatitis and aids in healing process.

NURSING DIAGNOSIS:	INFECTION, HIGH RISK FOR
Risk factors may include:	Thin, permeable skin, extra portals of entry (umbilical cord, circumcision), and immature immunologic response.

Possibly evidenced by:	[Not applicable; presence of signs/symptoms establishes an **actual** diagnosis.]
DESIRED OUTCOMES— NEONATE WILL:	Be free of signs of infection.
PARENT(S) WILL:	Identify individual risk factors and appropriate actions.

ACTIONS/INTERVENTIONS	RATIONALE

Independent

Demonstrate proper handwashing technique prior to handling infant. Ensure that only clean objects come in contact with infant.	Prevents spread of infection. Handwashing is especially important following maternal perineal pad changes and following contact with vaginal lochia, because some organisms, such as listerial or streptococcal organisms, may be present in the lochia for as long as 10 days following delivery.
Instruct parents to keep newborn away from crowds and from people with known contagious illnesses until newborn is at least 1 month of age.	Shields newborn from direct contact with infected persons, reducing cross-contamination.
Encourage parents to wash newborn's clothes separately from family laundry; to use hot water, mild detergents, and a double rinse; and to dry them in the sunshine if possible.	Prevents cross-infection; removes soap residue, feces, and urine that might irritate skin or cause skin breakdown.
Assess healing of umbilical cord stump; reinforce measures to promote healing and drying of stump through exposure to air and the use of astringents.	Stump usually heals and detaches by the 10th day of life. Small beads of blood may be present when infant strains while crying or passing stool.
Inspect penis of infant who has been circumcised.	Penis should be well healed by 7 days following circumcision.
Discuss home management of upper respiratory infections, including the use and cleaning of cool-mist humidifiers, vaporizers, and bulb syringes; upright positioning; and increasing fluid intake. Identify possible sequelae associated with otitis media, feeding problems, breathing difficulty, and coughing. (Refer to CP: Neonatal Assessment: 4 Weeks Following Birth, ND: Infection, high risk for.)	Enhances client's ability to meet infant's needs and promote health. (Note: Water reservoirs in humidifiers and vaporizers may harbor bacteria and require special care to prevent secondary health problems.)
Stress importance of refraining from medicating infant without first consulting healthcare provider; stress importance of using acetaminophen in place of aspirin products.	In general, safety of medications has not been determined/tested in the newborn population. The use of aspirin-containing products in presence of viral infection has been linked to Reye's syndrome.
Inspect skin for vesicular lesions surrounded by erythema (may be encrusted if ruptured).	May indicate impetigo caused by various strains of group A or B hemolytic streptococci, or by coagulase-positive *Staphylococcus aureus*.

ACTIONS/INTERVENTIONS

Independent

Review signs of generalized infection (e.g., pulmonary congestion, cough, and retractions, more than one episode of forceful vomiting, refusal of two feedings in a row) or sepsis (e.g., temperature instability, lethargy, restlessness, irritability, frequent vomiting over a 6-hr period; 2 consecutive green, watery stools; less than 6 wet diapers per day). Discuss when to notify healthcare provider.

Discuss advantages of breast milk for infant.

Inspect buccal cavity for white, curdy patches on tongue, palate, and inner aspects of cheeks; check for presence of fever and/or gastric distress.

Collaborative

Obtain/review complete blood count results and cultures as indicated.

Demonstrate proper administration of local systemic antibiotics or fungicides.

RATIONALE

Studies show that neonatal infections with late onset of signs, appearing from 2 to 12 weeks of age, are most frequently caused by cytomegalovirus and by organisms of *Chlamydia* and *Ureaplasma*.

Human milk contains iron-binding protein that exerts a bacteriostatic effect on *Escherichia coli*; macrophages and lymphocytes that promote a local inflammatory response; and passive transfer of maternal immunity to common mucosal pathogens, such as respiratory syncytial virus.

Newborn may have been contaminated by *Candida albicans* during descent through birth canal, or as a result of poor handwashing technique or contaminated bottles or nipples. Thrush typically causes gastrointestinal inflammation in addition to the "local" response.

May be necessary if temperature is elevated or presence of lesions/drainage warrants further evaluation.

Eradicates invading pathogen or infectious process. A fungicide such as nystatin (mycostatin) applied after feedings to surfaces of oral cavity is usually effective against *Candida albicans* infections.

NURSING DIAGNOSIS:	**PAIN [ACUTE], HIGH RISK FOR**
Risk factors may include:	Accumulation of gas in a confined space, with cramping of intestinal musculature.
Possibly evidenced by:	[Not applicable; presence of signs/symptoms establishes an **actual** diagnosis.]
DESIRED OUTCOMES— NEONATE WILL:	Be free of or display less frequent crying spells and episodes of colic.
PARENT(S) WILL:	Report parent-infant tension is relieved or easing.

ACTIONS/INTERVENTIONS

Independent

Evaluate infant's behavior.

RATIONALE

Colicky infant typically cries loudly, draws legs up to abdomen in pain, clenches fists, and sucks vigorously.

ACTIONS/INTERVENTIONS	RATIONALE

Independent

Obtain thorough, detailed history of normal daily events, household activity pattern, time of day in which attacks occur, and relationship of attacks to feeding.

Typically, attacks occur at a specific time of day. By determining the circumstances that possibly contribute to onset of attack and by manipulating those circumstances or environmental conditions, parents may be able to reduce overstimulation and tension that usually precipitate the attack.

Obtain 24-hour dietary recall when mother is breastfeeding. Suggest adoption of a milk-free diet for 5 days. Stress importance of reading food product labels; e.g., nondairy creamers may contain calcium caseinate, a cow's milk protein.

Gas-forming vegetables, spices, and chocolate may cause discomfort. Sensitivity to cow's milk products may precipitate colic attacks when milk products pass through the breast milk.

Observe feeding procedure. Analyze and discuss technique and behaviors with parents. Encourage burping infant in upright over-shoulder position before and after feedings. Recommend smaller, more frequent feedings and placing infant in upright position after feeding. Use slow bicycling of legs from extension to knee-chest position.

Excess air ingestion from too-rapid or improper bottle position and/or inadequate burping may result in gas accumulation. Overfeeding or excess carbohydrate ingestion may lead to excess fermentation and gas production. Upright position and bicycling maneuver promote gas expulsion.

Encourage parents to administer 1–2 oz of warm, diluted tea, then to place infant in prone position over heated towel or protected heating pad and to change infant's position frequently.

Helps stimulate peristalsis to relieve abdominal cramping.

Suggest use of collapsible bags in feeding bottles.

Reduces air ingestion.

Discuss infant's physical condition and well-being.

Gastric acidity reduces within first week of life, affecting digestion and/or development of colic, which usually resolves within 2–3 months. Despite colic attacks, infant normally thrives, gains weight, and tolerates feedings. However, the relationships between the parents/other family members may suffer the stressful effects of a crying, irritable infant; this may have a negative impact on the bonding process.

Assess parental response to colic attacks, methods used to relieve crying, and coping strategies. Initiate creative problem-solving to diminish impact of attacks.

Parental responses of anxiety and increased tension are transmitted to the newborn, escalating tension, irritability, and crying. Adoption of different strategies may stimulate a different response in the newborn.

Encourage parents to share feelings of frustration, anger, helplessness, and insecurity. Recommend that parents spend time in diversionary activities away from the house and the newborn.

Helps support parents through crisis of colic.

Collaborative

Provide information and demonstrations, as needed, for insertion of glycerin suppository using a well-lubricated finger.

Stimulates passage of flatus and feces.

Discuss and demonstrate technique for administering sedatives (phenobarbital elixir), anticholinergics (atropine), antispasmodics, and antiflatulents, if used.

Medications may be needed to reduce gastrointestinal motility and provide relief.

Neonatal Assessment: 4 Weeks Following Birth _____

NEONATAL ASSESSMENT DATA BASE

Review prior assessments for identified risk factors.

ACTIVITY/REST

Infant sleep pattern well-established.

CIRCULATION

Heart rate ranges from 70 to 170 bpm, with average rate of 120 bpm.

Blood pressure (obtained by using flush technique at wrist) ranges from 48 to 90 mm Hg, with a mean of 67 mm Hg; at ankle, 38 to 56 mm Hg, with a mean of 61 mm Hg.

EGO INTEGRITY

Regards faces, especially parents' faces, intently; may demonstrate beginning of social smile.

Responds to environmental stimuli: bright objects (which are best viewed 8–12 inches from face), sound, and touch.

ELIMINATION

Urine pale or straw-colored, with output of 6–10 wet diapers per day.

Abdomen soft, nondistended with bowel sounds present.

Individual bowel elimination pattern established, dependent on type of feeding.

FOOD/FLUID

Makes comfort noises during feeding, or may make small throaty noises.

Feeding generally 5 to 8 times per 24-hour period.

Height gain 2.5 cm (1 inch) monthly for first 6 months.

Weight gain of 3–5 oz/wk for first 6 months.

Drooling absent until 2 to 3 months of age, when salivary glands begin to function.

NEUROSENSORY

Begins to differentiate cry in relation to pain, discomfort, or hunger; uses cry to signal needs; quiets when picked up.

Head circumference increases 1.5 cm ($^{1}/_{2}$ inch) monthly for first 6 months.

Fontanels palpable and soft; posterior fontanel closes at 6 weeks of age.

Tears present, with tear glands beginning to function at 2–4 weeks of age.

Primitive reflexes present with strong, bilaterally equal responses.

Doll's eye and dance reflexes fading.

Crawling movements when prone.

Lifts head momentarily from bed while on abdomen, turns head from side to side when prone.

Demonstrates tonic neck reflex when supine.

Marked head lag when pulled from lying to sitting position (back is uniformly rounded), absence of head control in sitting position.

Strong grasp reflex: hand closes on contact with object.

PAIN/DISCOMFORT

Continuation of pain and cramping associated with colic may be reported.

RESPIRATION

Signs of aspiration (continued regurgitation associated with reverse peristalsis and immature or relaxed cardiac sphincter).

SAFETY

Axillary temperature stable between 36.5° and 37.0°C (97.7° to 98.6°F).

Perineal area clean and free of rashes.

DIAGNOSTIC STUDIES

Testing dependent on individual findings, risk factors.
Urine specific gravity: 1.008.

NURSING PRIORITIES

1. Promote newborn's growth and development.
2. Provide information appropriate to parents' learning needs.
3. Enhance home environment to promote infant's safety and stimulation.

DISCHARGE GOALS

1. Various indicators of growth and development show progression within normal limits (WNL).
2. Parent(s) understand individual needs of infant.
3. Parent(s) demonstrate proficiency in infant care activities.

NURSING DIAGNOSIS:	NUTRITION, ALTERED, LESS THAN BODY REQUIREMENTS, HIGH RISK FOR
Risk factors may include:	Failure to ingest/absorb adequate calories; e.g., biologic (insufficient intake, malabsorption, congenital problem, or neglect [failure to thrive]) or psychologic factors (emotional abuse).
Possibly evidenced by:	[Not applicable; presence of signs/symptoms establishes an **actual** diagnosis.]
DESIRED OUTCOMES— NEONATE WILL:	Display physical growth and weight gain appropriate for age and developmental stage.

ACTIONS/INTERVENTIONS	RATIONALE
Independent	
Measure infant's height and weight, and compare with measurements at birth and at 1 week of age.	Nutrients for infants are based on body weight. Most full-term, appropriate-for-gestational age infants regain birth weight within 10–14 days follow-

ACTIONS/INTERVENTIONS	RATIONALE

Independent

ing birth. Weight gain should be 3–5 oz/wk for first 6 months and may be as much as 1 oz/day in bottlefed infant. Gains less than 3–5 oz/wk may result in lifelong nutritional risks with potentially negative effects on infant development.

Assess infant for possible failure to thrive (FTT).

A breastfed infant who continues to lose weight after 10 days of life, does not regain the weight by 3 weeks of age, or gains weight at rate below 10th percentile after 1 month is probably an FTT infant and requires prompt evaluation relative to issues of lactation and infant capabilities. In the bottle-fed infant, formula preparation and appropriateness (tolerance) is evaluated. Finally, concerns regarding possible neglect must be addressed. Timely intervention and resolution may prevent permanent deficits.

Determine amount, type, and frequency of oral intake over last 24 hours.

Infants require about 115 kcal/kg for first 6 months of life or 54 kcal/lb. Fluid needs are approximately 530 ml/day. One third of energy is used for growth. Inadequate caloric and fluid intake results in nutritional inadequacies and poor weight gains. (Note: Adequate protein intake is critically important to provide brain growth during the hyperplasia and hypertrophy phase in the first 6 months of life. Inadequate protein ingestion during this phase can result in developmental delays.)

Assess hydration status, noting status of fontanels, production of mucus, skin turgor, and number of wet diapers per day.

Inadequate fluid intake results in dehydration, manifested by depressed fontanels, reduced urine output, poor skin turgor, and dryness of mucous membranes. (Note: Cases of hypernatremic dehydration have been associated with use of cow's milk feedings.)

Obtain 24-hour dietary recall in lactating mother. Note presence of illness, infection, or dietary inadequacies. Provide dietary teaching, as appropriate, to correct inadvertent or deliberate food restrictions. Identify adequate sources of calcium and protein; suggest supplementing maternal diet with brewer's yeast as appropriate.

Illness, infection, or marginal diet may affect mother's ability to nourish the infant adequately. Supplementing diet with brewer's yeast improves milk production significantly more than simply adding similar nutrients.

Evaluate lactating mother's sleep and rest, noting excess fatigue, family demands, and work or social commitments. Discuss individual needs and options to meet these needs.

Inadequate sleep resulting in excess fatigue is most common cause of inadequate milk supply, especially during first month, when milk supply is being established.

Evaluate effectiveness of let-down reflex in lactating mother. If mother smokes, suggest that she refrain or light cigarette after infant is sucking vigorously, rather than prior to feeding. Assist mother in evaluating stressors and using creative problem-solving.

Smoking and psychologic stress may inhibit let-down reflex.

509

ACTIONS/INTERVENTIONS	RATIONALE

Independent

Review techniques used in formula preparation and storage. Confirm that parents follow instructions for making powdered or concentrated formulas. Discourage home preparation of evaporated milk formula.

Many infant nutritional inadequacies are related to overdilution of commercial formulas, which results in inadequate calories and nutrients and FTT. Use of home-prepared evaporated milk formulas has been linked to problems associated with improper measurement and bacterial contamination.

Encourage continued use of formula for first 12 months of life. Discourage substitution of skim or whole cow's milk.

Skim milk contains about half the number of calories in breast or in commercial formulas; may not meet the infant's energy needs; and may cause deficiencies in iron, vitamin C, and fatty acids. Use of whole milk in the first 12 months may place the infant at risk for iron, vitamin C, and copper deficiencies.

Inspect infant for lesions; note swollen parotid glands.

May indicate poor nutritional state.

Determine color, frequency, consistency, and odor of stool.

Altered elimination pattern may suggest problem with digestion and absorption. Foul-smelling stool suggests parasitic infection. Diarrhea may reflect milk intolerance or ingestion of cathartics in lactating mother.

Auscultate bowel sounds; palpate abdomen. Note presence of loose stools, cramping, crying, reports of vomiting, or chronic blood loss in gastrointestinal tract.

Abdominal distention and gas accumulation may be associated with ingestion of gas-producing foods in lactating mother or with milk intolerance. Immaturity of the intestinal tract increases permeability to inadequately catabolized proteins, which produces an allergic response or milk intolerance in 1%–2% of infants.

Assess infant's color, gestational age and weight at birth, and current weight gains.

Iron stores are usually adequate until infant weight increases by $2\frac{1}{2}$ times. Pallor and inadequate weight gain, however, may indicate anemia.

Note excessive or forceful vomiting of nonbilious, possibly blood-tinged emesis; visible gastric waves moving right to left across epigastrium; and palpable olive-shaped mass in epigastric region.

May indicate hypertrophic pyloric stenosis, especially if infant appears alert and hungry, fails to gain weight, and has a history of recurrent vomiting.

Collaborative

Provide information as needed about prescribed alternatives to milk, such as soy milk formulas or hydrolyzed protein and amnio acid mixtures.

Alternative formulas relieve symptoms associated with cow's milk intolerance.

Refer to social services or Women, Infants, and Children (WIC) program, as indicated.

Additional assistance may be needed to meet infant/maternal nutritional needs if financial resources are limited.

Refer parents to pediatric nurse for assistance with surgical preparation and care if pyloric stenosis is confirmed.

Surgical management or pyloromyotomy is the standard treatment for hypertrophic pyloric stenosis; prognosis is excellent, and mortality is low.

NURSING DIAGNOSIS:	NUTRITION, ALTERED, HIGH RISK FOR MORE THAN BODY REQUIREMENTS
Risk factors may include:	Obesity in one or both parents, rapid transition across growth percentiles in infant.
Possibly evidenced by:	[Not applicable; presence of signs/symptoms establishes an **actual** diagnosis.]
DESIRED OUTCOMES— PARENT(S) WILL:	Identify and adopt appropriate infant feeding practices.
	Explain factors that promote excess weight gains and eating problems.

ACTIONS/INTERVENTIONS	RATIONALE

Independent

Assess measurement of newborn's weight/height for age and sex. Determine anthropometric assessment.	Weight greater than the 85th percentile in relation to height, age, sex, and body build is considered obese. Although anthropometric assessment is most accurate, serial weight and height measurements in relation to age are fairly good predictors of obesity or excess weight gain.
Review parental weight history.	Heredity and family feeding practices contribute to obesity. There is an 80% probability that if parents are obese, the child will also be obese. If parents are not obese, this probability is only 7%.
Note type of infant feeding (i.e., breast or bottle).	Breastfed infants are less likely to be obese than bottle-fed infants, because the breastfed infant regulates the feeding based on hunger needs. In a desire to empty the bottle, parents may overfeed the bottle-fed infant by continuing to feed even after satiation has been reached.
Determine amount and frequency of infant feedings.	Feedings in excess of infant caloric needs relative to energy expenditures result in excess weight gains, possibly leading to obesity.
Provide information about newborn's energy requirements; encourage mother to let infant regulate intake based on hunger needs.	Reduces likelihood of overeating.
Encourage mother to avoid introduction of solid foods until infant is at least 4 to 6 months of age.	Early addition of solid foods contributes to development of poor eating habits, excess food consumption, and infantile obesity. Mother may mistakenly think that addition of solids enhances newborn's chances of sleeping through the night, but such practices have been found to have no effect on infant sleep patterns.
Encourage mother to restrict the use of infant seat during waking hours and to allow infant to spend time on mat on floor.	Enhances activity and energy expenditure.

511

ACTIONS/INTERVENTIONS

Independent

Discuss mother's feeding of infant for emotional upsets or distress signals.

Discourage substitution of skim or whole milk for commercially prepared formula for first 12 months of life.

Discuss possible lifelong risks associated with overeating.

Review family eating patterns.

RATIONALE

Inappropriate use of food in response to newborn's distress encourages infant to associate food with emotional gratification rather than with hunger.

Such substitution may increase renal solute load as a result of excess protein and mineral ingestion. Use of whole milk may result in increased plasma osmolality, hyperphosphatemia, and hypernatremia.

Overeating increases risks of health problems related to cardiovascular system, hypertension, and diabetes.

Healthy eating habits and selection of appropriate amounts and types of foods can ultimately affect nutrition of the growing child.

NURSING DIAGNOSIS:	**KNOWLEDGE DEFICIT [LEARNING NEED], regarding infant care**
May be related to:	Lack of exposure/recall, misinterpretation, unfamiliarity with resources.
Possibly evidenced by:	Verbalization of problem/concern or misconceptions, inaccurate follow-through of instructions, development of preventable complications.
DESIRED OUTCOMES— PARENT(S) WILL:	Provide appropriate nutritional intake.
	Create safe, stimulating infant environment.
	Identify signs/symptoms requiring medical follow-up.
	Use healthcare system appropriately.
	Plan for short- and long-term child care.

ACTIONS/INTERVENTIONS

Independent

Reinforce or provide appropriate information about infant's nutritional needs for next few months.

Provide information about role of iron in body and the need for supplementation.

RATIONALE

Helps ensure normal growth patterns in height and weight, and may prevent overfeeding through too-early introduction of solid foods.

American Academy of Pediatrics recommends 1 mg of iron per kg of body weight per day for full-term infants, starting no later than 4 months of age. Iron-fortified commercial formula for bottle-fed infant offers most constant and predictable iron ingestion. By 4 to 6 months of age, breastfed infant should have supplemental iron in form of iron-fortified cereal or oral iron drops.

ACTIONS/INTERVENTIONS	RATIONALE

Independent

Discuss role of fluoride in body and in tooth development. Encourage parents to obtain fluoride supplements if appropriate.

Fluoride helps reduce incidence of tooth decay and improves quality of tooth enamel, making it more resistant to caries, if fluoride is ingested before eruption of teeth. Breastfed infants consume little or no water and should receive 0.25 mg of fluoride per 24 hours for first year of life. Although commercial formulas have minimal amounts of fluoride, supplementation is not necessary if home water supply used in formula preparation contains 0.3 parts per million (ppm) fluoride.

Review information for lactating mother, as needed, including increased infant appetite and caloric needs during growth spurts at 6 weeks and 3 months of age.

The "reward period" for the breastfeeding mother may not occur until 6 weeks after delivery, and she may need further encouragement and information to continue. (Note: Infant may need to nurse more frequently during periods of rapid growth.)

Determine how long mother plans to breastfeed. Discuss techniques of weaning from breast when desired and the process of introducing solids between 4 and 6 months of age. (Refer to NDs: Nutrition, altered, less than body requirements, high risk for; Nutrition, altered, high risk for more than body requirements.)

Anticipatory guidance related to the individual situation provides for anticipatory problem-solving and enhances optimal outcome.

Review signs of milk sensitivities, especially if lactating mother plans to wean infant to a bottle when she returns to work.

If milk sensitivity is present, infant may require use of soy or other formulas. (Refer to ND: Nutrition, altered, less than body requirements, high risk for.)

Discuss mother's plans for possible return to work and plans for child care and feeding practices. Provide anticipatory guidance for lactating mother to allow her to continue with breastfeeding and to maintain milk supply.

Allows mother to anticipate and plan for problems that may arise. Breastfeeding can be continued with adequate planning and management.

Identify factors to be considered and resources available when choosing child care. Stress importance of ongoing monitoring of care provided.

Placing infant in care of others can be difficult for parents relative to issues of trust and child well-being. Informed choice and vigilance enhance parent(s) level of comfort and promote optimal outcomes.

Provide oral or written anticipatory guidance related to infant safety, including discussion of potential accidental injury due to suffocation, falls, burns, motor vehicle accidents, or bodily trauma. (Refer to NDs: Suffocation, high risk for; Trauma, high risk for.)

Helps parents to recognize potential safety hazards and reduce risk of injury. Crawling reflex (which propels infant forward), rolling over, increasing eye-hand coordination, and voluntary grasp reflex increase risk of accidents in first 4 months of life.

Provide information about importance of recommended primary schedule for immunization.

Recommended primary schedule for immunization begins in infancy to reduce incidence of infectious disease due to diphtheria, tetanus, pertussis, polio, measles, mumps, and rubella. Although recommendations are to begin immunizations at 2 months of age, current discussion suggests immunizations should begin after the first year to avoid possible untoward responses.

ACTIONS/INTERVENTIONS	RATIONALE
Independent	
Discuss timing and importance of infant's regularly scheduled well-baby visits to physician or nurse practitioner.	Helps detect any deviations from normal growth and development and ensure early intervention if deviations are identified.
Discuss infant's physical, emotional, and developmental needs. Provide oral or written information about anticipated monthly progression of physical (gross and fine motor) development, sensory development, and vocalization and socialization.	Allows parents to monitor infant's growth and development during infancy.
Evaluate environment for its ability to provide appropriate infant stimulation. Assist parents as needed in planning for and providing appropriate visual, auditory, tactile, and kinetic stimulation. Discuss changing needs of infant play as development progresses during the first year. (Refer to ND: Sensory-Perceptual Alterations, high risk for.)	Helps parents to recognize and provide optimal environment for infant play and development. At 1 month of age, placing bright hanging objects 8 to 10 inches from infant's face or looking at infant from close range provides visual stimulation. Talking or singing to infant, or playing music box or radio, provides auditory stimulation. Holding, cuddling, and providing warmth offer tactile stimulation. Rocking infant in chair or cradle and using carriage provide kinetic stimulation.
Reassess mother-infant interaction. Discuss methods to foster mutually satisfying interactions and development of infant's trust.	Ongoing quality of emotional care is an important aspect in promoting optimal infant growth and development. Mutually satisfying mother-infant relationship fosters development of a sense of trust in newborn.
Encourage parents to pay attention to infant cues and to provide gratification soon after need is identified.	Allowing infant to feel physically comfortable, warm, emotionally loved, and secure aids in development of mutual trust and fosters development of healthy ego in the infant. Delayed gratification and/or meeting needs before infant signals them can lead to development of a sense of mistrust.
Review infant's sleep-wake patterns. Suggest ways to promote sleep through provision of warm, nonstimulating environment, position changes, and sleeping arrangements separate from parents' room.	Intervals of sleep at night range from 4 to 10 hours with frequent naps and increased periods of wakefulness without crying. By 3 months of age most infants have developed a nocturnal pattern; however, some do so much earlier.
Offer anticipatory guidance, as appropriate, regarding teething, shoes, use of pacifiers, thumb sucking, and so forth.	During first year of infant's life, both new and experienced parents may have concerns or questions, which if addressed early can foster positive coping, reduce anxiety, and increase problem-solving skills.

NURSING DIAGNOSIS:	**INFECTION, HIGH RISK FOR**
Risk factors may include:	Immature immunologic response, increased environmental exposure.
Possibly evidenced by:	[Not applicable; presence of signs/symptoms establishes an **actual** diagnosis.]

DESIRED OUTCOMES— NEONATE WILL:	Be free of infection.
PARENT(S) WILL:	Identify individual risk factors and appropriate interventions.
	List signs requiring medical intervention.

ACTIONS/INTERVENTIONS	RATIONALE

Independent

Discuss newborn development and individual risk factors.	By 4 weeks of age, the infant is usually out in public more often or may even be cared for outside the home. The infant is particularly susceptible to coryza, or the common cold, which is most frequently caused by a rhinovirus and an immature immunologic response. Because the infant has been an obligatory nose breather and is only beginning to learn to open mouth in response to an increase in mucus production and edema of nasal mucosa, respiratory problems and an increase in airway resistance may result. Possible complications such as otitis media, sinusitis, or lower respiratory tract infection may also develop.
Review signs of upper respiratory infection (e.g., poor feeding, breathing difficulty, cough, and nasal congestion) with parents.	Reinforces parental learning to assist them in identification of infant's respiratory problems.
Suggest elevating infant's head/shoulders by raising crib mattress to 30-degree angle when infant has trouble breathing.	Increases vertical chest capacity and lung expansion with descent of diaphragm. Facilitates drainage of mucus into stomach.
Recommend observing stool for passage of mucus.	Because infant cannot blow nose, excess mucus is excreted through the gastrointestinal tract with the stool.
Encourage giving infant sterile warm water between regular feedings twice a day.	Promotes hydration to liquefy secretions.
Provide information about benefits of humidifed air.	Liquefies secretions and prevents possible cracking of mucous membranes by keeping them moist.
Show parents how to inspect pharynx and to distinguish between viral and bacterial causative agent if area is reddened or inflamed. Discuss appropriate response.	Enlarged lymphoidal tissue and appearance of erythema (indicating viral cause) or white exudate (indicating bacterial or streptococcal cause) characterize pharyngitis and tonsillitis. Viral infections may resolve with only palliative measures, whereas bacterial infections usually require medication.
Discuss signs indicating a deterioration in newborn's status and necessitating evaluation by healthcare provider, such as pulling at ear (as child gets older), croupy cough, elevated temperature, cyanosis, and wheezing.	Involvement of lower respiratory structures or respiratory compromise requires further evaluation and treatment. Infant is prone to development of otitis media because of short, distensible eustachian tubes, which open inappropriately; an immature humoral defense system; and pooling of fluid in pharyngeal cavity when infant is in recumbent position.

ACTIONS/INTERVENTIONS	RATIONALE

Independent

Instruct parents not to medicate infant without discussing such action with healthcare provider.

Information about administration of medications, when to use them and when not to use them, helps parents know when to ask for assistance.

Demonstrate medication administration (e.g., antibiotics or ear or nose drops).

Enables parents to provide optimal care for infants individual needs. For example, saline nose drops instilled 15 min before feedings may improve oral intake at mealtime. (Note: Use of nose drops in newborn is somewhat controversial, because drops may lead to aspiration if they are improperly administered.)

Collaborative

Provide referral for laboratory studies (e.g., complete blood count [CBC], throat culture) if needed.

Helps confirm infectious process and identify pathogens, especially when causative organism may be beta-hemolytic streptococci.

NURSING DIAGNOSIS:	SUFFOCATION, HIGH RISK FOR; TRAUMA, HIGH RISK FOR
Risk factors may include:	Lack of ability to protect self (infant), lack of awareness of hazards (caregivers).
Possibly evidenced by:	[Not applicable; presence of signs/symptoms establishes an **actual** diagnosis.]
DESIRED OUTCOMES— NEONATE WILL:	Be free of injury.
PARENT(S) WILL:	Institute appropriate environmental adaptations or precautions to prevent accidental injury.
	Demonstrate concern for infant's well-being by responding to crying with soothing techniques, reacting appropriately during interactions with infant, and raising appropriate questions and concerns.

ACTIONS/INTERVENTIONS	RATIONALE

Independent

Provide oral or written information about infant's motor development between 1 and 4 months of age, its effect on mobility, and the increased risk of injury.

Allows parents to focus on age-appropriate safety measures. The major developmental changes that occur between birth and 4 months of age are increased eye-hand coordination, development of voluntary grasp, ability to roll over, and increased possibility of movement associated with crawling and with Moro reflex.

Review environmental factors that place infant at risk for suffocation.

Improper storage and use of plastic bags, loose-fitting bedding or mattress, opportunities for drowning, and strings around pacifiers/bibs (especially if they are worn at nap time or at night) place infant at risk for suffocation.

ACTIONS/INTERVENTIONS	RATIONALE

Independent

Discuss dangers associated with aspiration and proper use and storage of baby powder.

Aspiration dangers at 1 month are most often related to baby powder container, which because of its shape may be held like a bottle, thereby creating risk of inhalation, aspiration, and possibly fatal asphyxiation.

Provide anticipatory guidance regarding necessity of burping infant before placing in bed, proper positioning, keeping small objects out of infant's reach, avoiding use of clothing with buttons, avoiding balloons or toys with removable parts.

Regurgitation associated with reverse peristalsis and immature or relaxed cardiac sphincter increases risk of aspiration. As infant's coordination and strength increase, potential exists for infant's pulling toys and decorations apart and putting small pieces in mouth.

Reassess and discuss other home safety factors, including precautions for home layout and furniture used for infant care, cigarettes, hot liquids, and motor vehicles.

Reminds parents of situations that may present danger for their infant.

Re-evaluate parents' understanding and practices related to the potential for bodily harm to infant. Provide information as needed.

Keeping diaper pins closed and out of infant's reach and carefully putting away scissors, knives, and razors reduce risks associated with bodily injury from sharp or jagged-edged objects as infant matures and becomes more active.

Assess emotional tone and quality of parent-infant interaction. Note mother's response to infant's crying and nature of adjectives used to describe infant.

Failure of mother to have fun, talk, and make eye contact with infant; anger or frustration in response to crying episodes; and repeated use of negative adjectives to describe infant indicate a negative emotional bond between mother and infant, which may lead to emotional or physical abuse.

Evaluate infant for physical evidence of abuse.

Excessive bruising, pinch marks, handprints, lacerations, abrasions, malnutrition, FTT, or lack of subcutaneous fat indicates possible child abuse/neglect.

Collaborative

Make appropriate referrals to healthcare provider, community agencies, and support groups.

May be necessary to help parents develop positive parenting skills and reduce possibility of physical or emotional harm to infant.

Report suspected abuse to physician and appropriate social or child care agency.

Suspected child abuse may warrant further investigation before permanent injury or death occurs.

NURSING DIAGNOSIS:	**PAIN [ACUTE], HIGH RISK FOR**
Risk factors may include:	Accumulation of gas in a confined space with cramping of intestinal musculature.
Possibly evidenced by:	[Not applicable; presence of signs/symptoms establishes an **actual** diagnosis.]
DESIRED OUTCOMES— NEONATE WILL:	Be free of or display less frequent crying spells and episodes of colic.
PARENT(S) WILL:	Relieve newborn anxiety and tension.

ACTIONS/INTERVENTIONS	RATIONALE

Independent

Evaluate infant's behavior.	Helps differentiate cause of problem. For example, colicky infant typically cries loudly, draws legs up to abdomen in pain, clenches fists, and sucks vigorously.
Determine what parents have done previously and success of these interventions.	Assists in determining interventions that may be helpful at this time.
Reassess diet of lactating mother and infant feeding/formula preparation procedures.	Helps identify specific foods or errors in feeding process that may be causing discomfort.
Discuss physical condition and infant's well-being.	Gastric acidity reduces within first week of life, affecting digestion and development of colic, which often resolves within 2 to 3 months. Despite colic attacks, infant normally thrives, gains weight, and tolerate feedings.

(Refer to CP: Neonatal Assessment: 1 Week Following Discharge, ND: Pain [acute], high risk for.)

NURSING DIAGNOSIS:	SENSORY-PERCEPTUAL ALTERATIONS, HIGH RISK FOR
Risk factors may include:	Immature development of sensory organs, inappropriate/inadequate environmental stimuli; effects of disease, trauma, drugs.
Possibly evidenced by:	[Not applicable; presence of signs/symptoms establishes an **actual** diagnosis.]
DESIRED OUTCOMES— PARENT(S) WILL:	Identify impairments.
	Initiate appropriate interventions.

ACTIONS/INTERVENTIONS	RATIONALE

Independent

Repeat the Brazelton Neonatal Assessment Scale as appropriate, and compare with previous testing.	Measures cerebral and neurologic functioning and assesses interactive behavior. Although testing is usually done at 3 days of age, prolonged effects of intrapartal events/birth stress may affect initial results. Reevaluation provides opportunity for comparison and to verify appropriateness and progression of responses.
Observe responses to visual, auditory, or tactile stimuli; note motor function and reflexes.	The adequacy of sensory modes (e.g., visual, auditory, and tactile modes) in a 4-week-old infant is determined by eliciting responses and evaluating the age-specific response. Causes of deviations in sensory perception may be related to vascular or traumatic injury that develops over a period of hours; toxic, infectious, or electrolyte imbalances that peak in several days; or congenital or degenerative injuries that develop or worsen insidiously over days, weeks, and months.

ACTIONS/INTERVENTIONS	RATIONALE
Independent	
Assess occurrence of recent illnesses of infant or family members, prenatal or intrapartal complications and postnatal course.	Helps detect environmental infection and illness; may rule out mechanical causes of sensory-perceptual alteration.
Assess parents' behaviors and responses to infant using such measures as Cropley's Critical Attachment Tasks, Maternal Tasks, Mother-Infant Screening Tool (MIST), and Reiser Fathering Assessment Tool.	Helps to identify possible inadequacies in parent-infant interaction and establishes them as causative factors in infant's unresponsiveness to surroundings.
Encourage parents to stroke infant gently from head to toe with hand, washcloth, or cotton, and to hold, caress, cuddle, and swaddle infant.	Stimulates sense of touch; conveys feelings of warmth and protection.
Suggest parents place mobiles or bright, shiny objects within 20 to 25 cm (8 to 10 inches) of infant's face, to look at infant en face (face-to-face) at close range, and to decrease intensity of light and move objects slowly.	Stimulates visual development. At 4 weeks of age, infant can see shadows and outlines, showing preference for circular shapes, intricate patterns, and human faces.
Discuss placing ticking clock or radio playing soft music near infant, talking or singing to infant, and playing music box.	Provides auditory stimulation and may be soothing to infant; e.g., clock may simulate human heartbeat.
Encourage parents to rock infant, place infant in swing, gently cradle infant in arms, and take infant for walks in carriage or in backpack placed close to back or chest.	Provides kinetic stimulation.
Assess strength of muscles, finger grasp, limb recoil, and stretching. Institute age-appropriate exercises.	Provides parents with information about the infant's ability for reciprocal behavior. Specific exercises stimulate sensory development.
Refer to other resources (e.g., physician, nurse practitioner, physical therapy clinic, parenting classes, and support groups).	May be necessary for follow-up care and evaluation of identified problems. Facilitates role transition and skill acquisition.

NEONATAL ASSESSMENT DATA BASE

CIRCULATION

Apical pulse may be rapid and/or irregular within a normal range (120 to 160 bpm).

Audible heart murmur may indicate patent ductus arteriosus (PDA).

FOOD/FLUID

Weight less than 2500 g (5 lb 8 oz).

NEUROSENSORY

Body long, thin, limp with a slight potbelly.

Head size large in relation to body, sutures may be easily movable, fontanels may be large or wide-open.

May demonstrate twitching or eye rolling.

Edema of eyelids common, eyes may be fused shut (depending on gestational age).

Reflexes depend on gestational age; rooting well-established by 32 weeks' gestation; coordinated reflexes for sucking, swallowing, and breathing usually established by 32 weeks' gestation; first component of Moro reflex (lateral extension of upper extremities with opening of hands) appears at 28 weeks' gestation; second 2 components (anterior flexion and audible cry) appear at 32 weeks' gestation.

Dubowitz examination indicates gestational age between 24 and 37 weeks.

RESPIRATION

Apgar scores may be low.

Respirations may be shallow, irregular; diaphragmatic with intermittent or periodic breathing (40–60/min).

Grunting, nasal flaring, suprasternal or substernal retractions, or varying degrees of cyanosis may be present.

Auscultatory presence of "sandpaper" sound indicates respiratory distress syndrome (RDS).

SAFETY

Temperature fluctuates easily.

Cry may be weak.

Face may be bruised; caput succedaneum may be present.

Skin reddened or translucent; color may be pink/ruddy, acrocyanotic, or cyanotic/pale.

Lanugo widely distributed over entire body.

Extremities may appear edematous.

Sole creases may or may not be present on all or part of the foot.

Nails may be short.

SEXUALITY

Labor or delivery may have been precipitous.

Genitalia: Female labia minora may be larger than labia majora, with prominent clitoris; male testes may not be descended, rugae may be scant or absent on scrotum.

TEACHING/LEARNING

Maternal history may reveal factors that contributed to preterm labor, such as young age; low socioeconomic background; closely spaced pregnancies; multiple gestation; poor nutrition; previous preterm birth; obstetrical complication such as abruptio placentae, premature rupture of membranes (PROM), premature dilation of cervix, presence of infection; blood incompatibility associated with erythroblastosis fetalis; or use of prescription, over-the-counter, or street drugs.

DIAGNOSTIC STUDIES

Choice of tests and the expected results depend on presenting problems and secondary complications.

Amniotic fluid studies: For lecithin-to-sphingomyelin (L/S) ratio, fetal lung profile, and phosphatidylglycerol/phosphatidylinositol may have been performed during pregnancy to assess fetal maturity.

Complete blood count (CBC): Decreases in hemoglobin/hematocrit (Hb/Hct) may be associated with anemia or blood loss. White blood cell (WBC) count may be less than 10,000/mm^3 with a shift to the left (excess early neutrophils and bands), which is usually associated with severe bacterial disease.

Dextrostix: Reveals hypoglycemia. Serum glucose test may be required if Dextrostix result is less than 45 mg/ml.

Serum calcium: May be low.

Electrolytes (Na^{++}, K^+, Cl^-): Usually within normal limits initially.

Blood type: May reveal potential for ABO incompatibility.

Rh and direct Coombs' determination (if mother is Rh-negative and father is Rh-positive): Determines incompatabilities.

Arterial blood gases (ABGs): Po_2 may be low; Pco_2 may be elevated and reflect mild/moderate acidosis, sepsis, or prolonged respiratory difficulties.

Erythrocyte sedimentation rate (ESR): Elevated, indicating an acute inflammatory response. Diminishing ESR indicates resolution of inflammation.

C-reactive protein (a beta globulin): Present in serum in proportion to severity of infectious or noninfectious inflammatory process.

Platelet count: Thrombocytopenia may accompany sepsis.

Fibrinogen levels: May decrease during disseminated intravascular coagulation (DIC) or become elevated during injury or inflammation.

Fibrin split products: Present with DIC.

Blood cultures: Identify causative organisms associated with sepsis.

Urinalysis (on second voided specimen): Detects abnormalities, renal injury.

Urine specific gravity: Ranges between 1.006 to 1.013, elevated with dehydration.

Clinitest/Clinistix: Identifies presence of sugar in urine.

Hematest: Examines stools for blood; positive results suggest necrotizing enterocolitis.

Shake test on gastric aspirate: Determines presence or absence of surfactant. (Intermediate results if blood or meconium is present.)

Chest x-ray (PA and lateral) with air bronchogram: May have ground-glass appearance (RDS).

Serial cranial ultrasonography: Detects presence and severity of intraventricular hemorrhage (IVH).

Lumbar puncture: May be performed to rule out meningitis.

NURSING PRIORITIES

1. Promote optimal respiratory functioning.
2. Maintain neutral thermal environment.
3. Prevent or reduce risk of potential complications.
4. Maintain homeostasis through regulation of nutrition and hydration.
5. Foster development of healthy family unit.

DISCHARGE GOALS

1. Maintaining physiologic homeostasis with minimal support.
2. Weight 4$\frac{1}{2}$ lb or greater appropriate to age/condition.

3. Complications prevented/resolving or independently managed.
4. Family identifying and using resources appropriately.
5. Family demonstrates ability to manage infant care.

NURSING DIAGNOSIS:	GAS EXCHANGE, IMPAIRED
May be related to:	Ventilation perfusion imbalances, inadequate surfactant levels, immaturity of pulmonary arteriole musculature, immaturity of central nervous system (CNS) and neuromuscular system, ineffective airway clearance, anemia, and cold stress.
Possibly evidenced by:	Hypercapnia, hypoxia, tachypnea, cyanosis.
DESIRED OUTCOMES— NEONATE WILL:	Maintain Po_2/Pco_2 levels within normal limits (WNL).
	Suffer minimal RDS, with reduced work of breathing and no morbidity.
	Be free of bronchopulmonary dysplasia.

ACTIONS/INTERVENTIONS

Independent

Review information related to infant's condition, such as length of labor, type of delivery, Apgar score, need for resuscitative measures at delivery, and maternal medications taken during pregnancy or delivery, including betamethasone.

Note gestational age, weight, and sex.

Assess respiratory status, noting signs of respiratory distress (e.g., tachypnea, nasal flaring, grunting, retractions, rhonchi, or crackles).

Apply transcutaneous oxygen monitor or pulse oximeter. Record levels hourly. Change site of probe every 3–4 hr.

RATIONALE

Prolonged labor increases risk of hypoxia, and respiratory depression may follow maternal drug administration or usage. In addition, infants who required resuscitative measures at birth, or those with low Apgar scores, may require more intense interventions to stabilize blood gases and may have suffered CNS injury with damage to the hypothalamus, which controls respiratory functioning. (Note: Administration of corticosteroids to mother within 1 week of delivery fosters the infant's lung maturity and surfactant production.)

Neonates born before 30 weeks' gestation and/or weighing less than 1500 g are at higher risk for developing RDS. Additionally, males are twice as susceptible as females. (Note: The majority of deaths related to RDS occur in infants weighing less than 1500 g.)

Tachypnea indicates respiratory distress, especially when respirations are greater than 60/min after the first 5 hours of life. Expiratory grunting represents an attempt to maintain alveolar expansion; nasal flaring is a compensatory mechanism to increase diameter of nares and increase oxygen intake. Crackles/rhonchi may indicate pulmonary vasocongestion associated with PDA, hypoxemia, acidemia, or immaturity of muscles in arterioles, which fail to constrict in response to increased oxygen levels.

Provides constant noninvasive monitoring of oxygen levels. (Note: Pulmonary insufficiency usually worsens during the first 24–48 hours, then reaches a plateau.)

ACTIONS/INTERVENTIONS	RATIONALE

Independent

Suction nares and oropharynx carefully, as needed. Limit time of airway obstruction by catheter to 5–10 sec. Observe transcutaneous oxygen monitor or pulse oximeter before and during suctioning. Provide "bag" ventilation following suctioning.

May be necessary to maintain airway patency, especially in infant receiving controlled ventilation. Preterm infant does not develop the coordinated reflex for sucking, swallowing, and breathing until 32 to 34 weeks' gestation. Cilia may not be fully developed or may be damaged from use of endotracheal tube. Exudate phase associated with RDS at about 48 hours postpartum may contribute to infant's difficulty in handling secretions. Suctioning may stimulate vagus nerve, causing bradycardia, hypoxemia, or bronchospasm. Bag ventilation promotes rapid restoration of oxygen levels.

Maintain thermal neutrality with body temperature at 97.7°F (within 0.5°F). (Refer to ND: Thermoregulation, ineffective, high risk for.)

Cold stress increases infant's oxygen consumption, may promote acidosis, and may further impair surfactant production.

Monitor fluid intake and output; weigh infant as indicated by protocol.

Dehydration impairs ability to clear airways as mucus becomes thickened. Overhydration may contribute to alveolar infiltrates/pulmonary edema. Weight loss and increased urine output may indicate diuretic phase of RDS, usually beginning at 72–96 hr and preceding resolution of condition.

Promote rest; minimize stimulation and energy expenditure.

Reduces metabolic rate and oxygen consumption.

Position infant on abdomen if possible. Provide "rocker" mattress, as indicated.

Allows optimal chest expansion. Stimulates respirations and ventricular growth.

Observe for evidence and location of cyanosis.

Cyanosis is a late sign of low PaO_2 and does not appear until there are slightly more than 3 g/dl of reduced Hb in central arterial blood, or 4–6 g/dl in capillary blood, or until oxygen saturation is only 75%–85% with PO_2 levels of 32 to 41 mm Hg.

Investigate sudden deterioration in condition associated with cyanosis, diminished or absent breath sounds, shift of point of maximal impact (PMI), bulging of chest wall, hypotension, or cardiac dysrhythmias.

Sudden or unexplained deterioration of respiratory function may indicate onset of pneumothorax.

Monitor for signs of necrotizing enterocolitis. (Refer to ND: Constipation, high risk for; Diarrhea, high risk for.)

Hypoxia may cause shunting of blood to brain, thereby reducing circulation to the intestines, with resultant intestinal cell damage and invasion by gas-forming bacteria.

Collaborative

Monitor laboratory studies, as appropriate:

Graph serial ABGs.

Hypoxemia, hypercapnia, and acidosis reduce surfactant production. PaO_2 levels should be 50 to 70 mm Hg or higher, $PaCO_2$ levels should be 35 to 45 mm Hg, and oxygen saturation should be 92% to 94%.

ACTIONS/INTERVENTIONS	RATIONALE

Collaborative

Hb/Hct.

Decreased iron stores at birth, repeated blood sampling, rapid growth, and hemorrhagic episodes increase the likelihood that preterm infant will be anemic, thereby reducing the oxygen-carrying capacity of the blood. (Note: Administration of packed cells may be necessary to replace blood drawn for laboratory studies.)

Review serial chest x-rays.

Atelectasis, congestion, or air bronchogram suggests developing RDS.

Administer oxygen, as needed, by mask, hood, endotracheal tube, or mechanical ventilation using constant positive airway pressure (CPAP) and intermittent mandatory ventilation (IMV), or intermittent positive-pressure breathing (IPPB) and positive end-expiratory pressure (PEEP).

Hypoxemia and acidemia may further decrease surfactant production, increase pulmonary vascular resistance and vasoconstriction, and cause ductus arteriosus to remain open. Immaturity of the hypothalamus may necessitate ventilatory assistance to maintain respirations. Use of PEEP may reduce airway collapse, enhancing gas exchange and reducing the need for high levels of oxygen.

Monitor amount of oxygen administered and duration of administration.

Prolonged high levels of serum oxygen combined with prolonged high pressures resulting from IPPB and PEEP (barotrauma) may predispose infant to bronchopulmonary dysplasia.

Record fraction of oxygen in inspired air (FIO_2) every hour.

Amount of oxygen administered, expressed as FIO_2, is determined individually, based on transcutaneous monitoring or capillary blood samples. (Note: Prolonged high levels of oxygen [oxygen toxicity] may predispose infant to retinal damage [retrolental fibroplasia].)

Initiate postural drainage, chest physiotherapy, or lobe vibration every 2 hr, as indicated, noting infant's tolerance of procedure.

Facilitates removal of secretions. Length of time allotted to each lobe is related to infant's tolerance. (Infant usually cannot tolerate a full treatment regimen each time.)

Aspirate gastric contents for shake test.

Provides immediate information about presence or absence of surfactant. Surfactant, which is necessary to promote normal expansion and elasticity of alveoli, is usually not present in sufficient quantities until 32 to 33 weeks' gestation.

Provide feedings by nasogastric or orogastric tube instead of nipple feedings, as appropriate.

Reduces oxygen needs, promotes rest, conserves energy, and reduces risk of aspiration due to poorly developed gag reflex.

Administer medications as indicated:

Sodium bicarbonate.

If measures to increase respiratory rate or improve ventilation are not sufficient to correct acidosis, cautious use of sodium bicarbonate may help return pH to normal range.

Surfactant (artificial or exogenous).

May be given at birth or after diagnosis of RDS to decrease severity of condition and associated complications. Effect may last up to 72 hours.

ACTIONS/INTERVENTIONS	RATIONALE
Collaborative	
Assist with needle aspiration, thoracentesis, or chest tube insertion.	Reinflates lung through removal of trapped air or fluid, reestablishing negative pressure and enhancing gas exchange.

NURSING DIAGNOSIS:	**BREATHING PATTERN, INEFFECTIVE**
May be related to:	Immaturity of the respiratory center, limited muscular development, decreased energy/fatigue, drug-related depression, and metabolic imbalances.
Possibly evidenced by:	Dyspnea, tachypnea, periods of apnea, nasal flaring, use of accessary muscles, cyanosis, abnormal ABGs, tachycardia.
DESIRED OUTCOMES— NEONATE WILL:	Maintain periodic breathing pattern (apneic periods last 5–10 sec followed by short periods of rapid ventilation), with mucous membranes pink and heart rate WNL.

ACTIONS/INTERVENTIONS	RATIONALE
Independent	
Assess respiratory rate and breathing pattern. Note presence of apnea and changes in heart rate, muscle tone, and skin color associated with procedures or care. Institute continuous respiratory and cardiac monitoring.	Helps in distinguishing normal cyclic periodic breathing pattern from true apneic spells, which are particularly common prior to 30 weeks' gestation.
Suction airway as needed.	Removes mucus obstructing the airway.
Review maternal history for drugs that might contribute to respiratory depression in the infant.	Magnesium sulfate and narcotics depress respiratory center and CNS activity.
Position infant on abdomen or in supine position with rolled diaper beneath shoulders to produce slight hyperextension.	Such positioning may facilitate respiration and reduce apneic episodes, especially in the presence of hypoxia, metabolic acidosis, or hypercapnia.
Maintain optimal body temperature. (Refer to ND: Thermoregulation, ineffective, high risk for.)	Even a slight increase or decrease in environmental temperature can lead to apnea.
Provide prompt tactile stimulation (e.g., rub infant's back) if apnea occurs. Note presence of cyanosis, bradycardia, or hypotonia. Encourage parental contact.	Stimulates CNS to promote body movement and spontaneous return of respirations. Sometimes, infants experience fewer or no episodes of apnea or bradycardia if parents touch and talk to them.
Place infant on neowave mattress.	Movement provides stimulation, which may reduce apneic episodes.
Collaborative	
Monitor laboratory studies (e.g., ABGs, serum glucose, electrolytes, cultures, and drug levels) as indicated.	Hypoxia, metabolic acidosis, hypercapnia, hypoglycemia, hypocalcemia, and sepsis may contribute to apneic spells. Drug toxicity, which depresses respiratory function, may occur because of limited excretion and prolonged drug half-life.

ACTIONS/INTERVENTIONS

Collaborative

Administer oxygen, as indicated. (Refer to ND: Gas Exchange, impaired.)

Administer medications, as indicated:

    Sodium bicarbonate.

    Antibiotics.

    Calcium gluconate.

    Aminophylline.

    Pancuronium bromide (Pavulon).

    Glucose solutions.

RATIONALE

Correction of oxygen and carbon dioxide levels may improve respiratory function.

Corrects acidosis.

Treat respiratory infection or sepsis.

Hypocalcemia predisposes infant to apnea.

May increase activity of respiratory center and lower sensitivity to carbon dioxide, reducing frequency of apnea.

Induces skeletal muscle relaxation, which may be necessary if infant is to be mechanically ventilated.

Prevent hypoglycemia. (Refer to ND: Nutrition, altered, less than body requirements, high risk for.)

NURSING DIAGNOSIS:	THERMOREGULATION, INEFFECTIVE, HIGH RISK FOR
Risk factors may include:	Immature CNS development (temperature regulation center), decreased ratio of body mass to surface area, decreased subcutaneous fat, limited brown fat stores, an inability to shiver or sweat, poor metabolic reserves, muted response to hypothermia, and frequent medical/nursing manipulations and interventions.
Possibly evidenced by:	[Not applicable; presence of signs/symptoms establishes an **actual** diagnosis.]
DESIRED OUTCOMES— NEONATE WILL:	Maintain skin/axillary temperature within 95.9°F to 99.1°F (35.5°C to 37.3°C).
	Be free of signs of cold stress.

ACTIONS/INTERVENTIONS

Independent

Assess temperature frequently. Check rectal temperature initially; thereafter, check axillary temperature or use thermostat probe with open bed and radiant warmer. Repeat every 15 min during rewarming.

Place infant in warmer, isolette, incubator, open bed with radiant warmer, or open crib with appropriate clothing for larger or older infants. Use heating pad under infant as necessary, in conjunction with isolette or open bed.

RATIONALE

Hypothermia predisposes infant to cold stress, utilization of nonrenewable brown fat stores if present, and reduced sensitivity to increased levels of carbon dioxide (hypercapnia) or decreased oxygen levels (hypoxia). (Note: Too-rapid rewarming is associated with apneic states. This causes further respiratory depression instead of increased respiratory rate, leading to apnea and reduced oxygen uptake.)

Maintains thermoneutral environment, helps prevent cold stress.

ACTIONS/INTERVENTIONS	RATIONALE

Independent

Use heat lamps during procedures. Cover radiant warmers or the infant with plastic wrap or aluminum foil as appropriate. Warm objects coming in contact with infant's body, such as stethoscopes, linens, and clothing.

Decreases loss of heat to the cooler environment of the room.

Reduce exposure to drafts; avoid unnecessary opening of portholes in isolette.

Reduces heat losses due to convection/conduction. Limits heat losses from radiation.

Change clothing or bed linens when wet. Keep infant's head covered.

Decreases evaporative losses.

Monitor temperature-regulating system, radiant warmers, or incubators. (Maintain upper limit at 98.6°F, depending on infant's size or age.)

Hyperthermia—with resultant increases in metabolic rate, oxygen and glucose needs, and insensible water losses can occur when controlled environmental temperatures are too high.

Maintain relative humidity of 50%–80%. Warm humidified oxygen to 88°F to 93°F (31°C to 34°C).

Prevents excessive evaporation, reducing insensible fluid losses.

Note presence of tachypnea or apnea; generalized cyanosis, acrocyanosis, or mottled skin; bradycardia, poor cry, or lethargy. Evaluate degree and location of jaundice. (Refer to CP: Newborn: Hyperbilirubinemia.)

These signs indicate cold stress, which increases oxygen and caloric consumption and predisposes infant to acidosis associated with anaerobic metabolism. Hypothermia increases risk of kernicterus, as fatty acids released with brown fat metabolism compete with bilirubin for binding sites on albumin. (Note: Skin color may be bright red peripherally, with cyanosis noted centrally as a result of failure of dissociation of oxyhemoglobin.)

Provide gradual warming for infant with cold stress.

Rapid increase in body temperature may cause excessive oxygen consumption and apnea.

Assess urine output and specific gravity.

Reduced urine output and increased specific gravity of urine are related to reduced kidney perfusion during periods of cold stress.

Monitor serial weight gain. If weight gain is inadequate, increase environmental temperature as indicated.

Inadequate weight gain despite sufficient caloric intake may indicate that calories are being used to maintain body temperature, necessitating increased environmental temperature.

Note frequency and amount of food intake. Monitor Dextrostix. Assess infant for vomiting, abdominal distention, or apathy.

Poor feeding is common in infants with thermal instability. Dextrostix levels less than 45 mg/dl indicate hypoglycemia necessitating prompt intervention.

Assess infant's progressive ability to adapt to lowered temperatures in incubator or isolette, or to room temperature, while demonstrating appropriate weight gains.

Bassinet may be used when infant can maintain stable body temperature of 97.7°F in room air and still gain weight.

Monitor infant's temperature when out of warmed environment. Provide parents with information about thermoregulation.

Out-of-bed contact, especially with parents, may need to be brief, if allowed at all, to prevent cold stress. (Note: Hyperthermia can also occur when infant is held by parents.)

Note development of tachycardia, flushed color, diaphoresis, lethargy, apnea, coma, or seizure activity.

These signs of hyperthermia (body temperature greater than 99°F [37.2°C]) can progress to brain damage if untreated.

ACTIONS/INTERVENTIONS	RATIONALE

Independent

Evaluate external sources of heat (e.g., phototherapy, heat lamp, or sunlight), limit clothing, and provide tepid sponge bath. Verify proper positioning of temperature probe if used.

These measures are generally successful in correcting hyperthermia. (Note: If hyperthermia persists after assuring proper position and functioning of temperature probe, the possibility of a hypermetabolic state such as sepsis or narcotic withdrawal should be considered.)

Collaborative

Monitor laboratory studies, as indicated (e.g., ABGs, serum glucose, electrolytes, and bilirubin levels). (Refer to ND: Gas Exchange, impaired.)

Cold stress increases the needs for glucose and oxygen and may result in acid-base problems if infant resorts to anaerobic metabolism when sufficient oxygen levels are not available. Elevated indirect bilirubin levels may occur because of the release of fatty acids from brown fat metabolism, with fatty acids competing with bilirubin for binding sites on albumin. Metabolic acidosis may also occur with hyperthermia.

Administer $D_{10}W$ and volume expanders intravenously, as needed.

Administration of dextrose may be necessary to correct hypoglycemia. Hypotension due to peripheral vasodilation may require treatment in heat-stressed infant. Hyperthermia may cause a three-fold to fourfold increase in dehydration.

Provide supplemental oxygen as indicated.

If oxygen is not readily available to meet increased metabolic needs associated with efforts to increase body temperature, the infant will use anaerobic metabolism, resulting in acidosis due to lactic acid build up. Hypothermia reduces the preterm infant's response to hypoxia and hypercapnia, which causes further respiratory depression instead of increased respiratory rate, leading to apnea and reduced oxygen uptake. Hyperthermia caused by too-rapid warming is associated with apneic states, increased insensible water losses, and increased metabolic rates with increased demands for oxygen and glucose.

Administer medications, as indicated:

   Phenobarbital.

Helps prevent seizures associated with alterations in CNS function caused by hyperthermia.

   Sodium bicarbonate.

Corrects acidosis, which may occur with both hypothermia and hyperthermia.

NURSING DIAGNOSIS:	**FLUID VOLUME DEFICIT, HIGH RISK FOR**
Risk factors may include:	Extremes of age and weight (premature, under 2500 g), excessive fluid losses (thin skin, lack of insulating fat, increased environmental temperature, immature kidney/failure to concentrate urine).

Possibly evidenced by:	[Not applicable; presence of signs/symptoms establishes an **actual** diagnosis.]
DESIRED OUTCOMES— NEONATE WILL:	Be free of signs of dehydration or glycosuria with fluid intake approximating output and pH, Hct, and urine specific gravity WNL.
	Display weight gain of 20–30 g/day.

ACTIONS/INTERVENTIONS

Independent

Obtain daily serial weights using same scale at same time of day.

Compare fluid intake and output each shift and cumulative balance each 24-hour period. Maintain hourly records of infusing intravenous fluids. Assess output through measuring urine from collecting bag or through weighing/counting diapers. Maintain accurate records regarding amount of blood taken for laboratory testing.

Monitor urine specific gravity after each voiding, or every 2–4 hr, by aspirating urine from diaper if infant cannot tolerate adhesive or urine collecting bag.

Test urine with Dextrostix per protocol.

Minimize insensible fluid losses through use of clothing, thermoneutral temperatures, and warm or humidified oxygen.

Monitor blood pressure (BP), pulse, and mean arterial pressure (MAP).

Evaluate skin turgor, mucous membranes, and status of anterior fontanel.

RATIONALE

Weight is the most sensitive indicator of fluid balance. Weight loss should not exceed 15% of total body weight or 1%–2% of total body weight per day. Inadequate weight gain may be related to water imbalance or inadequate caloric intake.

Output should be 1–3 ml/kg/hr, while fluid therapy needs are approximately 80–100 ml/kg/day on the first day of life, increasing to 120–140 ml/kg/day by the third day post delivery. Removal of blood for testing causes reduction in Hb/Hct levels.

Although renal immaturity and inability to concentrate urine usually result in low specific gravity in the preterm infant (normal range is 1.006 to 1.013), urine specific gravity may vary, providing an indication of the level of hydration. Low levels indicate excessive fluid volume; levels greater than 1.013 indicate insufficient fluid intake and dehydration.

Even in cases of hypoglycemia, glycosuria occurs as immature kidneys begin excreting glucose, which may lead to osmotic diuresis, increasing risk of dehydration.

Preterm infant loses large amounts of water through skin, because blood vessels are close to surface and insulating fat levels are decreased or absent. Phototherapy or use of radiant warmer may increase insensible losses by 50% or by as much as 200 ml/kg/day. (Note: Infants weighing less than 1500 g (3 lb 5 oz) are most susceptible to insensible fluid losses.)

A loss of 25% of blood volume results in shock with MAP of less than 25 mm Hg indicating hypotension. (Note: BP is related to weight; i.e., the smaller the baby, the lower the MAP.)

Fluid reserves are limited in the preterm infant. Minimal fluid losses/shifts can quickly lead to dehydration, as noted by poor skin turgor, dry mucous membranes, and depressed fontanels.

ACTIONS/INTERVENTIONS	RATIONALE

Independent

Note lethargy, high-pitched cry, abdominal distention, increased apnea, twitching, hypotonia, or seizure activity.

These signs reflect hypocalcemia, which is most likely to occur during the first 10 days of life.

Assess intravenous site every hour. Note edema or failure of fluid infusion. Do not check needle position by lowering fluid below needle level.

Swelling may indicate that infiltration of fluid is occurring or that tape is too tight. Back-up of blood caused by lowering fluid may clog needle.

Collaborative

Monitor laboratory studies as indicated:

Hct.

Dehydration increases Hct level beyond the normal reading of 45%–53%.

Serum calcium and serum magnesium.

Preterm infant is susceptible to hypocalcemia (calcium level less than 7 mg/dl) because of low stores, depressed parathyroid stimulation, and stress due to hypoxia, sepsis, or hypoglycemia. Hypomagnesemia often accompanies hypocalcemia.

Serum potassium.

Hypokalemia may occur because of losses through nasogastric tube, diarrhea, or vomiting. Excessive levels of potassium (hyperkalemia) can result from replacement errors, potassium shifts from intracellular to extracellular compartments, acidosis, or renal failure.

Administer parenteral infusions in amounts greater than 180 ml/kg, especially in PDA, bronchopulmonary dysplasia (BPD), or necrotizing enterocolitis (NEC).

Fluid replacement expands blood volume; helps reverse vasoconstriction associated with hypoxia, acidosis, and right-to-left shunting through PDA; and has been helpful in reducing complications of necrotizing enterocolitis and bronchopulmonary dysplasia.

Administer potassium chloride, 10% calcium gluconate, and 50% magnesium sulfate, as indicated. Monitor infant for potential bradycardia via cardiac monitor; observe infusion site for signs of irritation or edema.

Correction of electrolyte imbalances is necessary to maintain or achieve homeostasis. Calcium administered through umbilical venous catheter may cause liver necrosis; if administered through umbilical artery, it may contribute to necrotizing enterocolitis. Early recognition and prompt intervention may limit untoward effects of infiltration of medication; such as sloughing, calcification, and necrosis. (Note: Calcium replacement is ineffective in presence of magnesium deficit.)

Administer blood transfusions.

May be necessary to maintain optimal Hb/Hct levels and replace blood losses.

Administer dopamine hydrochloride, as indicated.

May be used to counteract drops in blood pressure, especially when related to administration of Pavulon.

NURSING DIAGNOSIS:	INJURY, HIGH RISK FOR, central nervous system damage
Risk factors may include:	Tissue hypoxia, altered clotting factors, metabolic imbalances (hypoglycemia, electrolyte shifts, elevated bilirubin).
Possibly evidenced by:	[Not applicable; presence of signs/symptoms establishes an **actual** diagnosis.]
DESIRED OUTCOMES— NEONATE WILL:	Be free of seizures and signs of CNS impairment. Maintain homeostasis as evidenced by ABGs; serum glucose, electrolytes and bilirubin levels WNL.

ACTIONS/INTERVENTIONS	RATIONALE

Independent

Assess respiratory effort. Note presence of pallor or cyanosis.	Respiratory distress and hypoxia affect cerebral function and may damage or weaken walls of cerebral blood vessels, increasing risk of rupture. If untreated, hypoxia may result in permanent damage. (Refer to ND: Gas Exchange, impaired.)
Monitor Dextrostix levels, and observe infant for behaviors indicating hypocalcemia or hypoglycemia (e.g., convulsions, twitching, myoclonic jerks, or eye rolling). (Refer to ND: Nutrition, altered, less than body requirements, high risk for.)	Because of its demands for glucose, the brain may suffer irreparable damage when serum glucose levels are lower than 30–40 mg/dl. Hypocalcemia (serum calcium levels less than 7 mg/dl) often accompanies hypoglycemia and may result in apnea and seizures.
Observe infant for alterations in CNS function as manifested by behavior changes, lethargy, hypotonia, bulging or tense fontanel, eye rolling, or seizure activity. Investigate deteriorating status indicated by high-pitched cry, labored respirations, and cyanosis, followed by apnea, flaccid quadriparesis, unresponsiveness, hypotension, tonic posturing, and areflexia.	Birth trauma, fragile capillaries, and impaired coagulation processes place preterm infant at risk for IVH, especially those infants weighing less than 1500 g or under 34 weeks' gestation. Tense or bulging anterior fontanel may be first sign of IVH, hemorrhagic shock, or increased intracranial pressure (IICP), which can easily lead to death from circulatory collapse. Infant of less than 32 weeks' gestation may become lethargic or hypotonic and may manifest uncontrolled "roving-eye" movements and lack of visual tracking. (Note: Clinical signs of developing IVH may be absent, very subtle, or sudden and life threatening.)
Measure head circumference, as indicated.	Helps detect possible increased ICP or hydrocephalus, which may be a sequela of subdural hemorrhage. Only 35%–50% of infants with hydrocephalus develop normally.
Assess skin color, noting evidence of increasing jaundice associated with behavior changes such as lethargy, hyperreflexia, convulsions, and opisthotonos. (Refer to CP: Newborn: Hyperbilirubinemia.)	Preterm infant is more susceptible to kernicterus at lower serum bilirubin levels than full-term infant because of increased levels of unconjugated circulating bilirubin crossing the blood-brain barrier.

531

ACTIONS/INTERVENTIONS	RATIONALE
Collaborative	
Monitor laboratory studies, as indicated:	
Hb/Hct; ABGs.	Lowered Hb levels or anemia reduce oxygen-carrying capacity, increasing risk of permanent CNS damage associated with hypoxemia. Abrupt fall in Hct may be first indicator of IVH.
Bilirubin levels.	Rapidly rising levels may result in kernicterus if not treated.
Provide supplemental oxygen.	Hypoxemia increases the risk of impairment or permanent CNS damage.
Assist with diagnostic or therapeutic procedures, as indicated:	
Computerized tomography scanning, cranial ultrasonography.	Identifies presence/extent of hemorrhage, which is useful in predicting likelihood of long-term complications and in choice of treatment.
Lumbar puncture.	A bloody cerebrospinal fluid (CSF) specimen confirms IVH. Some hospitals carry out serial daily lumbar punctures to reduce ICP and prevent deleterious effects of hydrocephalus.
Exchange transfusion.	Elevated or rapidly rising bilirubin levels indicate the need for a double-volume exchange transfusion with O-negative blood to remove bilirubin and to prevent further hemolysis of red blood cells (RBCs).
Ventriculopuncture or taps.	May be used to remove excess blood from the ventricles, although studies have not indicated any corresponding improvement in outcome.
Placement of ventriculoperitoneal shunt.	Progressive ventricular dilation unresponsive to other measures may require surgical intervention to correct or prevent hydrocephalus.
Administer medications, as indicated:	
Calcium, magnesium, sodium bicarbonate, and/or glucose.	Correction of imbalances helps prevent neonatal seizure activity, which may occur in response to transient metabolic states.
Phenobarbital.	Helps to control acute convulsions and status epilepticus in newborn.
Phenytoin or diazepam.	May be used if other antiepileptic drugs are not successful in controlling seizure activity. (Note: Dosage should be based on blood levels.)
Furosemide, acetazolamide, or steroids.	Helps reduce intracranial pressure and treats secondary effects of bleeding.
Vitamin E.	Antioxidant property protects RBC membranes against hemolysis.
Indomethacin.	I.V. administration may correct hemodynamic imbalances through closure of patent ductus arteriosus.

ACTIONS/INTERVENTIONS

Collaborative

Assist with fluid replacement or restrictions.

RATIONALE

Cerebral perfusion depends on adequate circulatory volume. (Note: Fluids may need to be restricted in cases of hypertonicity, CNS damage with bleeding, or cerebral palsy.)

NURSING DIAGNOSIS:	NUTRITION, ALTERED, LESS THAN BODY REQUIREMENTS, HIGH RISK FOR
Risk factors may include:	Immaturity of enzymatic production; reduced production of hydrochloric acid (reduces absorption of fat and fat-soluble vitamins); immaturity of the cardiac sphincter; lax abdominal muscles; small stomach capacity; weak, absent, or unsynchronized reflexes associated with feeding; inadequate levels of stored nutrients.
Possibly evidenced by:	[Not applicable; presence of signs/symptoms establishes an **actual** diagnosis.]
DESIRED OUTCOMES— NEONATE WILL:	Maintain growth and weight gain in a normal curve, with steady weight gain at least 20–30 g/day.
	Maintain serum glucose WNL and positive nitrogen balance.

ACTIONS/INTERVENTIONS

Independent

Assess maturity of reflexes associated with feeding (i.e., sucking, swallowing, gag, and coughing).

Auscultate for presence of bowel sounds. Assess physical state and respiratory status.

Initiate intermittent or tube feedings as indicated.

Assess infant for proper placement of feeding tube; use appropriate clamping procedures to prevent entry of air into stomach.

Instill breast milk/formula slowly over 20 min at a rate of 1 ml/min.

RATIONALE

Determines appropriate feeding method for infant.

The first feeding in a stable infant with peristalsis can begin 6 to 12 hours following birth. If respiratory distress is present, parenteral fluids are indicated, and oral fluids should be withheld.

Gavage feedings may be necessary to provide adequate nutrition in infant who has a poorly coordinated suck and swallow reflex or who becomes fatigued during oral feedings.

Improper placement of tube in trachea can compromise respiratory function. When 1 ml or less is aspirated from the stomach, this sum should be subtracted from the feeding and reinstilled in tube. When more than 2 ml is aspirated, feeding schedule may need to be altered.

Too-rapid entry of feeding into stomach may cause rapid rebound response with regurgitation, increased risk of aspiration, and abdominal distention, all of which compromise respiratory status.

ACTIONS/INTERVENTIONS	RATIONALE

Independent

Assess energy level and expenditure, degree of fatigability, respiratory rate, and length of time needed for feedings.

Excessive expenditure of energy during feedings reduces calories available for normal growth and development. Total or intermittent use of tube feedings may be necessary to reduce fatigue. Oral feedings are not appropriate if respiratory rate is greater than 60/min.

Accommodate infant's need for sucking with use of pacifier during tube feedings. If baby is going to be breastfed eventually, mother may rub pacifier on breast, moistening it with a dab of breast milk to scent it. She may also hold the baby during feedings.

Provides oral satisfaction so that infant associates self-gratification in sucking with comfort of filling stomach.

Postpone postural drainage for at least 1 hour after feeding.

Allows optimal ingestion and absorption of feeding; helps prevent regurgitation associated with increased handling.

Note presence of diarrhea, vomiting, regurgitation, excessive gastric residual, or positive result of guaiac test. (Refer to ND: Constipation, high risk for; Diarrhea, high risk for.)

Indicates impaired gastric function. Gastric residual greater than 2 ml (aspirated via nasogastric [NG] tube before feedings) suggests a need to reduce amount of feedings and may indicate poor absorption or necrotizing enterocolitis.

Monitor Dextrostix levels and urine Clinitest per protocol.

Because the immature liver does not store or release glycogen well, risk of hypoglycemia is increased. Hypoglycemia can be diagnosed by a Dextrostix level less than 45 mg/dl. (Note: Infant may be asymptomatic even when Dextrostix results are as low as 20 mg/dl.)

Maintain thermoneutral environment and appropriate oxygenation of tissues. Disturb infant as little as possible.

Cold stress, hypoxia, and excessive handling increase infant's metabolic rate and caloric needs, possibly sacrificing growth and weight gains.

Monitor infant for local or systemic reactions to parenteral feeding (e.g., increased temperature, blood vessel thrombosis, dyspnea, vomiting, or cyanosis).

About 50% of complications associated with total parenteral nutrition (TPN) are due to sepsis, usually Candida septicemia. Other complications include fluid overload and obstruction or dislodgment of catheter.

Record growth by plotting daily weight and weekly measurements of body length and head circumference.

Growth and weight gain are criteria for establishing caloric requirements, for adjusting formula, and for determining frequency of feedings. Growth spurts increase caloric requirements and protein needs.

Collaborative

Start feedings of sterile water, glucose, and breast milk or formula, as appropriate.

Early feedings prevent depletion of reserves.

Feed as frequently as indicated based on infant's weight and estimated stomach capacity.

Infants less than 1250 g (2 lb 12 oz) are fed every 2 hr, infants between 1500 and 1800 g (3 lb 8 oz to 4 lb) are fed every 3 hr.

ACTIONS/INTERVENTIONS	RATIONALE

Collaborative

Use concentrated formula to provide 120–150 cal/kg/day or more, with 3–4 g/kg/day of protein. Add fortifiers to breast milk for gavage feeding as needed.

Calorie intake must be sufficient to prevent catabolism. Concentrated formulas supply more calories in less volume, which is necessary because of reduced gastric capacity and emptying, and the danger of stressing immature kidneys. (Note: Sick infants may require half-strength formula initially with volume/concentration advanced over 1–10 days as infant tolerates.)

Administer vitamins and minerals, especially vitamins A, C, D, and E, and iron, as indicated.

Replaces low nutrient stores to promote adequate nutrition and reduce risk of infection. Vitamin C may reduce susceptibility to hemolytic anemia and alleviate bronchopulmonary dysplasia and retrolental fibroplasia. Vitamin E helps prevent RBC hemolysis.

Maintain patency, assist with change of indwelling feeding tube (transpyloric, nasojejunal, nasoduodenal tubes).

Provides continuous infusion of formula in very small preterm infants who meet specific criteria; e.g., tachypnea, chronic lung disease, respirator dependence, recurrent aspiration, or repeated elevated gastric residuals with other feeding approaches. (Note: Potential risks accompanying use of these indwelling tubes must be weighed against benefits.)

Administer TPN feedings via infusion pump using indwelling catheter into vena cava or peripheral line. Infuse fat emulsions (intralipid) through peripheral line.

TPN infusion of protein hydrolysate, glucose, electrolytes, minerals, and vitamins may be necessary for infant with chronic diarrhea; malabsorption syndrome; surgical repair of gastrointestinal (GI) anomalies, obstruction, or necrotizing enterocolitis; or extreme prematurity. Intralipid infusion provides essential fatty acids to child receiving TPN. (Note: Benefits of using Intralipid must be weighed against possible risk of fat accumulation in the lungs.)

Monitor laboratory studies; e.g., serum glucose, electrolytes, total protein.

Measures appropriateness of TPN.

NURSING DIAGNOSIS:	INFECTION, HIGH RISK FOR
Risk factors may include:	Immature immune response, fragile skin, traumatized tissues, invasive procedures, environmental exposure (PROM, transplacental exposure).
Possibly evidenced by:	[Not applicable; presence of signs/symptoms establishes an **actual** diagnosis.]
DESIRED OUTCOMES— NEONATE WILL:	Maintain negative serum, CSF, urine, and nasopharyngeal cultures with CBC, platelets, pH level, and vital signs WNL.

ACTIONS/INTERVENTIONS	RATIONALE

Independent

Review record of delivery. Note whether resuscitative measures were required, length of rupture of membranes, and presence of chorioamnionitis.	Maternal factors such as PROM with preterm labor and delivery possibly caused by an infectious process predispose the preterm infant to ascending infection. Transplacentally acquired infections (which affect two thirds of all infected infants) are also a threat. Infant who has been resuscitated and has required invasive interventions is especially prone to introduction of pathogens and infection. Early-onset sepsis (occurring within the first 2 days of life) is affected by host defenses and duration of antepartal rupture of membranes.
Determine gestational age of fetus using Dubowitz criteria.	Delivery prior to 28 to 30 weeks' gestation increases infant's susceptibility to infection, because of reduced ability of WBCs to destroy bacteria, reduced transfer of immunoglobulin G (IgG is transported across the placenta primarily in the third trimester), lack of immunoglobulin A (IgA) if infant does not receive breast milk, and poorly keratinized skin with ineffective barrier qualities. (Note: Infant who suffers from intrauterine growth retardation is at greater risk for infection.)
Promote meticulous handwashing by staff, parents, and ancillary workers per protocol. Use antiseptic before assisting with surgical or invasive procedure.	Handwashing is the most important practice for preventing cross-contamination and controlling infection in the nursery.
Monitor staff and visitors for presence of skin lesions, draining wounds, acute respiratory infections, fever, gastroenteritis, active herpes simplex (oral, genital, or paronychial), and herpes zoster.	Transmission of disease to neonate by employees or visitors can occur directly or indirectly.
Provide adequate space between infants or between isolettes or individual units. Use separate isolation rooms and isolation technique as indicated.	Providing 4–6 ft of space between infants helps prevent spread of droplet or airborne infections.
Assess infant for signs of infection, such as temperature instability (hypothermia or hyperthermia), lethargy or behavior changes, respiratory distress (apnea, cyanosis, or tachypnea), jaundice, petechiae, nasal congestion, or drainage from eyes or umbilicus.	Useful in the diagnosis of infection; body temperature alone is an unreliable means of assessing infection in the preterm infant with impaired inflammatory response and WBC mobilization.
Establish a cohort of infants, when possible, and ensure that same nurse cares for the infants grouped together.	Infants who are born within the same time frame (usually 24 to 48 hours), or who are colonized/infected with the same pathogen, may be grouped together until discharge. Such grouping is an important measure in infection control in that it limits the amount of contact of one infant with other susceptible infants or personnel.
Perform care of umbilical cord according to hospital protocol.	Local application of alcohol, triple dye, and various antimicrobials helps prevent colonization.

ACTIONS/INTERVENTIONS	RATIONALE

Independent

Prepare site(s) of invasive procedures with alcohol (70%), tincture of iodine, or iodophor. Monitor intravenous infusion site(s) and sites of invasive monitoring lines per protocol.

Reduces incidence of possible phlebitis or bacteremia.

Use aseptic technique during suctioning. Date the opened solution for humidification, irrigation, or nebulization, and discard after 24 hours. Ensure routine cleaning or replacement of respiratory equipment.

Reduces opportunity for introduction of bacteria that could result in respiratory infection.

Treat arterial line, stopcocks, and catheter as sterile fields; draw all blood specimens at the same time.

Helps prevent bacteriemia associated with arterial line and its direct access to blood and deep tissues.

Monitor infant for signs of late-onset disease or infection.

Late-onset disease may occur as early as the fifth day, but it usually occurs after the first week of life. Signs of late-onset infection are likely to be caused by bacteria acquired from the maternal genital tract, or from human contact or contaminated equipment/supplies after birth.

Observe for signs of shock or disseminated intravascular coagulation (DIC), such as bradycardia, decreasing BP, temperature instability, listlessness, edema, or erythema of abdominal wall.

DIC may occur with gram-negative septicemia.

Provide breast milk for feeding, if available.

Breast milk contains IgA, macrophages, lymphocytes, and neutrophils, which provide some protection from infection.

Collaborative

Obtain specimens, as indicated (e.g., urine through suprapubic aspiration, blood, CSF, visible skin lesions, nasopharynx, or sputum if infant is intubated).

Cultures/sensitivity tests are necessary to diagnose pathogens and identify appropriate therapy.

Monitor laboratory studies, as indicated:

Serial WBC count and differential.

Prematurity reduces the immune response to infection. WBC count in preterm infant varies from 6,000 to 225,000/mm^3 and may change from day to day, limiting diagnostic reliability. A marked and sudden increase or decrease in WBCs or band cells may suggest infection.

Platelet count.

Sepsis causes platelet count to drop, but in the preterm infant, the normal platelet range may be 60,000 (in the first 3 days) to 100,000/mm^3.

Serum glucose and pH levels.

Hypoglycemia, hyperglycemia, or metabolic acidosis (with bicarbonate levels less than 21 mEq/L) suggests infection.

Administer antibiotics intravenously based on sensitivity reports.

Broad-spectrum antibiotic coverage with ampicillin and an amnioglycoside is usually initiated, pending results of culture and sensitivity tests. In-

Collaborative

discriminate or inappropriate use of systemic antibiotics may cause undesirable side effects, foster emergence of resistant bacterial strains, and alter the newborn's normal flora.

Assist with lumbar puncture, as needed.

Helps identify organism and site of infection when meningitis is suspected.

Assist with treatment for possible conditions associated with infection; e.g., hypoxemia, thermal abnormalities, electrolyte and acid-base imbalances, anemia, or shock.

Associated physiologic events and sequelae may be as life-threatening to the infant as the infection itself.

Administer intravenous immunoglobulin as appropriate.

Research suggests I.V. Ig may increase survival rates in septic infants. Additionally, prophylactic therapy for infants weighing less than 1500 g may reduce incidence of late-onset nosocomial infections.

NURSING DIAGNOSIS:	FLUID VOLUME EXCESS, HIGH RISK FOR
Risk factors may include:	Immature renal system and reduced glomerular filtration rate (inability to concentrate urine; to maintain acid-base, fluid, and electrolyte homeostasis; and to metabolize and excrete drugs).
Possibly evidenced by:	[Not applicable; presence of signs/symptoms establishes an **actual** diagnosis.]
DESIRED OUTCOMES— NEONATE WILL:	Maintain urine specific gravity, output, and pH WNL.

ACTIONS/INTERVENTIONS

RATIONALE

Independent

Monitor urine output, preferably by weighing diapers, or by assessing diaper saturation and number of diapers used per day. Measure urine specific gravity.

Output should be 1–3 ml/kg/hr and specific gravity should be 1.006 to 1.013. Hypovolemia and anuria or oliguria may follow severe hypoxia.

Calculate fluid balance (total intake minus total output) every 8 hr, and weigh infant per protocol.

Positive fluid balance and corresponding weight gain in excess of 20–30 g/day suggest fluid excess.

Evaluate hydration, noting presence of crackles, rhonchi, dyspnea, or tachypnea.

Limited ability of kidneys to excrete excess fluid increases risks of overhydration with cardiac or respiratory involvement.

Note presence, location, and degree of edema.

Excessive edema compromises circulatory and kidney volume as fluid shifts from plasma to tissues.

Institute measures to prevent infection. (Refer to ND: Infection, high risk for.)

Infection places increased demands on an already-compromised renal system.

ACTIONS/INTERVENTIONS	RATIONALE
Collaborative	
Monitor laboratory studies, as indicated:	
Electrolyte and pH levels.	Acidosis and altered electrolyte levels suggest renal inability to maintain homeostasis.
Blood urea nitrogen, creatinine, and uric acid levels.	Assesses severity of kidney involvement.
Provide feedings using breast milk, if possible; assure proper amount and concentration of supplemental formula.	Human milk contains less renal solute than does cow's milk. Kidney may be unable to handle formula with excess concentration of solute.
Correct fluid, electrolyte, and acid-base disturbances; correct hypoxic states.	Treatment may be necessary to restore glomerular filtration rate and renal blood flow following periods of hypoxia with lactic acid accumulation. Administration of sodium bicarbonate may be necessary, because buffering capacity of kidney predisposes preterm infant to metabolic acidosis.
Monitor infant for drug toxicity, especially if infant is receiving gentamicin or nafcillin.	Kidney immaturity inhibits or retards drug excretion, so that in the preterm infant, toxicity can occur more quickly and at lower levels than in the full-term infant.

NURSING DIAGNOSIS:	**CONSTIPATION, HIGH RISK FOR; DIARRHEA, HIGH RISK FOR**
Risk factors may include:	Dietary/fluid intake, physical inactivity, weak abdominal musculature, altered gastric motility.
Possibly evidenced by:	[Not applicable; presence of signs/symptoms establishes an **actual** diagnosis.]
DESIRED OUTCOMES— NEONATE WILL:	Establish customary bowel habits, dependent on type of feeding, with abdomen soft and nondistended.
	Be free of signs of necrotizing enterocolitis.

ACTIONS/INTERVENTIONS	RATIONALE
Independent	
Consider frequency and characteristics of stool in relation to infant's age and type of feeding. Auscultate bowel sounds. Measure abdominal girth, reporting any increase of 1 cm or more from previous measurement.	Decreased bowel functioning and GI motility result in infrequent stools and abdominal distention.
Note presence of risk factors, such as hypoxia, sepsis, or circulatory problems associated with PDA. (Refer to NDs: Gas Exchange, impaired; Infection, high risk for.)	These conditions can contribute to development of necrotizing enterocolitis. Recent findings suggest that the development of necrotizing enterocolitis is related to developmental and gestational age.

539

ACTIONS/INTERVENTIONS	RATIONALE

Independent

Assess hydration status and fluid intake and output. (Refer to NDs: Fluid Volume deficit, high risk for; Nutrition, altered, less than body requirements, high risk for.)

Inadequate hydration may contribute to dry or constipated stool.

Monitor for signs of necrotizing enterocolitis, such as abdominal distention, rigidity, or tenderness; shiny or taut abdominal skin; visible bowel loops; excessive spitting up, bile-stained emesis; failure of gavage feedings to be absorbed or excessive gastric residual; and absence of bowel sounds. Test stools (unless bloody diarrhea is present) using Hematest or guaiac. Test gastric residual.

Necrotizing enterocolitis is a potentially life-threatening complication that affects 3%–8% of preterm infants, usually presenting within the first 2 weeks of life.

Minimize handling of infant; provide stroking of face, hands, and feet. Talk to infant.

Avoids further abdominal trauma. Emotional and stroking needs can be met through touching extremities and head and through conversation.

Avoid use of diapers and rectal thermometers.

Diapers increase lower abdominal pressure and prevent or restrict observation of abdomen. Rectal thermometers may cause trauma to rectal mucosa.

Monitor infant for signs of sepsis, shock, or DIC (e.g., bradycardia, decreasing BP, temperature instability, listlessness, and edema or erythema of abdominal wall.)

Necrotizing enterocolitis can progress to bowel perforation with peritonitis, resulting in sepsis, shock, and DIC.

Maintain strict policy of handwashing after handling each infant.

Helps prevent an epidemic of necrotizing enterocolitis from occurring in the nursery.

Collaborative

Use breast milk for feedings whenever possible.

Breast milk is easily digested, produces softer stool, and may reduce risk of enteric infections or development of necrotizing enterocolitis.

Increase dilution of supplemental formula as indicated.

Diarrhea may indicate intolerance to formula concentration.

Monitor laboratory studies, as indicated; e.g., WBC count and differential, platelet count, prothrombin time, and partial thromboplastin time.

Increased or decreased WBC count or a shift to the left suggests sepsis. Thrombocytopenia or prolonged clotting times may indicate developing DIC.

Review abdominal x-rays.

Presence of distended loops of bowel, thickened walls, and ascites reflects necrotizing enterocolitis.

Send initial bloody or positive Hematest stool to the laboratory.

Alum precipitated toxoid test is required to differentiate infant from maternal blood.

Discontinue oral or NG feedings for 7 to 10 days, as indicated. Provide TPN feedings.

Allows the bowel to rest, promoting tissue healing while meeting fluid and nutritional needs.

Insert orogastric or NG tube, and connect to continuous low suction, as needed.

May be necessary for gastric decompression in cases of suspected necrotizing enterocolitis or following surgical intervention.

540

ACTIONS/INTERVENTIONS

Collaborative

Administer antibiotics, as indicated.

Prepare for surgery, if needed.

RATIONALE

Combat enteric infection; may promote healing of bowel.

Operative procedure may be necessary to remove segments of inflamed bowel.

NURSING DIAGNOSIS:	SKIN INTEGRITY, IMPAIRED, HIGH RISK FOR
Risk factors may include:	Thin skin, fragile capillaries near the skin surface, absence of subcutaneous fat over bony prominences, inability to change positions to relieve pressure points, use of restraints (protecting invasive lines/tubes), alterations in nutritional state.
Possibly evidenced by:	[Not applicable; presence of signs/symptoms establishes an **actual** diagnosis.]
DESIRED OUTCOMES— NEONATE WILL:	Maintain intact skin. Be free of dermal injury.

ACTIONS/INTERVENTIONS

Independent

Inspect skin, noting areas of redness or pressure.

Provide mouth care using saline or glycerin swabs. Apply petroleum jelly to lips.

Avoid application of harsh topical agents; carefully wash off povidone-iodine solutions after procedures.

Provide range-of-motion exercises, routine position changes, and fleece or flotation pad.

Minimize use of tape to secure tubes, electrodes, urine bags, I.V. lines, and so forth.

Bathe infant using sterile water and mild soap. Wash only grossly soiled body parts. Minimize manipulation of infant's skin.

Change electrodes only when necessary.

RATIONALE

Identifies areas of potential dermal breakdown, which can result in sepsis. (Refer to ND: Infection, high risk for.)

Helps prevent drying and cracking of lips associated with absence of oral intake or the drying effects of oxygen therapy.

Helps prevent skin breakdown and loss of protective epidermal barrier.

Helps prevent possible necrosis related to edema of dermis or lack of subcutaneous fat over bony prominences.

Removal of tape may accidentally remove epidermal layer, because cohesion is stronger between tape and stratum corneum than between dermis and epidermis.

After 4 days, skin develops some bactericidal properties due to acid pH. Frequent bathing using alkaline soaps or moisturizers may raise skin pH, compromising normal flora and natural defense mechanisms that protect against invading pathogens.

Frequent changing may contribute to skin breakdown.

ACTIONS/INTERVENTIONS

Collaborative

Apply antibiotic ointment to nares, mouth and lips if they are cracked or irritated.

RATIONALE

Promotes healing of cracking and irritation associated with administration of oxygen; may help prevent infection.

NURSING DIAGNOSIS:	SENSORY-PERCEPTUAL ALTERATIONS
May be related to:	Immaturity of neurosensory system, altered environmental stimuli (excessive/insufficient), effects of therapies.
Possibly evidenced by:	Changes in response to stimuli, apathy, irritability, change in muscle tension, measured change in sensory acuity.
DESIRED OUTCOMES—NEONATE WILL:	Respond appropriately to age-specific stimulation.
	Be free of signs of sensory overload.
	Demonstrate expected response to visual stimuli, free of signs of retinopathy of prematurity (ROP).

ACTIONS/INTERVENTIONS

Independent

Provide a primary nurse for each shift. (Assign one primary nurse per baby to provide information to parents.)

RATIONALE

Promotes continuity of care and follow-through with developmental program. Enhances recognition of subtle changes in infant's behavior and condition. Having one nurse responsible for giving information helps to reduce instances of parents' being uninformed or misunderstanding.

Change infant's position frequently (especially if infant has nasal CPAP or endotracheal tube).

Provides kinesthetic stimulation. Neuromuscularly immature infant is unable to reposition self or move about in the isolette.

Provide gentle stroking and caressing, especially at feeding time, introducing textures (tongue blade, washcloth), as appropriate.

Provides tactile stimulation, which is associated with weight gains and is especially critical when infant is 40 weeks' post conception or more. (Note: Slow, sure movements provide stimulation while reducing motor disorganization.)

Talk or sing to infant, call infant by name, play soft music in nursery, or play a tape of parent(s) voice.

Provides auditory stimulation. Playing tape of parents' voices may enhance infant's recognition of them.

Hold infant at face level, allowing eye contact. Provide colorful linens and changing designs or pictures on side of incubator, and encourage parents to make mobiles of construction paper and string once infant reaches post conception age of 40 weeks.

Visual stimulation is best provided by objects placed 7–9 inches from face. Black and white faces and a checkerboard design promote visual attention. Infant may become habituated to stimuli that does not change. Involving parents in creating stimuli for infant helps ensure that the process continues after discharge.

Hold infant in ventral position (e.g., baby held to shoulder to burp) when possible.

Stimulates visual orientation.

Assess infant for physiologic signs of sensory overload (e.g., apnea, color change, or bradycardia).

Overstimulation can result in physiologic changes.

ACTIONS/INTERVENTIONS	RATIONALE

Independent

Minimize social interaction stimuli other than those directly related to feeding if infant displays signs of sensory overload. Reduce stimuli prior to feedings.

Excessive stimulation may interfere with feeding, so that the necessary stimuli must be provided between feedings. Overstimulation prior to feedings may negatively affect sucking and GI motility and may cause vomiting or regurgitation.

Plan activities to allow periods of sleep. Prevent sudden position changes or loud noises, and reduce light intermittently by covering incubator with towel and/or by lowering room lighting.

Helps protect infant from overstimulation, which can negatively affect growth and physiologic status; promotes infant's sense of the day-night cycle. (Note: Research reveals cycled lighting lowers infant's heart rate and motor activity, promoting longer periods of quiet inactivity resembling quiet sleep and conserving energy.)

Uncover eyes periodically if infant is receiving phototherapy.

Protective eye patches needed in phototherapy severely reduce the opportunity for visual stimulation.

Assess infant's response to stimuli. Create individualized pattern of intervention based on infant's developmental age and needs.

Each infant responds uniquely to a pattern of interventions based on individual needs.

Weigh infant daily. Note feeding frequency and intake and frequency of stools.

Vagal stimulation produced by appropriate tactile and kinesthetic stimulation promotes weight gain, increases peristalsis and expulsion of waste products, reduces gastric retention, and increases feeding activity.

Measure head circumference.

Cerebral cortex is thought to increase in weight in response to stimulation in environment, and this increase, which continues into the later postnatal period, may enhance cognitive and intellectual development.

Note risk factors of birth weight, coexisting conditions, and associated therapies.

Retinopathy of prematurity is no longer believed to be exclusively the result of prolonged/high levels of oxygen therapy. Immaturity, presence of some congenital anomalies, and various therapies place the infant at risk. (Note: Infants with birth weight less than 1,000 g have an 88% incidence of retinopathy.)

Provide information to parent(s) regarding condition, prognosis, and infant's individual needs/responses.

Reduces anxiety/fears associated with unknowns, enhancing coping and problem-solving abilities. Awareness that visually impaired infant may not show recognition or feelings by changes in facial expression encourages parent(s) to observe body language/other cues reflecting self-expression, thereby strengthening the attachment bond.

Provide/encourage increased use of auditory and tactile stimulation.

Maintaining adequate and appropriate early stimulation may limit future cognitive and emotional problems related to environmental issues, including understimulation and parental responses/overprotectiveness.

ACTIONS/INTERVENTIONS	RATIONALE

Collaborative

ACTIONS/INTERVENTIONS	RATIONALE
Provide rocking or water beds, if indicated.	This kind of stimulation in preterm infants of less than 34 weeks' gestation has been shown to increase head size and biparietal diameter.
Monitor oxygen therapy closely, adjusting level and/or limiting duration as appropriate.	Helps prevent or limit development of retinopathy of prematurity. (Note: The retina has an immature vascular system that is susceptible to damage leading to vaso-obliteration. New vessels that are developing may rupture, creating retinal and vitreous hemorrhage leading to formation of scar tissue.)
Assist with procedures as needed:	
Indirect ophthalmoscopic fundal exam.	Recommended for all infants less than 36 weeks' gestation or under 2000 g and receiving oxygen therapy. Usually done between 4 and 8 weeks of age and repeated as indicated to diagnose/monitor progression of retinopathy of prematurity and determine therapy needs.
Laser therapy or cryotherapy.	May be useful in limiting adverse effects associated with acute stages of retinopathy of prematurity by obliterating newly forming vessels, reducing traction on the retina and subsequent detachment.

NURSING DIAGNOSIS:	**COPING, INDIVIDUAL, INEFFECTIVE**
May be related to:	Immaturity and/or CNS damage (low threshold for painful stimuli and stress), poor organizational ability, limited ability to control environment.
Possibly evidenced by:	Disorganized motor activity and sleep-wake cycles, irritability, inability to convey appropriate cues to caregiver so that stressors can be reduced or eliminated.
DESIRED OUTCOMES— NEONATE WILL:	Minimize/reduce behavioral cues indicating stress.
	Progress appropriately, according to individual pattern in growth and development.

ACTIONS/INTERVENTIONS	RATIONALE

Independent

ACTIONS/INTERVENTIONS	RATIONALE
Provide primary caregiver whenever possible.	Consistent and predictable care enables infant to develop trust in caregiver, environment, and self and facilitates coping. Multiple caretakers confuse the infant, increase distress during feeding, cause irritability, and upset visual attention.
Assess infant for behavioral cues indicating stress, noting causative factors and eliminating or reducing stressors when possible.	Familiarity with the infant's usual behavioral responses and personality traits is necessary for identifying subtle changes that indicate stress and the need for intervention to reduce such stress.

ACTIONS/INTERVENTIONS	RATIONALE

Independent

Create uterine-like atmosphere whenever possible by covering isolette for extended periods and playing recorded placental or maternal heart sounds.	Providing dark, quiet environment reduces stress, promotes adaptation, and has been found to correlate positively with weight gain, early weaning from oxygen or ventilators, and earlier discharge. Recorded maternal heart sounds tend to reduce or eliminate infant's perception of noise from the isolette.
Reposition infant using rolled diapers placed at the back and front if infant is in lateral position or at sides if infant can tolerate a prone position.	Neuromuscular immaturity can impair infant's ability to seek a position of comfort or to relieve stress through repositioning. Rolled diapers surrounding baby provide a sense of security and have a calming effect. Prone position promotes sleep and optimal relaxation.
Cover top of radiant warmer with plastic wrap, if appropriate.	Reduces environmental stress from air currents, which startle the infant as personnel move past the warmer.
Provide parents with information about infant's behavioral cues and responses to stressors. (Refer to ND: Sensory-Perceptual Alterations; Chapter 6, CP: The Parents of a Child With Special Needs, ND: Parenting, altered, high risk for.)	Parents must gain skill in recognizing subtle infant cues indicating stress so that they can effectively intervene to minimize stress and facilitate the infant's positive adaptation to extrauterine life.

Newborn: Deviations in Growth Patterns _____

Deviations in intrauterine growth patterns not only increase the risk of morbidity and mortality in the early newborn period, but may also have long-term implications for altered growth and development and for altered central nervous system (CNS) function and learning disabilities in childhood. This general plan of care is designed to facilitate optimal nursing management of the infant with deviations in intrauterine growth and is to be used in conjunction with the CPs: The Neonate at 2 Hours to 3 Days of Age and The Preterm Infant, as appropriate. The following are definitions for the terms small for gestational age/intrauterine growth retardation (SGA/IUGR), and large for gestational age (LGA).

SGA/IUGR—Any newborn whose birth weight falls at or below the 10th percentile on classification charts considering local factors (e.g., ethnicity, altitude).

LGA/macrosomic—Any newborn whose birth weight is at or above the 90th percentile on classification charts considering local population at any week in gestation or who at birth weighs more than 4000 g (8 lbs 13 oz).

NEONATAL ASSESSMENT DATA BASE

SGA Infant

ACTIVITY/REST

Activity level may be excessive with vigorous cry/hungry suck attributable to chronic intrauterine hypoxia.

ELIMINATION

Abdomen may appear scaphoid or concave.

FOOD/FLUID

All body parts may be below expected size for gestational age but in proportion/symmetric to each other (suggests a chronic or prolonged problem throughout gestation).

Disproportionate weight as compared to length and head circumference (appears long and thin with normal head circumference) suggests episodic vascular insufficiency in third trimester.

Dry, cracked and peeling skin present, with loose skin folds and absence of subcutaneous tissue.

Decreased muscle mass, especially in the cheeks, buttocks, and thighs.

May demonstrate metabolic instability associated with hypoglycemia/hypocalcemia.

NEUROSENSORY

Sparse scalp hair.

Skull suture and fontanels appear widened; bulging of fontanels due to inadequate bone growth may be evident.

Small head with protruding forehead, sunken nasal bridge, short upturned nose, thin upper lip, receding chin (indicative of fetal alcohol syndrome [FAS]).

Muscle tone may appear tight with flexion of upper and lower extremities, minor joint/limb abnormalities, and restricted movement (suggest FAS).

Wide-eyed appearance (associated with chronic hypoxia in utero).

RESPIRATION

Signs of respiratory distress may be present, especially in presence of meconium aspiration syndrome.

Mucus may be green tinged.

SAFETY

Meconium staining may be evident with greenish stains on fingernails and at base of umbilical cord.

Umbilical cord may have single artery and/or be thin, slightly yellow, dull, dry.

Congenital anomalies/malformations or infection may be present.

SEXUALITY

Higher incidence in females.

TEACHING/LEARNING

May be premature (and/or member of multifetus pregnancy).

MATERNAL FACTORS RESULTING IN SGA INFANT

CIRCULATION

Resides at high altitude.

Heart/lung disease; bleeding, severe anemia or sickle cell anemia; chronic hypertension or pregnancy-induced hypertension.

ELIMINATION

Pyelonephritis, chronic renal disease.

FOOD/FLUID

Small stature.

Advanced diabetes mellitus (Class D or above); malnutrition (chronic or during third trimester); phenylketonuria (PKU).

RESPIRATION

Heavy smoker.

SAFETY

Collagen disease; maternal infections such as rubella, syphilis, cytomegalovirus, toxoplasmosis; uterine tumors.

Irradiation and use of medications with teratogenic side effects (antimetabolites, anticonvulsants, trimethiadone).

SEXUALITY

Adolescent or advanced maternal age (younger than age 16 or older than age 40).

Primiparity, grand multiparity.

Placenta previa/separation, insufficiency, infarction, fibrosis, thrombosis, hemangioma, abnormal cord insertion and single umbilical artery with vascular anastomoses (twin-to-twin).

Chromosomal abnormalities, chronic intrauterine infections, congenital anomalies, multifetal pregnancy, inborn errors of metabolism.

SOCIAL INTERACTION

Low socioeconomic class.

Poor education.

Alcoholism, drug abuse.

Lack of prenatal care.

LGA Infant

CIRCULATION

Skin color ruddy (associated with polycythemia), jaundice (indicative of hyperbilirubinemia).

May have congenital anomalies such as transposition of the great vessels, Beckwith-Wiedemann syndrome, or erythroblastosis fetalis.

FOOD/FLUID

Macrosomia, excess fat deposits and reddened complexion, increased body size proportional (except in infant of diabetic mother, [IDM] whose weight may appear disproportionately large for length).

May demonstrate metabolic instability associated with hypoglycemia/hypocalcemia.

Weight may be 4000 g (8 lbs 13 oz) or more (dependent on gestational age).

NEUROSENSORY

Large amount of scalp hair.

RESPIRATION

Signs of respiratory distress may be present if stress of delivery has induced meconium aspiration/asphyxiation, or if delivered by cesarean section.

SAFETY

Birth injury(s) may be present; e.g. bruising, caput succedaneum, cephalhematomas; facial/phrenic nerve paralysis, brachial palsy; fractured clavicles, intracranial bleeding/depressed skull fracture(s); bulging fontanel indicative of neurologic problems, depressed fontanel suggestive of dehydration.

Intrapartal/delivery events may reveal fetal distress, meconium-stained amniotic fluid, oligohydramnios, late/variable decelerations, scalp pH levels less than 7.20, resuscitative measures if post-date infant.

Evidence of congenital malformations may involve the heart, CNS, kidney, lungs, gastrointestinal (GI) tract.

Long, hard nails extending beyond ends of toes and fingers.

Absence of vernix caseosa/lanugo, desquamation or epidermis.

SEXUALITY

Higher incidence in males.

TEACHING/LEARNING

May be preterm/post-term by clinical assessment.

May be post-term (42 weeks or more) due to postconceptional bleeding leading to a miscalculation of dates/prolonged pregnancy associated with menstrual cycle longer than 28 days.

MATERNAL FACTORS RESULTING IN LGA INFANT
FOOD/FLUID

Inappropriate/overnutrition, weight gain greater than 35 lb.

Large stature.

Diabetes mellitus (Class A, B, or C).

SEXUALITY

Birth of previous LGA infant.

Cesarean birth due to cephalopelvic disproportion or oxytocin-induced labor related to diabetes/fetal distress/prolonged pregnancy.

Multiparity.

DIAGNOSTIC STUDIES

Dextrostix glucose estimations: Less than 40 mg/dl in LGA infant or 25 mg/dl in SGA infant during first 3 days indicates hypoglycemia.

Serum glucose: Verifies Dextrostix value less than 40 mg/dl in LGA infant, less than 25 mg/dl in SGA infant.

Chest x-ray and arterial blood gases (ABGs): Determines cause/severity of respiratory distress if present.

Complete blood count (CBC): May reveal central venous hematocrit (Hct) elevated above 65%, central venous hemoglobin (Hb) 20 g/dl associated with polycythemia/hyperviscosity.

White blood cell count: May be elevated /depressed.

Platelet count: May be depressed if mother was preeclamptic or if infant was born with a congenital viral infection.

Coagulation studies (prothrombin time [PT], partial thromboplastin time [PTT], fibrinogen, fibrin split products [FSP]): May indicate disseminated intravascular coagulation (DIC), especially in the polycythemic or asphyxiated infant.

Blood type for ABO group, Rh factor and cross match: Plasma exchange may be necessary if Rh incompatibility exists.

Serum electrolytes (including ionized calcium): Assesses for hypocalcemia (level 7 mg/dl [3.5 mEq/L] or less in first 3 days of life); inappropriate antidiuretic hormone secretion, and instability related to metabolic complications.

Bilirubin: May be elevated secondary to polycythemia and resorption of bleeding associated with birth injury; e.g., intracranial hemorrhage, cephalhematoma.

Urinalysis on/after second voided specimen, including specific gravity and sugar/acetone: Assesses homeostasis.

Bacterial and viral cultures: Rule out/diagnose infection.

Electrocardiography, echocardiography, ultrasonography, angiography, and genetic studies: As appropriate with suspected FAS, congenital defects, and/or complications.

NURSING PRIORITIES

1. Maintain physiologic homeostasis.
2. Prevent and/or treat complications.
3. Identify/minimize effects of birth trauma.
4. Provide family with appropriate information/strategies for meeting short- and long-term problems associated with growth deviation.

NURSING DIAGNOSIS:	**GAS EXCHANGE, IMPAIRED**
May be related to:	Alveolar capillary membrane changes (decreased surfactant levels, retained pulmonary fluid, meconium aspiration), altered oxygen supply (diaphragmatic paralysis/phenic nerve paralysis, increased intracranial pressure).
Possibly evidenced by:	Restlessness/irritability, inability to move secretions, tachypnea, cyanosis, hypoxia.
DESIRED OUTCOMES— NEWBORN WILL:	Display spontaneous, unassisted regular respiratory effort with rate of 30–50/min; and ABGs within normal limits (WNL). Be free of apnea and complications of hypoxia/lung disease.

ACTIONS/INTERVENTIONS	RATIONALE
Independent	
Review history for abnormal prenatal growth patterns and/or reduced amounts of amniotic fluid, as detected by ultrasonography/fundal changes.	Low-birth-weight infant or infant with IUGR suffers chronic intrauterine asphyxia, resulting in hypoxia/malnutrition. Fetal contribution to the amniotic pool is reduced in the stressed infant. Macrosomia can be related to maternal diabetes, prolonged pregnancy, heredity, and inappropriate nutrition. Macrosomia in IDM results from excess release of growth hormone (thyroid stimulation), increasing the number of cells and/or organ size throughout the body.
Note type of delivery and intrapartal events indicative of hypoxia.	Infant with chronic hypoxia will be more susceptible to acidosis/respiratory depression/persistent fetal circulation (PFC) after delivery. Cesarean delivery increases risk of excess mucus because thoracic compression by the birth canal does not occur as in a vaginal delivery.
Note time/onset of breathing and Apgar scores. Observe ensuing respiratory patterns.	The infant with intrapartal asphyxia may present with a delayed onset of respirations and altered respiratory pattern. Apgar scores aid in evaluation of the degree of depression or asphyxia of the newborn at birth and are directly correlated with serum pH/degree of infant acidosis.
Assess respiratory rate, depth, effort. Observe and report signs and symptoms of respiratory distress, distinguishing from symptoms associated with polycythemia.	Infant with altered growth is more susceptible to respiratory distress associated with chronic asphyxia in SGA infant, inadequate surfactant levels in IDM, perinatal asphyxia, aspiration of meconium or amniotic fluid, and PFC. Diminished lung compliance may occur as a result of polycythemia.
Auscultate breath sounds regularly.	Presence of crackles/rhonchi reflect respiratory congestion and need for intervention.

ACTIONS/INTERVENTIONS	RATIONALE
Independent	
Suction nasopharynx/endotracheal tube as needed, after first providing supplemental oxygen.	Ensures patency of airway, removes excess mucus. Supplemental oxygen reduces hypoxic effect of procedure.
Auscultate apical pulse; note presence of cyanosis.	Tachypnea, bradycardia, and cyanosis may occur in response to altered oxygen levels.
Prevent iatrogenic complications associated with cold stress, metabolic imbalance, and caloric insufficiency.	Such complications increase metabolic demands and oxygen needs.
Ensure availability of resources in the event complications occur.	Equipment for oxygenation, suction, intubation, assisted ventilation, resuscitation, and chest tube placement must be readily available in the event of severe/prolonged respiratory distress.
Collaborative	
Monitor transcutaneous oxygen/pulse oximeter readings.	Identifies therapy needs/effectiveness.
Monitor laboratory studies, as indicated:	
Serum pH.	Detects possible metabolic acidosis occurring from inadequate oxygen intake/respiratory acidosis and anaerobic metabolism with acid end products. (Note: Normal values range from 7.35–7.44.)
ABGs.	Indicate degree of hypoxia/hypercapnia, as well as therapy needs/effectiveness. (Note: Normal newborn arterial Po_2 ranges from 60–80 mm Hg, arterial Pco_2 from 30–37 mm Hg.
Hct.	Polycythemia, which occurs in 50% of SGA infants related to excess red blood cell (RBC) production in response to chronic intrauterine hypoxia, typically increases capillary/venous Hct levels to greater than 60%, with resultant respiratory distress associated with diminished lung compliance.
Administer warm, humidified oxygen; provide assisted ventilation as indicated.	Corrects/prevents hypoxemia, hypercapnia, and respiratory acid-base imbalances.
Review chest x-rays.	May confirm meconium aspiration pneumonia, common in SGA or post-term infant, or respiratory distress syndrome, in IDM.
Provide chest physiotherapy as indicated.	Percussion and postural drainage promote mobilization of secretions, enhancing airway patency and gas exchange, especially in the presence of meconium aspiration. (Note: Contraindicated in preterm infant.)
Administer medications as indicated:	
Sodium bicarbonate.	Corrects metabolic imbalances/acidosis resulting from prolonged respiratory acidosis.
Xanthine derivatives; e.g., aminopylline (theophylline ethylenediamine).	Sympathomimetic bronchodilators may be useful in treating apnea of prematurity.

ACTIONS/INTERVENTIONS	RATIONALE
Collaborative	
Tolazolme HCl (Priscoline).	Potent vasodilator that relaxes smooth muscle to maximize circulatory effort/oxygenation in cases of meconium aspiration/PFC.
Dopamine.	Counteracts hypotensive effect of Priscoline administration.

NURSING DIAGNOSIS:	**NUTRITION, ALTERED, LESS THAN BODY REQUIREMENTS**
May be related to:	Decreased nutritional stores, increased insulin production and/or hyperplasia of the pancreatic beta cells.
Possibly evidenced by:	Weight deviation from expected, decreased muscle mass/fat stores, electrolyte imbalance.
DESIRED OUTCOMES— NEWBORN WILL:	Ingest adequate nutritional intake for weight gain (or weight loss less than 2%).
	Display serum glucose WNL.
PARENT(S) WILL:	Identify/treat/prevent short- and long-term complications of malnutrition.

ACTIONS/INTERVENTIONS	RATIONALE
Independent	
Assess weight in relation to gestational age and size. Document on growth chart. Weigh daily.	Identifies presence, degree, and risk of altered growth pattern. LGA infant with excess extracellular fluid is likely to lose up to 15% of birth weight. SGA infant may have already lost weight in utero or may suffer from reduced fat/glycogen stores.
Maintain thermoneutral environment, including use of incubator/radiant warmer as indicated. Monitor heat controls/temperature of infant and environment frequently, noting hypothermia or hyperthermia.	The SGA infant does not have adequate adipose tissue for insulation and has a large body surface area compared to body weight. Brown adipose tissue stores may be inadequate to maintain thermoregulation. Both hypothermia and hyperthermia increase metabolic demands, necessitating increased intake in an already-compromised infant. (Note: Thermal instability may be iatrogenically induced by improperly operated heating equipment used to maintain thermogenesis in dysmature infant.) (Refer to CP: The Preterm Infant, ND: Thermoregulation, ineffective.)
Initiate early and frequent feedings and advance as tolerated.	Assists in maintaining fluid/electrolyte balance and meeting caloric needs to support metabolic process. Helps prevent hypoglycemia associated with inadequate body stores in SGA infant or continued pancreatic secretion of insulin in IDM.

ACTIONS/INTERVENTIONS	RATIONALE

Independent

Assess tolerance to feedings. Note stool color, consistency, and frequency; presence of reducing substances; abdominal girth; vomiting, and gastric residuals.

Advances in amount and caloric composition of feedings are dependent on tolerance. (Note: Poor sucking reflex and recurrent vomiting or persistent regurgitation may be seen in FAS, requiring further evaluation/intervention.) (Refer to CP: The Infant of an Addicted Mother.)

Monitor intake and output. Calculate daily caloric and electrolyte consumption.

Provides information about actual intake in relation to estimated needs for use in readjustment of dietary prescription.

Assess hydration level, noting fontanels, skin turgor, urine specific gravity, condition of mucous membranes, and weight fluctuations.

Increased metabolic demands of the SGA infant may increase fluid requirements. Hyperglycemic states may produce diuresis in the infant. Intravenous administration of fluids may be required to meet increased demands but must be conscientiously managed to avoid fluid excess.

Monitor Dextrostisx levels immediately after birth and routinely until serum glucose is stabilized.

Hypoglycemia may occur after birth due to limited glucose stores in the SGA infant and from hyperplasia/continued release of insulin in the LGA infant. Symptoms in the SGA infant usually appear between 24 and 72 hours of age, but may begin as early as 3 hours or as late as 7 days. Hyperglycemia may result from infusion of solutions containing glucose.

Assess for signs of hypoglycemia; e.g., tachypnea and irregular respirations, apnea, lethargy, flaccidity, cyanosis, temperature fluctuations, diaphoresis, poor feeding, jitteriness, high-pitched cry, tremors, eye-rolling, seizure activity.

Because glucose is a major source of fuel for the brain, deficits may cause permanent CNS damage. Hypoglycemia significantly increases morbidity and mortality, and severity of long-term effects is dependent on duration of such episodes. Untreated symptomatic infants have a higher incidence of neurologic abnormalities and/or lower mean IQ later in childhood than treated infants.

Note signs of hypocalcemia; e.g., neuromuscular irritability (tremors, twitching, seizing, clonus), hypotonia, vomiting, high-pitched cry, cyanosis, apnea, and cardiac dysrhythmias with prolonged Q-T interval.

Peak incidence of early hypocalcemia is during first 48–72 hours of life and is often related to temporary abdominal distension, neonatal hypoparathyroidism in premature infant, or prenatal asphyxia in SGA infant or IDM. Late hypocalcemia (at 6–10 days) may be due to ingestion of milk formulas containing a higher ratio of phosphorus to calcium.

Collaborative

Monitor laboratory studies as indicated:

   Serum glucose.

Hypoglycemia may occur as early as 3 hours after birth in the SGA infant as glycogen reserves are quickly depleted and gluconeogenesis is inadequate due to reduced stores of muscle protein and fat.

ACTIONS/INTERVENTIONS	RATIONALE

Collaborative

Calcium.	Frequency of screening dependent on risk group; i.e., IDM, intrapartal asphyxia, or preterm infants. (Note: Levels less than 7 mg/dl require further evaluation/intervention.)
Sodium, potassium, chloride, phosphorus and magnesium.	Electrolyte instability may be a consequence of deviations in growth, inadequate placental transfer, or altered maternal mineral balance. (Note: Hypomagnesemia/hyperphosphatemia are usually associated with hypocalcemia.)
Blood urea nitrogen, creatinine, serum/urine osmolality, urine electrolytes.	Detects altered kidney function associated with reduced nutrient stores and fluid levels resulting from acute malnutrition/asphyxia.
Triglyceride/cholesterol levels, and liver function tests.	Useful in determining nutritional deficits and therapy needs/effectiveness.
Provide electrolyte supplementation as indicated; e.g., 10% calcium gluconate.	Metabolic instability in the SGA/LGA infant may necessitate supplements to maintain homeostasis, especially calcium, sodium, and occasionally magnesium.
Establish intravascular access as indicated.	Intravenous access allows for fluid and electrolyte administration. Intra-arterial access allows for ease in monitoring laboratory values.
Administer parenteral nutrition.	The severely compromised infant with deviations in intrauterine growth may be unable to consume fluids and nutrients via an enteral route.
Discuss long-term complications of malnutrition in SGA infant and obesity in LGA infant; discuss importance of protein during phase II of brain growth.	Chronic protein deficiencies in the SGA infant make child prone to learning difficulties and cerebral dysfunction, characterized by short attention span, poor fine motor coordination, hyperactivity behavior problems, and speech defects. Excess fat cells in the LGA/macrosomic infant may create life-long problems associated with obesity (e.g., diabetes, cardiovascular disease, stroke). Adequate protein during hyperplasia/hypertrophy phase of brain growth during the first 6 months of life helps to overcome insults that occurred in early gestational period of brain development.

NURSING DIAGNOSIS:	**TISSUE PERFUSION, ALTERED, HIGH RISK FOR**
Risk factors may include:	Interruption of arterial or venous blood flow (hyperviscosity associated with polycythemia).
Possibly evidenced by:	[Not applicable; presence of signs/symptoms establishes an **actual** diagnosis.]
DESIRED OUTCOMES— NEWBORN WILL:	Maintain normal vital signs, with adequate peripheral pulses and Hct WNL.
	Be free of complications associated with polycythemia.

ACTIONS/INTERVENTIONS	RATIONALE

Independent

Note presence of polycythemia.

Polycythemia resulting from increased erythropoietin production in response to chronic intrauterine hypoxia may occur in both the SGA/LGA infant. In many cases, infants of diabetic mothers are polycythemic. Although the pathophysiology of the hyperviscosity is not fully understood, it may be related to decreased extracellular fluid volume or increased bone marrow stimulation associated with hypoxia.

Assess skin color for ruddiness or pallor. Note hyperthermia, respiratory distress, hypertension or hypotension, tachycardia, decreased pulses, oliguria, hematuria, or altered neurologic findings.

Helps detect/prevent possible complications of polycythemia; e.g., myocardial, cerebral, and renal ischemia; cardiopulmonary congestion; hyperbilirubinemia; thromboemboli, and convulsions.

Monitor temperature, intake/output, and urine specific gravity. Note skin turgor, condition of mucous membranes, and fontanels.

Prevention or correction of dehydration decreases the risks of hyperviscosity.

Collaborative

Monitor CBC and bilirubin. Send blood for type, crossmatch, and Rh. (Refer to CP: Newborn: Hyperbilirubinemia.)

Indicates degree of polycythemia/hyperviscosity. Hyperbilirubinemia often results from polycythemia (central Hct is greater than 65%, Hb is greater than 22 g/dl) as excess RBCs break down.

Establish intravascular access, preferably through umbilical catheterization.

Provides for fluid administration to correct hyperviscosity and exchange transfusion if necessary.

Prepare for/assist with exchange transfusion as necessary.

Fresh frozen plasma replaces infant's blood in equal amounts, thereby diluting infant's remaining blood volume. Usually 10% of the infant's blood volume is removed/exchanged at one time.

Monitor for complications of procedure, including transfusion reactions, catheter complications, and hepatitis.

Provides for early detection/intervention.

NURSING DIAGNOSIS:	INJURY, HIGH RISK FOR, multiple factors
Risk factors may include:	Immature immune response, abnormal blood profile, altered growth patterns, delayed CNS/neurologic development.
Possibly evidenced by:	[Not applicable; presence of signs/symptoms establishes an **actual** diagnosis.]
DESIRED OUTCOMES— NEWBORN WILL:	Be free of complications.

ACTIONS/INTERVENTIONS	RATIONALE

Independent

Assess all LGA infants for birth injuries. Note bulging/tense fontanels; muscle spasticity, twitching, or flaccidity; high-pitched, weak, constant cry; tremors or seizure activity; changes in pupil size/reaction; or asymmetric chest movement.

Because of disproportion between fetal size and maternal pelvis, LGA infants have a high incidence of birth injuries/trauma such as increased intracranial pressure (IICP)/CNS damage, cervical/brachial plexus palsy, fractured clavicle/humerus, diaphragmatic paralysis, and cephalhematoma.

Monitor for signs and symptoms of infection (e.g., changes in temperature, color, muscle tone and activity, feeding tolerance, cardiopulmonary status; or presence of petechiae, rash, jaundice).

Poor resistance to infection, cracks in epidermis, and possible exposure to infectious agents in utero place the SGA/post-term infant at risk for infection, which may be life-threatening, especially if not detected in its earliest phases. (Refer to CP: The Preterm Infant, ND: Infection, high risk for.)

Assess for signs of bleeding at invasive sites, in urine/stool, nasogastric drainage, and pulmonary secretions. Note petechiae/bruising, changes in responsiveness/activity level or muscle tone, nystagmus, opisthotonic posturing, or convulsions.

Early recognition promotes timely intervention. Septicemia, congenital syphilis, cytomegalic inclusion disease, and rubella may result in DIC resulting in pulmonary, cerebral, or intraventricular hemorrhage (IVH).

Measure occipital frontal circumference as indicated.

Hydrocephalus may develop following IVH.

Monitor vital signs. Note peripheral capillary refill and color and temperature of skin.

Hypotension, bradycardia, apnea, hypothermia, delayed capillary refill, and pallor reflect developing shock requiring prompt assessment/intervention.

Collaborative

Monitor laboratory studies as indicated:

CBC with differential.

Dropping Hct may reflect hemorrhage; a shift of the differential may suggest infection.

Coagulation studies: PTT/APTT, PT, fibrinogen levels, FSP, platelets.

Alterations in clotting times, presence of FSP reflects developing coagulopathies.

Blood type, crossmatch, and Rh factor.

Blood replacement may be required. Verifies presence, etiology, severity of infectious process.

Bacterial and viral cultures and sensitivities.

Verifies presence, etiology, severity of infectious process.

Provide supplemental oxygen, constant positive airway pressure (CPAP), and/or mechanical ventilation as needed. (Refer to ND: Gas Exchange, impaired.)

Aids in correcting hypoxemia, acidemia, and hypotension; reduces risk of IVH/increased ICP.

Administer antibiotics as indicated. Monitor drug levels routinely. Repeat cultures and sensitivities as indicated.

Treats infections and guides pharmacologic administration/management.

Administer blood products, albumin and coagulants, as necessary.

Replaces losses/enhances circulating volume; may help control bleeding.

Administer anticonvulsants (e.g., phenobarbital) as indicated.

May be necessary to quiet cerebrum and reduce electrical stimuli that precipitate convulsions.

ACTIONS/INTERVENTIONS

Independent

Assist with diagnostic studies as indicated; e.g., lumbar puncture, computerized tomography (CT) scan, or ultrasound scan.

Note presence of conditions that may have long-term sequelae, such as birth injury or CNS damage, which may result in convulsions or altered reflex responses. Refer to appropriate community resources.

RATIONALE

Bloody spinal fluid indicates IVH. Scans are useful in identifying site/extent of cerebral hemorrhage.

Ensures early identification and optimal management of long-term effects of injury. Fetal malnutrition/hypoxia play a significant role in late or subnormal CNS functioning.

NURSING DIAGNOSIS:	SENSORY-PERCEPTUAL ALTERATIONS
May be related to:	Functional limitations related to growth deviations (restricting neonate's opportunity to seek out, recognize, and interpret stimuli), therapeutically restricted environments (incubator, special care nursery), neurologic complications, electrolyte imbalance, and psychologic stress.
Possibly evidenced by:	Changes in or decreased response to stimuli, apathy, irritability, change in muscle tension.
DESIRED OUTCOMES—NEWBORN WILL:	Respond appropriately to age-specific stimulation. Be free of signs of sensory overload.
PARENT(S) WILL:	Identify/minimize sensory overload and/or deprivation.

ACTIONS/INTERVENTIONS

Independent

Assess infant's capacity for stimulation, noting behavioral responses involving gross and fine motor movement, presence of irritability, restlessness, crying, eye contact, and facial expressions.

Monitor sensory stimulation. Minimize/remove inappropriate or hazardous stimuli.

Provide stimuli consistent with chronologic and developmental capabilities.

Provide parents with information regarding the newborn's sensory capabilities/needs.

Promote ongoing assessment of neurodevelopmental gains/deficits. Plan future interventions accordingly.

Collaborative

Refer to/discuss early stimulation program if available/indicated.

RATIONALE

Allows provision of stimuli consistent with infant's capabilities and with cues reflecting sensory overload.

Demands of environmental stimuli may overtax SGA/LGA infant.

Size of the infant/child with deviations in growth may be a false indicator of capacity for stimulation.

Parents who are informed of their newborn's capabilities can provide appropriate stimulation to optimize the newborn's development.

Prevents/minimizes complications and optimizes growth and development.

Optimizes infant development/interactional skills (affective, cognitive, social).

(Refer to CP: The Preterm Infant, ND: Sensory-Perceptual Alterations.)

NURSING DIAGNOSIS:	COPING, INDIVIDUAL, INEFFECTIVE
May be related to:	Immaturity or CNS damage (low threshold for stress), low energy reserves, poor organizational ability, limited ability to control environment.
Possibly evidenced by:	Disorganized motor activity and sleep-wake cycles, irritability.
DESIRED OUTCOMES— NEWBORN WILL:	Minimize/reduce behavioral cues indicating stress.
	Progress appropriately, according to individual pattern in growth and development.

ACTIONS/INTERVENTIONS	RATIONALE
Independent	
Assess infant's physiologic and behavioral responses to stress.	These responses communicate valuable information about coping abilities.
Identify etiology and eliminate/reduce causes of infant stressors.	Control of stressors can reduce infant's energy demands, aiding in maintenance of homeostasis.
Encourage parental involvement in identification of coping strategies/deficits of infant, including control of behavioral state and temperament. (Refer to CP: The Preterm Infant, ND: Coping, Individual, ineffective.)	Fosters continued support of the infant's capacities in the acute care setting and at home. Identifies role for parents in managing ineffective coping.
Collaborative	
Refer for long-term neurodevelopmental assessment and intervention as indicated.	Sequelae of morbidity associated with deviations in intrauterine growth may affect long-term coping.

NURSING DIAGNOSIS:	KNOWLEDGE DEFICIT [LEARNING NEED], regarding condition, prognosis, and treatment needs
May be related to:	Lack of exposure, misinterpretations, unfamiliarity with resources.
Possibly evidenced by:	Verbalization of problem, misconception, request for information.
DESIRED OUTCOMES— PARENT(S) WILL:	Identify newborn's short- and long-term needs.
	List available resources.
	Participate in discharge planning.

ACTIONS/INTERVENTIONS	RATIONALE
Independent	
Provide appropriate anticipatory guidance regarding implications of growth deviations.	Malnutrition in SGA infant may result in subnormal CNS/intellectual development as well as hearing/speech deficits. LGA infant is susceptible to malnutrition problems associated with obesity. (Refer to ND: Nutrition, altered, less than body requirements.)

ACTIONS/INTERVENTIONS	RATIONALE

Independent

Review short- and long-term needs for care of the SGA/LGA infant. Assist with follow-up in discharge planning.

Provides information for parents to understand need for ongoing physical, neurodevelopmental, and psychosocial assessment needed for long-term follow-up. (Refer to Chapter 6 CP: The Parents of A Child With Special Needs, NDs: Knowledge Deficit [Learning Need]; Family Coping, ineffective: compromised, high risk for.)

Identify community/governmental resources as appropriate.

Presence of specific needs such as feeding problems, resolving complications, or congenital anomalies will require ongoing monitoring and problem-solving to foster optimal growth and development.

Circumcision _____

Circumsion is a surgical procedure in which the prepuce (foreskin) of the penis is separated from the glans and a portion is excised. This elective procedure is performed in the United States based on parental choice for reasons related to hygiene, religion, tradition, social norms, and culture. It is usually performed at 12 to 24 hours of age or when the infant is considered physically stable.

NEONATAL ASSESSMENT DATA BASE

CIRCULATION

Vital signs within normal limits (WNL), no signs of cold stress.

Administration of vitamin K.

FOOD/FLUID

Weight at least 2500 g (5 lb 8 oz).

SAFETY

Temperature WNL.

Free of congenital anomalies; no family history of bleeding disorders or history of "proud flesh" scar formation (especially in black families).

SEXUALITY

Infant full-term (based on Dubowitz criteria).

Genitalia normal, with no evidence of hypospadias or epispadias; testes descended, and scrotal sac free of hydrocele; prepuce, still developing at birth, normally nonretractable.

DIAGNOSTIC STUDIES

Complete blood count (CBC): Rules out presence of anemia.

Clotting studies: Identify coagulation problems.

NURSING PRIORITIES

1. Provide parents with sufficient information to make an informed choice.
2. Promote comfort and healing.
3. Identify and minimize postoperative complications.
4. Instruct parent(s) in proper care of circumcised infant.

NURSING DIAGNOSIS:	KNOWLEDGE DEFICIT [LEARNING NEED], regarding surgical procedure, prognosis, and treatment
May be related to:	Lack of exposure, misinterpretation, unfamiliarity with information resources.
Possibly evidenced by:	Request for information, verbalization of concerns/misconceptions, inaccurate follow-through of instructions.

DESIRED OUTCOMES— PARENT(S) WILL:	Make informed decision.
	Demonstrate proper technique of care following procedure.
	Verbalize understanding of signs of complications.

ACTIONS/INTERVENTIONS	RATIONALE
Independent	
Assess parents' level of knowledge.	Provides a basis for discussion and identifies need for further information. Some circumcisions are performed for religious reasons. Some studies have shown that many women do not know the meaning of the word or whether their husbands are circumcised.
Review information about the advantages and disadvantages of circumcision.	The routine practice of circumcision has been questioned, and the position of the American Academy of Pediatrics (1989) is that there are both potential medical benefits and advantages as well as disadvantages and risks. Proponents believe that circumcision may reduce risk of cancer of the penis and prostate in men and of the cervix in women; that it has prophylactic effects against a number of diseases, including herpes; that it facilitates hygiene; and that an uncircumcised boy may feel different from his peers. Opponents believe that the cancer link is not proven by scientific studies and that hygiene is more of a factor in cancer prevention than is circumcision; that the long-term effects of pain and stress are not known; and that complications are a significant concern.
Note any special requests made by parents.	Parents may want to be present during the procedure or may have specific religious or cultural preferences.
Provide information about the healing process and proper care (e.g., cleaning, diapering, positioning, use of petroleum gauze dressing or bacterial ointment). Discuss the need to check infant frequently to prevent gauze from drying out and sticking to site of circumcision. Suggest soaking gauze with warm sterile water before removing it.	Prevents complications associated with infection; promotes infant's comfort. (Refer to ND: Pain [acute].) (Note: If plastic bell method is used to cover the glans, petroleum gauze is not needed.)
Discuss potential complications, e.g., hemorrhage, infection, or other signs warranting notification or healthcare provider.	Ensures prompt identifications and treatment of problems.

561

NURSING DIAGNOSIS:	PAIN [ACUTE]
May be related to:	Trauma to/edema of tender tissues.
Possibly evidenced by:	Crying, irritability, changes in sleep pattern, refusal to eat.
DESIRED OUTCOMES— NEONATE WILL:	Appear relaxed, appropriately consolable.
	Resume normal sleeping and eating patterns.

ACTIONS/INTERVENTIONS	RATIONALE

Independent

Provide pacifier, stroke lightly, and talk gently to infant during procedure.

Provides distraction and sense of reassurance to soothe the infant.

Remove infant from restraints immediately following procedure. Calm infant by holding, cuddling, dressing, and talking to him. Encourage parents to feed and cuddle infant.

A sense of uneasiness occurs due to positioning and restraint. Discomfort occurs at the time of surgical procedure, because the foreskin contains numerous nerve endings. Change of position, freedom of movement, and tactile activities refocus infant's attention and comfort infant. Feeding may promote relaxation.

Apply petroleum jelly and gauze dressing loosely around glans. Leave in place for at least 24 hours.

Protects against adherence to diaper and direct contact with urine.

Position infant on side or back, not on abdomen. Loose diaper or use no diaper at all for 24–72 hr following procedure. Note continued placement of plastic rim following circumcision with plastic bell.

Prevents friction or pressure on the penis. Plastic rim remains in place for 5 to 7 days. Plastic bell falls off by itself when glans is healed. (Note: Removal of the bell by the healthcare provider may be required.)

Avoid use of soaps on penis; clean with clear water.

Soap may cause irritation, increasing discomfort, and may cause plastic bell to fall off prematurely.

Protect the surgical site from alcohol when caring for umbilicus.

Alcohol may cause stinging, adding to infant's discomfort.

Apply a small amount of bland or petroleum-based ointment on the affected area or on the dressing that may be covering the site at each diaper change or at least 4 to 5 times a day for 24 to 48 hours.

Prevents the area from sticking to diaper.

Note infant's behavior following procedure.

Pain following the procedure may last for up to 7 days until healing is completed. Discomfort during this time is related to trauma, edema, and irritation from clothing. Changes in sleep patterns, fussiness, and/or refusal of feedings usually persist for 2–3 hr following procedure because of discomfort. However, studies indicate that elevated cortisol levels are associated with stress of the procedure and can interfere with the newborn's ability to regulate sleep-wake cycles for some time following circumcision.

Assist with dorsal penile nerve block with 1% lidocaine without epinephrine.

Although it is not used routinely, anesthesia abolishes the pain and distress manifested in the unmedicated infant by vigorous crying, attempts to wriggle from restraints, and trembling.

NURSING DIAGNOSIS:	URINARY ELIMINATION, ALTERED
May be related to:	Tissue injury/inflammation, or development of urethral fistula.
Possibly evidenced by:	Edema, difficulty voiding.
DESIRED OUTCOMES—NEONATE WILL:	Void within 6 to 8 hours following circumcision.
	Establish normal elimination pattern.
PARENT(S) WILL:	Prevent/minimize edema.

ACTIONS/INTERVENTIONS	RATIONALE

Independent

Record time of first voiding following procedure. Note amount and adequacy of stream and presence of hematuria.	Trauma to the urinary meatus from the procedure may result in delayed voidings, blocked urinary passage, or interrupted stream.
Loosely diaper the newborn and position on side or back.	Reduces pressure on affected site.
Avoid placing petroleum jelly over the meatus.	Excessive amounts of petroleum jelly may block meatus, requiring greater effort to empty bladder.
Place warm wet washcloth over the bladder area if voiding has not occurred within 6–8 hr following procedure.	Relaxes musculature and may encourage voiding.
Notify physician if infant fails to void within 12 hr following procedure.	Failure to void may indicate urethral fistula, necessitating further evaluation.

NURSING DIAGNOSIS:	INJURY, HIGH RISK FOR, hemorrhage
Risk factors may include:	Decrease in clotting factors immediately after birth (do not return to prebirth levels until the end of the first week), previously unidentified problems with bleeding and clotting.
Possibly evidenced by:	[Not applicable; presence of signs/symptoms establishes an **actual** diagnosis.]
DESIRED OUTCOMES—NEONATE WILL:	Be free of injury, no evidence of hemorrhage.

ACTIONS/INTERVENTIONS	RATIONALE

Independent

Delay surgical procedure until at least 12–24 hr following birth.	Postponing circumcision from the time immediately following birth to 12 or more hours following birth helps prevent complications associated with physiologic instability, cold stress, undetected congenital anomaly, and illness.

563

Independent

Observe infant every hour for first 12 hours after the procedure.

Aids in early detection of excess blood loss. (Note: Excess blood loss may be an initial indicator of bleeding and coagulation problems such as hemophilia.)

Apply gentle direct pressure to bleeding site, using a sterile gauze pad.

Promotes vasoconstriction to stop bleeding.

Apply sterile petroleum gauze dressing to site immediately following procedure and with each diaper change. Moisten gauze with water if it adheres to surgical site. (Gauze is not needed if plastic bell method is used.)

Acts as a pressure dressing to control bleeding and prevent surgical site from adhering to the diaper, which could cause further irritation or loss of stable clot.

Collaborative

Apply Gelfoam to bleeding areas.

Gelfoam acts as a local hemostatic agent to promote platelet adhesion and clotting.

Assist with placement of suture(s), as needed.

May be necessary to control bleeding.

NURSING DIAGNOSIS:	INFECTION, HIGH RISK FOR
Risk factors may include:	Immature immune system, invasive procedure/tissue trauma, environmental exposure.
Possibly evidenced by:	[Not applicable; presence of signs/symptoms establishes an **actual** diagnosis.]
DESIRED OUTCOMES— NEONATE WILL:	Display timely healing of circumcision site within 1 week.
	Be free of signs of infection.

Independent

Clean penis gently with warm sterile water or hydrogen peroxide, and apply fresh sterile petroleum gauze with each diaper change.

Removes urine/feces from penis; helps promote healing. (Note: Excessive scrubbing may irritate the site and provide entry for bacteria.)

Note appearance of whitish yellow exudate around the glans. Do not remove.

Exudate is usually noted 24–48 hr following procedure. It is a normal sign of the granulation process and eventually disappears on its own.

Observe for signs of infection (e.g., erythema or purulent exudate at site of circumcision) with each diaper change. Ensure that plastic bell is still firmly attached if used.

Early detection of infection can prevent generalized sepsis from occurring.

Collaborative

Obtain culture of exudate if present.

May be necessary to identify pathogens.

Monitor results of laboratory studies; e.g., CBC.

Confirms presence or resolution of infectious process.

Administer local or systemic antibiotic as indicated.

Treats infection; prevents systemic involvement.

Newborn: Hyperbilirubinemia

Elevation of serum bilirubin levels is related to hemolysis of red blood cells (RBCs) and subsequent resorption of unconjugated bilirubin from the small intestines. The condition may be benign or may place the neonate at risk for multiple complications/untoward effects.

CLIENT ASSESSMENT DATA BASE

ACTIVITY/REST

Lethargy, listlessness.

CIRCULATION

May be pale, indicating anemia.

Residing at altitudes above 5000 ft.

ELIMINATION

Bowel sounds hypoactive.

Meconium passage may be delayed.

Stools may be loose/greenish-brown during bilirubin excretion.

Urine dark, concentrated; brownish black (bronze baby syndrome).

FOOD/FLUID

History of delayed/poor oral feeding, more likely to be breastfed than bottle fed.

Abdominal palpation may reveal enlarged spleen, liver.

NEUROSENSORY

Large cephalhematoma may be noted over one or both parietal bones related to birth trauma/vacuum extraction delivery.

Generalized edema, hepatosplenomegaly, or hydrops fetalis may be present with severe Rh incompatibility.

Loss of Moro reflex may be noted.

Opisthotonos with rigid arching of back, bulging fontanels, shrill cry, seizure activity (crisis stage).

RESPIRATION

History of asphyxia.

Crackles, pink-tinged mucus (pleural edema, pulmonary hemorrhages).

SAFETY

Positive history for infection/neonatal sepsis.

May have excessive ecchymosis, petechiae, intracranial bleeding.

May appear jaundiced initially on the face with progression to distal parts of the body; skin brownish black in color (bronze baby syndrome) as a side effect of phototherapy.

SEXUALITY

May be preterm, small-for-gestational-age (SGA) infant, infant with intrauterine growth retardation (IUGR), or large-for-gestational age (LGA) infant, such as infant of diabetic mother.

Birth trauma may have occurred associated with cold stress, asphyxia, hypoxia, acidosis, hypoglycemia, hypoproteinemia.

Occurs more often in male than female infants.

TEACHING/LEARNING

May have congenital hypothyroidism, biliary atresia, cystic fibrosis (inspissated bile).

Family factors; e.g., ethnic descent (Oriental, Greek, or Korean), history of hyperbilirubinemia in previous pregnancies/siblings, liver disease, cystic fibrosis, inborn errors of metabolism (galactosemia), blood dyscrasias (spherocytosis, glucose-6-phosphate dehydrogenase [G-6-PD] deficiency).

Maternal factors, such as maternal diabetes; ingestion of medications (e.g., salicyclates, oral sulfonamides late in pregnancy or nitrofurantoin (Furadantin); Rh/ABO incompatibility; infectious illness (e.g., rubella, cytomegalovirus, syphilis, toxoplasmosis).

Intrapartal contributing factors, such as preterm labor, delivery by vacuum extraction, oxytocin induction, delayed clamping of umbilical cord, or traumatic delivery.

DIAGNOSTIC STUDIES

Coombs' test on newborn cord blood: Positive results of indirect Coombs' test indicate the presence of Rh-positive, anti-A, or anti-B antibodies in mother's blood. Positive results of direct Coombs' test indicate presence of sensitized (Rh-positive, anti-A, or anti-B) RBCs in neonate.

Infant and maternal blood type: Identifies ABO incompatibilities.

Total bilirubin: Direct (conjugated) levels are significant if they exceed 1.0–1.5 mg/dl, which may be associated with sepsis. Indirect (unconjugated) levels should not exceed an increase of 5 mg/dl in 24 hours, or should not be greater than 20 mg/dl in a full-term infant or 15 mg/dl in a preterm infant (dependent on weight).

Total serum protein: Levels less than 3.0 g/dl indicate reduced binding capacity, particularly in preterm infant.

Complete blood count: Hemoglobin (Hb) may be low (less than 14 g/dl) because of hemolysis. Hematocrit (Hct) may be elevated (greater than 65%) with polycythemia, decreased (less than 45%) with excess hemolysis and anemia.

Glucose: Dextrostix level may be less than 45% whole blood glucose less than 30 mg/dl, or serum glucose less than 40 mg/dl if newborn is hypoglycemic and begins to use fat stores and release fatty acids.

Carbon dioxide combining power: Decreased level reflects hemolysis.

Transcutaneous jaundice meter: Identifies infants requiring serum bilirubin determination.

Reticulocyte count: Elevation (reticulocytosis) indicates increased production of RBCs in response to hemolysis associated with RH disease.

Peripheral blood smear: May reveal abnormal or immature RBCs, erythroblasts in Rh disease, or spherocytes in ABO incompatibility.

Betke-Kleihauer test: Evaluation of maternal blood smear for fetal erythrocytes.

NURSING PRIORITIES

1. Prevent injury/progression of condition.
2. Provide support/appropriate information to family.

NURSING DIAGNOSIS:	INJURY, HIGH RISK FOR, central nervous system involvement
Risk factors may include:	Prematurity, hemolytic disease, asphyxia, acidosis, hypoproteinemia, and hypoglycemia.
Possibly evidenced by:	[Not applicable; presence of signs/symptoms establishes an **actual** diagnosis.]
DESIRED OUTCOMES— NEWBORN WILL:	Display indirect bilirubin levels below 12 mg/dl in term infant at 3 days of age.
	Resolution of jaundice by end of the first week of life.
	Be free of CNS involvement.

ACTIONS/INTERVENTIONS	RATIONALE
Independent	
Note infant/maternal blood group and blood type.	ABO incompatibilities affect 20% of all pregnancies and most commonly occur in mothers with type O blood, whose anti-A and anti-B antibodies pass into fetal circulation, causing RBC agglutination and hemolysis. Similarly, when an Rh-negative mother has previously been sensitized by Rh-positive antigens, maternal antibodies cross the placenta and attach to fetal RBCs, causing immediate or delayed hemolysis.
Review intrapartal record for specific risk factors, such as low birth weight (LBW) or IUGR, prematurity, abnormal metabolic processes, vascular injuries, abnormal circulation, sepsis, or polycythemia.	Certain clinical conditions may cause a reversal of the blood-brain barrier, allowing bound bilirubin to separate either at the level of the cell membrane or within the cell itself, increasing the risk of CNS involvement.
Note use of vacuum extractor for delivery. Assess infant for presence of cephalhematoma and excessive ecchymosis or petechiae.	Resorption of blood trapped in fetal scalp tissue and excessive hemolysis may increase the amount of bilirubin being released and cause jaundice.
Review infant's condition at birth, noting need for resuscitation or evidence of excessive ecchymosis or petechiae, cold stress, asphyxia, or acidosis.	Asphyxia and acidosis reduce affinity of bilirubin to albumin.
Keep infant warm and dry; monitor skin and core temperature frequently.	Cold stress potentiates release of fatty acids, which compete for binding sites on albumin, thereby increasing the level of freely circulating (unbound) bilirubin.

567

ACTIONS/INTERVENTIONS

Independent

Initiate early oral feedings within 4 to 6 hours following birth, especially if infant is to be breastfed. Assess infant for signs of hypoglycemia. Obtain Dextrostix levels, as indicated.

Evaluate maternal and prenatal nutritional levels; note possible neonatal hypoproteinemia, especially in preterm infant.

Observe infant in natural light, noting sclera and oral mucosa, yellowing of skin immediately after blanching, and specific body parts involved. Assess oral mucosa, posterior portion of hard palate, and conjunctival sacs in dark-skinned newborns.

Note infant's age at onset of jaundice; differentiate type of jaundice (i.e., physiologic, breast milk-induced, or pathologic).

Apply transcutaneous jaundice meter.

Assess infant for progression of signs and behavioral changes: Stage I involves neurodepression (e.g., lethargy, hypotonia, or diminished/absent reflexes). Stage II involves neurohyperreflexia (e.g., twitching, convulsions, opisthotonos, or fever). Stage III is marked by absence of clinical manifestations. Stage IV involves sequelae such as cerebral palsy or mental retardation.

RATIONALE

Establishes proper intestinal flora necessary for reduction of bilirubin to urobilinogen; decreases enterohepatic circulation of bilirubin (bypassing liver with persistence of ductus venosus); and decreases resorption of bilirubin from bowel by promoting passage of meconium. Hypoglycemia necessitates use of fat stores for energy-releasing fatty acids, which compete with bilirubin for binding sites on albumin.

Hypoproteinemia in the newborn may result in jaundice. One gram of albumin carries 16 mg of unconjugated bilirubin. Lack of sufficient albumin increases the amount of unbound circulating (indirect) bilirubin, which may cross the blood-brain barrier.

Detects evidence/degree of jaundice. Clinical appearance of jaundice is evident at bilirubin levels greater than 7–8 mg/dl in full-term infant. Estimated degree of jaundice is as follows, with jaundice progressing from head to toe: face, 4–8 mg/dl; trunk, 5–12 mg/dl; groin, 8–16 mg/dl; arms/legs, 11–18 mg/dl; and hands/feet, 15–20 mg/dl. Yellow underlying pigment may be normal in dark-skinned infants.

Physiologic jaundice usually appears between the second and third days of life, as excess RBCs needed to maintain adequate oxygenation for the fetus are no longer required in the newborn and are hemolyzed, thereby releasing bilirubin, the final breakdown product of heme. Breast milk jaundice usually appears between the fourth and sixth day of life, affecting only 1%–2% of breastfed infants. The breast milk of some women is thought to contain an enzyme (pregnanediol) that inhibits glucuronyl transferase (the liver enzyme that conugates bilirubin), or to contain several times the normal breast milk concentration of certain free fatty acids, which are also thought to inhibit the conjugation of bilirubin. Pathologic jaundice appears within the first 24 hours of life and is more likely to lead to the development of kernicterus/bilirubin encephalopathy.

Provides noninvasive screening of jaundice, quantifying skin color in relation to total serum bilirubin.

Excessive unconjugated bilirubin (associated with pathologic jaundice) has an affinity for extravascular tissue, including the basal ganglia of brain tissue. Behavior changes associated with kernicterus usually occur between the 3rd and 10th days of life and rarely occur prior to 36 hours of life.

ACTIONS/INTERVENTIONS	RATIONALE

Independent

Evaluate infant for pallor, edema, or hepato-splenomegaly.

These signs may be associated with hydrops fetalis, Rh incompatibility, and in utero hemolysis of fetal RBCs.

Collaborative

Monitor laboratory studies, as indicated:

Direct and indirect bilirubin.

Bilirubin appears in two forms: direct bilirubin, which is conjugated by the liver enzyme glucuronyl transferase, and indirect bilirubin, which is unconjugated and appears in a free form in the blood or bound to albumin. The infant's potential for kernicterus is best predicted by elevated levels of indirect bilirubin. Elevated indirect bilirubin levels of 18–20 mg/dl in full-term infant, or greater than 13–15 mg/dl in preterm or sick infant, are significant. (Note: Stressed or preterm infant is susceptible to deposition of bile pigments within brain tissue at far lower levels than nonstressed full-term infant.)

Direct/indirect Coombs' test on cord blood.

Positive results of indirect Coombs' test indicate presence of antibodies (Rh-positive or anti-A, anti-B) in mother's and newborn's blood; positive results of direct Coombs' test indicate presence of sensitized (Rh-positive, anti-A, or anti-B) RBCs in neonate.

Carbon dioxide (CO_2) combining power.

A decrease is consistent with hemolysis.

Reticulocyte count and peripheral smear.

Excessive hemolysis causes reticulocyte count to increase. Smear identifies abnormal or immature RBCs.

Hb/Hct.

Elevated Hb/Hct levels (Hb greater than 22 g/dl; Hct greater than 65%) indicate polycythemia, possibly caused by delayed cord clamping, maternal-fetal transfusion, twin-to-twin transfusion, maternal diabetes, or chronic intrauterine stress and hypoxia, as seen in LBW infant or infant with compromised placental circulation. Hemolysis of excess RBCs causes elevated levels of bilirubin with 1 g of Hb yielding 35 mg of bilirubin. Low Hb levels (14 mg/dl) may be associated with hydrops fetalis or with Rh incompatibility occurring in utero and causing hemolysis, edema, and pallor.

Total serum protein.

Low levels of serum protein (less than 3.0 g/dl) indicate reduced binding capacity for bilirubin.

Calculate plasma bilirubin-albumin binding capacity.

Aids in determining risk of kernicterus and treatment needs. When total bilirubin value divided by total serum protein level is less than 3.7, the danger of kernicterus is very low. However, the risk of injury is dependent on degree of prematurity, presence of hypoxia or acidosis, and drug regimen (e.g., sulfonamides, chloramphenicol).

ACTIONS/INTERVENTIONS	RATIONALE

Collaborative

Initiate phototherapy per protocol, using fluorescent bulbs placed above the infant or bile blanket (except for newborn with Rh disease). (Refer to NDs: Injury, high risk for, side effects of phototherapy treatment; Injury, high risk for, complications of exchange transfusions.)

Causes photo-oxidation of bilirubin in subcutaneous tissue, thereby increasing water solubility of bilirubin, which allows rapid excretion of bilirubin in stool and urine. Rate of hemolysis in Rh disease usually exceeds rate of bilirubin reduction related to phototherapy, so that an exchange transfusion is the only appropriate treatment.

Discontinue breastfeeding for 24–48 hr, as indicated. Assist mother as needed with pumping of breasts and reestablishment of breastfeeding.

Opinions vary as to whether discontinuing breastfeeding is necessary when jaundice occurs. However, formula ingestion increases gastrointestinal motility and excretion of stool and bile pigment, and serum bilirubin levels do begin to fall within 48 hr after discontinuation of breastfeeding.

Administer enzyme induction agent (phenobarbital, ethanol) as appropriate.

Stimulates hepatic enzymes to enhance clearance of bilirubin.

Assist with preparation and administration of exchange transfusion. Use same type of blood as infant's, but Rh-negative or type O-negative blood, if results of direct Coombs' test on cord serum are greater than 3.5 mg/dl in the first week of life, serum unconjugated bilirubin levels are greater than 20 mg/dl in the first 48 hr of life, or Hb is less than 12 g/dl at birth in infants with hydrops fetalis. (Refer to ND: Injury, high risk for, complications of exchange transfusions.)

Exchange transfusions are necessary in cases of severe hemolytic anemia, which are usually associated with Rh incompatibility, to remove sensitized RBCs that would soon lyse; to remove serum bilirubin; to provide bilirubin-free albumin to increase binding sites for bilirubin; and to treat anemia by providing RBCs that are not susceptible to maternal antibodies.

NURSING DIAGNOSIS:	INJURY, HIGH RISK FOR, side effects of phototherapy treatment
Risk factors may include:	Physical properties of therapeutic intervention and effects on body regulatory mechanisms.
Possibly evidenced by:	[Not applicable; presence of signs/symptoms establishes an **actual** diagnosis.]
DESIRED OUTCOMES—NEWBORN WILL:	Maintain body temperature and fluid balance within normal limits.)
	Be free of skin/tissue injury.
	Demonstrate expected interaction patterns.
	Display decreasing serum bilirubin levels.

ACTIONS/INTERVENTIONS	RATIONALE

Independent

Note presence/development of biliary or intestinal obstruction.

Phototherapy is contraindicated in these conditions because the photoisomers of bilirubin produced in the skin and subcutaneous tissues by exposure to light therapy cannot be readily excreted.

ACTIONS/INTERVENTIONS	RATIONALE

Independent

Measure quantity of photoenergy of fluorescent bulbs (white or blue light) using photometer.

The intensity of light striking skin surface from blue spectrum (blue lights) determines how close to the light source the infant should be placed. Blue and special blue lights are considered more effective than white light in promoting bilirubin breakdown, but they create difficulty in evaluating the newborn for cyanosis.

Document type of fluorescent lamp, total number of hours since bulb replacement, and the measured distance between lamp surface and infant.

Light emission may decay over time. Infant should be placed approximately 18–20 inches from light source for maximal benefit. (Note: Use of fiberoptic blanket connected to an illuminator [light source] allows infant to be "wrapped" in therapeutic light without risk to corneas. Additionally, infant can be held and fed without interrupting therapy.)

Apply patches to closed eyes; inspect eyes every 2 hr when patches are removed for feedings. Monitor placement frequently.

Prevents possible damage to the retina and conjunctiva from high-intensity light. Improper application or slipping of patches can cause irritation, corneal abrasions, and conjunctivitis, and compromise breathing by obstructing nasal passages.

Cover testes and penis of male infant.

Prevents possible testicular damage from heat.

Place Plexiglas shield between baby and light.

Filters out ultraviolet radiation (wavelengths less than 380 nm) and protects infant if bulb breaks.

Monitor neonate's skin and core temperature every 2 hr or more frequently until stable (e.g., axillary temperature of 97.8°F, rectal temperature of 98.8°F). Regulate incubator/isolette temperature, as appropriate.

Fluctuations in body temperature can occur in response to light exposure, radiation, and convection.

Reposition infant every 2 hr.

Allows equal exposure of skin surfaces to fluorescent light, prevents excessive exposure of individual body parts, and limits pressure areas.

Monitor fluid intake and output; weigh infant twice a day. Note signs of dehydration (e.g., reduced urine output, depressed fontanels, dry or warm skin with poor turgor, and sunken eyes). Increase oral fluid intake by at least 25%.

Increased water losses through stools and evaporation can cause dehydration. (Note: Infant may sleep for longer periods in conjunction with phototherapy, increasing risk of dehydration if frequent feeding schedule is not maintained.)

Note color and frequency of stools and urine.

Frequent, greenish, loose stools and greenish urine indicate effectiveness of phototherapy with breakdown and excretion of bilirubin.

Carefully wash perianal area after each passage of stool; inspect skin for possible irritation or breakdown.

Helps prevent irritation and excoriation from frequent or loose stools.

Bring infant to parents for feedings. Encourage stroking, cuddling, eye contact, and talking to infant during feedings. Encourage parents to interact with infant in nursery between feedings.

Fosters attachment process, which may be delayed because of separation required by phototherapy. Visual, tactile, and auditory stimulation helps infant overcome sensory deprivation. Intermittent phototherapy does not negatively affect photo-oxidation process.

ACTIONS/INTERVENTIONS	RATIONALE

Independent

Note behavioral changes or signs of deteriorating condition (e.g., lethargy, hypotonia, hypertonicity, or extrapyramidal signs).

Such changes may signify deposition of bile pigment in the basal ganglia and developing kernicterus.

Evaluate appearance of skin and urine, noting brownish black color.

An uncommon side effect of phototherapy involves exaggerated pigment changes (bronze baby syndrome), which may occur if conjugated bilirubin levels rise. The changes in skin color may last for 2–4 months, but are not associated with harmful sequelae.

Collaborative

Monitor laboratory studies, as indicated:

Bilirubin levels every 12 hr.

Decreases in bilirubin levels indicate effectiveness of phototherapy; continued increases suggest continued hemolysis and may indicate the need for exchange transfusion. (Note: Blood sample drawn for bilirubin determination should be protected from light to prevent continued photo-oxidation.)

Hb levels.

Continued hemolysis is manifested by continued decreases in Hb level.

Platelets and white blood cells (WBCs).

Thrombocytopenia during phototherapy has been reported in some infants. Decrease in WBCs suggests a possible effect on peripheral lymphocytes.

Administer fluids parenterally as indicated.

May be necessary to correct or prevent severe dehydration.

NURSING DIAGNOSIS:	INJURY, HIGH RISK FOR, complications of exchange transfusions
Risk factors may include:	Invasive procedure, abnormal blood profile, chemical imbalances.
Possibly evidenced by:	[Not applicable; presence of signs/symptoms establishes an **actual** diagnosis.]
DESIRED OUTCOMES— NEWBORN WILL:	Complete exchange transfusion without complications.
	Display decreasing serum bilirubin levels.

ACTIONS/INTERVENTIONS	RATIONALE

Independent

Note condition of infant's cord prior to transfusion if umbilical vein is to be used. If cord is dry, administer saline soaks for 30–60 min prior to procedure.

Soaks may be necessary to soften cord and umbilical vein prior to transfusion for I.V. access and to ease passage of umbilical catheter.

Maintain NPO (nothing by mouth) status for 4 hr prior to procedure, or aspirate gastric contents.

Reduces risk of possible regurgitation and aspiration during procedure.

Ensure availability of resuscitative equipment.

To provide immediate support if necessary.

ACTIONS/INTERVENTIONS	RATIONALE

Independent

Maintain infant's temperature prior to, during, and after procedure. Place infant under radiant warmer with servomechanism. Warm blood prior to infusion by placing in incubator, warm basin of water, or blood warmer.

Helps prevent hypothermia and vasospasm, reduces risk of ventricular fibrillation, and decreases blood viscosity.

Verify infant's and mother's blood type and Rh factor. Note blood type and Rh factor of blood to be exchanged. (Exchanged blood will be the same type as the baby's, but will be Rh-negative or type O-negative blood that has been cross-matched with mother's blood beforehand.)

Exchange transfusions are most often associated with Rh incompatibility problems. Using Rh₀ (D)-positive blood would only increase hemolysis and bilirubin levels, because antibodies in infant's circulation would destroy new RBCs.

Ensure freshness of blood (not more than 2 days old). Heparinized blood is preferred.

Older blood is more likely to hemolyze, thereby increasing bilirubin levels. Heparinized blood is always fresh, but must be discarded if not used within 24 hr.

Monitor venous pressure, pulse, color, and respiratory rate/ease before, during, and after transfusion. Suction as needed.

Establishes baseline values, identifies potentially unstable conditions (e.g., apnea or cardiac dysrhythmia/arrest), and maintains airway. (Note: Bradycardia may occur if calcium is injected too rapidly.)

Carefully document events during transfusion, recording amount of blood withdrawn and injected (usually 7–20 ml at a time).

Helps prevent errors in fluid replacement. Amount of blood exchanged is approximately 170 ml/kg of body weight. A double volume exchange transfusion ensures that between 75%, and 90% of circulating RBCs are replaced.

Monitor for signs of electrolyte imbalance (e.g., jitteriness, seizure activity, and apnea; hyperreflexia; bradycardia; or diarrhea).

Hypocalcemia and hyperkalemia may develop during and following exchange transfusion.

Assess infant for excessive bleeding from i.v. site following the transfusion.

Infusion of heparinized blood (or citrated blood without calcium replacement) alters coagulation for 4–6 hr following the exchange transfusion and may result in bleeding.

Collaborative

Monitor laboratory studies, as indicated:

Hb/Hct levels prior to and following transfusion.

If Hct is less than 40% prior to transfusion, a partial exchange with packed RBCs may precede full exchange. Dropping levels following the transfusion suggest the need for a second transfusion.

Serum bilirubin levels immediately following procedure, then every 4–8 hr.

Bilirubin levels may decrease by half immediately following procedure, but may rise shortly thereafter, necessitating a repeat transfusion.

Total serum protein.

Multiplying level by 3.7 determines the degree of elevation of bilirubin necessitating exchange transfusion.

Serum calcium and potassium.

Donor blood containing citrate as an anticoagulant binds calcium, thereby decreasing serum calcium levels. In addition, if blood is more than 2 days old, RBC destruction releases potassium, creating a risk of hyperkalemia and cardiac arrest.

573

ACTIONS/INTERVENTIONS	RATIONALE

Collaborative

Glucose.	Low glucose levels may be associated with continued anaerobic glycolysis within donor RBCs. Prompt treatment is necessary to prevent untoward effects/CNS damage.
Serum pH levels.	Serum pH of donor blood is typically 6.8 or less. Acidosis may result when fresh blood is not used and infant's liver cannot metabolize citrate used as an anticoagulant, or when donor blood continues anaerobic glycolysis, with production of acid metabolites.
Administer albumin prior to transfusion if indicated.	Although somewhat controversial, administration of albumin may increase the albumin available for binding of bilirubin, thereby reducing levels of freely circulating serum bilirubin. Synthetic albumin is not thought to increase available binding sites.
Administer medications, as indicated:	
5% calcium gluconate.	From 2 to 4 ml of calcium gluconate may be administered after every 100 ml of blood infusion to correct hypocalcemia and minimize possible cardiac irritability. (Note: Some controversy exists as to the purpose and effectiveness of this practice.)
Sodium bicarbonate.	Corrects acidosis.
Protamine sulfate.	Counteracts anticoagulant effects of heparinized blood.

NURSING DIAGNOSIS:	**KNOWLEDGE DEFICIT [LEARNING NEED], regarding condition, prognosis, and treatment needs**
May be related to:	Lack of exposure, misinterpretation, unfamiliarity with information resources.
Possibly evidenced by:	Statement of problem/misconceptions, request for information, inaccurate follow-through of instructions.
DESIRED OUTCOMES— PARENT(S) WILL:	Verbalize understanding of cause, treatment, and possible outcomes of hyperbilirubinemia.
	Demonstrate appropriate care of infant.

ACTIONS/INTERVENTIONS	RATIONALE

Independent

Provide information about types of jaundice and pathophysiologic factors and future implications of hyperbilirubinemia. Encourage questions; reinforce or clarify information, as needed.	Corrects misconceptions, promotes understanding, and reduces fear and feelings of guilt. Neonatal jaundice may be physiologic, breast milk-induced, or pathologic, and protocol of care depends on its cause and contributing factors.

ACTIONS/INTERVENTIONS	RATIONALE

Independent

Review means of assessing infant for increasing bilirubin levels (e.g., observing blanching of skin over bony prominence or behavior changes), especially if infant is to be discharged early. Provide parents with 24-hour emergency telephone number and name of contact person, and stress importance of reporting increased jaundice.

Enables parents to recognize signs of increasing bilirubin levels.and to seek timely medical evaluation.

Discuss home management of mild or moderate physiologic jaundice, including increased feedings, direct exposure to sunlight, and follow-up serum testing program.

Parents' understanding helps foster their cooperation once infant is discharged. Information helps parents to carry out home management safely and appropriately and to recognize the importance of all aspects of management program.

Provide information about maintaining milk supply through use of breast pump and about reinstating breastfeeding when jaundice necessitates interruption of breastfeeding.

Helps mother to maintain adequate milk supply to meet infant's needs when breastfeeding is resumed.

Review rationale for specific hospital procedures (e.g., phototherapy, exchange transfusions) and treatment and changes in bilirubin levels, especially in the event that neonate must remain in hospital for treatment while mother is discharged.

Assists parents in understanding importance of therapy. Keeps parents informed about infant's status. Promotes informed decision making.

Discuss need for Rh immune globulin (Rh-Ig) within 72 hr following delivery for Rh-negative mother who has an Rh-positive fetus/infant and who has not been previously sensitized.

In RH$_0$ (D)-negative client with no Rh antibodies, who has given birth to an Rh$_0$ (D^u)-positive infant. Rh-Ig may reduce incidence of maternal isoimmunization in nonsensitized mother and may help to prevent erythroblastosis fetalis in subsequent pregnancies.

Assess family situation and support systems. Provide parents with appropriate written explanation of home phototherapy, listing technique and potential problems.

Home phototherapy is recommended only for full-term infants after the first 48 hr of life, whose serum bilirubin levels are between 14 and 18 mg/dl with no increase in direct reacting bilirubin concentration.

Provide appropriate referral for home phototherapy program if necessary.

Lack of available support systems and education may necessitate use of visiting nurse to monitor home phototherapy program.

Make appropriate arrangements for follow-up testing of serum bilirubin at same laboratory facility.

Treatment is discontinued once serum bilirubin concentrations fall below 14 mg/dl, but serum levels must be rechecked in 12–24 hr to detect possible rebound hyperbilirubinemia.

Discuss possible long-term effects of hyperbilirubinemia and the need for continued assessment and early intervention.

Neurologic damage associated with kernicterus includes death, cerebral palsy, mental retardation, sensory difficulties, delayed speech, poor muscle coordination, learning difficulties, and enamel hypoplasia or yellowish-green staining of teeth.

(Refer to Chapter 5, CP: The Parents of a Child With Special Needs, ND: Knowledge Deficit [Learning Need].)

The Infant of an Addicted Mother _____

From 80% to 90% of infants born to addicted mothers are physiologically addicted and experience passive signs of drug withdrawal, commonly referred to as neonatal withdrawal syndrome or neonatal abstinence syndrome. An additional 3000 to 5000 infants are found yearly to be suffering from fetal alcohol syndrome (FAS).

NEONATE ASSESSMENT DATA BASE

ACTIVITY/REST

High-pitched cry, wakefulness, short or unquiet sleep patterns, yawning.

Difficulty maintaining alert states.

CIRCULATION

Tachycardia.

EGO INTEGRITY

Poor state organization (cocaine use).

Facial abnormalities (FAS, toxic vapor abuse).

ELIMINATION

Diarrhea.

FOOD/FLUID

May be low-birth-weight (LBW) or small-for-gestational age (SGA) infant, may have intrauterine growth retardation (IUGR) (maternal use of heroin, alcohol, or cocaine, or maternal malnutrition); or may be large-for-gestational age (LGA) infant (maternal use of methadone).

Poor feeding with uncoordinated frantic sucking, drooling, hiccups, hyperphagia; possible cleft lip.

Weight decrease or failure to gain weight.

Vomiting/regurgitation.

Dry mucous membranes, poor skin tugor, sunken fontanels.

NEUROSENSORY

Apgar score may be low (e.g., intrauterine asphyxia or medication given to mother during intrapartal period).

Small head circumference (nicotine); microcephaly (FAS, cocaine use, toxic vapor abuse).

Hyperirritability (including increased startle response), hyperactivity, hypertonicity may be present.

Hyperacusis (abnormal sensitivity to sound), tremors, persistent or rhythmic myoclonic jerks, or convulsions may be noted.

Increased or exaggerated reflexes (e.g., sucking, rooting, deep tendon, and Moro reflex) may be noted.

RESPIRATION

Periods of apnea, tachypnea, increased tearing, rhinorrhea, stuffy nose, or sneezing may be present.

Tracheoepiglottal abnormalities (FAS).

SAFETY

Temperature variations.

Sweating, mottling, and flushing may be seen.

Rub marks on face and knees related to constant "mouthing/crawling" motions.

Sclera, skin may be jaundiced.

Congenital anomalies (associated with cardiovascular or genitourinary systems) may be present.

Signs of infection or sepsis (acquired in utero), history of premature rupture of membrane, impaired immunologic mechanisms (marijuana).

SOCIAL INTERACTION

May exhibit poor tolerance for being held, decreased interactive behavior (difficulty responding to human voice/face, environmental stimuli).

SEXUALITY

Female more commonly affected, ratio 2:1 (FAS).

Genital abnormalities in females (FAS).

TEACHING/LEARNING

May be premature.

Mother may have received no prenatal care (literature suggests that 75% of women who abuse drugs during pregnancy do not seek prenatal care until the onset of labor), or may report prenatal problems associated with preterm labor, abruptio placentae, or placenta previa; infections such as pneumonia, endocarditis, sexually transmitted disease, or hepatitis; pregnancy-induced hypertension; and anemia.

DIAGNOSTIC STUDIES

Toxicology or drug screen (maternal/infant blood and urine, and fetal meconium): Identifies current substance exposure. Cocaine metabolites may persist in urine for 4–7 days after use, or even longer in infant.
Serum electrolytes: Demonstrates hypocalcemia.
Serum glucose: May be decreased.
Complete blood count (CBC) and blood cultures: For differential diagnosis associated with sepsis.
Platelet count: May be decreased (tranquilizers).
Bilirubin levels: Increased risk of jaundice (especially in infant of methadone user).
Electroencephalogram (EEG): May be abnormal, demonstrating cerebral irritation, in cocaine-exposed infant. Normalization of EEG noted by 3 to 12 months of age.

NURSING PRIORITIES

1. Facilitate and support drug withdrawal in infant.
2. Prevent injury, and reduce risk of short- and long-term complications.
3. Foster parent-infant interaction and attachment.
4. Provide information and support to parent(s) during rehabilitation process.

DISCHARGE GOALS

1. Gaining weight appropriately.
2. Free of injury, complications resolving.
3. Parent-infant interactions progressing satisfactorily.
4. Parent(s) understand condition, prognosis, infant's needs.

ACTIONS/INTERVENTIONS	RATIONALE
Independent	
Determine maternal history of addiction, noting duration, type of drug(s) used (including alcohol), and time and strength of last dose before delivery.	Degree of infant narcosis and withdrawal is related to the amount of mother's regular drug intake, the length of time mother has been addicted to drug(s), and the drug level at time of delivery. The closer the drug ingestion is to the time of delivery, the longer it takes for the infant to develop withdrawal and the more severe the manifestations are. (Note: An addicted mother frequently uses more than one substance; e.g., alcohol, cocaine, heroin, and phencyclidine [PCP].)
Review prenatal/intrapartal record, and note any anesthesia or analgesia administered during intrapartal period.	The newborn is susceptible to possible long-term effects from fetal asphyxia associated with placental insufficiency, fetal drug withdrawal in utero (secondary to maternal withdrawal), and increased incidence of strokes and intracerebral hemorrhage. Medications administered to the mother during the intrapartal period, acidosis, and hypoxia associated with meconium aspiration may also contribute to temporary or permanent alterations in CNS function.
Observe infant for initial signs of acute withdrawal (e.g., tremors, restlessness, hyperactive reflexes, sneezing, high-pitched shrill cry, and hypertonicity).	Although these signs usually appear soon after delivery (6 to 24 hours), the mean is 72 hours after birth, with delay of onset for as long as 10 to 14 days following delivery, especially if mother was on methadone maintenance during prenatal period. (Note: Frequency of withdrawal signs is significantly less if methadone dose at time of delivery was less than 20 mg.)
Monitor withdrawal using an evaluative tool or a seizure withdrawal chart (e.g., Neonatal Abstinence Score).	Consistent use of an objective tool provides a cumulative record that is useful in judging progress of withdrawal and/or effectiveness of supportive care and in determining need to institute or alter pharmacologic therapy. Early identification of infants requiring medical or pharmacologic intervention decreases incidence of mortality and morbidity. Subacute effects of narcotic drug withdrawal may last 4–6 months.

ACTIONS/INTERVENTIONS	RATIONALE

Independent

Place infant on abdomen. Provide pacifier.

Encourages hand-mouth contact, which facilitates quieting and behavior organization. Pacifier may reduce tension levels, may decrease crying and irritability, and may actually reduce amount of drug treatment needed.

Swaddle infant in prone fetal (flexed) position. Provide quiet, dimly lit area and scheduled periods of uninterrupted sleep.

Decreases external stimuli, reducing CNS stimulation. (Note: Infant may need to be positioned on side when risk of vomiting or regurgitation is present.)

Observe sleep patterns and degree and timing of irritability.

Excessive jitteriness and irritability interrupt sleep cycle, possibly necessitating initiation or alteration of pharmacologic therapy. Withdrawal prevents adequate periods of deep sleep, but therapy promotes rapid-eye-movement and deep sleep cycles.

Place baby in infant carrier, play soft music, and provide gentle rocking during periods of arousal.

Mimics intrauterine posture, helps soothe infant; provides body closeness.

Monitor effects of handling; decrease handling as indicated.

Holding infant and providing close contact usually reduces hyperactivity and quiets child, although some infants become more irritable when they are held.

Monitor vital signs and neurologic status.

Early detection and treatment of potential complications such as meningitis, intracranial hemorrhage, and pyrexia reduce risk of long-term sequelae. Prematurity and liver immaturity, especially when associated with use of methadone, increase the risk of jaundice and kernicterus.

Observe infant for change in withdrawal signs and/or for side effects of drug therapy.

Changes in withdrawal signs may necessitate alteration in medication dosage to produce the best effect at the lowest dose without the side effects of excessive CNS depression, impaired sucking, or delayed bonding. (Note: The greater the number and severity of withdrawal signs, the higher the probability of infant mortality or morbidity.)

Observe infant for signs of seizure activity, such as twitching (rhythmic movements not decreased when limbs are held), rigidity, arching of back, nystagmus, and tongue thrusting or sucking motions. Institute seizure precautions.

Newborns experiencing passive withdrawal from addiction are subject to convulsions associated with CNS stimulation, which increases risk of injury.

Suction airway, and provide resuscitative measures, as indicated.

Maintains airway patency and supports vital functions.

Collaborative

Monitor laboratory values, as indicated:

Glucose.

Useful in differentiating signs of withdrawal from those of hypoglycemia. (Note: Increased risk of hypoglycemia exists in FAS infants, who are often SGA with limited nutritional reserves.)

ACTIONS/INTERVENTIONS	RATIONALE

Collaborative

Arterial blood gases (ABGs).	Hypoxia and acidosis may develop, requiring prompt intervention.
CBC, sodium, calcium, and blood cultures.	Alterations in electrolytes and presence of sepsis or meningitis can produce signs similar to those of withdrawal.
Administer medications, as indicated:	Note: Infant experiencing cocaine withdrawal usually does not require pharmacologic support.
Paregoric (administered orally).	Paregoric is the drug of choice for pharmacologic management of drug withdrawal in the infant because of its sedative effect and lack of adverse effects.
Phenobarbital.	Sedatives may prevent or control seizure activity and modify hyperactive movement by depressing cerebrum, reducing CNS stimuli, and controlling irritability and insomnia.
Chlorpromazine.	Controls CNS and gastrointestinal (GI) effects of withdrawal, but may be associated with prolonged excretion time and hypothermia.
Diazepam.	Rapidly suppresses narcotic withdrawal effects, but is poorly metabolized and excreted by infant and may require as long as 1 month for total elimination. Parenteral administration may displace bilirubin and is contraindicated in jaundiced or premature infant.
Administer supplemental oxygen, as needed.	Corrects hypoxia and may prevent associated CNS damage.
Refer to foster care or child protection agency. (Refer to ND: Parenting, altered, high risk for.)	Psychosocial environment of home setting may predispose infant to neglect, addiction, or personality problems in later life. Some state laws require that all addicted mothers be reported to a child protection agency.

NURSING DIAGNOSIS:	**AIRWAY CLEARANCE, INEFFECTIVE; GAS EXCHANGE, IMPAIRED**
May be related to:	Excess production of mucus, depression of cough reflex and respiratory center, intrauterine asphyxia.
Possibly evidenced by:	Tachypnea, tachycardia, cyanosis, nasal flaring, grunting respirations, hypoxia, acidosis.
DESIRED OUTCOMES— NEWBORN WILL:	Display ABGs and respiratory rate WNL, with pink mucous membranes.
	Be free of signs of respiratory distress.

ACTIONS/INTERVENTIONS	RATIONALE

Independent

Note respiratory rate and effort, color, heart rate, presence of cough reflex, and signs of respiratory distress.

Narcotic may depress respiratory center and cough reflex. Transient tachypnea (greater than 60 respirations/min) secondary to excess fluid resorption in the lungs may occur. Tachycardia, cyanosis, nasal flaring, or grunting indicates hypoxia and respiratory failure. Mottling may occur as a vasomotor response during withdrawal and may be unrelated to peripheral oxygenation.

Review and record fetal status during prenatal and intrapartal periods, and at delivery, for evidence of stress, hypoxia, or meconium-stained amniotic fluid.

Provides data about infant's respiratory status and indicates occurrence and degree of hypoxic insults.

Place infant on side or in semi-Fowler's position.

Reduces risk of aspiration.

Note nasal stuffiness; suction prior to feedings, as indicated.

Increased nasal stuffiness and production of mucus interfere with breathing, especially during feedings.

Monitor infant's temperature. Control environment to promote cooling if infant's temperature is elevated.

Pyrexia associated with CNS stimulation increases metabolic rate and oxygen needs.

Collaborative

Monitor and graph serial ABGs.

Drug withdrawal causes an increase in oxygen consumption. In addition, respiratory depression or failure may result in hypoxia and acidosis. Although narcotic-addicted infants are usually delivered prematurely, chronic intrauterine stress, especially when associated with heroin addiction, can increase surfactant production, thereby reducing risk of respiratory distress syndrome.

Administer oxygen if indicated.

Increased oxygen demands and respiratory depression are associated with withdrawal and may compromise respiratory function, causing hypoxia and respiratory acidosis and alkalosis.

Avoid use of narcotic antagonists, such as naloxone hydrochloride (Narcan) and naltrexone hydrochloride (Trexan).

These drugs are contraindicated in narcotic-addicted infants because they may precipitate acute withdrawal.

Place infant on cardiopulmonary monitor. Initiate resuscitative measures as appropriate.

May be necessary in cases of severe respiratory interference. (Note: Increased incidence of sudden infant death syndrome [SIDS] has been reported in cocaine-exposed infants, possibly due to altered neurotransmitter content and disruption of brain structures regulating respiration.)

NURSING DIAGNOSIS:	NUTRITION, ALTERED, LESS THAN BODY REQUIRE-MENTS
May be related to:	Inability to ingest/digest/absorb adequate nutrients to meet metabolic needs (e.g., poor/uncoordinated sucking and swallowing, frequent GI irritation with vomiting, diarrhea, and repeated regurgitation; frequent hyperactivity).
Possibly evidenced by:	Failure to gain weight or weight loss, decreased adipose tissue.
DESIRED OUTCOMES—NEWBORN WILL:	Tolerate feedings, free of aspiration. Maintain adequate nutritional intake as evidenced by normal weight gain and customary stool cycle.

ACTIONS/INTERVENTIONS

Independent

Determine infant's gestational age. Note maternal prenatal nutritional state and evidence of maternal prenatal care.

Monitor strength and coordination of sucking and swallowing reflexes.

Assess infant for nasal congestion, stuffiness, or sneezing. Suction prior to feedings as indicated.

Encourage mother to feed infant, and assist her with activity as appropriate. Note effects of drugs and withdrawal syndrome on infant's feeding behaviors.

Provide small, slow, or frequent feedings. Encourage mother to avoid overfeeding.

Position infant on right side; do not disturb after feedings.

Monitor infant's intake and output, including frequency and consistency of stools.

RATIONALE

IUGR and delivery of LBW infant can result from heroin use, which decreases cellular multiplication and growth hormone production in utero. Many addicted mothers are malnourished throughout the pregnancy, leading to birth of a preterm SGA/LBW infant having low protein, iron, and glucose stores. Approximately 75% of women who abuse drugs during pregnancy do not seek prenatal care until labor begins.

CNS hyperactivity may negatively affect feeding behaviors and oral intake of nutrients.

Clears respiratory passage of excess mucus, allowing newborn to breathe more easily while eating, which may improve oral intake.

Hyperactive or sedated newborn is difficult to feed and put to the breast. In addition, FAS infants may display feeding problems and persistent vomiting for 6–7 months and have difficulty adjusting to solid foods.

Reduces risk of abdominal distention with resultant regurgitation. Slow feedings may allow infant to coordinate sucking and swallowing reflexes, improving intake. In many cases, mothers overfeed, offering milk whenever the newborn cries, which may actually prolong the GI dysfunction.

Facilitates emptying of stomach; promotes absorption. Disturbances may increase likelihood of regurgitation.

Identifies imbalances, permitting early intervention. GI irritability is associated with frequent loose or watery stools, vomiting, and regurgitation with resultant dehydration and malnutrition.

ACTIONS/INTERVENTIONS	RATIONALE

Independent

Weigh infant as indicated. Graph weight gains and losses.

Excessive or steady weight loss may indicate that caloric intake is inadequate for amount of energy being expended.

Institute a calorie count.

Inadequate weight gain may require use of higher-calorie formula and supplements, especially in LBW/SGA infant.

Note dryness of skin and mucous membranes, sunken fontanels, poor skin turgor, fever, diaphoresis, and increased urine specific gravity.

Dehydration can occur quickly in newborns because of fluid/electrolyte losses through diarrhea, vomiting, fever, and sweating.

Provide pacifier between feedings.

Satisfies infant's need for sucking, promotes self-quieting, and may decrease metabolic demands.

Reduce external stimuli, and swaddle infant. (Refer to ND: Injury, high risk for, CNS damage.)

Reduces activity level, metabolic needs, and energy expenditure.

Test stool for presence of reducing substances.

Identifies possible lactose intolerance or poor nutritional state, necessitating use of soy-based formula.

Collaborative

Monitor laboratory studies, as indicated:

  Hemoglobin/hematocrit.

Identifies anemia.

  White blood cell count with differential; blood cultures.

Infection/sepsis may be acquired in utero.

  Serum glucose.

Hypoglycemia may develop as a result of poor feeding, hyperactivity with increased metabolic demands, or GI disturbances resulting in faulty utilization of formula.

  Serum electrolytes.

Electrolyte imbalances may result from profuse diaphoresis, diarrhea, and inadequate fluid and nutrient intake.

Administer supplemental fluids parenterally.

May be necessary to prevent dehydration and to correct fluid and electrolyte imbalances associated with diarrhea, sweating, and vomiting.

Provide gavage feedings as indicated.

Conserves energy and decreases risk of regurgitation and aspiration. Gavage may be necessary if sucking and swallowing reflexes are ineffectual or uncoordinated and result in slower difficult feedings, or if tachypnea or respiratory distress is present.

Administer antispasmodics (e.g., paregoric, tincture of opium) between feedings, as indicated.

Reduces GI irritation, controls loose or watery stools, and helps prevent dehydration.

583

NURSING DIAGNOSIS:	SKIN INTEGRITY, IMPAIRED, HIGH RISK FOR
Risk factors may include:	Mechanical factors (continual rubbing of face and knees against bedding, scratching of the face with hands) presence of excretions.
Possibly evidenced by:	[Not applicable; presence of signs/symptoms establishes an **actual** diagnosis.]
DESIRED OUTCOMES— NEWBORN WILL:	Maintain intact skin.

ACTIONS/INTERVENTIONS

Independent

Inspect skin for abrasion or excoriation, especially on face, nose, knees, elbows, and shoulders, and under buttocks.

Provide soft bedding or sheepskin; cover hands with mitts.

Reposition infant at least every 2 hr.

Swaddle infant; place in infant carrier.

Provide skin care and meticulous cleansing of diaper area.

RATIONALE

Changes in tissue color and integrity indicate increased irritation and need for intervention.

Decreases risk of dermal injury.

Avoids prolonged pressure on body parts.

Confines infant; reduces activity level and risk of dermal irritation.

Prevents breakdown in diaper area, which is more susceptible to excoriation because of loose excretions/moisture and lack of air circulation.

NURSING DIAGNOSIS:	PARENTING, ALTERED
May be related to:	Lack of available role model or ineffective role model, lack of support between/from significant other(s), unmet emotional maturation needs of parent, interruption in bonding process, lack of knowledge, lack of appropriate response of child to relationship.
Possibly evidenced by:	Verbalization of role inadequacy, inability to care for infant, inattention to infant needs, inappropriate caretaking behaviors, lack of parental attachment behaviors.
DESIRED OUTCOMES— PARENT(S) WILL:	Demonstrate appropriate attachment behaviors.
	Verbalize realistic perception of the maternal/parental role.
	Verbalize insight into own dependency needs.
	Contact/use support resources effectively.

ACTIONS/INTERVENTIONS	RATIONALE

Independent

Evaluate mother's prenatal and current physical and emotional status. Assess family stressors. Note mother's involvement in prenatal care, childbirth classes, and drug or alcohol rehabilitation programs.

Provides data necessary to evaluate parenting capabilities and the family/home situation. Because of her own emotional state, the addicted mother is often unable to assume the overwhelming task of unselfish giving and nurturing, so that the potential for infant abuse or neglect exists.

Discuss mother's perception of herself, noting realistic and unrealistic appraisals and her desire to change. Maintain nonjudgmental attitude.

Fosters mother's desire to provide data about drug dependence, to discuss her emotional status, and to look realistically at her own ability to cope with the stress of childrearing and with the infant's withdrawal behaviors. The drug-addicted mother is usually dependent and depressed, and has low self-esteem and inadequate support systems stemming from an inability to form lasting intimate relationships. Her drug dependence has resulted from her inadequate coping skills. Fear and guilt associated with her observation of infant's physiologic withdrawal may reinforce her negative self-image and may negatively affect her ability to cope and care for the infant.

Encourage mother to express anxieties, fears, and anger. Discuss ways to release frustrations and manage stress (e.g., stating concern directly or use of physical exercise).

Helps mother to ventilate her concerns. Abusive behavior, guilt, and fear may reinforce feelings of incompetence.

Discuss current status of substance abuse. Initiate plans for enrollment in drug or alcohol rehabilitation program.

Mother's insight into her dependency needs and her ability to use resources to promote change may affect the decision regarding newborn placement with parents or in foster care.

Ascertain maternal/paternal perceptions of parenting role and state of the family.

Provides realistic appraisal of parenting capabilities. Aids in predicting the amount of follow-up needed, and influences decisions regarding custody of newborn.

Encourage frequent visits/telephone contact as appropriate.

Minimizes separation between mother and newborn, reducing interruption in bonding process.

Recommend bringing infant to eye contact gradually while speaking slowly and softly.

May limit infant irritability and enhance interactive behavior. (Note: Limited ability to tolerate visual activity may result in infant taking a time-out by averting eyes after only 30–60 sec of interaction. Parent may erroneously interpret this as rejection by the infant.)

Observe attachment behaviors and quality of parent-infant interaction.

Previous lifestyles, a potential lack of knowledge regarding child care and the needs of a growing infant, and the possibility of the infant experiencing problems of withdrawal can interfere with the attachment process. Poor maternal interactional capabilities increase risk for a disturbed mother-child relationship. Furthermore, separation related to the infant's withdrawal, treatment, and hospitalization of the infant required after discharge of the mother may negatively affect the acquaintance process.

ACTIONS/INTERVENTIONS	RATIONALE

Independent

Assess parents' ability and desire to keep child.

Subtle cues of parental anxiety may be apparent in parents' behavior or in the expression of their concerns. The child may need to be placed in foster care if the mother/couple is unable to care for infant for a protracted period of time.

Support parents' efforts to understand and care for child.

Many parents require constant emotional support to build confidence.

Encourage performance of infant care tasks by mother and father.

Fosters positive adaptation to parenting role; facilitates the parent-newborn acquaintance process.

Provide information about the signs of acute newborn withdrawal, anticipated behaviors, and the therapeutic measures to be employed. Let parents know that these signs are usually temporary; however, infants with FAS can have subacute or long-term withdrawal effects, as well as mental retardation.

Prepares parents for management of withdrawal. Information about therapy may help relieve feelings of guilt, fear, and ambivalence. Feeding problems, excessive crying, irritability, inconsolability, and sleep disturbances may further reinforce parents' low self-esteem, may create potential negative feedback patterns (e.g., avoidance or rough handling of infant), and may interfere with or prevent positive attachment.

Provide names, phone numbers, and addresses of supportive resources providing 24-hour availability. Encourage use of these resources.

Allows parents to obtain help and information to help them to cope with stressful situations.

Schedule home visit within 7 to 10 days of infant's discharge from hospital.

Helps to monitor home setting and to assess the possibility of substance abuse, poor parenting, and infant neglect or abuse.

Collaborative

Refer parents to community resources such as addiction counselor, social service, visiting nurse services, or peer/support group.

Ongoing support and assistance in a protective or therapeutic environment such as a halfway house or the use of ongoing services in the home may help parents develop appropriate parenting skills and promote well-being of the infant.

Make appropriate referral to foster care or child care agency.

Some state laws require notification of such agencies if mother is a known substance abuser. Maternal maturation associated with pregnancy may be insufficient to meet increasing demands of infant care. (Note: Studies show an increased incidence of illness in the offspring of substance abusers believed to be directly related to poor parenting.)

Refer mother to drug assistance program, as indicated (e.g., Narcotics Anonymous or Alcoholics Anonymous).

Mother needs to take care of herself before she can assume responsibility for another person.

NURSING DIAGNOSIS:	**KNOWLEDGE DEFICIT [LEARNING NEED], regarding infant condition, prognosis, and care**
May be related to:	Lack of exposure/unfamiliarity with information resources, misinterpretation, lack of recall.

Possibly evidenced by:	Request for information, statement of misconceptions, inaccurate follow-through of instructions.
DESIRED OUTCOMES—PARENT(S) WILL:	List behaviors/signs associated with substance withdrawal.
	Verbalize/demonstrate appropriate infant care activities.

ACTIONS/INTERVENTIONS	RATIONALE
Independent	
Provide information to parents about infant's behavior and physiologic signs of withdrawal. Discuss rationale of treatment plan.	Fosters cooperation and understanding of interventions; promotes safety of infant. Promotes informed decision-making.
Review altered responses of infant during withdrawal (increased sensitivity to auditory stimuli, depressed visual orientation and response, increased lability, and reduced alertness). Encourage mother to provide early visual input and pattern stimulation.	Information helps parent(s) understand infant's needs, optimizing infant's capabilities and interactional qualities, which can increase parents' self-esteem and provide reinforcement for efforts.
Identify long-term physiologic effects of addiction on infant.	Although most infants are free of withdrawal signs by 10 days of age, mild patterns of irritability may persist for 3 to 4 months, and sleep problems may persist for as long as 1 year, creating stress for parents. Use of opiates, methadone, and possibly other drugs has been correlated with SIDS, feeding problems (failure to thrive), hyperactivity, and brief attention span (which may be manifested with apparent long-term growth retardation and disturbed behavior patterns, especially in the FAS infant). In addition, smaller head size associated with cocaine use can lead to neurologic impairment and difficulties with language skills as the infant matures.
Discuss passage of drugs (e.g., nicotine, narcotic, or alcohol) through breast milk.	Alternative feeding method may need to be considered if maternal withdrawal program includes prescribed pharmacologic agents. Mother needs to be aware that any drugs she takes can be passed on to the infant. (Note: Cocaine may remain in breast milk for up to 60 hours following maternal use.)
Provide information about infant's needs following discharge (e.g., food, clothing, and equipment). (Refer to CP: Neonatal Assessment: 1 Week Following Discharge, ND: Knowledge Deficit [Learning Need]; CP: Neonatal Assessment: 4 Weeks Following Birth, ND: Knowledge Deficit [Learning Need].)	Helps ensure that parents have necessary articles in the home to care for the child.

ACTIONS/INTERVENTIONS

Independent

Recommend that parent(s) learn infant CPR.

RATIONALE

Research suggests a fivefold increased incidence of SIDS in cocaine-exposed infants.

NURSING DIAGNOSIS:	**FAMILY COPING, INEFFECTIVE: DISABLING**
May be related to:	Significant person with chronically unexpressed feelings of guilt, anxiety, hostility, despair, and so forth; dissonant discrepancy of coping styles for dealing with adaptive tasks by/among significant person(s).
Possibly evidenced by:	[Not applicable; presence of signs/symptoms establishes an **actual** diagnosis.]
DESIRED OUTCOMES— FAMILY WILL:	Verbalize realistic understanding and expectations of family members.
	Participate positively in care of infant, within limits of family's abilities.
	Express feelings and expectations openly and honestly, as appropriate.

ACTIONS/INTERVENTIONS

Independent

Discuss parents' expectations of themselves and of infant, noting realistic and unrealistic perceptions.

Assess family stressors, history, and situation, and available support systems. Involve other family members in plan of care if appropriate.

Observe parent-infant interaction and child care skills. Evaluate parents' level of knowledge and decision-making skills in regard to keeping and raising the infant. (Refer to ND: Parenting, altered, high risk for.)

Ascertain long-range plans and mother's commitment to seeking assistance and making necessary lifestyle changes to achieve and maintain drug-free life.

RATIONALE

Increases parents' awareness of common problems that may arise and helps them to have a more realistic view of parenting.

A stable relationship, the presence in the home of adults who are not substance abusers, and previous success in childrearing increase chance of positive outcome for infant. Family disorganization and disruption, with absence of strong, consistent father figure or a history of sexual abuse of female who is addicted, may negatively affect mothering qualities.

Identifies areas of weakness or misunderstanding. Anxiety, depression, low self-esteem and self-confidence, and poor interpersonal skills typically render parents ineffective as primary caregivers and may foster intergenerational problems of child abuse or child neglect and predispose family members to substance abuse.

Mother's drug problem and treatment status, together with her poor coping skills and lack of family support, may interfere with integration of infant into the family, necessitating alternative placement.

ACTIONS/INTERVENTIONS

Collaborative

Provide referrals, as indicated, to meet physical, emotional, and financial needs (e.g., visiting nurse services, group homes, halfway houses, drug programs, and counseling or psychotherapy).

RATIONALE

May be necessary to provide ongoing care, to reduce incidence of recidivism, and to foster optimal growth and development of parent(s) and infant.

The Infant of an HIV-Positive Mother _____

Frequently, the newborn who is subsequently determined to be human immunodeficiency virus (HIV)-positive will be asymptomatic during the nursery stay. The Centers for Disease Control and Prevention (CDC) classifies HIV-positive newborns as indeterminate, asymptomatic, or symptomatic. Only 20%–40% of infants born to HIV-positive mothers are themselves infected.

This plan of care is to be used in conjunction with the previous newborn plans of care.

NEONATE ASSESSMENT DATA BASE

As a rule, neonate is asymptomatic at birth, although a few may show signs of opportunistic infections at or within several days of birth. Additionally, effects of maternal substance use/abuse and/or prematurity may be present.

FOOD/FLUID

Low birth weight.

NEUROSENSORY

Neurologic deficits.

Microcephaly.

TEACHING/LEARNING

Prematurity.

Developmental delays.

History of parental i.v. drug use.

DIAGNOSTIC STUDIES

Current tests do not distinguish between mother's/infant's antibodies, and the infant may test negative by 9 to 15 months of age. Research is trying to develop an inexpensive readily available procedure to differentiate infant vs. maternal antibody response.

Complete blood count (CBC) and total lymphocyte count: Nondiagnostic in newborns but provides baseline immunologic data.

EIA or ELISA and Western Blot test: May be positive, but invalid.

HIV cultures (with peripheral blood mononuclear cells and, if available, plasma).

Polymerase chain reaction testing with peripheral blood leukocytes: Detects viral DNA in presence in small quantities of infected peripheral mononuclear cells.

Serum or plasma p24 antigen: Increased quantitative values can be indicative of progression of infection (may not be detectable during very early stages of HIV infection).

Quantitative serum immunoglobin G, M, and A (IgG, IgM, and IgA) determinations: Nondiagnostic in newborns but provide baseline immunologic data.

NURSING PRIORITIES

1. Prevent/minimize infections.
2. Maximize nutritional intake.
3. Promote attachment, growth, and development.
4. Provide information to parent(s) about disease process/prognosis and treatment needs.

DISCHARGE GOALS

1. Free of opportunistic/nosocomial infection.
2. Gaining weight appropriately.
3. Perform skills typical of age group within scope of present developmental level.
4. Parent/caregiver understands condition/prognosis and treatment needs.

Refer to previous newborn plans of care for customary infant needs.

NURSING DIAGNOSIS:	INFECTION, HIGH RISK FOR
Risk factors may include:	Immature immune system, inadequate acquired immunity, suppressed inflammatory response, invasive procedures, malnutrition, chronic disease (infections).
Possibly evidenced by:	[Not applicable; presence of signs/symptoms establishes an **actual** diagnosis.]
DESIRED OUTCOMES— INFANT WILL:	Be free of opportunistic infection.
PARENT/CAREGIVER WILL:	Verbalize understanding of individual risk factors. Identify interventions to reduce risk of infection. Provide safe environment for infant.

ACTIONS/INTERVENTIONS	RATIONALE
Independent	
Use mechanical suction or bulb syringe in place of oral mucus extractors (e.g., DeLee trap) to clear airways. Avoid mouth-to-mouth contact for resuscitation.	Prevents exposure of healthcare provider to virus.
Wash neonate at time of delivery. Minimize exposure to maternal blood and body fluids. Prepare skin with soap and water and then alcohol prior to injections/heel-sticks.	The neonate is considered potentially uninfected and should be protected from additional contamination.
Provide customary physical care of neonate (e.g., skin care, eye care, vitamin K administration) as for all newborns, using universal precautions.	Universal precautions are routinely required for contact with body fluids/blood products to protect the healthcare provider from potential infection.
Stress need for care providers/family members washing hands before and after contact with infant. Wear gloves for contact with secretions (e.g., diapering, cord care, injections, handling of blood/blood by-products).	Reduces risk of cross-contamination and risk to care providers.
Notify laboratory of HIV status and mark specimens accordingly.	Proper preparation and handling reduces risk of cross-contamination.

591

ACTIONS/INTERVENTIONS	RATIONALE

Independent

Note maternal HIV status/presence of high-risk behaviors.

Anti-HIV antibodies are transmitted across the placenta and are present in all infants of HIV-seropositive mothers. However, only 20% to 40% of these infants will themselves eventually test positive for HIV. (Note: Maternal antibodies may not be cleared from infant's system until 9 to 15 months of age.)

Apply mittens; file infant's nails as indicated.

Protects skin from injury that can provide additional portals of entry for infectious agents.

Monitor/limit contact with care providers and family members as appropriate.

Reduces number of pathogens presented to the infant's immune system and decreases possibility of infant contracting a nosocomial infection.

Provide for complete isolation as indicated.

Presence of enteritis, congenital syphilis, or cytomegalovirus (CMV) or other viral infections increases risk of cross-contamination to other infants.

Monitor temperature and secretions. Auscultate breath sounds. Note behavioral changes; e.g., irritability, lethargy. Palpate lymph node chains.

HIV-seropositive infants have increased risk for developing recurrent upper respiratory infection, otitis media, thrush, CMV, erythematous rash, and lymphadenopathy. (Note: Although *Pneumocystis cannii* pneumonia [PCP] is common in both infants and adults, lymphocytic interstitial pneumonitis [LIP] is rarely seen in adults and is the second most common indicator disease for diagnosing acquired immune deficiency syndrome [AIDS] in infants.)

Seal soiled tissues, paper wipes/trash, and disposable diapers in plastic bags per protocol.

Reduces risk of cross-contamination and alerts appropriate personnel/departments to exercise specific hazardous materials procedures.

Investigate sudden fever, dyspnea, dry cough, hypoxia, abnormal breath sounds, use of accessory muscles, retractions, and nasal flaring.

Up to 50% of HIV-infected infants develop PCP during first year of life.

Observe infant for seizure activity, neck stiffness, muscle rigidity, irritability or lethargy, or positive Kernig's sign.

Suggests meningitis or opportunistic CNS infection. (Note: If symptoms develop slowly over weeks, may reflect HIV effect on CNS rather than acute infectious process.)

Collaborative

Monitor laboratory studies as indicated:

Urine screening.

Increased risk of CMV in utero or during hospital stay necessitates routine microscopic evaluation. (Note: Once discharged, exposure to CMV is a risk in day-care setting as well.)

IgG, IgM, IgA.

Elevated serum immunoglobins are a hallmark of pediatric HIV infections and may develop before the decrease in CD_4 (T helper cells) is noted. (Note: Polyclonal hypergammaglobulinemia occurs in approximately 80% of infected infants, usually in first months of life.)

592

ACTIONS/INTERVENTIONS	RATIONALE
Collaborative	
CD$_4$ counts.	Decline reflects immunologic compromise and need for institution of zidovudine therapy. CD$_4$ counts of 3000/mm^3 or more are normal in healthy infants and gradually decline to adult levels. Counts below 1500/mm^3 in first year place infant at increased risk of developing PCP.
Administer medications as appropriate:	
Zidovudine (AZT).	Useful in preventing replication of HIV in infants older than 3 months of age; however, side effects may limit its usefulness.
Didanosine (Videx).	May be used to treat HIV strains resistant to zidovudine.
Ketoconazole (Nizoral).	Effective treatment for systemic yeast infections.
Trimethoprim-sulfamethoxazole (Bactrim) prophylaxis.	Instituted for symptomatic infants or asymptomatic infants with CD$_4$ counts below 500/mm^3 to prevent PCP.
Triple dye, bacitracin.	Antimicrobial agents used in cord care to reduce risk of infection.
Ganciclovir.	Treatment of choice for CMV infection to prevent blindness/life-threatening dissemination.
Recommend/coordinate periodic ophthalmologic examinations as appropriate.	Early detection of retinitis in presence of CMV infection allows for prompt intervention.

NURSING DIAGNOSIS:	**NUTRITION, ALTERED, LESS THAN BODY REQUIREMENTS, HIGH RISK FOR**
Risk factors may include:	Inability to ingest, digest, or absorb nutrients (e.g., impaired suck/swallow, gastrointestinal [GI] infection, malabsorption, diarrhea).
Possibly evidenced by:	[Not applicable; presence of signs/symptoms establishes an **actual** diagnosis.]
DESIRED OUTCOMES— INFANT WILL:	Demonstrate progressive weight gain toward goal.
	Display laboratory values within normal limits.
	Be free of signs of malnutrition/failure to thrive (FTT).
PARENT/CAREGIVER WILL:	Demonstrate understanding of feeding techniques and infant's specific needs.

ACTIONS/INTERVENTIONS	RATIONALE

Independent

Obtain baseline weight. Establish regular schedule for weighing following discharge. Identify resources if scale is not available in home setting.	These infants are at increased risk for FTT as evidenced by weight loss or little weight gain from birth. Early recognition provides opportunity for prompt intervention. (Note: If infant is eating well, but not gaining weight, evaluate for GI infection.)
Observe coordination of sucking and swallowing reflexes.	Abnormal oral motor patterns may impair feeding.
Inspect oral cavity. Review procedure with caregivers.	Development of oral sores (e.g., thrush) impairs ability to feed, and, if untreated, can spread to the esophagus, necessitating alternative feeding techniques.
Counsel mother regarding risk of breastfeeding. Encourage alternative feeding.	HIV is present in colostrum and breast milk and although limited, does present some risk to the infant.
Note infant tolerance of feedings.	Feeding difficulties, gastric distress, or signs of fatigue may require small frequent feedings for optimal intake.
Hold infant during feedings.	Provides human contact/stimulation and may enhance intake.
Investigate presence of diarrhea.	May indicate lactose intolerance requiring lactose-free formula or reflect GI manifestations of HIV infection (e.g., diarrhea, malabsorption, impaired gastric motility, and liver dysfunction).
Observe feeding techniques of caregivers. Provide assistance and encouragement.	Attention to positioning and handling may be required to normalize postural tone while feeding and to maximize sucking/swallowing efforts.
Stress importance of close monitoring for infectious processes.	Infant is prone to parotitis, as well as frequent episodes of rapid-onset pneumonia, interfering with both appetite and feeding. Additionally, presence of infectious process greatly increases metabolic rate and thereby nutritional needs.
Review age-appropriate diet and addition of solid foods considering developmental abilities.	Provides optimal nutrition based on individual needs following discharge.

Collaborative

Administer nystatin as indicated.	Effective treatment for oral yeast infection.
Provide enteral/parenteral feedings as appropriate.	Motor impairments and/or presence of infection may necessitate alternative feeding techniques to meet dietary needs.
Obtain stool specimens as indicated.	Stool cultures; tests for ova/parasites, cryptosporidium, c. dificil (toxin produced by bacteria), acid-fast bacillus and Gram stain may identify causes for gastric distress/diarrhea and weight loss or failure to gain.

NURSING DIAGNOSIS:	GROWTH AND DEVELOPMENT, ALTERED, HIGH RISK FOR
Risk factors may include:	Separation from significant others, inadequate caretaking, inconsistent responsiveness/multiple caretakers, environmental and stimulation deficiencies, effects of chronic condition/disabilities.
Possibly evidenced by:	[Not applicable; presence of signs/symptoms establishes an **actual** diagnosis.]
DESIRED OUTCOMES— INFANT WILL:	Respond to parent/caregiver interactions.
	Perform motor, social, and/or expressive skills typical of age group, within scope of present capabilities.
PARENT/CAREGIVER WILL:	Verbalize understanding of developmental status and plans for intervention.
	Demonstrate skills in handling infant needs.

ACTIONS/INTERVENTIONS	RATIONALE
Independent	
Determine individual status using Denver Developmental or similar screening tool.	Provides baseline to note future progress/changes and identify therapy needs. Cognitive impairments vary, may be present at birth or develop as a result of environmental deprivation or viral infections affecting the CNS. Additionally, some infants may have delayed sensorimotor development while others display abnormal muscle tone and movement patterns with delayed development of righting and equilibrium reactions.
Identify developmental milestones and anticipated time frames for achievement.	Reinforces belief that infant may progress with appropriate support and interventions. (Note: Lack of development or regression is an indicator of need for further evaluation and may reflect effect of infectious process.)
Discuss caregiver's perceptions of infant's capabilities and plan for growth.	Increased illness, prolonged/recurrent hospitalizations, neglect/overprotection by caregivers may limit sensory/movement stimuli and motivation.
Observe infant-parent interactions.	Eye contact, reaching out of infant promotes adult response. Effect of maternal drug use, presence of illness, or developmental delays may prevent or limit infant interactions, impairing bonding.
Encourage verbalization of feelings by parent(s)/ family members.	Frequently, feelings of guilt and despair may be expressed as hostility, denial, or defensiveness regarding diagnosis. Awareness of these feelings provides opportunity to work through them and develop a positive relationship with the infant.

595

ACTIONS/INTERVENTIONS

Independent

Avoid confronting denial, which may be very strong when the infant is asymptomatic. Counsel without lecturing, provide information without patronizing, and support and give hope without making false promises.

Encourage/support family efforts to care for infant.

Discuss ways to provide a normal atmosphere (e.g., spending time outdoors, using support systems effectively).

Collaborative

Coordinate multidisciplinary team conference to include pediatrician, primary nurse, social worker, nutritional support, psychologist or psychiatrist, physical/occupational therapists, and speech therapists.

Stress importance of frequent screening and formal evaluations by developmental specialists.

RATIONALE

Parent(s) need to progress at their own rate. Providing information, Active-listening, and acceptance of the person in nonjudgmental ways promotes more positive progression and resolution.

Personal interactions, even after a period of abandonment, enhance the bonding process. (Note: Volunteers may be required to support staff efforts in the absence of family involvement or ineffective family involvement.)

Enhances sense of control and provides encouragement for enjoying the present and possibilities of the future.

Necessary to address complex issues and maximize infant's potential because all areas are interrelated to growth and development.

Identifies developmental delays and effectiveness of therapy (e.g., early intervention program [EIP]).

NURSING DIAGNOSIS:	KNOWLEDGE DEFICIT [LEARNING NEED], regarding condition, prognosis, and treatment needs
May be related to:	Lack of exposure, misinterpretation, unfamiliarity with resources, lack of recall.
Possibly evidenced by:	Request for information, statement of misconceptions, inaccurate follow-through of instructions, development of preventable complications.
DESIRED OUTCOMES— PARENT/CAREGIVER WILL:	Verbalize understanding of condition and treatment needs.
	Identify signs/symptoms requiring intervention.
	Perform necessary procedures correctly and explain reasons for the actions.
	Establish plan for ongoing therapy and evaluations.

ACTIONS/INTERVENTIONS

Independent

Determine parent(s)'/caregivers' understanding of condition and prognosis.

RATIONALE

Provides starting point for information and opportunity to clarify misconceptions. Incubation period of initial HIV infection to progressive encephalopathy varies from 2 months to 5 years. HIV directly affects CNS, cardiovascular, GI, and renal func-

ACTIONS/INTERVENTIONS	RATIONALE
Independent	tion. Median age for appearance of opportunistic infections is 9 months. Impaired brain growth, loss of developmental milestones, and progressive motor dysfunction indicate a very poor prognosis. (Note: Children rarely develop Kaposi's sarcoma, tuberculosis, toxoplasmosis, cryptococcosis, or histoplasmosis.)
Provide realistic, optimistic information during each contact with parent.	Enhances attachment process and reduces likelihood of abandonment. Many people have been exposed to media information about AIDS or have friends/lovers who have died of the disease, and parent/caregiver may be pessimistic about outcome for infant.
Note response to contact with infant by parent(s)/family, and other caregivers. Discuss individual concerns.	Interactions may be affected by fear of contamination and of personal judgments regarding suspected high-risk behaviors of parents. (Note: To date, there have been no documented cases of individuals contracting AIDS from routine care of infected infants when following established CDC precautions.)
Note roles of family members and availability of extended family.	HIV infection is frequently a multigenerational disease, directly affecting mothers, offspring, and other family members. As mother must deal with her own chronic illness, awareness of the role of the father and grandparents is necessary in determining family needs or necessity of alternative placement.
Review current medication/treatment options.	Research is ongoing and often openly discussed in the media, sometimes raising false hopes that must be clarified to enhance the decision-making process. Current studies suggest monthly intravenous immunoglobulins (IV-Ig) may reduce infections and incidence of hospitalization. Additionally, trials of experimental vaccines for asymptomatic HIV-seropositive infants are presently being tried in the hopes of enhancing the response of the immune system.
Identify ways to protect infant from exposure to common infections, diseases, or contact with recently vaccinated individuals.	Impairment of immune system reduces infant's ability to ward off disease.
Stress importance of routine immunization as appropriate.	Provides protection from some infectious agents. (Note: Infant should receive injectable [Salk] instead of oral [Sabin] polio vaccine, which contains live virus. Additionally, asymptomatic infants do not require influenza vaccine.)
Review side effects of therapy, e.g., zidovudine.	Nausea/vomiting, abnormalities of liver function, and suppression of bone marrow limit therapy/drug dosage.

597

ACTIONS/INTERVENTIONS	RATIONALE

Independent

Review living conditions, physical care, prevention of spread of infection, and prevention of opportunistic infections.

Mother's lifestyle/condition may preclude her providing appropriate care for infant. Other family members (e.g., grandparents, aunt/uncle) may be providing care for mother and/or other involved family members and be unable to care for infant too.

Discuss placement options as appropriate.

Chronically ill/impaired mother and extended family members who may be overtaxed with caring for ill family members may not be able to meet the needs of even a well infant. Residential or foster home may be indicated at least for a period of time until family or parent(s) are able to assume responsibility for infant. (Note: Many foster homes refuse HIV-infected infants, and as a rule, these children are not usually available for adoption.)

Stress frequency and content of follow-up care, especially with health professionals experienced in caring for HIV-seropositive women and infants.

Knowledgeable providers are better equipped to deal with the complex health issues and use newly developed treatment options to promote optimal outcomes for the infant/family.

Discuss significance of HIV and other testing.

Regular testing to age 2 is necessary to verify HIV status in absence of opportunistic infections. Viral cultures, polymerase chain reaction, IgA, IgM, p24 antigen assay, and evaluation of CD_4 lymphocyte count monitor presence/progression of infection. Additionally some resources believe *all* infants born to HIV-risk women require vigilant pediatric follow-up for early diagnosis of true HIV infection.

Identify signs/symptoms requiring notification of healthcare provider; e.g., fever, pain, altered activity level, difficulty breathing, poor appetite, weight loss, vomiting, diarrhea, skin rashes, oral thrush, or developmental regression.

Prompt evaluation and intervention may limit process and progression to AIDS.

Encourage parents/caregivers to care for their own health and to make time to meet their own needs for rest and relaxation.

As they learn to take time for themselves, parents/caregivers can better manage long-term care of a chronically ill child.

Identify sources for family counseling, community support groups, and other resources (e.g., visiting nurse services, home care agency, social services, respite care).

Mother-infant dyads are at increased risk for impaired bonding. Physical illness, financial stressors, depression, maternal drug use, and poor support systems interfere with parenting abilities, placing infant at risk for physical and emotional neglect/abuse. Additionally, family members will require assistance in coping with chronic illness and future prognosis for family members.

Bibliography

General Reference Books

Berkow, R, (ed) *The Merck Manual*, ed 16, Merck & Co., Rahway, NJ, 1992.

Bobak, IM, and Jensen, MD: *Maternity & Gynecologic Care, The Nurse and the Family*, ed 5, CV Mosby, St. Louis, 1993.

Cella, J, and Watson, J: *Nurse's Manual of Laboratory Tests.* FA Davis Co., Philadelphia, 1989.

Cox, HC, et al.: *Clinical Applications of Nursing Diagnosis*, ed 2, FA Davis, Philadelphia, 1993.

Deglin, JH, and Vallerand, AH: *Davis's Drug Guide for Nurses*, ed 3, FA Davis, Philadelphia, 1993.

Doenges, ME, and Moorhouse, MF: *Application of Nursing Process and Nursing Diagnosis: An Interactive Text*, FA Davis, Philadelphia, 1992.

Doenges, ME, and Moorhouse, MF: *Nurse's Pocket Guide: Nursing Diagnoses with Interventions*, ed 4, FA Davis, Philadelphia 1993.

Fischback, R: *A Manual of Laboratory & Diagnostic Tests.* JB Lippincott, Philadelphia, 1992.

Ladewig, P, London, M, and Olds, S: *Essentials of Maternal-Newborn Nursing*, ed 2, Addison-Wesley, Redwood City, CA, 1990.

Olds, S, London, M, and Ladewig, P: *Maternal Newborn Nursing, A Family-Centered Approach.* ed 4, Addison-Wesley, Redwood City, CA, 1992.

Professional Guide to Diseases, ed 3, Springhouse Corp., Springhouse, PA, 1989.

Suddarth, DS: *The Lippincott Manual of Nursing Practice*, ed 5, JB Lippincott, Philadelphia, 1991.

Chapter 1: Articles

Chasnoff, IJ: Drugs, alcohol, pregnancy, and the neonate. JAMA 266(11):1567, 1991.

Chez, RA: *Identifying maternal/fetal risks before pregnancy.* Medical Aspects of Human Sexuality 25(4):54, April 1991.

Lucas, VA: *Birth: Nursing's role in today's choices*, RN 56(6):38, 1993.

Chapter 2: Articles

Zylke, J: *Maternal, child health needs noted by two major national study groups.* JAMA, 261(12):1687–1688, 1989.

Starn, J, and Neiderhauser, V: *An MCN model for nursing diagnosis to focus interventions.* MCH, 15:180–183, 1990.

Chapter 3: Articles

Chez, RA: *Identifying maternal/fetal risks before pregnancy*, Medical Aspects of Human Sexuality, 25(4):54, 1991.

Edmond, S: *Preeclampsia—baby aspirin*, Harvard Health Letter, 16(2):4, 1990.

Sibai, BM: *Low-dosage aspirin may prevent preeclampsia.* Perinatal Outlook, 2(1):2, 1991.

Chapter 4: Articles

Acosta, YM, et al: *HIV disease and pregnancy: Antepartum and intrapartum care*, part 2, JOGNN, 21(2):97–103, 1992.

Anderson, J: *HIV in women: factors that increase their risk*, Medical Aspects of Human Sexuality, 25(5):20–27, 1991.

Apuzzio, JJ, and Leo, MV: *Herpes in the pregnant woman*, Medical Aspects of Human Sexuality, 25(6):54, 1991.

Beckmann, CR, and Beckmann, CA: *Effect of a structured antepartum exercise program on pregnancy and labor outcome in primiparas*, The Journal of Reproductive Medicine, 35:704–709, 1990.

Berkowitz, RS, and Goldstein, DP: *Diagnosis and management of the primary hydatidiform mole*, Obstetrics and Gynecology Clinics of North America, 15:491–503, 1988.

Blakemore, KJ: *Prenatal diagnosis by chorionic villus sampling.* Obstetrics and Gynecologic Clinics of North America, 15:179–213, 1988.

Bullock, LF, and McFarlane, J: *The birth-weight battering connection*, AJN, 89(9):1153.

Catlin, AJ: *Early pregnancy loss; What you can do to help*, Nursing89, 19(11):43.

Chavkin, W, and St. Clair, D: *Beyond prenatal care: A comprehensive vision of reproductive health.* Journal of the American Medical Women's Association, 45:55–57, 1990.

Chez, R: *Identifying maternal/fetal risks before pregnancy*, Medical Aspects of Human Sexuality. 25(4):54–58, 1991.

Christmas, JT: *The risks of cocaine use in pregnancy*, Medical Aspects of Human Sexuality, 26(2):36, 1992.

Coste, J, Job-Spina, N, Fernandez, H: *Increased risk of ectopic pregnancy with maternal cigarette smoking.* Am J Pub Health 81:199, 1991.

Craft, K: *Pregnant? Take these precautions.* Nursing89, 19(1):63.

Craig, DI: *The adaptation to pregnancy of spinal cord injured women*, Rehabilitation Nursing, 15(1):6, 1990.

Eicher, D: Birth *anxiety loses its fearful image, pregnant teens learn basics about delivery.* The Denver Post, Sat., March 23, 1991.

Fulroth, R, et al: *Perinatal outcome of infants exposed to cocaine and/or heroin in utero.* AJDC, 143:905–910, Aug. 1989.

Gill, P, Smith, M, and Katz, M: *Tocolysis for preterm labor.* Tokos Medical Corp., Santa Ana, CA.

Gill, P, and Katz, M: *Let's prevent preterm birth,* Tokos Medical Corp., Santa Ana, CA.

Graeber, L: *Beyond ultrasound.* Parenting, 76–81, March 1991.

Green, D, and Malin, J: *Prenatal diagnosis: When reality shatters parents' dreams.* Nursing88, 18(2):61.

Hadeed, AJ, and Siegel, SR: *Maternal cocaine use during pregnancy: Effect on the newborn infant.* Pediatrics, 84:205–210, 1989.

Helton, AS: *A buddy system to improve prenatal care.* MCN, 15:234–237, 1990.

Kern, V: *Action Stat: Ruptured ectopic pregnancy.* Nursing89, 19(10):33.

Kitzmiller, JL, et al: *Preconception care of diabetics: Glycemic control prevents congenital anomalies.* JAMA 265:731, 1991.

Kivikoski, AI, Martin, CM, and Smeltzer, JA: *Transabdominal and transvaginal ultrasonography in the diagnosis of ectopic pregnancy.* Am J Obstet Gynecol, 163:123–128, 1990.

Kritz-Silverstein, D, Barrett-Connor, E, and Wingard, D: *The effect of parity on the later development of non-insulin-dependent diabetes mellitus or impaired glucose tolerance.* N Engl J Med 321:1214, 1989.

Langer, A, and Kudart, E: *Construction of a family pedigree in genetic counseling before amniocentesis.* Journal of Reproductive Medicine, 35:715–718, 1990.

Longobucco, DC, and Freston, MS: *Relation of somatic symptoms to degree of paternal-role preparation of first-time expectant fathers.* JOGNN, 18:482–288, 1989.

Naeye, RL: *Maternal body weight and pregnancy outcome.* Am J Clin Nutr, 52:273–279, 1990.

Patient guide, When diabetes develops during pregnancy, Medical Aspects of Human Sexuality, 91:45–46, 1991.

Paulson, RJ: *Conservative surgical treatment of ectopic pregnancy,* The Journal of Reproductive Medicine, 35:22–24, 1990.

Peters, H, and Theorell, CJ: *Fetal and neonatal effects of maternal cocaine use,* JOGNN, 20:121–126, Mar/Apr 1991.

Pitts, KS, and Weinstein, L: *Cocaine and pregnancy-A lethal combination.* Journal of Perinatology, 10(2):180–182, 1990.

Plessinger, MA, and Woods, JR: *The cardiovascular effects of cocaine use in pregnancy.* Reproductive Toxicology, 5:99–113, 1990.

Silverman, S: *Scope, specifics of maternal drug use, effects on fetus are beginning to emerge from studies.* JAMA, 261(12):1688–1689, 1989.

Shah, DM, et al: *Cordocentesis for rapid karyotyping.* Am J Obstet Gynecol, 162:1548–1550, 1990.

Stirrat, GM: *Common causes of recurrent miscarriage,* Medical Aspects of Human Sexuality, 25(7):36–44, 1991.

Stringer, MR: *Chorionic villi sampling: A nursing perspective.* JOGNN, 17:19–22, 1987.

Taysi, K: *Preconceptional Counseling,* Obstetrics and Gynecology Clinics of North America, 15:167–178, 1988.

Wilkins-Haug, L, Gabow, PA: *Toluene abuse during pregnancy: Obstetric complications and perinatal outcomes.* Obstetrics and Gynecology, 77(44):504–509, 1991.

Woods, M: *Mother's intake of folic acid reduces birth defects in infants.* Rocky Mountain News, Wed, Nov. 13, 1991.

Zacharias, JF: *The new genetics.* JOGNN 19:122–128, 1990.

Chapter 5: Intrapartal: Articles

Acosta, YM, et al: *HIV disease and pregnancy: Antepartum and intrapartum care, part 2,* JOGNN 21(2):97–103, 1992.

Cassidy, J: *A picture birth,* RN, 56(6):45–6, 1993.

Doe, J: *Tunnel vision,* Nursing91, 21(10):55–56.

Roan, S: *Childbirth still a pain,* The Denver Post, Sun., Aug 18, 1991.

Lynch, M, and McKeon, A: *Cocaine use during pregnancy: Research findings and clinical implications.* JOGNN, 19(4):285–292, 1990.

Chapter 6: Postpartal: Articles

Acosta, YM, et al: *HIV disease and pregnancy: Antepartum and intrapartum care, part 2.* JOGNN 21(2):97–103, 1992.

Bastin, N, et al: *HIV disease and pregnancy: Postpartum care of the HIV-positive woman and her newborn, part 3.* JOGNN 21(2):105–11, 1992.

Eaton, AP: *Current controversies in infant feeding: Why breast is best,* Pediatric Rounds, 2(1):7–9, 1993.

Fertility and contraception: Some diabetics can use OCs safely. Medical Aspects of Human Sexuality, 25(3):16, 1991.

Haines, F: *The sensual mom.* Parenting, 68–72, October 1991.

Hoeman, SP: *A research-based transdisciplinary team model for infants with special needs and their families.* Holistic Nurse Pract 7(4):63–72, 1993.

Kreck, C: *Breastfeeding conditions on mend.* The Denver Post, July 10, 1992.

Rentschler, DD: *Correlates of successful breastfeeding.* Image, Journal of Nursing Scholarship, 23(3):151–154, 1991.

Wiener, L: *No sex please, we're mothers.* Parenting, 45–49, August 1989.

Chapter 7: Newborn: Articles

Anderson, J, et al: *Occupational therapy for children with perinatal HIV infection.* American Journal of Occupational Therapy 44(3):249–55, 1990.

Bastin, N, et al: *HIV disease and pregnancy: Postpartum care of the HIV-positive woman and her newborn, part 3.* JOGNN 21(2):105–11, 1992.

Boland, MG, and Czarniecki, L: *Starting life with HIV.* RN 54:54–59, Jan 1991.

Butz, A, Hutton, N, and Larson, E: *Immunoglobulins and growth parameters at birth of infants born to HIV-seropositive and seronegative women.* American Journal of Public Health 81(10):1323–1326, 1991.

Chez, R: *Identifying maternal/fetal risks before pregnancy.* Medical Aspects of Human Sexuality, 25(4):54–58, 1991.

Christmas, JT: *The risks of cocaine use in pregnancy.* Medical Aspects of Human Sexuality, 26(2):36, 1992.

Doan-Johnson, S, and McGinley, E: *Filling the void—Boarder babies and the nurses who love them.* Nursing90, 20(2):44.

Dusick, AM, et al: *Risk of intracranial hemorrhage and other adverse outcomes after cocaine exposure in a cohort of 323 very low birth weight infants.* The Journal of Pediatrics, 122(3):438–445, 1993.

Free, T, Russell, F, Mills, B, and Hathaway, D: *A descriptive study of infant and toddlers exposed prenatally to substance abuse,* MCN, 15:245–248, 1990.

Fulroth, R, et al: *Perinatal outcome of infants exposed to cocaine and/or heroin in utero,* AJDC, 143:905–910, Aug 1989.

Green, A: *Intravenous immunoglobulin for neonates,* MCH: American Journal of Maternal-Child Nursing, 16(4):208–11, 1991.

Gingras, JL, et al: *Cocaine and development: Mechanisms of fetal toxicity and neonatal consequences of prenatal cocaine exposure.* Early Human Development, 31:1–24, 1992.

Jones, VN: *When pregnant women drink.* Rocky Mountain News, Tues, April 16, 1991.

Karthas, NP, and Chanock, S: *Clinical management of HIV infection in infants and children.* Family and Community Health 13(2):8–20, 1990.

Lynch, M, and McKeon, A: *Cocaine use during pregnancy: Research findings and clinical implications.* JOGNN, 19(4):285–292, 1990.

Lissauer, T: *Impact of AIDS on neonatal care.* Archives of Disease in Childhood, 64(1):4–7, 1989.

Marlow, JR: *They're saving babies.* Parade Magazine, Exosurf Neonatal Uninsured Patient Program, Burroughs Wellcome Co., Department P, 3030 Cornwallis Road, Research Triangle Park, NC 27709.

Meintz, SL, and Lynch, RD: *The human right of bonding for warehoused "AIDS babies."* Family and Community Health, 12(2):60–64, 19   89.

Peters, H, and Theorell, CJ: *Fetal and neonatal effects of maternal cocaine use.* JOGNN 20(2):121–126, 1991.

Plessinger, MA, and Woods, JR: *The cardiovascular effects of cocaine use in pregnancy.* Reproductive Toxicology, 5(2):99–113, 1991.

Porcher, FK: *HIV-infected pregnant women and their infants: Primary health care implications.* Nurse Practitioner: American Journal of Primary Health Care, 17(11):46, 49–50, 53–54, 1992.

Shiao, S: *Fluid and electrolyte problems of infants of very low birth weight.* AACN Clinical Issues in Critical Care Nursing, 3(3):698–704, 1992.

Singer, L, et al: *Neurodevelopmental effects of cocaine.* Clinics in Perinatology, 20(1):245–261, 1993.

Smith, J: *Bringing Theresa home.* Nursing91, 21(3):94.

Smith, M, Gill, PJ, and Katz, M: *The premature baby.* Tokos Medical Corp, Irvine, CA, 1987.

WHO/UNICEF issue statement on HIV and breastfeeding, International Nursing Review, 39(4):108, 1992.

Wilfert, CM: *HIV infection in maternal and pediatric patients,* Hospital-Practice, 26(5):55–62, 65–67, 1992.

Wise, N: *Putting babies to the test.* Parenting, 76–77, May 1993.

Zuckerman, B, et al: *A preliminary report of prenatal cocaine exposure and respiratory distress syndrome in premature infants.* AJDC 145:696–698, June 1991.

Index of Nursing Diagnoses

604